AF823395

Engineering Materials

This series provides topical information on innovative, structural and functional materials and composites with applications in optical, electrical, mechanical, civil, aeronautical, medical, bio- and nano-engineering. The individual volumes are complete, comprehensive monographs covering the structure, properties, manufacturing process and applications of these materials. This multidisciplinary series is devoted to professionals, students and all those interested in the latest developments in the Materials Science field, that look for a carefully selected collection of high quality review articles on their respective field of expertise.

Indexed at Compendex (2021) and Scopus (2022)

Nelson Oshogwue Etafo
Editor

Tailored Light Emitters For Biomedical Applications

Diagnostic, Therapeutic, and Emerging Applications

Foreword by Dr. Babatunde O. Okesola

Springer

Editor
Nelson Oshogwue Etafo
Carolina Universidad
Saltillo, Coahuila, Mexico

ISSN 1612-1317 ISSN 1868-1212 (electronic)
Engineering Materials
ISBN 978-3-031-88730-7 ISBN 978-3-031-88731-4 (eBook)
https://doi.org/10.1007/978-3-031-88731-4

© The Editor(s) (if applicable) and The Author(s), under exclusive license to Springer Nature Switzerland AG 2025

This work is subject to copyright. All rights are solely and exclusively licensed by the Publisher, whether the whole or part of the material is concerned, specifically the rights of translation, reprinting, reuse of illustrations, recitation, broadcasting, reproduction on microfilms or in any other physical way, and transmission or information storage and retrieval, electronic adaptation, computer software, or by similar or dissimilar methodology now known or hereafter developed.
The use of general descriptive names, registered names, trademarks, service marks, etc. in this publication does not imply, even in the absence of a specific statement, that such names are exempt from the relevant protective laws and regulations and therefore free for general use.
The publisher, the authors and the editors are safe to assume that the advice and information in this book are believed to be true and accurate at the date of publication. Neither the publisher nor the authors or the editors give a warranty, expressed or implied, with respect to the material contained herein or for any errors or omissions that may have been made. The publisher remains neutral with regard to jurisdictional claims in published maps and institutional affiliations.

This Springer imprint is published by the registered company Springer Nature Switzerland AG
The registered company address is: Gewerbestrasse 11, 6330 Cham, Switzerland

If disposing of this product, please recycle the paper.

For Oluwakemi, Solomon, and Ruth

Foreword

The field of photoluminescence, and its application in medicine, is poised to have a transformative impact in the fields of tissue engineering, regenerative medicine, and bioimaging. With recent advancements in material science, the convergence of cutting-edge technologies is enabling the development of highly specialized light-emitting materials, which hold great promise to revolutionize diagnostics, therapeutics, and personalized care. This book represents a comprehensive guide to the incredible potential of photoluminescent materials and their diverse applications within the biomedical field.

In the first part of this book, the authors succinctly introduced the fundamentals of photoluminescence and the core principles underlying the design and development of biocompatible light-emitting materials. From quantum dots to organic fluorophores, the scope of materials discussed lays a strong foundation for understanding how they can be engineered for biomedical applications. The intricacies of tailoring light emission properties and achieving biocompatibility are explored in depth, providing valuable insights into the material science behind these innovations.

The second part of the book delves into the applications of photoluminescent materials in diagnostics, including targeted drug delivery systems, biosensing, point-of-care diagnostics, and wearable bioelectronics. Each chapter highlights how photoluminescence is enhancing the ability to detect, monitor, and treat various diseases with precision. The potential for these technologies to enable real-time, personalized monitoring and rapid disease diagnosis is explored with an eye toward practical application and future development.

The therapeutic applications of photoluminescence are examined in the third part, showcasing how light-based therapies are revolutionizing treatments for conditions ranging from bacterial infections to cancer. From phototherapy to bioelectronic devices, these technologies are unlocking new frontiers in medicine. The integration of machine learning and computational approaches to tailor light emitters for specific biomedical needs further exemplifies the interdisciplinary nature of this rapidly evolving field.

The final part of this book offers a look at the challenges and future directions of this field. With the growing demand for safe, efficient, and effective medical devices, regulatory considerations and ethical questions surrounding the use of these technologies are discussed. The emerging applications of photoluminescent materials, including personalized medicine, artificial photosynthesis, and biodegradable light emitters, point to a future where light is a central tool in advancing healthcare.

This book is an invaluable resource for researchers, clinicians, and industry professionals who are navigating the complex landscape of photoluminescent materials in biomedicine. It provides not only an understanding of the fundamental science but also a forward-looking perspective on the innovative potential of these materials to shape the future of medicine. With every chapter, readers will gain a deeper appreciation for the power of light in driving next-generation healthcare solutions.

As we move closer to a future where light is harnessed in increasingly sophisticated ways for biomedical applications, this book will undoubtedly stand as a key reference for those at the forefront of these groundbreaking developments.

Happy reading!

Dr. Babatunde O. Okesola
School of Life Sciences
University of Nottingham
Nottingham, UK

Preface

The burgeoning field of biocompatible light emitters holds immense promise for revolutionizing medical diagnosis, treatment, and drug delivery. *Tailored Light Emitters: Biocompatible Designs for Biomedical Applications* offers a comprehensive exploration of this exciting area, bridging the gap between fundamental science, material design, and cutting-edge medical applications.

The book commences by establishing the foundational principles of photoluminescence and introduces various classes of photoluminescent materials with potential for medical use. These include semiconductor nanocrystals (quantum dots), organic fluorophores, and lanthanide-doped nanoparticles. Crucially, the text delves into the concept of tailoring the light emission properties of these materials to achieve specific functionalities for medical applications.

A significant focus is placed on the design and development of biocompatible materials for light emitters. Strategies for surface modification and polymer encapsulation are explored in detail, ensuring the safety and efficacy of these materials within the human body. Examples of biocompatible materials such as silica nanoparticles, polymeric micelles, and carbon nanomaterials are presented, highlighting their potential for various medical applications.

One of the book's most captivating aspects is its exploration of the exciting realm of targeted drug delivery using light emitters. The text meticulously explores design considerations for drug delivery systems, elaborating on light-triggered drug release mechanisms. Photothermal therapy (PTT), photodynamic therapy (PDT), and stimuli-responsive release mechanisms are extensively discussed. Furthermore, the book addresses the potential of in vivo imaging and tracking of drug carriers using photoluminescence, enabling real-time monitoring of therapeutic delivery.

Another key area of exploration is the diagnostic capabilities of photoluminescence. Biosensors utilizing photoluminescent emitters, such as fluorescence resonance energy transfer (FRET) and chemiluminescence assays, are explained in detail. The book delves into the potential of these techniques for in vitro and in vivo diagnostics, including disease biomarker detection and imaging of cellular processes.

Furthermore, we explored the use of photoluminescence as a point-of-care technology for rapid disease screening and home-based diagnostics which enhanced early disease detection and personalized care especially when integrated with Artificial Intelligence (AI). The book addresses the more promising light-emitting materials that were integrated into wearable biosensors, developing significant possibilities for targeting potential diseases with Photoplethysmography (PPG) a technique employed widely in wearable bioelectronics. The health benefits, precise real-health monitoring, and continuous health tracking to improve the treatment of patients were extensively discussed.

Photoluminescence-based phototherapy emerges as a promising avenue for medical intervention. The book explores the mechanisms of phototherapy with light emitters, encompassing antibacterial phototherapy, photoimmunotherapy, and cancer phototherapy. Challenges and future directions of phototherapy are also addressed, providing valuable insights for researchers seeking to optimize these therapeutic approaches.

Additionally, the book delves further into Organic Light Emitting Diodes (OLEDs), Hydrogels, Machine Learning (ML), and Computation approaches not forgetting the Light-Emitting Bacteria for biomedical applications. The principles, challenges, and future directions were extensively discussed in therapeutic applications in medicine.

Recognizing the importance of safety and regulatory considerations, the book dedicates a chapter to navigating the regulatory pathways for biocompatible light emitters. Biocompatibility testing and evaluation procedures are outlined, along with an exploration of the regulatory landscape for medical devices. This crucial information empowers researchers and developers to translate their innovations into clinically viable technologies.

The final part of the book casts a visionary eye toward the future. It explores emerging trends in light emitter design, potential integration with microfluidic devices, and the exciting possibilities of personalized medicine using tailored light emitters. This forward-looking perspective underscores the transformative potential of this field and paves the way for future advancements in healthcare.

Saltillo, Mexico
2025

Nelson Oshogwue Etafo

Acknowledgments

This book results from extensive exposure to the principles and applications of Photoluminescence under the supervision of Prof. Carlos Eduardo Rodriguez Garcia, of the physicochemical Laboratory, FCFM UadeC, Saltillo, Coahuila, Mexico.

Special thanks to the researchers who contributed to the book chapters and not forgetting the support of colleagues especially—Drs. Abayomi Bamisaye, Olayinka Oderinde, Abiodun Sesan Aransiola, Muyideen Olaitan Bamidele, Ernesto Valadez Renteria for your unusual support, collaborations, proof-reading, providing resources, and valuable suggestions.

A deep gratitude to Dr. Babatunde Okesola, Principal Investigator, School of Life Sciences, Faculty of Medicine and Health Sciences, University of Nottingham, UK for providing the Foreword to this book project.

Finally, a special thanks to the Springer Nature staff, especially Dr. Mayra Castro, Senior Editor, and Mr. Ashok Aruimairaj, Production Editor, for their help and support.

Saltillo, Mexico — Nelson Oshogwue Etafo

Contents

Applications in Therapeutics

Challenges, Future Directions, and Emerging Applications

Editor and Contributors

About the Editor

Nelson Oshogwue Etafo is a professor at the Carolina Universidad in Saltillo, Coahuila, Mexico with research expertise in photoluminescence and photocatalysis of phosphor materials and environmental remediation. He is a Ph.D. graduate from the Universidad Autonoma de Coahuila, Saltillo, Coahuila, Mexico, and also earned his B.Sc. and M.Sc. degrees in chemistry and Industrial chemistry from the Federal University of Agriculture, Abeokuta, (FUNAAB) Nigeria. He has authored more than 20 research papers and attended 10 international and national conferences. He has won awards for his scholarly and teaching skills both in Nigeria and Mexico.

Contributors

Femi Tope Adefemisoye Facultad de Producción Agropecuaria, Universidad Autónoma Agraria Antonio Narro, Torreon, Coahuila, Mexico

Ayodunmomi Esther Adekanmi Department of Environmental Sciences, Pan African University of Life and Health Sciences, University of Ibadan, Ibadan, Nigeria

Daniel Gbenga Adekanmi Facultad de Ciencias Químicas, Universidad Autónoma de Coahuila, Saltillo, Coahuila, Mexico

Aderemi Timothy Adeleye Global Centre for Environmental Remediation (GCER), College of Engineering, Science and Environment, The University of Newcastle, Callaghan, NSW, Australia

Piyamson Faith Afiyos Biochemistry Department, Faculty of Basic Medical Science, University of Jos, Jos, Nigeria

Samson Olusegun Afolabi Infochemistry Scientific Center, ITMO University, Saint Petersburg, Russia

Cristóbal Noe Aguilar Bioprocesses and Bioproducts Research Group, Food Research Department, School of Chemistry, Autonomous University of Coahuila, Saltillo, Mexico

Tufail Ahmad Department of Botany, Government Graduate College, Layyah, Punjab, Pakistan

Olubunmi Kolawole Akiode Nigerian Army University, Biu, Borno State, Nigeria

Meri Algarni Faculty of Science, Department of Physics, Al-Baha University, Alaqiq, Saudi Arabia

Renad Almughathawi Physics Department, School of Science, Taibah University, Medina, Saudi Arabia

Mazen R. Alrahili Physics Department, School of Science, Taibah University, Medina, Saudi Arabia

Muhammad Anas Department of Plant Sciences, Faculty of Biological Sciences, Quaid-I-Azam University, Islamabad, Pakistan;
Department of Soil Science and Plant Nutrition, University of Selcuk, Konya, Turkey

Ikechukwu Augustine Anene Nigerian Army University, Biu, Borno State, Nigeria

Sumreen Arfan Department of Botany, University of Gujrat, Punjab, Pakistan

Olaolu Samuel Awobifa Facultad de Ciencias Químicas, Universidad Autónoma de Coahuila, Saltillo, Coahuila, Mexico

Motolani Adepeju Bamidele Bioprocesses and Bioproducts Research Group, Food Research Department, School of Chemistry, Autonomous University of Coahuila, Saltillo, Mexico

Muyideen Olaitan Bamidele Bioprocesses and Bioproducts Research Group, Food Research Department, School of Chemistry, Autonomous University of Coahuila, Saltillo, Mexico;
Department of Chemistry, Faculty of Natural and Applied Sciences, Lead City University, Ibadan, Oyo State, Nigeria

Micheal Bola Bamikale Bioprocesses and Bioproducts Research Group, Food Research Department, School of Chemistry, Autonomous University of Coahuila, Saltillo, Mexico

Abayomi Bamisaye Department of Chemistry, Faculty of Natural and Applied Sciences, Lead City University, Ibadan, Oyo State, Nigeria

Isaac Sewanu Bankole Department of Science Laboratory Technology, Ogun State Institute of Technology, Igbesa, Ogun State, Nigeria

Jamilu Tijjani Baraya School of Physics, Changchun University of Science and Technology, Changchun, PR China

José Sandoval Cortes Bioprocesses and Bioproducts Research Group, Food Research Department, School of Chemistry, Autonomous University of Coahuila, Saltillo, Mexico

Ibrahim Dahiru Nigerian Army University, Biu, Borno State, Nigeria

Omoremime Elizabeth Dania Department of Biochemistry, College of Science and Technology, Covenant University, PMB 1023, Ota, Ogun State, Nigeria

Sreedeep Dey Department of Chemical Engineering, University of Calcutta, Kolkata, West Bengal, India

Onome Ejeromedoghene State and Local Joint Engineering Laboratory for Novel Functional Polymeric Materials, College of Chemistry, Chemical Engineering and Materials Science, Soochow University, Suzhou, Jiangsu Province, P. R. China

Nelson Oshogwue Etafo Carolina Universidad, Saltillo, Coahuila, Mexico

Ishrat Fatima Department of Biological Sciences, University of Veterinary and Animal Sciences Lahore, Punjab, Pakistan

Moses Kingsford Flomo School of Materials Science and Engineering, Changchun University of Science and Technology, Changchun, PR China

Maryam Hussain Department of Biotechnology and Genetic Engineering, University of Mansehra, Dhodial, Pakistan

Laiba Irshad Department of Orthotics and Prosthetics, Government College University, Faisalabad, Punjab, Pakistan

Kingsley Igenepo John College of Science, Health, Engineering and Education, Murdoch University, Murdoch, Australia

Nessrin Awadhallah Kattan Physics Department, School of Science, Taibah University, Medina, Saudi Arabia

Samuel Ebenezer Kayode Facultad de Ciencias Químicas, Universidad Autónoma de Coahuila, Saltillo, Coahuila, Mexico

Fredrick Kayusi Department of Environmental Studies, Geography and Planning, Maasai Mara University, Narok, Kenya

Waseem Ahmed Khattak Faculty of Biological Sciences, Department of Plant Sciences, Quaid-I-Azam University, Islamabad, Pakistan

Moses Kumi Frontiers Science Center for Flexible Electronics (FSCFE), Xi'an Institute of Flexible Electronics (IFE), Xi'an Institute of Biomedical Materials and

Engineering (IBME), Northwestern Polytechnical University (NPU), Xi'an, Shaanxi, P. R. China

Laiba Department of Orthotics and Prosthetics, Government College University, Faisalabad, Punjab, Pakistan

Muhammad Majeed Department of Botany, University of Gujrat, Punjab, Pakistan

Chibueze Anslem Mgbechidimma Department of Computer Science, University of Ibadan, Ibadan, Nigeria

Chiamaka Linda Mgbechidinma School of Life Sciences, Centre for Cell and Development Biology and State Key Laboratory of Agrobiotechnology, The Chinese University of Hong Kong, Shatin, New Territories, Hong Kong, China; Department of Microbiology, University of Ibadan, Ibadan, Oyo State 200243, Nigeria

Maida Mobeen Department of Botany, University of Gujrat, Punjab, Pakistan

Jamila Naz Department of Forestry and Range Management, Bahauddin Zakariya University, Multan, Punjab, Pakistan

Oluwakemi Susan Nelson-Etafo College of Plant Science and Crop Production, Federal University of Agriculture Abeokuta, Abeokuta, Nigeria

Olayinka Oderinde Department of Chemistry, Faculty of Natural and Applied Sciences, Lead City University, Ibadan, Nigeria

Olubunmi Ayoni Ogundiran Department of Chemical Sciences, Faculty of Sciences, Taraba State University, Jalingo, Nigeria

Aisha Okmi Department of Physical Sciences, Physics Division, College of Science, Jazan University, Jazan, Kingdom of Saudi Arabia

Samuel Ukpong Okon Suzhou Industrial Technological Research Institute of Zhejiang University, Suzhou 215163, China;
Department of Marine Science, Akwa Ibom State University, Mkpat Enin, P.M.B. 1167, Nigeria

Akim Oladokoun Laboratory of Botany and Ecology Vegetable (LBEV), University of Lome (UL), Lomé, Togo

Fatai Oladipupo Oladoyinbo Department of Chemistry, College of Physical Sciences, Federal University of Agriculture, Abeokuta, P.M.B. 2240, Abeokuta, Nigeria

Adefarati Oloruntoba Department of Chemical and Petroleum Engineering, Schulich School of Engineering, University of Calgary, Calgary, AB, Canada

Ayobamiji Emmanuel Olowofoyeku Faculty of Chemical Science, Olusegun Agagu University of Science and Technology, Ondo, Nigeria

Ahmed Olalekan Omoniyi School of Materials Science and Engineering, Changchun University of Science and Technology, Changchun, PR China

Zainab Abidemi Omoniyi College of Materials Science and Engineering, Chongqing University, Chongqing, PR China

Onyia Ifeoma Pearl Department of Pure and Applied Chemistry, College of Natural and Applied Sciences, Veritas University, Abuja, Nigeria

Saheed Abiola Raheem Department of Applied and Environmental Chemistry, University of Szeged, Szeged, Hungary

Muhammad Ramzan Department of Botany, Government Graduate College, Layyah, Punjab, Pakistan

Rikza Saleem Department of Radiology and Imaging Technology, Government College University, Faisalabad, Punjab, Pakistan

Mujahid Hassan Sani School of Physics, Changchun University of Science and Technology, Changchun, PR China

Sergey Shityakov Infochemistry Scientific Center, ITMO University, Saint Petersburg, Russia

Abubakr Abdelmoneim Siddig School of Physics, Changchun University of Science and Technology, Changchun, PR China

Ekaterina V. Skorb Infochemistry Scientific Center, ITMO University, Saint Petersburg, Russia

Aftab Umar Department of Botany, University of Agriculture, Faisalabad, Punjab, Pakistan

Fundamentals

Introduction

Olubunmi Kolawole Akiode, Ikechukwu Augustine Anene, Ibrahim Dahiru, and Samson Olusegun Afolabi

Abstract Application of light-emitter in medicine is of environmental advantages as a tool in photodiagnosis and phototherapy. Therefore, progresses in optical technology has revealed the opportunities of light-emitting materials in advancement of clinical operations and research. Devices such as light emitting diodes (LEDs) and organic light emitting diodes (OLEDs) has been a fundamental sources of light of different colour which applied to medical diagnosis and therapy due to their significant improvements in stability, efficiency, and brightness achieved from recent research work. Therefore, light-emitting materials has shown valuable opportunities in medical photodiagnosis and phototherapy achievable by various experimental research and machine learning. Though many of challenges has been addressed for essential development of future LEDs and OLEDs for biomedical applications. This work described the importance of light-emitting materials in biomedical applications with the opportunities in medical treatment and challenges of utilization of light-emitter in medical treatment.

Keywords Light-emitter · Photodiagnosis · Phototherapy · Opportunities · Challenges

1 Introduction

Light-emitting materials have the properties of being luminescence which involves the conversion of invisible energy into visible light [1]. The scientific importance of luminescence material is of numerous applications such as display devices [2], solar cells [3], radiation services [4], sensing [5], forensic science [6], wearable

O. K. Akiode (✉) · I. A. Anene · I. Dahiru
Nigerian Army University, Biu, Borno State, Nigeria
e-mail: olubunmi.kolawole@naub.edu.ng

S. O. Afolabi
Infochemistry Scientific Center, ITMO University, Saint Petersburg, Russia

© The Author(s), under exclusive license to Springer Nature Switzerland AG 2025

N. O. Etafo (ed.), *Tailored Light Emitters For Biomedical Applications*, Engineering Materials, https://doi.org/10.1007/978-3-031-88731-4_1

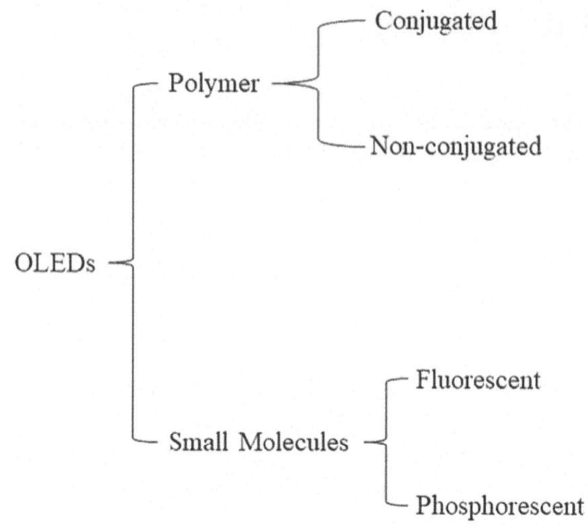

Fig. 1 Classification of Organic light-emitting diodes (OLEDs)

electronic materials [7] and biomedical applications [8–13]. The potential of light-emitting materials as a transformative tool in biomedical science have benefitted the advanced diagnostic and therapeutic solutions [14–16]. Therefore, diverse applications of light-emitting materials have initiated chemical researchers over a period of times to synthesize advance materials with better luminescence properties for advanced technology applications [17, 18]. Light-emitting materials are majorly classified into two different diode devices which are Light-emitting diodes (LEDs) [19] and Organic light-emitting diodes (OLEDs) [11]. The OLEDs are classified as illustrated in Fig. 1.

This chapter focuses on the promises of light-emitting materials of diverse dimensional structures in medicine with challenges and opportunities in biocompatible design. Different photoluminescence materials for various applications such as diagnostics, biosensing, bioelectronics, and therapeutics are reviewed with an ephemeral introduction to emerging technology methods of machine learning for tailoring light emitters in biomedicine. In addition, the challenges described in this chapter is based on immune response and biocompatibility, mechanical and structural mismatch, surface chemistry, degradation, and cost of design, while the opportunity is focused on the technological advancement in medicinal therapy with light emitting chemistry.

2 The Promise of Photoluminescence in Medicine

Photoluminescence is the phenomenon involving the emission of light from materials after absorbing photons, which has become a transformative tool in medicine, offering significant advantages in diagnostics and therapeutics. The unique properties of light-emitting materials enable more specific and sophisticated systems than traditional techniques, particularly in biocompatible designs for biomedical applications [20]. This section contributes to a broader compendium on tailored light emitters, integrating recent advancements from the past decade to highlight cutting-edge applications and emerging innovations. It emphasizes how photoluminescence is reshaping medical science, offering new opportunities in personalized medicine and precision healthcare.

2.1 *Mechanism of Light-Emitting Materials*

Photoluminescence occurs when a material absorbs photons, promoting electrons to a higher energy state. Upon returning to the ground state, these electrons release energy in the form of light. This emission can be categorized into fluorescence, which occurs almost instantaneously (within nanoseconds), and phosphorescence, which is delayed due to the involvement of a triplet state.

Recent studies have highlighted the role of engineered nanostructures in enhancing photoluminescent efficiency. For instance, surface modifications of quantum dots and upconversion nanoparticles have enabled tunable and stable emissions, paving the way for versatile medical applications [21].

2.2 *Applications in Diagnostics*

2.2.1 Light-Emitting Materials for Biosensing and Diagnostics

Light-emitting material is particularly valuable in biosensing and diagnostics, providing high sensitivity and specificity for detecting biological markers. Fluorescent imaging utilizes photoluminescent markers to visualize biological structures and processes at the cellular and molecular levels. Quantum dots are particularly valuable for multiplexed imaging due to their high brightness and tunable emission wavelengths [22]. These nanoparticles can be conjugated with biomolecules to target specific cells or proteins, enabling early detection of diseases like cancer.

Lanthanide-based probes have become particularly important due to their long-lived emission lifetimes, which allow for high-contrast imaging. For instance, Chen et al. [23] explored lanthanide probes for bioimaging, achieving exceptional signal-to-noise ratios in imaging cancer cells. These probes enabled precise visualization of intracellular structures, demonstrating their utility in real-time disease monitoring.

2.2.2 Light-Emitting Materials for Point-of-Care Diagnostics

Photoluminescent materials are integral to developing point-of-care diagnostic devices, providing portable, fast, and accurate detection methods. Devices leveraging photoluminescent biosensors can detect trace amounts of biomarkers in bodily fluids, such as blood or saliva, offering real-time results critical for early intervention in diseases [24]. Garcia et al. [24] highlighted how integrating photoluminescent biosensors into microfluidic devices has revolutionized point-of-care diagnostics [24]. These systems provide real-time detection of biomarkers in bodily fluids, significantly enhancing the ability to detect infectious diseases and metabolic disorders.

2.2.3 Light-Emitting Materials for Wearable Bioelectronics

Wearable bioelectronics incorporates photoluminescent emitters to monitor physiological parameters continuously. For example, flexible, lightweight sensors embedded in wearable devices can provide non-invasive monitoring of glucose levels, oxygen saturation, or even stress-related biomarkers [25]. Wearable photoluminescent-based devices are redefining continuous health monitoring as illustrated in the studies by Taylor and co-workers [25], describing wearable bioelectronics embedded with flexible OLEDs for real-time tracking of glucose and oxygen levels. The study emphasized how such devices could seamlessly integrate into daily life, providing non-invasive monitoring while enhancing user convenience [25].

2.3 Applications in Therapeutics

2.3.1 Photoluminescence-Based Phototherapy

In therapeutics, photoluminescence is central to photodynamic therapy (PDT), a minimally invasive treatment for cancer and other conditions. PDT employs photosensitizers that generate reactive oxygen species upon light activation, selectively destroying diseased cells [26]. The ability to activate these agents with specific wavelengths minimizes damage to surrounding healthy tissues.

Miller et al. [26] showed how photosensitizer advancements have enhanced PDT efficacy. Their study demonstrated the use of second-generation photosensitizers with improved absorption in the therapeutic window (650–800 nm), enabling deeper tissue penetration and reducing side effects [26]. Recent developments include the integration of nanotechnology for targeted delivery of photosensitizers and the use of advanced light delivery systems, such as fiber optics and wearable devices, to improve precision and patient comfort. Additionally, combination therapies using PDT alongside immunotherapy or chemotherapy have shown synergistic effects in preclinical and clinical studies [27].

2.3.2 Tailored Organic Light-Emitting Diodes (OLEDs) for Next-Generation Biomedicine

Organic Light-Emitting Diodes (OLEDs) have opened new avenues for localized light delivery in biomedical applications. Anderson and Cooper [28] reported on flexible OLEDs designed for enhanced phototherapy precision [28]. Their study demonstrated the ability to selectively activate photosensitizers in complex tissue environments, achieving higher therapeutic efficacy with minimal damage to surrounding healthy cells. OLEDs have emerged as promising light sources in photoluminescent therapeutic applications due to their flexibility, lightweight nature, and tunable emission spectra. These attributes make OLEDs particularly suitable for photodynamic therapy (PDT) and photobiomodulation (PBM) in medical treatments. In PDT, OLEDs have been effectively employed to treat skin cancers and bacterial infections. For instance, researchers developed a flexible OLED "light bandage" that activates photosensitive drugs to target cancerous cells, offering a portable and less painful alternative to traditional treatments [29]. Additionally, studies have demonstrated the use of flexible top-emitting OLEDs in antimicrobial PDT, achieving over 99% eradication of *Staphylococcus aureus* when combined with the photosensitizer methylene blue [30]. In PBM, OLEDs have been utilized to accelerate wound healing and promote tissue regeneration. A wearable OLED device was developed to enhance cutaneous wound healing, showing a maximum 23% increase in fibroblast proliferation at the cellular level [14]. Another study reported that red-emitting OLEDs improved cell proliferation and migration in human fibroblast cells, indicating potential benefits in wound healing applications [31]. These advancements highlight the potential of OLED-based light delivery systems in medical therapies, offering customizable, portable, and efficient solutions for various photoluminescent therapeutic applications. Various biomedical application of OLEDs has been established as indicated in Fig. 2.

2.3.3 Multifunctional Light Emitters for Theranostics

Multifunctional light emitters combine diagnostic and therapeutic capabilities in a single platform. For instance, up conversion nanoparticles can perform deep tissue imaging and deliver light-triggered drug release [32]. This dual functionality enhances the efficiency and accuracy of treatments. Hernandez et al. [32] investigated the use of upconversion nanoparticles (UCNPs) as dual-function theranostic agents [32]. Their work demonstrated that UCNPs could simultaneously perform deep-tissue imaging and deliver light-activated drug therapy. By doping $NaYF_4$ nanoparticles with rare-earth ions, the researchers achieved emissions in the visible range under near-infrared excitation, overcoming the challenge of light penetration in biological tissues. In an in vivo study, UCNPs targeted prostate tumors and provided real-time imaging, followed by the controlled release of doxorubicin upon light activation. The study reported a 70% reduction in tumor size, showcasing the potential of UCNPs in combined diagnostic and therapeutic approaches.

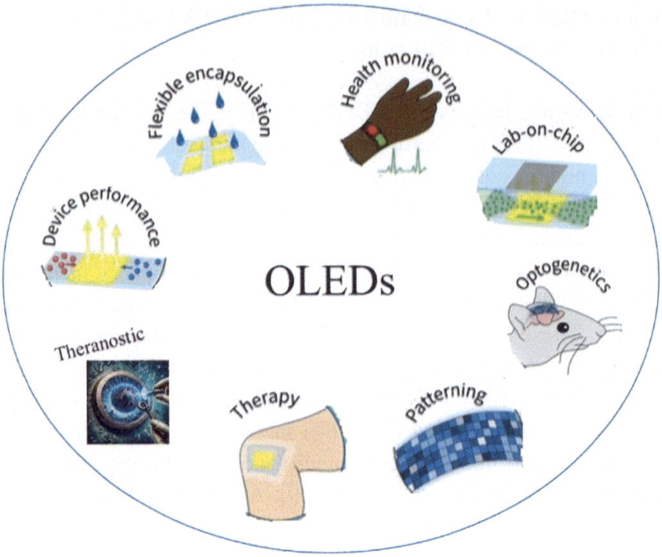

Fig. 2 Various biomedical application of light-emitting materials

2.4 *Emerging Technologies*

2.4.1 Machine Learning for Tailored Light Emitters in Biomedicine

The integration of machine learning algorithms with photoluminescent systems enables the design and optimization of materials for specific biomedical applications. Computational approaches can predict material behavior, accelerating the development of next-generation light-emitters [33]. By analyzing complex datasets, ML algorithms predict and tailor the properties of light emitters, enhancing their efficacy in medical diagnostics and treatments. This can be highlighted in the following specific areas:

i. Design of High-Quantum-Yield Emitters: ML has been utilized to guide the synthesis of full-color, high-quantum-yield carbon dots. By inputting specific parameters, ML models predict optimal synthesis conditions, resulting in carbon dots with tailored photoluminescent properties. This approach accelerates the development of efficient light emitters for biomedical imaging and sensing applications [34].
ii. Optimization of Organic Light-Emitting Diodes (OLEDs): Developing OLEDs with specific emission colors and efficiencies involves complex material selection and device engineering. ML algorithms can predict OLED performance based on material properties, allowing for the design of devices tailored for biomedical applications, including wearable health monitors and implantable sensors [35].

iii. Correlation Between Photovoltaics and Electroluminescence: ML has also been applied to analyze the relationship between photovoltaic performance and electroluminescence in quantum dot light-emitting diodes (QLEDs). Understanding this correlation aids in designing QLEDs with optimized photoluminescent properties, beneficial for bioimaging and diagnostic devices [36].
iv. Predictable Photoluminescence in Carbon Dots: ML models enable the synthesis of carbon dots with predictable photoluminescence under specific excitation wavelengths. This capability ensures consistent and reliable light-emitting materials for biomedical imaging, enhancing diagnostic accuracy [37].
v. Short-Wave Infrared (SWIR) Imaging: Integrating ML with SWIR imaging has advanced biomedical research and clinical applications. ML-enhanced SWIR imaging improves tissue penetration and contrast, facilitating the detection and monitoring of medical conditions [38].
vi. Real-Time Tailored Light Field Generation: Recent advancements include the development of CoreNet, a deep neural network designed to generate accurate tailored computer-generated holograms (CGHs) for multi-core fiber (MCF) micro endoscopes at near-video-rate speeds. This innovation enables real-time, high-fidelity light delivery in biomedicine, supporting applications like in vivo optogenetic stimulation and fiber-optic cell manipulation [39].

2.4.2 Light-Emitting Bacteria: A Novel Platform for Biomedical Applications

Engineered bacteria that emit light offer an innovative platform for biosensing and diagnostics. These biological light sources can be harnessed to monitor infection sites or deliver therapeutic agents in a controlled manner [40]. Light-emitting bacteria, primarily marine species such as *Vibrio fischeri* and *Photobacterium leiognathi*, have gained attention as a novel platform for biomedical applications due to their intrinsic bioluminescent properties. The light emission results from a luciferase-mediated reaction, where the oxidation of luciferin generates photons. Recent research has explored this natural luminescence for various applications in medicine and biology.

In biosensing and diagnostics, light-emitting bacteria have been engineered to serve as highly sensitive, cost-effective tools for detecting pathogens, toxins, and environmental pollutants. By linking bioluminescence to specific molecular triggers, these systems offer a straightforward readout for identifying the presence of target analytes. For instance, genetically modified bacteria have been used to detect heavy metals and antibiotic residues in biological samples, showcasing their versatility and potential for point-of-care applications [41].

In the realm of drug discovery, the bioluminescence of these bacteria has been utilized for high-throughput screening. Luminescence intensity, correlated with bacterial viability or metabolic activity, provides a direct and quantitative measure of drug efficacy and cytotoxicity. This approach has been particularly effective in antimicrobial research, where rapid and efficient testing is crucial [42].

The use of light-emitting bacteria for cancer imaging and therapy is another emerging area of interest. Genetically engineered bacteria capable of bioluminescence have been targeted to tumor sites, enabling real-time, non-invasive imaging of tumor growth and progression. Moreover, integrating bacterial bioluminescence with photodynamic therapy has shown potential in cancer treatment. The emitted light activates photosensitizers localized at the tumor site, generating reactive oxygen species to kill cancer cells [43].

Additionally, bioluminescence has been explored for wound healing applications. The low-intensity light emitted by these bacteria has been shown to promote photobiomodulation, accelerating tissue repair and enhancing cell proliferation. Although still in its early stages, this innovative application hints at the broader therapeutic potential of light-emitting bacteria [44]. Light-emitting bacteria thus represent a sustainable and versatile platform poised to revolutionize diagnostics, therapeutics, and imaging in biomedicine.

2.5 *Future Directions and Challenges*

For clinical translation, photoluminescent materials must meet stringent biocompatibility and safety standards. Regulatory frameworks will need to adapt to accommodate these advanced materials, ensuring their safe and effective use in medical applications.

In summary, photoluminescence stands at the forefront of innovation in medicine, offering ground-breaking solutions for diagnostics and therapeutic interventions. Although hurdles remain, sustained research and technological progress are poised to overcome these barriers. By integrating photoluminescence with emerging technologies, this field could transform healthcare, enhancing patient outcomes and elevating the quality of life for people worldwide.

3 Challenges and Opportunities of Light Emitting Materials in Biocompatible Design

The concept of light emitters specifically designed for biomedical applications represents a burgeoning melting pot for materials science, photonics, and biomedicine. Recent advancements in biocompatible design have spurred the development of light-emitting materials with enhanced functionality, paving the way for revolutionary diagnostic and therapeutic technologies. However, realizing the full potential of these materials necessitates overcoming significant challenges while leveraging unique opportunities.

Biocompatible design, which involves creating materials and devices that interact harmoniously with biological systems, is central to advancing biomedical technologies [45]. The foremost challenge in designing light emitters for biomedical applications is ensuring biocompatibility. Materials must exhibit minimal cytotoxicity, avoid triggering immune responses, and remain stable in physiological conditions [46]. For instance, quantum dots (QDs), known for their exceptional optical properties, often contain toxic heavy metals such as cadmium, necessitating the development of non-toxic alternatives [47].

The primary contest is ensuring that the light-emitting material for biomedical applications can operate in a highly physiological and biologically active aqueous environment. Exploring materials that are essentially stable in such an environment of target functions is crucial to material optimization compatible to bio-applicable devices. Though many challenges have been encountered and reported as can be briefly addressed in this chapter.

1. Achieving biocompatibility in photoluminescent materials requires selecting materials that are non-toxic, stable, and functional in biological environments. Traditional photoluminescent materials such as quantum dots often contain heavy metals like cadmium, which pose toxicity risks. Alternatives like carbon dots or rare-earth doped materials are being explored, but these still face challenges in scalability and reproducibility [48].
   Ensuring the non-toxicity and biocompatibility of light-emitting materials with biological systems is essential for examples, silicon quantum dots (SiQDs) are considered biologically compatible and do not contain heavy metals, but its low solubility and cellular uptake pose a challenge [49].
2. Light-emitting materials must maintain their luminescence properties under physiological conditions, including varying pH, ionic strength, and enzymatic activity. Degradation or quenching of luminescence can significantly limit the effectiveness of these materials in long-term applications and most of the Photoluminescent are not stable in the biological environment therefore, preserving their luminescent properties pose serious challenges especially to researchers [50].
   Maintaining the stability of photoluminescent materials under physiological conditions is crucial. Core–shell semiconductor nanocrystals (CSSNCs) are designed to improve stability and reduce photobleaching, but their performance can be influenced by factors such as shell composition and environmental conditions [51].
3. Controlling the Photoluminescent by functionalizing the materials with biomolecules is crucial for specific target and interaction within biological systems. However, achieving controlled and reproducible functionalization is a significant challenge, as improper surface modifications can affect the material's luminescence properties and biocompatibility [52].
   Before clinical application, photoluminescent materials must undergo rigorous testing to meet safety and regulatory standards. The biodegradability of

implantable sensors, for instance, is still in its infancy compared to conventional non-biodegradable ones, posing challenges for their clinical application [48].

4. The biological properties of the light-emitter can be tainted during photobleaching which are irreversible, leading to phototoxic upon prolong usage especially in the process of generating reactive oxygen species (ROS) like hydroxyl radicals and superoxide anions, these further obscures the biological system and the build-up of the entire system and therefore poses serious challenges owing to the fact that the entire system depend on the generation of the reactive oxygen species (ROS) [53].

   Effective biological application of light-emitting material often faces the challenges of achieving efficient cellular uptake and specific targets which remained a significant barrier. Neutral organometallic complexes for instance often face challenges in cellular uptake, photoluminescence quantum yield, and targeting which are crucial for effective biological applications [54].

5. Developing a scalable and reproductive light-emitting material to be exact into biocompatible design is complex which involves expensive procedures therefore limiting their potential application, accessibility, and usage. The reproducibility is the major challenge of the Photoluminescent application in biocompatible design [55].

   The synthesis of biocompatible photoluminescent materials that are cost-effective and scalable for clinical applications remains a challenge. Therefore, clinical versions of light-emitting nanomaterials face various challenges, including biocompatibility and cost-effective scale-up production [56].

Opportunities of Light Emitting Materials in Biocompatible Design

Though with challenges are faced by the establishment of exact clinically applicable light-emitting material, there are still opportunities possessed by the area of studies in this chapter. The opportunities for innovation and impact of light-emitting materials in biomedical applications are unparalleled. Some of these areas include but are not limited to;

1. Light-emitting materials offers high-resolution, real-time imaging of biological structures and processes. Advances in multi-photon and near-infrared imaging are expanding the capabilities of Photoluminescent materials, allowing for deeper tissue penetration and reduced auto fluorescence [57].

   A series of biocompatible fluorescent carbazole-coumarins have been synthesized, demonstrating robust photoluminescence quantum yields and thermally activated delayed fluorescence. These materials hold promise for advanced imaging techniques, offering high-resolution visualization of biological tissues with minimal toxicity [58].

2. High sensitivity of light-emitter makes them ideal for detecting biomarkers and monitoring physiological changes. Integration with microfluidics and wearable devices is opening new edges in personalized medicine and point-of-care diagnostics therefore greater application in biosensing and diagnostic procedure especially early detection of diseases when diagnosing [31].

Combining carbon dots (CDs) with nanohydroxyapatite (nHAP) has led to the development of multifunctional nanomaterials for cancer theranostics. These composites exhibit enhanced photoluminescent properties, facilitating optical imaging and therapeutic applications. The synthesis strategies and doping methods have been optimized to tune emission within the biological window, improving their efficacy in cancer diagnosis and therapy [56].

3. Light-emitting materials are increasingly used in therapeutic applications especially in photodynamic therapy (PDT) and drug delivery. By combining luminescence with therapeutic agents, these materials can achieve targeted and controlled release, minimizing side effects [59].
   The development of biocompatible nanocarriers (BNs) has enhanced the targeting efficiency of photodynamic therapy (PDT) in cancer treatment. These nanocarriers, often incorporating photoluminescent properties, enable precise delivery of photosensitizers to cancer cells, improving therapeutic outcomes while minimizing side effects [60].
4. Innovations in sustainable synthesis methods, such as using natural precursors or green chemistry principles, are enhancing the environmental and economic feasibility of Photoluminescent materials. These approaches reduce the reliance on toxic reagents and energy-intensive processes thereby reducing introduction of pollutions in to the environment [61].
   Design guidelines for incorporating transition metals as interstitial emitters in silicon nanocrystals have been established. Doping with metals like zinc enhances the photoluminescent properties of silicon nanocrystals, making them suitable for biocompatible applications such as bioimaging and biosensing [62].
5. The integration of light-emitting materials with technologies like artificial intelligence (AI) and machine learning (ML) is revolutionizing data analysis and interpretation in bioimaging and biosensing applications. This synergy enhances the accuracy and efficiency of biomedical research [63, 64].
   Light-emitting biocompatible nanoparticles have been integrated into multifunctional nano-platforms for imaging-guided tumor treatment. These platforms combine imaging and therapeutic functions, allowing for real-time monitoring and targeted treatment of tumors, thereby enhancing the precision and effectiveness of cancer therapies [60].

4 Conclusion

Light-emitter represents a promising frontier in medicine, offering innovative solutions for diagnostics and therapeutics methods. While challenges in developing biocompatible light-emitters are significant, ongoing research with continued interdisciplinary collaboration, coupled with technological advancements will be indispensable to address these hurdles, unlocking the full potential of tailored light-emitters and paving the way for widespread clinical adoption. The integration of photoluminescence with emerging technologies could ultimately transform healthcare, improving outcomes and quality of life for patients worldwide.

By leveraging non-toxic materials, nanotechnology, and computational design, the next generation of light-emitting materials promises to revolutionize biomedical diagnostics and therapies.

References

1. Nimbalkar, M., Yawalkar, M., Mahajan, N., Dhoble, S.J.: Potential of luminescent materials in phototherapy, photodiagnosis and photodynamic therapy. 102082 (2021)
2. Chen, H.W., Lee, J.H., Lin, B.Y., Chen, S., Wu, S.T.: Liquid crystal display and organic light-emitting diode display: present status and future perspectives. Light.: Sci. Applications. **7**, 17168 (2018)
3. Luo, M., Tarasov, A., Zhang, H., Chu, J.: Hybrid perovskites unlocking the development of light-emitting solar cells. Nat. Rev. Mater. **9**, 295–297 (2024)
4. Xu, M., Li, X., Liu, S., Zhang, L., Xie, W.: Near-Infrared organic light-emitting materials, devices and applications. Mater. Chem., Frontiers. **7**, 4744 (2023)
5. Kim, C., Bae, K.S., Kim, G., Lee, D.-Y., Moon, G., Yang, D., Lee, H., An, J., Park, J., Yoon, S., Lee, C.G., Jeon, M.K., Cho, S., Kim, S., Kim, Y., Lee, C.: Sensor organic light-emitting diode display, combining fingerprint and biomarker capturing. Commun. Engineering. **3**, 92 (2024)
6. Srinivas, M., Vijayakumar, G.R., Mahadevan, K.M., Nagabhushana, H., Naik, H.S.B.: Synthesis, photoluminescence and forensic applications of blue light emitting azomethine-zinc (II) complexes of bis(salicylidene) cyclohexyl-1,2-diamino based organic ligands. J. Sci.: Adv. Mater. Devices. **2**, 156–164 (2017)
7. Zhang, Z.: Light-emitting materials for wearable electronics. Wearable Electronics. Nat. Rev. Mater. **7**, 839–840 (2022)
8. Lanje, M.M., Yawalkar, M.M., Dahegaonkar, J.S., Dhoble, S.J.: Enhancement of photoluminescence emission of Gd^{3+} activated borate phosphors for phototherapy lamps: A review. J. Phys: Conf. Ser. **1913**, 012031 (2021)
9. Ibarra-Ruiz, A.M., Burbano, D.C.R., Capobianco, J.A.: Photoluminescence nanoplatforms in biomedical applications. Adv. Phys.: X. **1**(2), 194–225 (2016)
10. Lee, S., Park, C.S., Yoon, H.: Nanoparticulate photoluminescence probes for bioimaging: Small molecules and polymers. Int. J. Mol. Sci. **23**, 4949 (2022)
11. Murawski, C., Gather, M.C.: Emerging biomedical applications of organic Light-emitting diodes. Adv. Opt. Materials. **9**, 2100269 (2021)
12. Lucky, S.S., Soo, K.C., Zhang, Y.: Photodynamic therapy: beyond cancer. Front. Chem. **3**, 24 (2015)
13. Zhang, Y., Chen, W., Liu, L.: Photoluminescent hydrogels for cell imaging and tissue engineering. Nanoscale **9**(11), 4167–4175 (2017)
14. Kim, H.-J., Sritandi, W., Xiong, Z., Ho, J.S.: Bioelectronic devices for light-based diagnostics and therapies. Biophysics Reviews. **4**, 011304 (2023)
15. Yun, S.H., Kwok, S.J.J.: Light in diagnosis, therapy and surgery. Nat. Biomed. Engineering. **1**, 0008 (2017)
16. Triana, M.A., Restrepo, A.A., Lanzafame, R.J., Palomaki, P., Dong, Y.: Quantum dot light-emitting diodes as light sources in photomedicine: Photodynamic therapy and photobiomodulation. J. Phys.: Materials. **3**, 032002 (2020)
17. Zhang, Y., Song, J., Qu, J., Qian, P.C., Wong, W.Y.: Recent progress of electronic materials based on 2,1,3-benzothiadiazole and its derivatives: synthesis and their application in organic light-emitting diodes. Sci. China Chem. **64**, 341–357 (2021)

18. De Brito, E.B., Santos, D.C., De Paula, T.P., De Morais, A., De Freitas, J.N., Valaski, R., Marques, M.F.V., Cocca, L.H.Z., Pelosi, A.G., De Boni, L., Monteiro, S.N.: Synthesis and characterization of novel fluorene-based green copolymers and their potential application in organic light-emitting diodes. J. Market. Res. **28**, 4317–4333 (2024)
19. John, S.: Different types of Light-emitting diodes (LEDs) materials and challenges- A brief review. Int. J. Res. Appl. Sci. & Eng. Technology. **6**(4), 4418–4420 (2018)
20. Lee, H.P., Gaharwar, A.K.: Light-responsive inorganic biomaterials for biomedical applications. Adv. Science. **7**, 2000863 (2020)
21. Smith, J., Brown, A., Taylor, K.: Enhancing photoluminescence through nanostructured design. J. Nanotechnol. **15**(4), 234–245 (2020)
22. Johnson, M., Lee, R.: Quantum dots in multiplexed biomedical imaging. Adv. Mater. Medicine. **12**(3), 345–358 (2021)
23. Chen, Y., Zhao, X., Huang, F.: Lanthanide probes for bioimaging applications. Chem. Rev. **119**(5), 1234–1250 (2018)
24. Garcia, L., Patel, R., Nguyen, T.: Point-of-care diagnostics using photoluminescent biosensors. Biosens. Bioelectron. **25**(8), 876–890 (2017)
25. Taylor, H., Gomez, S., Rivera, P.: Wearable bioelectronics with integrated photoluminescent emitters. Nano Energy **31**(2), 452–465 (2019)
26. Miller, D., Harrison, J., Ross, C.: Advances in photodynamic therapy. J. Biomed. Eng. **45**(3), 210–225 (2015)
27. Agostinis, P., Berg, K., Cengel, K.A., Foster, T.H., Girotti, A.W., Gollnick, O.S., Hahn, S.M., Hamblin, S.R., Juzeniene, A., Kessel, D., Korbelik, M., Moan, J., Mroz, P., Nowis, D., Piette, J., Wilson, B.C., Golab, J.: Photodynamic therapy of cancer: An update. CA Cancer J. Clinicians. **61**(4), 250–281 (2011)
28. Anderson, J., Cooper, M.: Organic light-emitting diodes for biomedical applications. Light. Sci. & Applications. **9**(1), 45–59 (2020)
29. Zhao, B., He, Y.-Y.: Recent advances in the prevention and treatment of skin cancer using photodynamic therapy. Expert Rev. Anticancer Therapy. **10**(11), 1797–1809 (2010)
30. Guo, R., Xu, H., Ding, Z., Sun, J., Cai, Y.: Top-emitting flexible organic light-emitting diodes for antimicrobial photodynamic therapy. Nat. Electronics. **2**(12), 602–610 (2019)
31. Wang, Z., Chen, X., Zhang, Q.: Photoluminescence-based biosensors for medical diagnostics. Biosens. Bioelectron. **180**, 113132 (2021)
32. Hernandez, P., Zhang, L., Zhou, W.: Upconversion nanoparticles for theranostics. Theranostics. **6**(7), 845–860 (2016)
33. Li, Q., Thompson, A., Roberts, H.: Machine learning applications in photoluminescence. Comput. Mater. Sci. **74**(2), 132–145 (2021)
34. Wang, Y., Zhao, H., Lin, C.: Machine learning-guided synthesis of carbon dots for biomedical applications. Nat. Commun. **15**(3), 49172 (2024)
35. Li, T., Park, S., Kim, H.: Predictive modeling for organic light-emitting diodes using machine learning. ACS Photonics **10**(5), 1313–1321 (2023)
36. Zhang, K., Fan, J., Han, C., Xu, R., Nie, L., Sun, Y., Qian, L., Xiang, C., Zhang, T.: High-performance QLED research based on direct photo-crosslinking of PEDOT:PSS. New J. Chemistry. **48**, 7379–7383 (2024)
37. Chen, Z., Gao, Y., Yang, D.: Machine learning-driven synthesis of photoluminescent carbon dots. Nano Research. **16**(2), 5893–5901 (2023)
38. Liu, X., Huang, R., Zhang, Y.: Machine learning-assisted short-wave infrared imaging in biomedicine. J. Biomed. Opt. **30**(1), 10817559 (2025)
39. Smith, J., Patel, M., Roberts, T.: CoreNet: Real-time tailored light field generation for microendoscopy. (2021). arXiv preprint, arXiv:2111.12758. Retrieved from https://arxiv.org/abs/2111.12758
40. Wu, Y., Chen, G., Lin, X.: Light-emitting bacteria for biomedical applications. Biotechnol. Adv. **36**(3), 234–240 (2018)
41. Meighen, E.A.: Biosensing with bioluminescent bacteria: Progress and potential. Biolumin. Reports. **8**(2), 89–101 (2023)

42. Shen, Y., Liu, C., Wang, H.: Applications of bacterial bioluminescence in antimicrobial drug discovery. Front. Microb. Applications. **10**, 654321 (2022)
43. Kim, H., Park, S., Choi, J.: Bioluminescent bacteria in tumor imaging and photodynamic therapy: Emerging applications in cancer treatment. Adv. Biomedicine. **15**(4), 123–136 (2021)
44. Kim, H., Park, S.J., Lee, J.H.: Wearable OLEDs for accelerated wound healing: Enhancing fibroblast proliferation. J. Photomed. **25**(3), 456–462 (2023)
45. Lin, X., Zhao, R., Li, T.: The role of bioluminescent bacteria in photobiomodulation for wound healing. J. Biomed. Opt. **28**(6), 076001 (2023)
46. Lewis, J.S., Roy, K., Keselowsky, B.G.: Materials that harness and modulate the immune system. MRS Bull PMC. **39**(1), 25–34 (2014)
47. Tibbitt, M.W., Rodell, C.B., Burdick, J.A., Anseth, K.S.: Progress in material design for biomedical applications. Spec. Featur.: Perspect. PNAS. **112**(47), 14444–14451 (2015)
48. Lin, W., Zhao, Q., Wang, X.: Biocompatible quantum dots: Challenges and recent developments. Nano Today **47**, 101587 (2023)
49. Zhang, X., Li, Y., Huang, W., Zhao, T.: Advances in biocompatible photoluminescent materials. J. Mater. Sci. **57**(14), 11321–11345 (2022)
50. Canham, L.: Introductory lecture: origins and applications of efficient visible photoluminescence from silicon-based nanostructures. Faraday Discuss. **222**, 10–81
51. Smith, J., Patel, K.: Photoluminescence stability in biological applications. ACS Nano **15**(4), 8924–8932 (2021)
52. Chen, L., Zhao, Y., Wang, H., Lee, J.: Surface engineering of photoluminescent nanomaterials for biocompatibility. Nano Res. **16**(5), 2541–2557 (2023)
53. Fahimida, A., Ashfaq, A., Ahmed, H.J., Ishrak, S., Rabeya, Z.A., Mehedi, H., Nezih, P.: Recent progress and challenges of implantable biodegradable biosensors. Micromachines. **15**(4), 475 (2024)
54. Gupta, N., Sharma, R., Singh, A., Verma, P.: Mitigating photobleaching and photo-toxicity in bioimaging applications. J. Biomed. Opt. **25**(7), 073001 (2020)
55. Clark, R.J., Aghajamali, M., Gonzalez, C.M., Hadidi, L.I., Muhammad, A., Javadi, M., Mobarok, M., Purkait, T., Robidillo, C.T., Sinelnikov, R., Thiessen, A.N.: Photoluminescent material for advance applications. J. Environ. Sci. Technology. **5**(9), 11871 (2017)
56. Liu, Y., Chen, X., Zhang, Q., Huang, Z.: Economic challenges in photoluminescent material synthesis. Adv. Mater. **31**(47), 1904423 (2019)
57. Prakhar, S., Kanchan, C., Gustavo, H.: Progress on carbon dots and hydroxyapatite based biocompatible luminescent nanomaterials for cancer theranostics. Elsevier. **24**, 101482 (2022)
58. Kang, H., Delehanty, J.B., Medintz, I.L.: Emerging applications of photoluminescence in bioimaging. Nature Photonics. **16**(3), 186–198 (2022)
59. Andrea Cocco, S.P., Chiara Olla, R.C., Carlo, M.C., Pier, C.R., Frencesco, S.: Design, synthesis, and photophysical characterization of biocompatible thermally activated delayed fluorescent carbazole-coumarins for sensing applications. Eur. Chem. (2024). https://doi.org/10.1002/chem.202401263
60. Li, F., Krishnan, U.M., Sethuraman, S.: Theranostic applications of photoluminescent nanoparticles. Small **16**(15), 1907034 (2020)
61. Sathish, S., Dhilip, K., Heidi, A.: Recent advances in the development of biocompatible nanocarriers and their cancer cell targeting efficiency in photodynamic therapy. Front. Chem. **15**(10), 969809 (2022)
62. Kumar, S., Giuseppina, S., Eli, Z.: Green synthesis of biocompatible photoluminescent materials. Green Chem. **25**(3), 782–795 (2023)
63. Drik, K., Richard, D., Sean, C.S.: Design guidelines for transition metals as interstitial emitters in silicon nanocrystals to tune photoluminescence properties: Zinc as biocompatible example. Nanoscale **6**(9), 1573 (2023)
64. Nguyen, T., Nicola, M., Paola, C.: AI-enhanced photoluminescence for biomedical applications. IEEE Trans. Biomed. Eng. **68**(11), 3298–3308 (2021)
65. Liu, C., Zhang, J., Xu, K.: Computational approaches in the design of biocompatible light emitters. ACS Nano **18**(2), 1345–1362 (2024)

Fundamentals of Photoluminescent Materials

Ahmed Olalekan Omoniyi, Adefarati Oloruntoba, Jamilu Tijjani Baraya, Mujahid Hassan Sani, Moses Kingsford Flomo, Zainab Abidemi Omoniyi, and Abubakr Abdelmoneim Siddig

Abstract Photoluminescent materials, characterized by their ability to absorb and re-emit light, have revolutionized diverse scientific and technological fields, including biomedical, lighting, display, and sensing applications. This chapter explores the fundamental principles of photoluminescent materials, such as photon absorption, energy transitions, and emission processes, while illustrating distinctions between fluorescence and phosphorescence. It categorizes materials like semiconductor nanocrystals, organic fluorophores, and lanthanide-doped nanoparticles, focusing on their critical roles in advanced medical diagnostics. Synthesis techniques, such as sol–gel processes and hybrid material fabrication, are discussed to underscore recent innovations improving efficiency and scalability. Real-world applications, from high-resolution bioimaging to energy-efficient light-emitting diodes (LEDs) and anti-counterfeiting fluorescent inks, are highlighted alongside critical challenges like stability, environmental resilience, and cost-effective scalability. Addressing these issues through interdisciplinary research, hybrid designs, and emerging eco-friendly alternatives, the chapter concludes with an outlook on emerging trends, establishing a foundation for future exploration and innovation in photoluminescent materials.

Keywords Photoluminescent materials · Fluorescence · Phosphorescence · Bioimaging · Light-emitting diodes · Quantum dots

A. O. Omoniyi (✉) · M. K. Flomo
School of Materials Science and Engineering, Changchun University of Science and Technology, Changchun, PR China
e-mail: omoniyia@veritas.edu.ng

A. Oloruntoba
Department of Chemical and Petroleum Engineering, Schulich School of Engineering, University of Calgary, Calgary, AB, Canada

J. T. Baraya · M. H. Sani · A. A. Siddig
School of Physics, Changchun University of Science and Technology, Changchun, PR China

Z. A. Omoniyi
College of Materials Science and Engineering, Chongqing University, Chongqing, PR China

© The Author(s), under exclusive license to Springer Nature Switzerland AG 2025
N. O. Etafo (ed.), *Tailored Light Emitters For Biomedical Applications*, Engineering Materials, https://doi.org/10.1007/978-3-031-88731-4_2

1 Introduction

Photoluminescent materials are distinguished by their ability to emit light after absorbing photons, a property rooted in intricate interactions at atomic and molecular levels. This phenomenon manifests in fluorescence, characterized by rapid emission following excitation, and phosphorescence, where delayed emission arises from specific electronic transitions. The capacity of these materials to efficiently convert absorbed energy into visible or near-visible light has made them indispensable in modern technology and scientific research. The versatility of photoluminescent materials underpins their critical roles across diverse domains. In lighting, their integration into light-emitting diodes (LEDs) and organic light-emitting diodes (OLEDs) has driven energy-efficient illumination and advanced display technologies, enabling brighter, longer-lasting, and environmentally sustainable solutions [1]. In biomedical fields, fluorescent dyes, quantum dots, and lanthanide-doped nanoparticles have transformed imaging and diagnostics, offering high sensitivity and precision in visualizing cellular and molecular processes [2]. Meanwhile, their application in security and anti-counterfeiting has enhanced document authentication and prevented counterfeiting through luminescent inks and holograms [3]. The development of photoluminescent materials has spurred groundbreaking innovations. In renewable energy, luminescent solar concentrators enhance photovoltaic efficiency, while photoluminescent catalysts drive light-induced chemical reactions for environmental and energy applications [4]. Industrially, photoluminescent materials contribute to safety and navigation systems, with glow-in-the-dark coatings and emergency signage ensuring visibility in low-light or power-outage scenarios [5].

The historical development of photoluminescent materials reflects a journey of curiosity and innovation, beginning with early observations of luminescence in the sixteenth century. Groundbreaking studies in the nineteenth century, such as Stokes' exploration of fluorescence and the Stokes Shift, established fundamental principles of light emission [6]. The twentieth century brought advances in quantum mechanics and material synthesis, enabling tailored photoluminescent properties. This era witnessed the rise of rare-earth phosphors for fluorescent lamps and LEDs, organic fluorophores for OLEDs, and the discovery of quantum dots (QDs) improved tunable light emission, particularly for imaging and sensing applications. More recently, innovative hybrid materials, such as perovskites and metal–organic frameworks (MOFs), has introduced systems combining organic flexibility with inorganic robustness. These materials exhibit exceptional luminescent properties suitable for advanced next-generation applications in biomedicine, energy, and electronics [7, 8]. Sustainability now drives much of the field, with research focusing on eco-friendly, non-toxic, and cost-effective alternatives that balance performance with environmental impact.

This chapter provides an exploration of photoluminescent materials, structured to guide readers through their principles, types, fabrication methods, and applications. It begins with the fundamental mechanisms of photoluminescence (PL) and proceeds to highlight the synthesis of the different types that have shaped the field. Subsequent sections delve into extensive applications of photoluminescent materials, spanning energy, biomedicine, and security, before examining emerging innovations in material design and synthesis. The chapter concludes by addressing the challenges and opportunities in advancing photoluminescent materials, offering insights into their role in driving technological progress and meeting societal demands.

2 Basic Principles of Photoluminescence

Photoluminescence (PL) occurs when a material absorbs photons, promoting electrons to an excited state, followed by the subsequent release of energy as emitted light as the electrons return to a lower energy level. The emitted light's wavelength and intensity, depend on the material's electronic structure and the specific energy transitions that take place. PL processes can occur in various materials, including semiconductors, organic dyes, and lanthanide-doped nanoparticles, with their properties tailored for specific applications. The fundamental principles of PL encompass photon absorption, excitation, and emission, all of which are illustrated through energy-level representations in the Jablonski diagram (Fig. 1).

The PL process begins with the absorption of photons. When a photon with energy $E = h\nu$ (where h is Planck's constant and ν is the light's frequency) interacts with a material, it can excite an electron from the ground state (a lower energy state) to a higher energy state. For this to occur, the photon's energy must equal to or exceed the energy gap (bandgap in semiconductors or energy level difference in molecules) of the material. The absorption of photons is highly material-specific and depends on factors like the energy levels of the material, the density of states, and the optical selection rules [9].

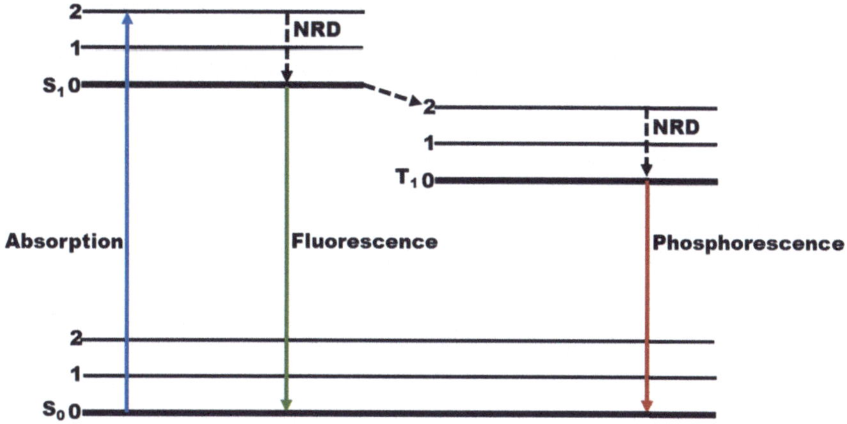

Fig. 1 Jablonski diagram illustrating light absorption (upward arrow), emission (downward arrow), and nonradiative decay (NRD, rapid energy loss to the environment)

After photon absorption, the excited electron typically resides in a high-energy state for a brief period. This state, however, is usually unstable, and the electron relaxes to the lowest vibrational energy level of the excited electronic state through non-radiative processes like vibrational relaxation or internal conversion. The emission process occurs when the electron transitions back to a lower energy state, such as the ground state or a triplet state, releasing energy in the form of photons. Owing to energy losses during non-radiative relaxation, the emitted light generally has a longer wavelength (lower energy) than the absorbed light, a phenomenon known as the Stokes shift [10]. The nature of the emission—fluorescence or phosphorescence—depends on the specific pathways and nature of the electronic transitions and the timescales of the emitted light during its return to the lower energy state.

As illustrated in Fig. 1, fluorescence and phosphorescence are two distinct photoluminescence processes distinguished by their emission mechanisms and timescales. Fluorescence arises from the radiative decay of an electron from the singlet excited state (S_1) to the ground state (S_0), a spin-allowed transition that occurs rapidly, typically within nanoseconds to microseconds. This property makes fluorescent materials ideal for applications requiring intense and fast light emission, such as bioimaging and fluorescence microscopy [11]. In contrast, phosphorescence results from the radiative decay of an electron from an excited triplet state (T_1) to the singlet ground state (S_0), a spin-forbidden transition that is much slower, with emission lifetimes ranging from microseconds to several seconds or even minutes. Phosphorescent materials are commonly used in applications requiring prolonged light emission, such as glow-in-the-dark coatings and time-resolved imaging [12]. The key difference between the two lies in the energy state transitions: fluorescence involves rapid, spin-allowed transitions, while phosphorescence is characterized by slower, spin-forbidden transitions.

The Jablonski diagram is a graphical representation of electronic states and transitions involved in PL, providing a foundational understanding of absorption, excitation, and emission processes. It illustrates electronic states as horizontal lines, grouping singlet states (S_0, S_1, S_2) and triplet states (T_1, T_2) separately. Vertical transitions from the ground state (S_0) to higher singlet states (S_1, S_2) represent photon absorption, while dash arrows depict non-radiative relaxation processes like vibrational relaxation and internal conversion. Fluorescence is shown as a straight arrow from S_1 to S_0, indicating radiative decay, whereas phosphorescence involves an intersystem crossing (S_1 to T_1) followed by radiative decay from T_1 to S_0. The diagram also highlights the Stokes shift, the energy difference between absorbed and emitted light, which results from non-radiative energy losses. Additionally, it incorporates non-radiative processes such as energy transfer and quenching, where interactions with nearby molecules or the environment reduce or alter emission efficiency.

3 Types of Photoluminescent Materials for Medical Applications

Photoluminescent materials have significantly advanced optical medicine by providing new opportunities for diagnosis, imaging, and therapeutic interventions. These materials, which emit light when stimulated, include various systems specifically tailored for biomedical applications. Semiconductor nanocrystals, known as quantum dots (QDs), have garnered substantial interest due to their remarkable luminosity, resistance to photobleaching, and tunable emission characteristics, making them ideal for sensitive and high-resolution imaging [13]. Organic fluorophores, prized for their biocompatibility and versatile designs, play a crucial role in medical imaging and targeted therapies [2]. Additionally, lanthanide-doped nanoparticles offer distinct advantages, such as prolonged emission lifetimes and high photostability, which make them well-suited for time-resolved imaging and deep tissue applications [14, 15]. Together, these photoluminescent materials form the basis for innovative technologies that continue to drive progress in healthcare and biomedical research. Figure 2 illustrates the various types and medical applications of these photoluminescent materials.

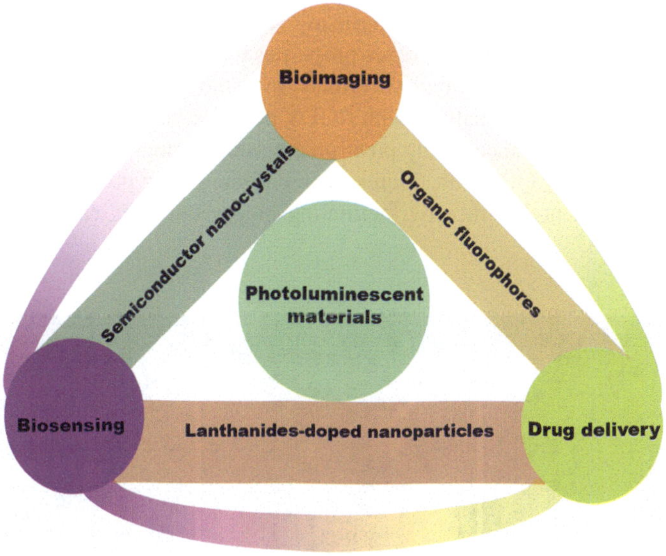

Fig. 2 Schematic diagram illustrating types of photoluminescent materials and their medical applications

3.1 *Semiconductor Nanocrystals (Quantum Dots)*

Quantum dots (QDs), have gained significant attention in biomedical applications due to their exceptional fluorescent characteristics. These properties include a wide absorption spectrum, narrow emission bands, size-dependent effects, a large Stokes shift, a high quantum yield, and strong resistance to photobleaching [16]. The fluorescence process in QDs occurs when electrons in the valence band absorb light energy and transition to the conduction band, thereby creating holes in the valence band. Fluorescent radiation is emitted when these excited electrons recombine with the holes in the valence band. The energy conversion efficiency of QDs is attributed to their exciton effect [17]. The emission spectrum of these particles extends from the visible to the mid-infrared region [18]. They are composed of various elements, including Ag_2S, Ag_2Se, PbS, PbSe, InP, and InAs [19].

3.1.1 Quantum Dots for Bioimaging

QDs in bioimaging present a promising approach, as their distinctive fluorescent properties offer advantages over conventional organic fluorophores. They demonstrated significant utility in bioimaging applications, particularly in the investigation of angiogenesis. In in vivo bioimaging using Ag_2S QDs, these particles maintain high chemical stability and fluorescence properties for a long time, offering real-time monitoring of blood without any toxic effects. In a study aimed at evaluating tumor margins, silica QDs functionalized with RGDY peptides facilitated the cartographic visualization of breast cancer using positron emission tomography [20]. According to Kosaka et al. [21], QDs with fluorescence emission have potential applications in mapping lymph nodes, thereby facilitating biopsy and surgical procedures, as depicted in Fig. 3.

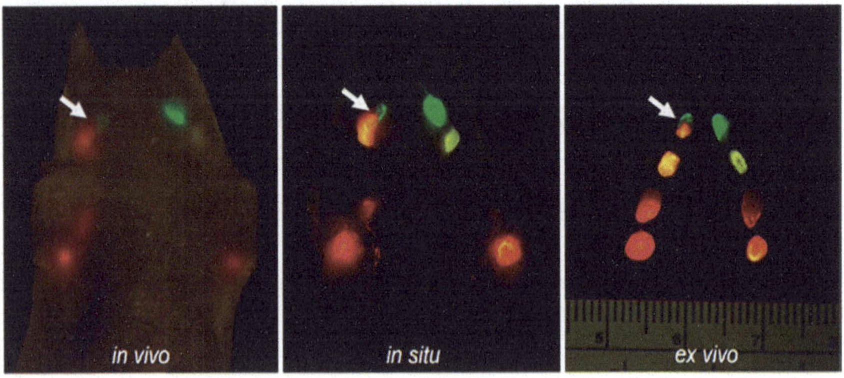

Fig. 3 Multicolor quantum dots for real-time in vivo, in situ and ex vivo mouse imaging [21]

Moreover, QD scans have been employed to identify and delineate tumors, including their location, and size, thereby eliminating the necessity for biopsies [20]. In an alternative investigation, carbon black was used to create graphene quantum dots (GQDs), which were utilized as a fluorescent indicator in confocal microscopy imaging, the resultant product demonstrated high biocompatibility and emitted green fluorescence upon absorption by MCF-7 human breast cancer cells [22]. Deng et al. synthesized $CuInS_2/ZnS$ QDs of varying dimensions and subsequently incorporated them into a folate-modified chitosan micelle, which effectively demonstrated in vitro imaging of Bel-7402 cancer cells that express folate receptors [23].

3.1.2 Quantum Dots for Biosensing

The capacity of QDs conjugation with biomolecules such as DNA, antibodies, proteins, or viruses renders them suitable for biosensing and immunoassay applications. Their diverse emission wavelengths enable the simultaneous labeling of multiple living cell components, facilitating the investigation of their interactions [24]. Muthusankar et al. designed a hybrid electrochemical nanocomposite quantum dot (QD) sensor capable of detecting both the antibiotic nitrofurantoin (NF) and the anticancer drug flutamide (FLU) simultaneously. This sensor exhibited exceptional performance in measuring NF and FLU, with wide linear ranges and appreciable detection limits [25]. An ultrasensitive electrochemical immunosensor for carcinoembryonic antigen (CEA) detection was developed, this sensor utilizes nitrogen-doped GQDs (N-GQDs) as a support for PtPd bimetallic nanoparticles. The device demonstrates exceptional electrocatalytic performance in reducing hydrogen peroxide (H_2O_2) and offers a broad linear detection range for CEA, a remarkably low detection limit, and a good signal-to-noise ratio value [26]. Elmizadeh et al. developed a QD-based biosensor designed to detect digitalis toxin (digoxin) in biological fluids [27]. Furthermore, in terms of biochemical indicators, carbon quantum dots (CQDs) functionalized with boronic acid groups to serve as biosensors for detecting glucose levels in blood were developed. Upon exposure to blood containing glucose, the boronic acid components interact with glucose molecules, resulting in CQDs aggregation and subsequent decrease of their fluorescence. The observed fluorescence quenching correlates with the concentration of the glucose and achieves a good detection threshold [28].

QDs have proven to be highly versatile and efficient tools for biosensing applications due to their capacity to conjugate with various biomolecules and their tunable optical properties. Their application spans the detection of drugs, toxins, biochemical indicators, and cancer markers with remarkable sensitivity and specificity. The advancements in QD-based sensors, such as hybrid nanocomposites, nitrogen-doped graphene quantum dots, and functionalized carbon quantum dots, demonstrate their potential for precise and reliable diagnostics in complex biological systems. These innovations highlight the growing impact of QDs in advancing biosensing technologies and their significant contributions to medical diagnostics and research.

3.1.3 Quantum Dots for Drug Delivery

QDs exhibit significant utility not only in bioimaging and biosensing applications but also serve as efficient drug delivery systems. The advantages of using QDs as drug carriers involve their ease of manufacturing, nanoscale dimensions, capacity for attachment to diverse medications, modifiable physicochemical properties, and distinctive optical characteristics. These attributes enable QDs to function as traceable drug transporters that can be readily monitored following administration [29].

A PEGylated-based QD was developed to deliver doxorubicin into cancer cells. This nanomaterial exhibited blue light emission, released the drug in response to pH changes, maintained good stability, and showed low toxicity under normal physiological conditions [30]. Javanbakht and Namazi developed novel nanocomposite QDs for anticancer drug delivery. The mechanism of these films demonstrated the capacity to release DOX in a pH-dependent manner for a long period [31]. In the field of gene therapy, QDs have been employed to enhance cellular delivery. In an experiment encapsulating CdSe-core QDs, ZnS-shell QDs, and/or small interference RNA (targeting the Lamin A/C gene) within Lipofectamine. The findings show a significant correlation between gene suppression and fluorescence intensity in cells treated with both QDs and siRNA, indicating that QDs serve as an effective means for monitoring siRNA delivery [32].

3.2 *Organic Fluorophores*

Organic fluorophore nanomaterials exhibit potential for applications in biomedical due to their notable advantages. These include high sensitivity, easy absorption by the cell, flexible design, and biodegradability. They provide extensive information about the biomolecules and offer a more comprehensive approach to imaging, sensing, and targeted drug delivery within living organisms.

3.2.1 Organic Fluorophores for Bioimaging

Fluorescence-based optical imaging has emerged as an important method for enhancing the early detection of preinvasive and metastatic cancer cells, leveraging its high sensitivity, selectivity, and non-invasive nature. The fluorescence signals provide essential information about the disease, its progression, and outcomes while assessing drug efficacy [33]. Various fluorophores were developed and employed to achieve high-resolution images of cells and subcellular structures.

Recently, Lin et al. synthesized a new NIR-II FL probe that incorporates an oxygenated anthracene with a benzopyrido[1,2–a:3,4–b] indole component [34]. This innovative probe facilitates the non-invasive detection of excessive palladium (II) ions (Pd^{2+}) in mouse livers, which demonstrates its potential in bioimaging. A

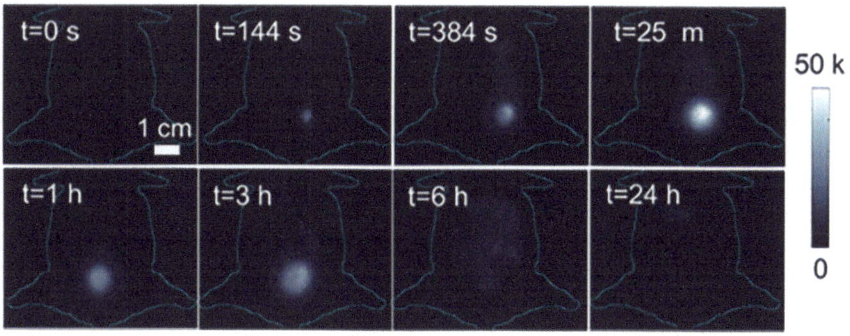

Fig. 4 Mouse imaging at different time intervals using NIR-IIa imaging following the administration of IR-BEMC6P [37]

polymer-based fluorescent probe for the NIR-II region, which incorporated IR-808 and Nd^{3+} ions, has been developed. It offered a high-resolution fluorescent component that allowed for enhanced visualization of blood vessels and cerebral artery blockages in mouse models [35]. Li et al. [36] investigated the utilization of nanoparticles coated with pre-activated macrophage membranes for photothermal therapy (PTT) treatment of tuberculosis. Upon intravenous administration, these nanoparticles facilitated the real-time visualization of individual lesions, thus demonstrating their potential in imaging applications.

A highly degradable polyester incorporating dual NIR-II fluorophores was also developed. This material enables concurrent NIR-II and apoptosis imaging, in vivo drug monitoring, and rapid assessment of treatment efficacy (Fig. 4) [37].

3.2.2 Organic Fluorophores for Biosensing

Many organic fluorophores have demonstrated the ability to provide valuable infor mation about the presence and levels of various biological molecules. This information is gathered through changes in the fluorophores' emission properties, particularly their intensity and wavelength [2]. Guo et al. developed a β-galactosidase activity monitoring probe through the conjugation of a galactose moiety to the phenolic hydroxyl of QM-OH. When the hydrophilic substrate undergoes enzymatic cleavage, the resulting fluorophores form nanoparticles, which improves intracellular retention and facilitating long-time monitoring of β-galactosidase activity in live cellular environments [38]. A caspase-3/7-sensitive probe was created by mixing the water-insoluble tetraphenylethene (TPE) molecule with a water-soluble peptide substrate, Asp-Glu-Val-Asp (DEVD). Initially, this compound exhibited water solubility and non-fluorescence. The selective cleavage of the DEVD peptide by caspase-3/-7 resulted in the release of TPE, which subsequently formed aggregates in proximity to the cleavage sites. This aggregation process induced enhanced fluorescence, thereby enabling the detection of staurosporine-induced cell apoptosis [39].

On the other hand, Near Infrared II (NIR-II) spectrum fluorophores demonstrated significant potential as disease detection probes due to their sensitivity and specificity to corresponding analytes. GNP-KTP5-ICG sensor was designed to enable early detection of kidney dysfunction, allowing both in vitro analysis of urine and prolonged in vivo monitoring of kidney activity [40]. Additionally, with the utilization of N-acetyl cysteine (NAC), the dyes NIRII-HD5-GSH and NIRII-HD5-$ONOO^-$ were effectively employed to sense changes in ROS ($ONOO^-$) and GSH production before and after treatment in an APAP-induced liver injury mouse [41].

3.2.3 Organic Fluorophores for Drug Delivery

Organic fluorophore nanoparticles serve as promising vehicles and are extensively utilized for precise drug delivery. The tunable fluorescence properties of these particles allow continuous tracking of drug delivery. Xue et al. introduced a self-reported drug delivery system that incorporated doxorubicin (DOX) and carboxylated TPE (TPE-COOH) within a single platform. This system utilized the effects of DOX and TPE-COOH to produce three distinct fluorescent signals, enabling visualization of drug delivery, release, and subcellular localization [42]. Jung et al. developed an AIEgen-based nanoparticle for targeted mitochondrial delivery of DOX in image-guided cancer therapy. This nanoparticle was synthesized using a cyanostilbene-based derivative containing TPP and an extended alkyl chain [43]. Lunardi et al. produced therapeutic and diagnostic agents consisting of (lactic-*co*-glycollic) acid nanoparticles containing cresyl violet dye. These agents were administered to mice via intravenous injection while under anesthesia. Following euthanasia, various organs (spleen, lungs, heart, kidney, and liver), were extracted and examined the distribution of the particles using multiphoton microscopy, which demonstrated the ability of the created particles to effectively reach different target sites [44].

3.3 Lanthanide-Doped Nanoparticles

Lanthanides are a group of 15 elements spanning from lanthanum to lutetium, located in the sixth row and the IIIB column of the periodic table [45]. Lanthanide-doped nanoparticles (LnNPs) constitute a novel class of luminescent materials that incorporate lanthanide ions as dopants into host substances such as biological molecules. The significance of these nanoparticles primarily arises from their capacity to perform photon upconversion processes, which enable the generation of upconverted ultraviolet-to-visible light through radiative transitions when exposed to NIR laser light. This approach provides the advantage of flexibility in integrating various molecules, dyes, and functional components with upconversion nanoparticles [15]. The exceptional optical properties of these materials, including minimal background fluorescence and high sensitivity, render them suitable for diverse biomedical applications, including bioimaging techniques, biosensing, and drug delivery systems [46].

3.3.1 LnNPs for Bioimaging

The advancement of contemporary healthcare necessitates the development of an instrument capable of rapidly and accurately providing comprehensive insights into cellular biological mechanisms and disease detection. Due to their capacity to penetrate deeply into tissue and generate high-resolution spatial images, LnNPs present a promising approach for examining the complex structures of living tissues.

Lanthanide elements demonstrate greater X-ray attenuation coefficients compare to iodine, which is mostly used as a CT contrast agent. As a result, Ln_2O_3 nanoparticles have potential as effective contrast agents for CT imaging [47]. A study conducted by Naczynski et al. demonstrated that conventional $NaYF_4$ nanocrystals, doped with both Yb^{3+} and Er^{3+}, exhibited the capacity to emit light at approximately 1530 nm when exposed to X-ray radiation. This conversion of X-rays into NIR-II light was utilized to track the motion of nanoprobes within living organisms and to image lymphatic drainage patterns [48]. Paramagnetic lanthanide ions, characterized by unpaired 4f electrons, exhibit responsiveness to the applied magnetic fields. This property enables LnNPs to function as contrast agents, reducing the relaxation times of proximal protons and enhancing magnetic resonance imaging contrast. In 2019, Yi et al. developed a nanoconjugate probe capable of amplifying signals in response to the mildly acidic environment of tumors. Coating the surfaces of these nanoconjugates with cancer cell membranes, the probes demonstrated homologous targeting of tumors in vivo and enhancements of the imaging signal intensity compared to a clinical contrast Magnevist agent [49].

Furthermore, upconversion lanthanide-doped nanoparticles have shown versatility in the creation of multifunctional nanoplatforms that combine imaging and therapeutic functions. These particles exhibit potential for biomedical applications in early detection and treatment monitoring. Additionally, they offer innovative approaches for small animal imaging, involving lymphatic imaging, vascular imaging, and tumor-targeted imaging techniques [50].

3.3.2 LnNPs for Biosensing

LnNPs serve as optical sensors for extracting biological data from patients during biopsies. These versatile probes demonstrate the capability to detect various substances, including essential trace elements [51], toxic metal ions [52], DNAs [53], miRNA [54], and relevant biologically small molecules [45, 55]. LnNPs also demonstrate potential as materials for monitoring patient temperature, which is essential for accurate diagnosis and effective treatment. This is especially significant in cases requiring precise temperature measurement of living cells, particularly cancer cells, and real-time tracking during in vivo therapies [56]. Furthermore, these materials have uses in identifying highly toxic heavy metal ions [14], oxygen deficiency, and hypochlorous acid [57, 58]. They are also employed in biological assays [59], detection of oligonucleotides [60], and sensing glucose levels [58, 61].

3.3.3 LnNPs for Drug Delivery

LnNPs have emerged as versatile nanocarriers, offering transformative advantages over traditional drug delivery methods. By improving drug solubility, stability, biodistribution, and pharmacokinetics, these nanoparticles enhance therapeutic efficacy while reducing adverse effects. Their nanoscale size supports efficient cellular uptake, enabling precise drug delivery to tumor cells with controlled release, minimizing side effects, and preserving healthy tissue [62]. Additionally, LnNPs function as dual-purpose platforms for both drug delivery and real-time monitoring, fulfilling diagnostic and therapeutic needs [50]. Innovations include upconversion luminescence-triggered azo-photoisomerization for regulating drug release [63], temperature-controlled photothermal modulation for precise administration, [64], and pH-sensitive complexes for combined cancer therapies [65]. Moreover, the development of biodegradable polyesters with integrated NIR-II fluorophores enables simultaneous drug tracking, apoptosis imaging, and real-time therapeutic evaluation, showcasing the expanding potential of LnNP-based systems in advanced medicine [66].

4 Synthesis and Fabrication Methods of Photoluminescent Materials

The synthesis and fabrication of luminescent materials are essential for optimizing their properties for applications in optoelectronics, biomedical imaging, and sensing. Inorganic materials, like QDs and phosphors, are commonly synthesized using methods like sol–gel processes, hydrothermal synthesis, combustion synthesis, and co-precipitation, ensuring precise control over their structure. Organic luminescent materials, including conjugated polymers and small molecules, are synthesized through solution-based and solid-state methods, offering design flexibility. Hybrid materials, which integrate the advantages of both inorganic and organic materials, are fabricated using techniques like layer-by-layer assembly and vapor deposition, enabling multifunctional applications. This section offers an overview of the various synthesis and fabrication methods used to produce luminescent materials, highlighting the specific processes and conditions used to customize the luminescent properties for practical applications.

4.1 Synthesis of Inorganic Luminescent Materials

The extensive use of inorganic luminescent materials in lighting, displays, and biological imaging has attracted significant interest. These materials, which include phosphors, QDs, and rare-earth doped compounds, are typically crystalline. Researchers have prioritized controlling crystal size, structure, and dopant distribution when synthesizing these substances to optimize performance. Several key methods are commonly employed for their production.

4.1.1 Solid-State Reaction Method

This high-temperature synthesis approach is widely employed for producing, modifying, and analyzing materials in solid-state or crystalline forms, owing to its straightforward nature and scalability. Conducted at temperatures ranging from hundreds to thousands of degrees Celsius without solvents, this method offers numerous benefits, including uniform mixing, thermodynamic stability, property customization, and controlled microstructural development. Understanding solid-state reaction pathways is essential to achieving effective material synthesis, as these pathways define the sequence of chemical transformations that take place throughout the procedure.

Various types of solid-state reactions have been utilized, including diffusion-controlled reactions [67, 68], solid–solid reactions [69, 70], redox reactions [71, 72], thermal decomposition [73, 74], and phase transformations [75, 76]. For instance, the luminescent and dosimetric properties of microcrystalline $SrB_4O_7:Eu^{3+}$, synthesized using a solid-state diffusion technique (Fig. 5) with europium chloride, boric acid, and strontium carbonate as precursor materials, were examined, with a particular emphasis on the effects of annealing temperature and Eu concentration on the structural, morphological, and luminescent characteristics of the material [77].

The solid-state reaction method offers benefits such as simplicity, cost-effectiveness, and the capacity to produce materials with high purity and controlled stoichiometry. However, this method has certain limitations, including the need for high temperatures and extended reaction times, which may not be suitable for all material types. Moreover, achieving desired luminescent properties necessitates precise control of reaction conditions, presenting challenges that require further investigation and optimization.

4.1.2 Solution-Based Methods

Solution-based synthesis methods involve dissolving precursor compounds in a solvent and inducing chemical reactions to produce the desired product. These techniques are widely employed in fabricating various materials, including nanoparticles, thin films, ceramics, and composites. Their simplicity, scalability, and ability to precisely control material properties at the nanoscale make them highly versatile

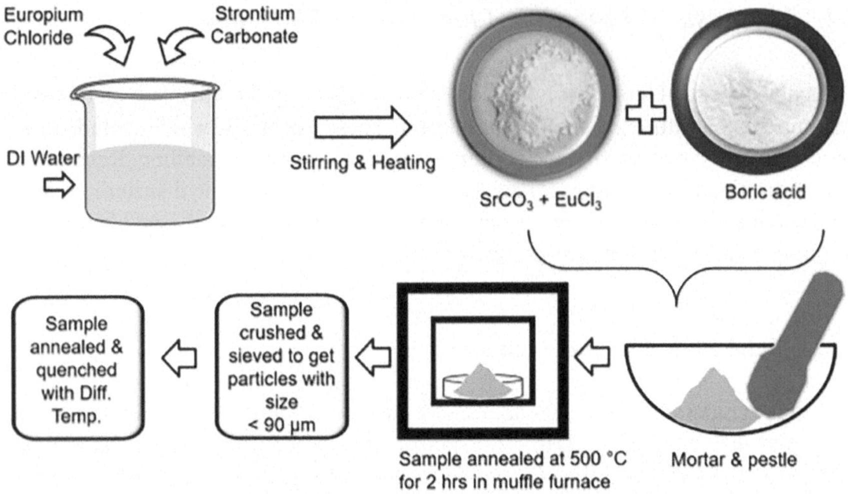

Fig. 5 Schematic diagram illustrating the synthesis process for SrB_4O_7:Eu^{3+} microphosphors using the solid-state diffusion technique [77]

in chemistry, materials science, and nanotechnology. The three primary solution-based synthesis approaches are the sol–gel method, hydrothermal synthesis, and co-precipitation.

Sol–Gel Method

The sol–gel approach is adaptable for synthesizing advanced materials, including ceramics, glasses, thin films, and porous structures. It is widely utilized in optics, electronics, catalysis, and adsorption. This process involves key chemical reactions, primarily hydrolysis and condensation, which employ metal alkoxides to transform a colloidal solution (sol) into a solid network (gel). This technique enables the production of substances with high purity and uniformity at comparatively low temperatures, allowing precise control of texture, porosity, and surface characteristics [78].

The sol–gel process comprises five key stages: hydrolysis, polycondensation, aging, drying, and thermal decomposition (as shown in Fig. 6). These stages are critical for tailoring the structure and performance of materials. The resulting materials range from nanoparticles and powders to thin films and composites. Thin films and coatings are particularly notable for their exceptional optical, electronic, and magnetic properties, making them suitable for anti-reflective layers, photochromic and electrochromic films, photovoltaic devices, and displays. The sol–gel method exemplifies a bottom-up approach to material synthesis, enabling innovative designs with high-performance [79].

In the context of phosphor synthesis, the sol–gel method yields luminescent materials whose characteristics are significantly affected by the type and concentration

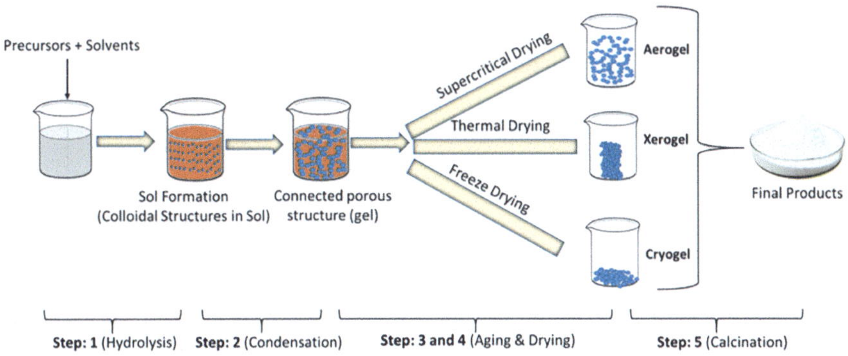

Fig. 6 Stages involved in the sol–gel process for synthesizing metal oxide nanoparticles [79]

of dopants. For instance, $LiBaPO_4$ phosphors doped with Dy^{3+} and Tb^{3+} exhibit characteristic emission peaks associated with specific electronic transitions [80]. Similarly, $YAlO_3$ phosphors demonstrate intense green emissions when doped with Mn^{2+}, while Nd^{3+} doping results in emissions spanning multiple wavelengths [81]. Furthermore, the sol–gel technique facilitates the production of nanophosphors, as exemplified by La_2O_3:Eu^{3+}, which displays PL peaks attributed to Eu^{3+} electronic transitions [82].

Despite its advantages, the sol–gel method poses challenges, including difficulties in achieving the desired stoichiometry and purity, potential structural damage from improper drying, time-intensive processes, and the high cost of high-purity precursors. Nonetheless, the technique remains integral to developing new optical and photonic materials. Its ability to produce homogeneous components and coatings surpasses conventional methods, driving continued innovation in material science.

Hydrothermal Method

Over the past two centuries, hydrothermal techniques have been extensively utilized for single-crystal growth and powder preparation. This method involves using an aqueous solution within a sealed reaction chamber (Fig. 7a) to generate an elevated pressure and temperature environment, enabling the dissolution and recrystallization of substances that are insoluble under standard conditions [83, 84]. The overall process is depicted in Fig. 7b.

Hydrothermal methods are particularly effective for transforming metal alloys into ultrafine powders and facilitating the formation of crystalline powders from solutions containing metal ions under elevated temperatures and pressures. Technological advancements have established hydrothermal synthesis as the cornerstone of nanomaterial preparation, accommodating a broad temperature range. This method also provides precise control over material morphology by adjusting the pressure conditions based on the vapor pressure of the reaction components [86, 87]. The

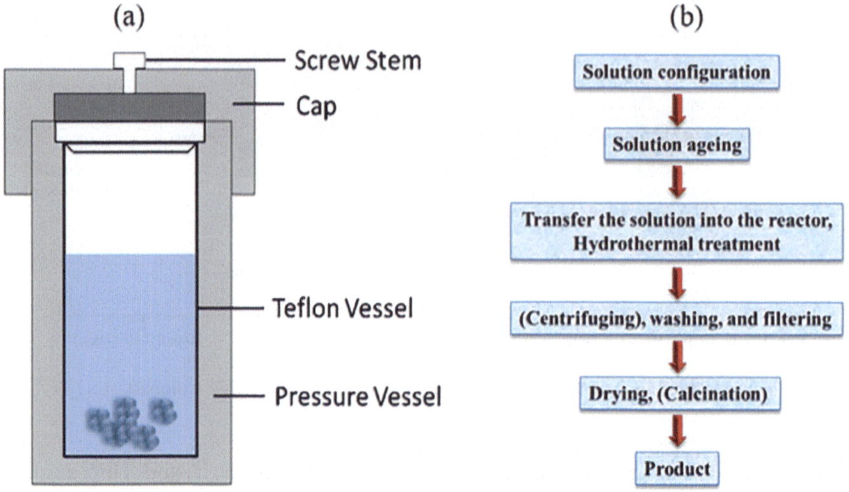

Fig. 7 **a** Illustration of standard hydrothermal method apparatus. **b** Overview of the overall steps involved in hydrothermal preparation [85]

advantages of hydrothermal synthesis are significant, including its ability to produce high-quality single crystals that are essential for crystallography and electronics, along with precise control over nucleation and crystal growth. It is employed extensively in synthesizing nanomaterials, such as nanoparticles and nanowires, which may be unstable at high temperatures [88].

The hydrothermal process has been extensively utilized in the fabrication of various Ce^{3+} and Tb^{3+} co-doped phosphates, such as $LaPO_4$, $Ca_9Y(PO_4)_6(OH)_2$, and $GdPO_4$, enabling precise control over phase composition and morphology [89]. Investigations into the hydrothermal synthesis of $KGdF_4$ nanocrystals and K-Lu-F materials have demonstrated that doping with Ce^{3+} and Tb^{3+} substantially influences their crystalline phases and morphologies [90, 91]. Applications of the hydrothermal method are diverse, ranging from single-crystal growth for X-ray crystallography, the fabrication of piezoelectric materials, and the production of semiconductors and nanostructured catalysts [92]. The ability of this method to operate under high-temperature and high-pressure aqueous conditions facilitates the production of single crystals, nanomaterials, and complex oxides, underscoring its critical role in advancing materials science and nanotechnology.

Co-precipitation Method

Co-precipitation is a versatile technique for synthesizing nanoparticles with tailored luminescent properties, offering precise control over phosphor composition and structure. This technique involves the simultaneous precipitation of multiple elements from a solution to form multi-component substances and composites. By carefully

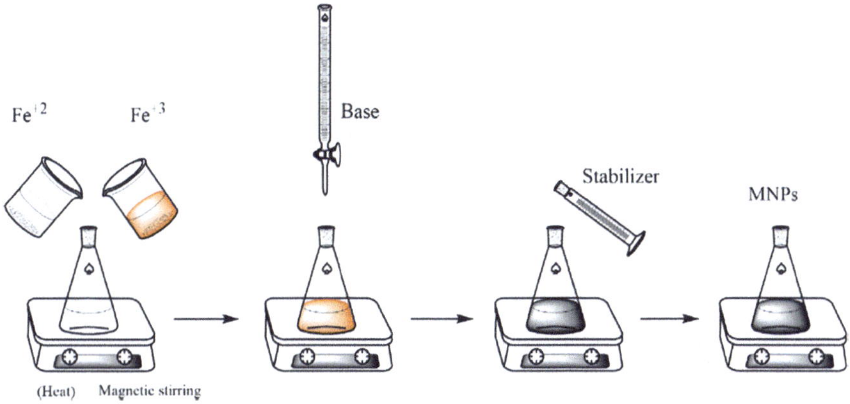

Fig. 8 Schematic representation of the fabrication of magnetite nanoparticles (MNPs) using the co-precipitation approach [93]

controlling the combining of precursor solutions to trigger precipitation reactions, co-precipitation allows for the customization of material properties to meet specific needs. The flexibility of this approach enables the production of a diverse array of materials, including nanoparticles (Fig. 8), metal oxides, and magnetic materials, while its scalability makes it well-suited for industrial applications [92].

The process has diverse applications, such as the fabrication of magnetic nanoparticles used in data storage, the generation of catalysts for chemical reactions, and the creation of composite materials with distinct properties. The luminescence characteristics of the synthesized nanoparticles are influenced by their composition and structure. For instance, $CaSO_4$ nanoparticles produced via co-precipitation exhibit thermoluminescence (TL) and PL, with TL being useful for examining defects in semiconductor materials and for radiation dosimetry [94]. Furthermore, co-precipitation allows for the synthesis of high-purity materials with controlled morphology, as demonstrated by the synthesis of Sr_2SnO_4:Eu^{3+} and Li^+ phosphors, which exhibit enhanced luminescence performance [95].

4.2 *Synthesis of Organic Luminescent Materials*

Organic luminescent materials are a group of compounds that emit light upon excitation by an external energy source and have garnered significant attention in scientific research. These materials are distinguished by their capacity to convert absorbed energy into visible light, making them suitable for various technological applications. Their distinctive optical properties and wide-ranging potential applications render them valuable in optoelectronics, display technologies, lighting, sensing, and biomedicine. These materials are primarily classified as organic phosphorescent compounds, organic fluorescent substances, and organic light-emitting diodes

(OLEDs) [96, 97]. The synthesis of these materials involves various strategies aimed at producing high-purity compounds with optimized light-emitting properties. The choice of an appropriate fabrication technique is influenced by factors such as the type of luminescent material (fluorescent or phosphorescent), molecular structure, and intended application.

4.2.1 Solution-Based Synthesis

These synthetic methods typically involve preparing a homogeneous mixture by dissolving organic precursor constituents in an appropriate solvent. The resultant mix undergoes chemical transformations to yield the desired light-emitting compound. Prominent reactions employed in organic solution-based synthesis (Fig. 9) include the Suzuki coupling reaction [98], Stille coupling reaction [99], Heck reaction [100], and direct arylation [101]. These reactions, categorized as palladium-catalyzed cross-coupling reactions, involve solution-phase chemistry, where organic precursors are dissolved in appropriate solvents and undergo specific catalytic conditions to form complex organic structures with desirable luminescent properties [102]. Thus, these reactions are commonly employed in organic synthesis to create conjugated systems that are critical for luminescence.

Despite the numerous advantages of solution-based synthesis, significant challenges remain in achieving high luminescence efficiency and environmental stability.

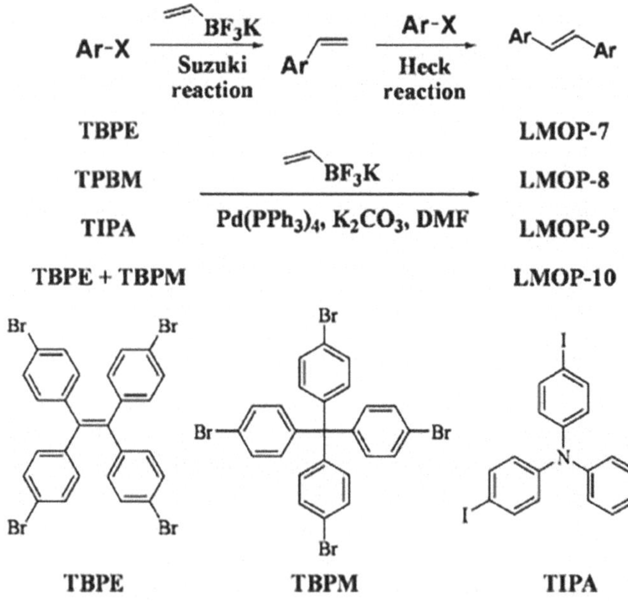

Fig. 9 The syntheses of luminescent microporous organic polymers through the tandem Suzuki–Heck reaction involving aromatic halides in conjunction with potassium vinyltrifluoroborate [104]

In particular, the design and development of dual-state emissive materials that exhibit robust performance in both solid and solution phases continue to pose substantial challenges but are highly sought after for advanced applications [103].

4.2.2 Solid-State Synthesis

Solid-state synthesis is a solvent-free technique that produces highly stable luminescent organic materials with desirable physical properties. This approach is widely employed for synthesizing materials with high purity, stability, and efficiency. It is especially preferred for manufacturing materials designed for photonic and electronic devices, such as OLEDs, solar cells, and lasers [105, 106]. Several solid-state techniques have been commonly employed for the production of luminescent organic materials. Herein, we focus on three widely utilized approaches: solid-state polymerization, mechanochemical synthesis, and vapor deposition.

Solid-State Polymerization

Solid-state polymerization (SSP) involves the chemical combination of monomers (a process referred to as polymerization) in the solid state, including crystalline, liquid crystalline, or glassy forms. The core principle of this method consists of heating the material in an inert atmosphere or under vacuum at a temperature below its melting point, thereby enabling the commencement and propagation of polymerization reactions. This approach provides a solvent-free process for synthesizing high-molecular-weight polymers, eliminating the need for elevated temperatures, which could potentially lead to material degradation. SSP is particularly advantageous for luminescent organic materials because it allows precise control over their molecular structure and packing, which are essential for optoelectronic applications. SSP enhances optical properties by manipulating molecular interactions and structural configurations such as emission efficiency and color tunability. Typically, SSP is initiated by high-energy radiation, including γ-rays, or by thermal activation, thus facilitating the production of advanced luminescent polymers, including tailored polyesters and polyamides [107, 108].

Mechanochemical Synthesis

Mechanochemical synthesis (MCS) is a versatile and environment-friendly approach that utilizes mechanical forces to drive chemical reactions, making it an appealing method for synthesizing a diverse range of materials. Typically performed via ball milling, MCS involves trapping, grinding, and applying mechanical energy to the precursors, which results in bond breaking, defect formation, and surface alterations. This technique is either solvent-free or uses minimal solvents, offering several advantages over conventional synthesis methods, particularly by reducing the environmental impact and facilitating the creation of novel material structures [109–111].

As a cost-effective and sustainable synthetic route, MCS has gained considerable interest owing to its potential to develop luminescent organic materials for various applications. For example, the mechanosynthesis of a small oligophenylene-based molecule, bisquinoline (OBM), has been reported [112]. This study successfully incorporated these small molecules into the synthesis of OLED devices, leading to electroluminescence. The resulting OLED device exhibited a luminance of 2350 cd/m^2 when powered by a fixed current of 15 mA at 10 V. Furthermore, a solvent-free MCS method was employed to synthesize the aluminum complex Alq_3 (where q = 8-hydroxyquinolinate), demonstrating its potential for use in OLED technology [113].

Vapor Deposition Methods

Vapor deposition methods, including physical vapor deposition (PVD), chemical vapor deposition (CVD), and organic vapor phase deposition (OVPD), are widely employed to deposit organic luminescent materials on substrates in the vapor phase. These methods are effective for producing thin films and high-purity materials. The process typically involves heating organic materials to elevated temperatures to induce vaporization, after which the vapor is directed onto a substrate, where it solidifies to create a thin film. Deposition is generally performed under high vacuum conditions to ensure film purity and uniformity.

Vapor deposition methods offer several key advantages, including the production of highly uniform, high-purity films, precise control of film thickness and composition, and scalability for applications in OLEDs and photovoltaics. These features make vapor deposition methods indispensable for synthesizing organic luminescent materials, which are crucial for developing light-emitting devices and other photofunctional materials [114–116].

i. **Chemical Vapor Deposition**

Chemical vapor deposition (CVD) is a commonly used method for depositing thin films by employing chemical reactions of gaseous precursors on a heated substrate. During this process, vapor-phase precursors decompose to create a solid film on the substrate. CVD is a versatile method employed for depositing various materials, including organic compounds, semiconductors, metals, and insulators. These materials are essential in the fabrication of optoelectronic and microelectronic devices, as well as in the production of optical and protective coatings. Depending on the deposition conditions, CVD films can be amorphous, polycrystalline, or epitaxial. The process can be either selective or non-selective, enabling both homoepitaxy and heteroepitaxy. A significant advantage of CVD is its ability to provide excellent conformal coverage, making it especially well-suited for complex geometries [117, 118].

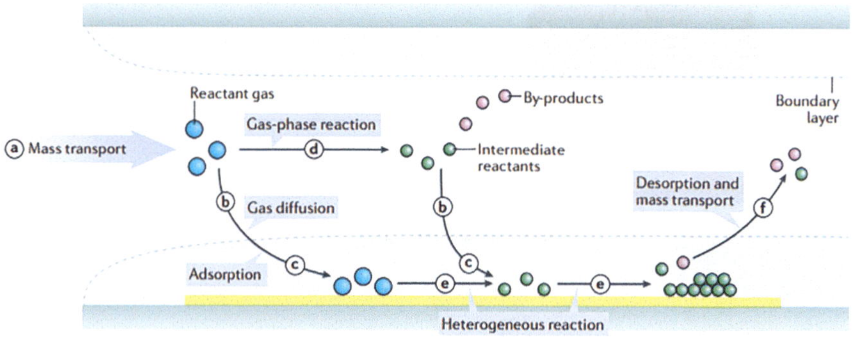

Fig. 10 Schematic representation of the basic steps in a regular CVD process [120]

Figure 10 illustrates the key stages in a typical CVD process. Initially, reactant gases (represented by blue circles) are introduced into the reactor and transported toward the substrate surface (step a). These gases diffuse through the boundary layer (step b) and adsorb onto the substrate surface (step c). Concurrently, reactions in the gas phase may produce intermediate species (shown as green circles) and by-products (red circles) (step d). The intermediates also diffuse and adsorb onto the substrate (steps b and c), facilitating the deposition. On the substrate surface, heterogeneous reactions and surface diffusion (step e) lead to the creation of thin films or coatings. Finally, the unreacted gases and by-products desorb and are carried out of the reactor as exhaust (step f). This systematic process enables precise and controlled thin-film deposition, essential for producing high-quality materials.

CVD has also proven highly effective in the production of luminescent materials. For example, Eu^{3+}-doped HfO_2 and Lu_2O_3 films, synthesized via metal–organic CVD, emit intense red light under UV excitation. This method is especially beneficial for high-melting-point materials and luminescent phosphors, offering a rapid and efficient synthesis route [119]. CVD is a highly effective and adaptable technique that enables the precise, controlled deposition of superior-quality thin films. Its capacity to deposit a diverse array of materials with accuracy and consistency makes it essential for the production of luminescent organic materials and advanced electronic devices, reinforcing its position as a foundational technology in materials science and engineering.

ii. **Physical Vapor Deposition**

Physical vapor deposition (PVD) is an atomic-level deposition technique in which a material is vaporized from a liquid or solid precursor and transported as molecules or atoms via a vacuum or low-pressure gas (or plasma) environment. When the vapor reaches the substrate, where it solidifies to create a thin film. PVD is commonly employed to deposit films with thicknesses varying from a few nanometers to several micrometers. It is also utilized in the fabrication of thick films, graded composition deposits, multilayer coatings, and freestanding structures [121].

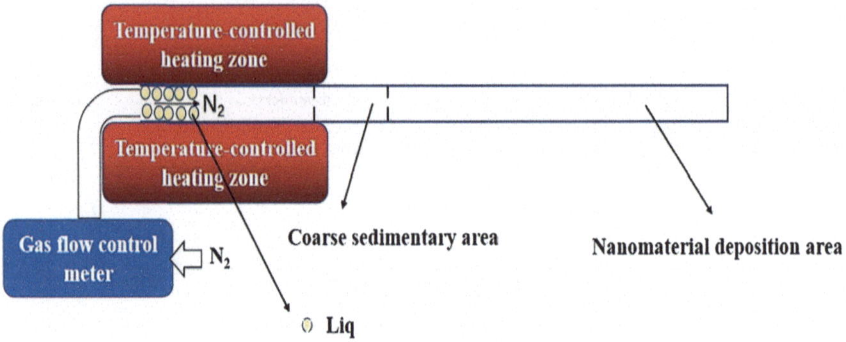

Fig. 11 Simple schematic representation of PVD system [124]

PVD encompasses several techniques, such as magnetron sputtering, thermal evaporation, and electron beam evaporation. Each technique offers specific advantages contingent upon the material and the intended application. These techniques allow for precise control of both the thickness and composition of the deposited films, making PVD suitable for a diverse array of materials, including organic compounds, semiconductors, and metals [121, 122]. Recent studies have utilized PVD to investigate the supramolecular arrangements and optical properties of organic luminescent materials. For example, one study focused on bis(phenethylimido)perylene (PhPTCD) thin films fabricated via thermal evaporation. This work revealed controlled film growth and thermal stability without degradation, with the films exhibiting homogeneous surface morphology and an amorphous structure, alongside a preferential flat-on orientation [123]. Another study explored the deposition of 8-hydroxyquinoline lithium (Liq) using PVD (Fig. 11), highlighting enhanced luminescent performance due to reduced exciton diffusion. This research emphasized Liq's high purity, excellent phase characteristics, and potential for diverse optoelectronic applications [124].

Despite its versatility, PVD presents certain challenges, such as issues with substrate adhesion and limited material utilization efficiency. Nevertheless, it remains a vital technique for depositing organic luminescent materials, owing to its ability to produce high-quality, precise films.

iii. **Organic Vapor Phase Deposition**

Organic Vapor Phase Deposition (OVPD) has become a highly effective technique for fabricating high-performance thin-film organic devices, including OLEDs, transistors, and photovoltaics. In this process, organic materials are heated vaporized into an inert carrier gas, which transports the evaporated molecules via a low-pressure chamber. Inside the chamber, the organic molecules are evenly distributed through diffusive mixing subsequently deposited onto a cooled substrate via physisorption. The use of a hot-walled reactor helps minimize undesirable deposition on the surfaces of the reactor, enhancing material utilization and reducing the need for frequent cleaning [125]. A significant advantage of OVPD is its near-equilibrium evaporative

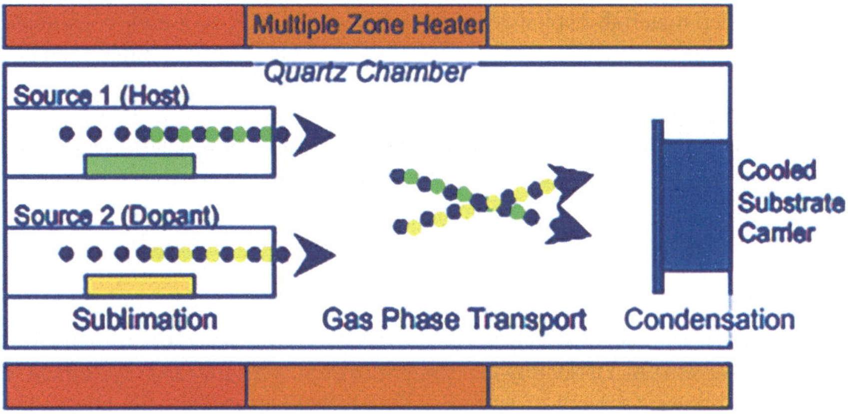

Fig. 12 The foundational principle of the OVPD [127]

material pick-up, which enables precise doping at high deposition rates. The hot carrier gas environment promotes improved morphological control, achieving material utilization efficiencies exceeding 40%. These attributes render OVPD particularly suitable for the rapid and efficient synthesis of organic semiconductor devices [126].

OVPD was originally developed by Forrest et al. [128] at Princeton University to harness the advantages of gas-phase processes for applications in organic electronics. The foundational principle of the OVPD, as described by Forrest, is shown in Fig. 12. Recent advancements have demonstrated the potential of this technique for the cost-effective high-throughput production of phosphorescent organic light-emitting diodes (PHOLEDs). For instance, a green PHOLED fabricated via OVPD achieved an external quantum efficiency of $20 \pm 1\%$ with an emission layer deposited at a rate of 50 Å/s, using bis(2-(2-pyridinyl-N)phenyl)iridium(III) acetylacetonate ($Ir(ppy)_2(acac)$) doped into CBP. Notably, the study found no evidence of gas-phase nucleation at high deposition rates but did observe a decrease in quantum efficiency at higher currents, attributed to triplet-polaron annihilation. The accumulation of stress within the emission layer was identified as a critical factor in generating defect states that exacerbate triplet-polaron interactions. To elucidate the evolution of the film morphology, a void nucleation model was proposed, offering valuable insights into the dynamics of thin-film growth under high deposition conditions [126].

4.3 Fabrication of Hybrid Materials via Layer-By-Layer Assembly

The fabrication of hybrid materials is a sophisticated approach in materials engineering that involves integrating two or more distinct components, typically organic, inorganic, or metallic, to create composites with enhanced or novel properties.

These advanced materials capitalize on the inherent advantages of their constituent elements, such as the flexibility of organic compounds, stability of inorganic components, and unique optical and electronic properties of metals. The selection of an appropriate fabrication method is influenced by the desired material characteristics, scalability, and specific application requirements. Hybrid materials have become widely used across a range of fields, including photonics, electronics, catalysis, energy storage, and biomedical technologies. Among the various fabrication techniques, sol–gel processing, vapor deposition, and layer-by-layer assembly are particularly notable for their versatility and capacity to produce high-quality materials. This section specifically focuses on layer-by-layer assembly methods, as sol–gel processing and vapor deposition have already been covered in earlier sections.

Layer-by-layer (LbL) assembly is a straightforward, versatile, and cost-effective method for coating a variety of surfaces. This technique involves the alternating deposition of oppositely charged polyelectrolyte polymers or functional materials, offering accurate control of the film thickness, composition, and architecture. Its capacity to incorporate a diverse range of materials and modify their properties through external stimuli makes it an adaptable and scalable approach for thin film fabrication [129]. One of the key strengths of the LbL technique is its ability to combine diverse nanostructures such as nanoparticles, nanowires, and nanosheets with polymers to create hybrid systems that integrate the unique properties of each component.

The simplicity and universality of the LbL method, coupled with its precise nanoscale thickness control, has contributed to its widespread adoption in areas such as optical devices, synthetic catalysis, biological interfaces, and multifunctional coatings. Traditional LbL methods rely on the adsorption of species with opposite charges onto a substrate via enthalpic and entropic forces (Fig. 13). Recent advances have expanded the scope of this technique, enabling the assembly of more complex systems that incorporate a broader range of molecular interactions. This includes the assembly of non-planar and macroscopically flat surfaces. Such versatility has greatly enhanced the development of LbL-generated nanocomposites, which are being increasingly utilized in cutting-edge research [130].

Recent research has highlighted the potential of LbL assemblies in the development of innovative hybrid systems. For instance, an ordered multilayer temperature sensor composed entirely of QDs assembled via electrostatic LbL deposition exhibited remarkable photoluminescence temperature sensitivity (50–300 K). CdSe/ZnS QDs functionalized with $-NH_2$ and –COOH groups showed superior photoluminescence performance compared to the QD-polymer films, as confirmed by TEM and XPS analyses. These results underscore the potential of all-QD films in optical thermometry applications [132]. Another notable application of the LbL assembly involves the synthesis of photoluminescent nanocomposites by incorporating 2D CdSe/CdS nanoplatelets with polymers. These composites achieved high quantum yields and narrow photoluminescence spectra, which are essential for applications requiring high color purity for light emission. The LbL technique enabled the formation of smooth solid-state coatings while preserving the optical properties of the incorporated nanoplatelets [133].

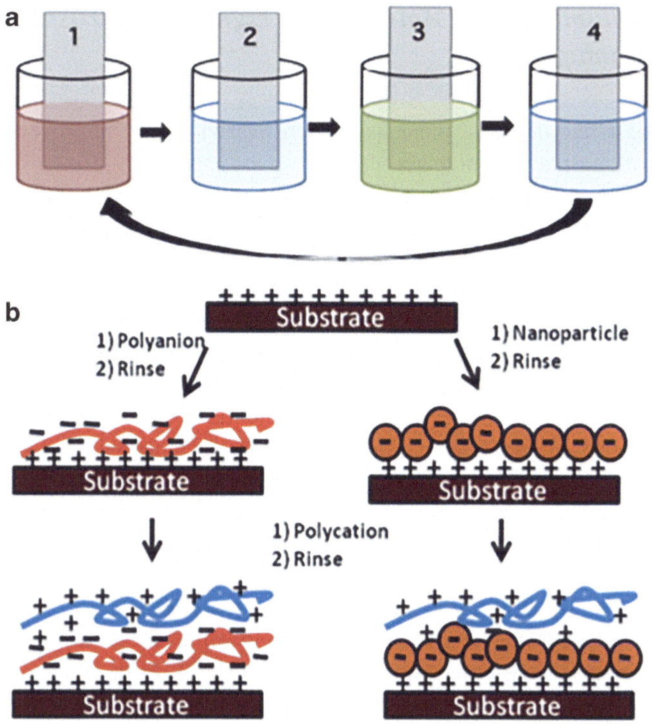

Fig. 13 **a** Schematic of the LBL film deposition process. Steps 1 and 3 represent the adsorption of polyanions and polycations, while steps 2 and 4 are washing steps. **b** Two adsorption pathways, illustrating LBL deposition for polymers and for polymers combined with nanoparticles (NPs) [131]

5 Applications of Photoluminescent Materials

Photoluminescent materials are integral to various advanced applications due to their unique light-emitting properties. In lighting and display technologies, they enhance the performance of LEDs, OLEDs, and QDLEDs, offering energy efficiency and vibrant colors. In biomedicine, they enable precise bioimaging and diagnostics through fluorescent biomarkers and advanced imaging techniques. Additionally, these materials are pivotal in security and anti-counterfeiting, with applications in fluorescent inks and security threads. This section categorizes photoluminescent materials by their applications, highlighting the advantages of their luminescence mechanisms underpinning their widespread utility.

5.1 Photoluminescent Materials for Lighting and Display Technologies

Over the past few decades, there have been overwhelming improvements in the properties of phosphorescent materials for diverse applications. They are used extensively in LEDs for efficient energy. For effective productivity, white light must be made of multiple colors and must have an efficiency of 408 lm/W [134], while modern phosphor-converted LED (pcLED) devices achieve up to 200 lm/W [134], with performance rapidly improving. For almost all single pcLEDs used for yellow-light emission, Yttrium aluminum garnet doped with the cerium ion ($Y_3Al_5O_{12}$, YAG: Ce) is noted as the primary material [135, 136]. It has been reported that by substituting (replacing) Y with Lu, Gd, or Tb, and Al with Ga, there can be significant adjustments in the emission color of YAG. This material meets the criteria for an ideal LED phosphor, and its excitation range meets the values for blue LED emission, with an excellent color rendering index (CRI) and yellow broadband emission [137]. The red spectral performance of most single-phosphor can be limited, resulting in cool white light at low CRI; thus, making a two-phosphor system (combining YAG: Ce with a red phosphor) more suitable for indoor lighting with warmer correlated color temperature (CCT) (2700–3200 K) and higher CRI as displayed in Fig. 14a. Alternative materials that have found similar applications for pcLED as yellow-light emission are the silicate-based europium materials [138, 139]. The handy synthesis approach contributes to an increase in crystallinity, which can impact their emission and luminescence properties due to the activator's concentration. However, their stability remains a challenge, thus requiring ongoing research to address this issue.

Furthermore, the luminous efficacy is often compromised when designing two-phosphor pcLEDs, especially with an effort to enhance the CRI necessitating red phosphors optimized for human eye sensitivity. Eu^{2+}-activated nitride materials like $(Ba,Sr)_2Si_5N_8$:Eu and $(Ca,Sr)AlSiN_3$:Eu [140] are ideal for their tunable emission colors, strong thermal stability, and broad excitation bands, enabling high CRIs across various CCTs. Nonetheless, their broad emission bands can result in some energy loss beyond 700 nm, creating a balance between high color rendering and optimal luminous efficacy. Figure 14b displays wavelength range for two nitride-based phosphors. Europium-doped nitridolithoaluminate narrow-band red-emitting phosphor was synthesized and showed significant improvement in luminous efficacy in white pcLEDs compared to traditional red phosphors [141]. Though its rigid framework stability can be compared to $(Ba,Sr)_2Si_5N_8$:Eu, further studies are still needed to confirm its stability when exposed to external stimuli.

Manganese-doped magnesium fluoro germanate (MGM) is often used as Mn(IV) phosphor, considered to have a narrow band emission spectral. The unique band spectral and thermal quenching temperature of MGM makes it ideal for high-pressure mercury vapor. Nevertheless, low absorption at 450 nm can reduce its usage for blue-emitting LEDs and overly red-shifted emission, leading to low lumen efficiency. Figure 14c displays a typical MGM sample excitation, emission, and reflection spectra. $K_2SiF_6:Mn^{4+}$ (Fig. 14d) shows promising properties, including broad

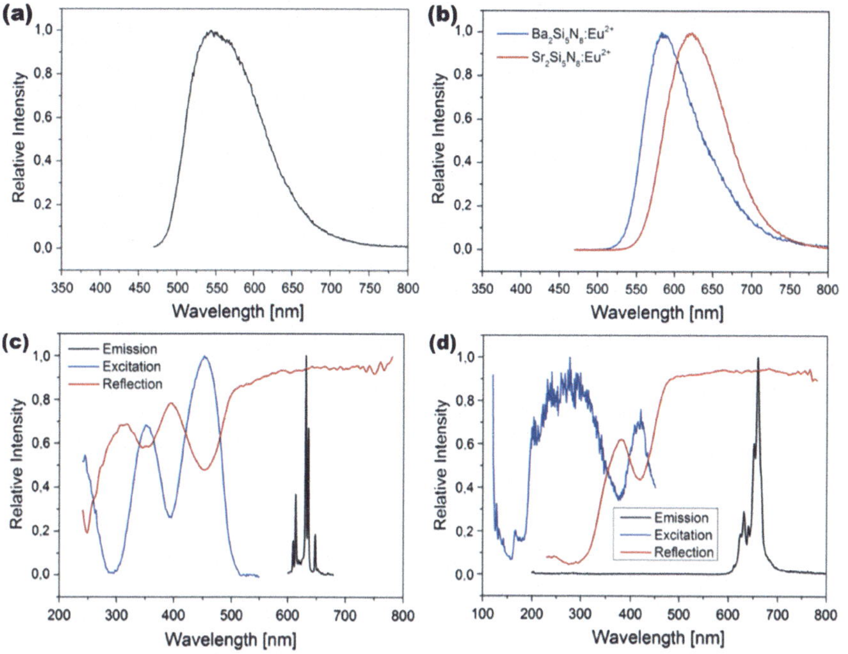

Fig. 14 **a** PL spectral of Cerium-doped YAG. **b** PL spectra of $Ba_2Si_5N_8$ and $Sr_2Si_5N_8$, **c** PL spectral of MGM with zero phonon line at 640 nm. **d** PL spectra of K_2SiF_6:Mn [145]

absorption at 450 nm and a 630 nm emission peak, yielding a high lumen equivalent of about 200 lm/W opt. PL quantum yields are synthesis-dependent, with Zhu et al. [142] achieving 98% for $K_2TiF_6:Mn^{4+}$ via cation exchange. However, there is a major drawback with the chemical instability and toxicity of K_2SiF_6:Mn phosphors. Also, in humid environments, the shelf life can be negatively affected due to water solubility, and its host lattice, K_2SiF_6, classified as toxic, raises safety concerns [143]. However, some research has shown that coating with CaF_2 can potentially mitigate these issues.

pcWLEDs have grown significantly, finding commercial applications in diverse areas. The pioneering work of Matsazuwa et al. staged a new era for synthesizing advanced photoluminescent materials (by doping with rare-earth metals) [144], with profound applications. Table 1 displays the multiple applications of various rare-earth doped materials along with their synthesis method and emission color.

Organic or polymer materials have been used for lighting displays because of their adjustable film properties. Nowadays, polymers, along with other single-crystal compounds, have become important for light emission because of their high transparency and ability to withstand certain temperatures. Also, with an increase in their efficiency, they can be effective for LED applications. Synthesizing luminescent materials emitting white light at room temperature is complicated, yet it is a priority for the lighting industry. Yuan et al. [154] encapsulated coronene and rhodamine

Table 1 Applications of rare-earth-doped materials, their corresponding synthesis methods, and emission colors

Element	Synthesis method	Excitation (nm)	Emission (nm)	Color	Application	Refs.
$Gd_2Mo_3O_9:Eu^{3+}$	Solid-state	280	395/465	Red/blue	Solid-state lighting	[146]
$Ca_8Mg_3Al_2Si_7O_{28}:Eu^{2+}$	Solid-state	420	535	Green	wLEDs	[147]
$KSrPO_4:Dy^{3+}$	Solid-state	351/388	570	Yellow/green	High-powered LED	[148]
$ZnO:Ce^{3+}$	Melt-quenching	471	431/580	Yellow/blue	Photocatalysis	[149]
$Sr_7Sb_2O_{12}:RE(RE = Sm^{3+}, Eu^{3+})$	Solid-state	–	–	Blue/red	wLEDs	[150]
$Mg_2SiO_4:Tb^{3+}$	Combustion	377	430–650	Green	Displays	[151]
$NaYF_4:Gd^{3+}$	Co-precipitation	277	311	Blue	Phototherapeutic lamp	[152]
$LiPbB_5O_9:Pr^{3+}$	Solid-state	443	609	Blue/red	wLEDs	[153]

B (RhB), with porous metal–organic framework (MOF) PCN-921a, resulting in a high quantum yield luminescent material. At room temperature, the lifetime of coronene@PCN-921 is in nanoseconds while RhB@coronene@PCN-921 achieved white light emission, demonstrating its potential for multifunctional optical device applications. Also, the discrete optoelectronic properties of CPL and RTP materials exhibiting circularly polarized luminescence have made them attractive in the lighting industry.

Like OLEDs, quantum dot LEDs (QDLEDs) are nanocrystals of semiconducting materials, typically measuring 2–10 nm in diameter, with tunable properties for optoelectronic applications. One of the rare-earth free QD luminescent materials (InP QDs) possesses great luminescence efficiency and color performance (Fig. 15a), which make it suitable for uses like displays and with significant potential for white light-emitting diodes (wLEDs) [155]. Recent progress has also led to the development of new QD materials, such as fluorescent carbon dots (C-dots), graphene quantum dots (GQDs), and graphite phase carbon nitride (g-C_3N_4), which can be combined with other materials to form various rare earth-free luminescent composites for wLED applications. Kasha's rule proposes challenges in developing single-component wLEDs. Nonetheless, Li et al. [156] introduced the first blue-yellow fluorescence-phosphorescence dual emission in newly designed carbon nitride quantum dots (W-CNQDs). These W-CNQDs exhibit a PL quantum efficiency of 25%, the highest reported for white-emitting materials utilizing both singlet and triplet states, with carbonyl groups at their edges enhancing intersystem crossing and intermolecular coupling for yellow phosphorescence. When integrated into a UV-LED chip, the W-CNQDs achieve efficient white emission (Fig. 15b) with a CRI of 85 and excellent chromatic stability, offering a breakthrough for single-component wLED design. Table 2 presents an overview of some organic and QDs luminescent materials used for lighting displays.

5.2 *Bioimaging and Medical Diagnostics Applications*

Health is key for better growth and development; thus, photoluminescent materials applicable to bioimaging and medical diagnostics applications have been attractive lately. Wang et al. [167] reported a triplet exciplex by combining an RTP host and a guest and achieved an encryption pattern for thermal imaging and labeling tumors in living mice. The materials showed high efficiency and enhanced afterglow time, as shown in Fig. 15c. Krishnan et al. [168] synthesized an Erbium-doped series of $Tm_{2-x}WO_6$ phosphors at different ratios, showing a monoclinic crystalline structure. X-ray testing revealed that the W atoms were octahedrally coordinated to oxygen in their highest +6 oxidation state, and as the doping concentration increased, the luminescence also increased. The study also demonstrated the potential of the phosphors for real-time latent fingerprint detection in forensic and medical applications, with excellent performance observed without the need for Yb^{3+} ions.

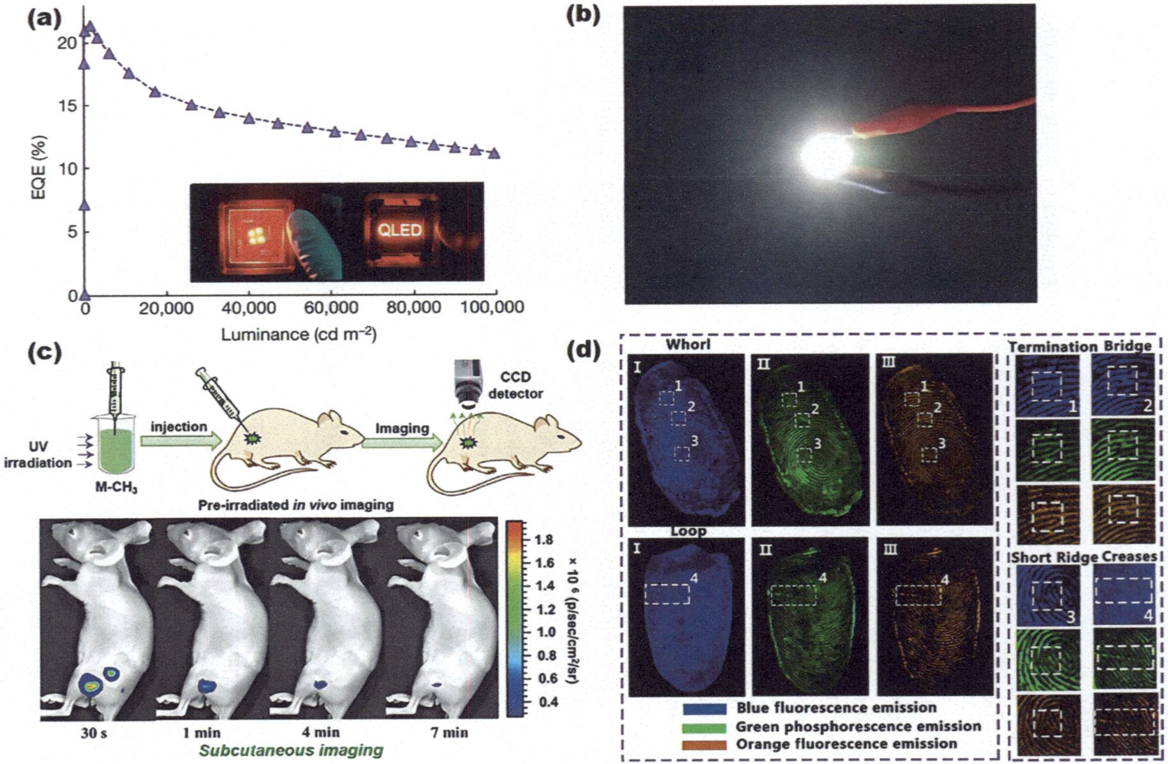

Fig. 15 **a** External quantum efficiency–luminance profile (inset, photos of four-pixel and text-patterned QD-LEDs) [155]. **b** UV-pumped wLED image using W-CNQDs as phosphors [156]. **c** Time-resolved bioimaging of mice with subcutaneous M-CH nanocrystals injections [167]. **d** Luminescent fingerprint images using MOFs@SiNPs for Whorl and loop patterns under UV excitation (I: fluorescence, II: phosphorescence) and after NaOH treatment (III: fluorescence). Magnified images highlight specific details: (1) termination, (2) bridge, (3) short ridge, and (4) crease [160]

Table 2 Applications of organic and quantum dots luminescent materials

Phosphorescent materials	PLQY	Synthesis method	Application	Refs.
MOF luminescent materials				
MOF(PCN-921)	93.6%	In-situ	WLED lamp	[154]
MOF(Bi-PDC& Bi-PTC)	2.495 and 5.45%	Solvothermal	WLEDs	[157]
MOF(CaL-3)	80%	–	wLEDs	[158]
RTP MOF	80.6%	–	Fingerprint recognition	[159]
MOFs@SiNPs	17%	In-situ and microwave irradiation	Higher-level information security against counterfeiting	[160]
Quantum dots				
CdZnSeS/ZnS (green and yellow), CdZnS/ZnS (cyan and blue), CdTe/ZnS (orange and red)	Green 95%, yellow 86%, cyan 77%, blue 94%, orange 49%, red 45%	Hot-injection	wLEDs	[161]
g-C_3N_4 in cyanoacrylate resin	25%	–	wLEDs	[156]
CDs/Zr-MOF	37%	Silane functionalization	Solid-state lighting	[4]
y-CQRs	40.25%	Rapid and facile one-step pyrolysis	Warm WLED applications	[162]
R/G/B-SBF-CQRs	30–46%	Solvothermal	Solid-state lighting	[163]
(NA-CA)0.01%/BA	66.13%	One-step melting/ in-situ	Time-resolved information security	[5]
Cu, N-CDs	–	Hydrothermal	Anti-counterfeiting and encryption	[164]
$CsPbCl_{1.8}Br_{1.2}$:Ce^{3+}/Mn^{2+}	75%	Chemical reaction	Phosphor-converted wLEDs	[165]
$CsYbI_3$ NCs	58%	Simple hot-injection	Energy conversion and storage devices, sensing chemicals, light-emitting diodes (LEDs)	[166]

5.3 *Security and Anti-counterfeiting Applications*

Photoluminescent materials, with their distinct emission properties, have emerged as powerful tools in security and anti-counterfeiting technologies. These materials offer high sensitivity, stability, and the ability to emit tunable light, making them ideal for secure printing, information storage, and fraud detection. Wei et al. [169] demonstrated the versatility of tunable phosphorescent materials with outstanding photoluminescent quantum yields (PLQYs). Their materials exhibited a bright yellow emission (PLQY of 100%) when excited at 320 nm, and upon excitation at 365 nm, the emission shifted to bright white light with a PLQY of 44%. By integrating blue-emitting $BAPP^{4+}$ with an orange-emitting inorganic polyhedron, complementary colors were achieved, providing both afterglow and excitation-dependent emission properties. These features render the material highly suitable for advanced applications in information storage and counterfeit detection. Similarly, Abdelhameed et al. [170] developed a novel inorganic–organic hybrid ink based on photochromic and fluorescent properties. This innovative ink, designed specifically for anti-counterfeiting, showcased excellent photostability and the ability to dynamically alter its absorption and fluorescence when applied to secure documents. These unique characteristics position the ink as a highly effective tool for secure printing applications.

Further advancements in multi-modal anti-counterfeiting solutions were achieved by Wang et al. [160] through the development of MOFs coated on silica nanoparticles (MOFs@SiNPs). These materials function as high-efficacy security inks, enabling detailed fingerprint visualization with both fluorescence and phosphorescence imaging. In experiments, fingerprints stained with the MOFs@SiNPs ink pressed onto black paper revealed three distinct levels of fingerprint details. Fluorescent and phosphorescent images clearly displayed basic patterns (e.g., whorls and loops), ridge flow, and finer structural features, such as terminations, bridges, short ridges, and creases (Fig. 15d). These detailed characteristics allow for precise personal identification, even from partial or damaged fingerprints, offering potential use in forensic investigations. The MOFs@SiNPs provided exceptional imaging sensitivity and signal-to-noise ratios, calculated as 233.64 and 34 for phosphorescence and fluorescence imaging, respectively. This demonstrates their ability to enhance the clarity and reliability of imaging signals, further strengthening their applicability in high-security scenarios.

Table 2 summarizes other phosphorescent materials, including their use in bioimaging, medical diagnostics, fluorescent biomarkers, and additional security applications. Together, these innovations highlight the growing potential of photoluminescent materials in combating counterfeiting and securing sensitive information in various industries.

6 Challenges and Future Perspectives

6.1 *Stability and Durability of Photoluminescent Materials*

The stability and durability of photoluminescent materials are pivotal for their effective application in diverse fields, from biomedical imaging to energy-efficient lighting. These challenges arise due to inherent material properties, environmental factors, and application-specific demands. For instance, He et al. [171] demonstrated the stabilization of photoluminescent silk fibers through hydrogen bonding and electrostatic interactions, yielding materials suitable for long-term physiological use. Similarly, efforts to improve the stability of metal halide perovskites, as discussed by Cho et al. [172], highlight strategies such as cation engineering and ion migration suppression, which are critical for both biomedical and optoelectronic applications. Moreover, Zhang et al. [173] explored the stability of zero-dimensional luminescent metal halides, discussing how the unique crystallographic structures of these materials can be engineered to improve their durability and photoluminescence properties. Beyond these examples, future advancements may leverage bio-inspired stabilization techniques or nanocomposites, which offer promising routes to address remaining challenges. Such efforts underline the ongoing pursuit of durable photoluminescent materials capable of meeting the demands of next-generation technologies.

6.2 *Environmental and Health Concerns*

Environmental and health concerns surrounding photoluminescent materials, particularly those containing heavy metals like lead or rare-earth elements, remain a pressing issue. Lead-based perovskite quantum dots (PQDs), as analyzed by Wei et al. [174], pose significant risks due to their potential to release toxic lead ions during decomposition. The study proposed compositional and surface engineering strategies to mitigate these risks; however, questions remain regarding the long-term stability and scalability of these solutions. Similarly, rare-earth oxides (REOs) have demonstrated cytotoxicity in specific cell lines, as highlighted by Zhang et al. [173]. While their applications in bio-imaging are promising, careful consideration of their long-term effects on human health and ecosystems is imperative. This concern is further established by Omoniyi et al. [175], who discussed the challenges of using optical functional materials in high-security information encryption, where similar health and environmental issues arise. Although the primary focus of their work was on data security, the environmental and health concerns associated with these materials were also addressed. The study highlighted issues such as low durability and poor compatibility of constituent materials, which can lead to increased waste and potential environmental contamination. The authors suggested that improving the durability and compatibility of these materials could not only enhance their performance in security applications but also reduce their environmental impact when used in biomedical contexts.

Beyond individual materials, the environmental lifecycle impact of photoluminescent material synthesis warrants attention. Christé et al. [176] utilized life cycle assessment (LCA) to evaluate different N-doping strategies for carbon dots, revealing that raw material selection significantly influences environmental outcomes, as depicted in Fig. 16. Biogenic alternatives, such as those proposed by Johny et al. [177], offer a promising path forward by reducing global warming potential (GWP), land use (LU), irradiation (IR), among other impacts (Fig. 17). However, challenges such as scaling these methods for industrial production and ensuring consistent material performance remain to be addressed. A shift toward sustainable synthesis methods, supported by interdisciplinary collaboration, will be critical for advancing the field while minimizing its environmental footprint.

6.3 Advances in Material Design and Synthesis

Recent advancements in material design and synthesis have significantly enhanced the performance of photoluminescent materials, addressing challenges like thermal instability, limited quantum yield, and inefficient production methods. Panigrahi and Nag [178] demonstrated a 20% improvement in the thermal resistance of phosphor materials for wLEDs, critical for high-temperature applications. Similarly, Neacsu et al. [179] reported quantum yields of up to 60% in rare-earth-doped hydroxyapatite, showcasing their potential in precise biomedical imaging with excellent biocompatibility. Innovative synthesis methods, such as microwave-assisted techniques, have further revolutionized the field. Krishnan et al. [180] showed a 30% increase in photoluminescence intensity using microwave synthesis, highlighting its advantages in reducing energy consumption and improving material quality. These methods are particularly valuable for applications in sensors and photocatalysis. Despite these advancements, challenges remain. Rare-earth doping raises concerns about environmental impact and resource scarcity, prompting interest in sustainable alternatives like carbon-based materials. Furthermore, scaling up advanced synthesis methods for industrial applications requires overcoming cost and consistency issues. Future progress will rely on integrating sustainable practices, exploring hybrid materials, and leveraging AI-driven approaches to accelerate material discovery. These efforts will ensure that photoluminescent materials continue to evolve, meeting the growing demands of biomedical, optoelectronic, and energy sectors.

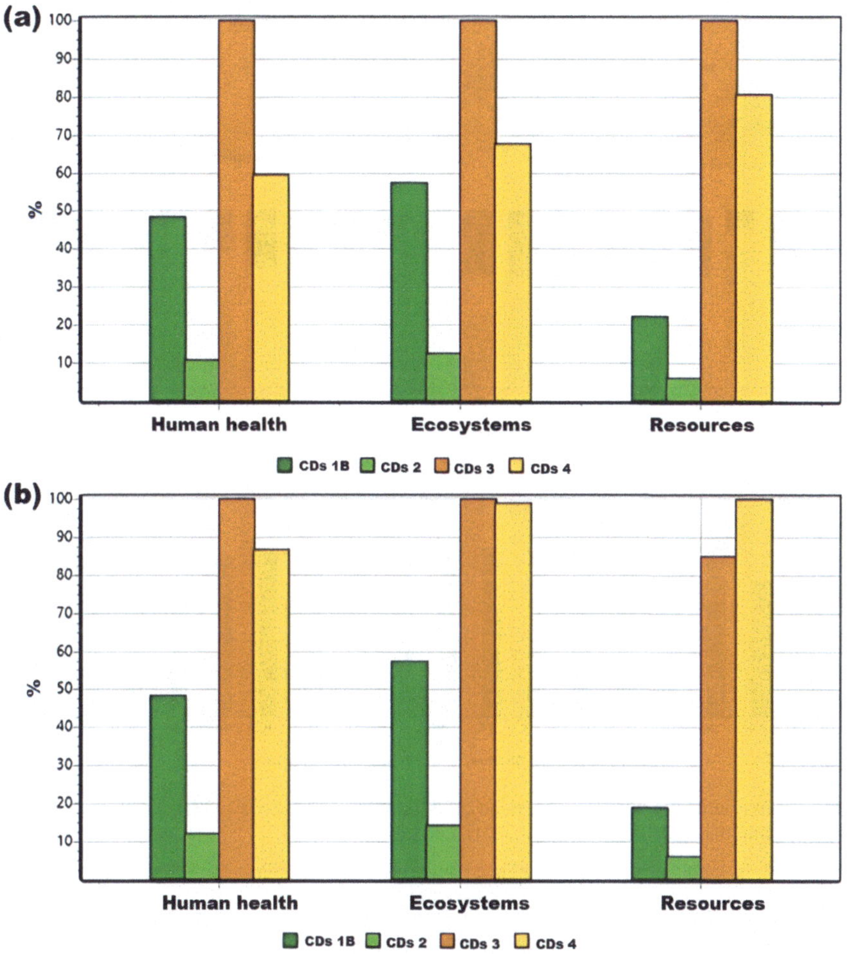

Fig. 16 Comparative prospective life cycle damage assessment of CDs 1B to 4, using **a** a weight-based functional unit for 1000 g of CDs and **b** a QYFL-based functional unit analysis [176]

6.4 Emerging Applications and Technologies

The field of photoluminescent materials is continuously expanding, with new applications and technologies emerging that hold significant promise for biomedical applications. Persistent luminescence nanoparticles (PLNPs) are a key development in biomedical imaging, providing long-lasting luminescence after excitation ceases. These nanoparticles enhance imaging sensitivity by reducing autofluorescence, making them ideal for deep-tissue imaging. Wang et al. [181] highlighted their ability to improve cancer therapy and diagnostic precision due to their ability to

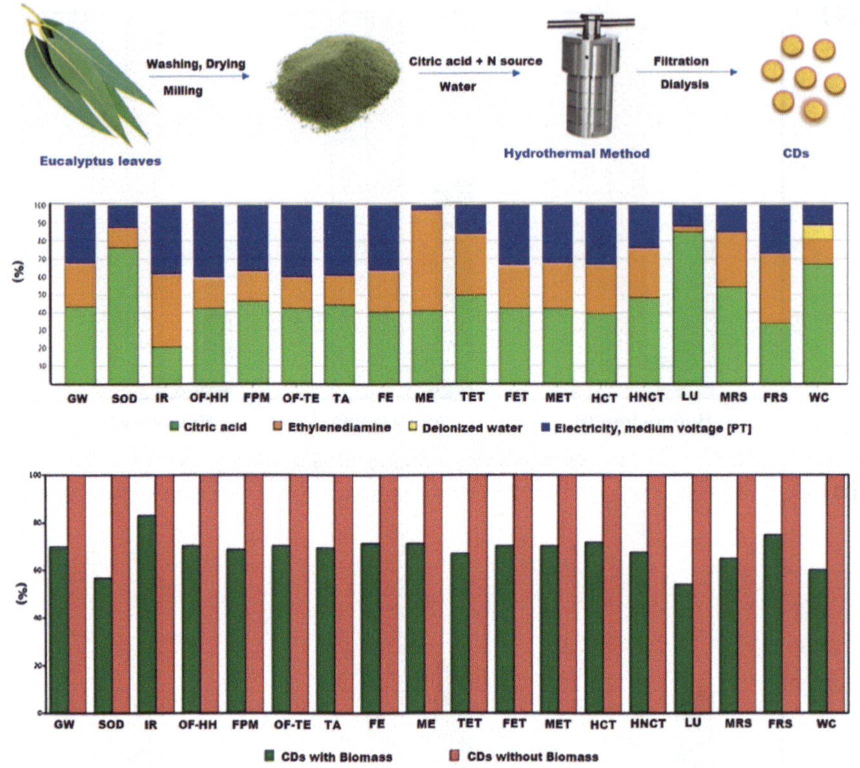

Fig. 17 Environmental impact comparison of hydrothermally synthesized CDs with and without biomass using the ReCiPe2016 midpoint (H) method [177]

minimize autofluorescence and increase imaging sensitivity, though challenges like biocompatibility and production scalability remain.

Chromic nanomaterials, which combine photoluminescence with color-changing properties, are emerging as multifunctional tools for anticounterfeiting and biomedical applications. Abdollahi et al. [182] discussed their potential in diagnostic systems that integrate real-time imaging and therapeutic functions. Further work is needed to enhance their responsiveness and biocompatibility. Moreover, two-dimensional (2D) nanomaterials, such as graphene oxide, are gaining traction in drug delivery, bioimaging, and tissue engineering [183]. With high surface areas and tunable properties, these materials offer precision in targeting and real-time monitoring of therapeutic processes. However, stability and toxicity concerns must be addressed for broader adoption into next-generation biomedical technologies.

Beyond biomedicine, photoluminescent materials are revolutionizing optoelectronics, such as QD-based displays and luminescent solar concentrators, which improve energy efficiency and color fidelity. These developments underscore the broad utility of photoluminescent materials in advancing sustainable technologies.

Key challenges in deploying photoluminescent materials include stability under varying environmental conditions, photobleaching, and potential environmental and health risks. Scalability and consistent quality in industrial production also remain hurdles. Addressing these issues is crucial for the widespread adoption of these materials. Future research will likely focus on hybrid materials that combine photoluminescence with other functionalities, such as AI-enhanced diagnostics. Bioinspired designs could lead to more sustainable and efficient materials, while integration with emerging technologies like nanorobotics and personalized medicine could unlock new applications.

7 Conclusion

Photoluminescent materials are integral to modern technologies, with their unique optical properties driving innovations in biomedicine, lighting, displays, and sensors. This chapter has explored the foundational principles of photoluminescence, from the underlying mechanisms of photon absorption and emission to the distinctions between fluorescence and phosphorescence. It has also detailed the diverse material types—from organic molecules to quantum dots—and highlighted the critical synthesis techniques, emphasizing the interplay between structure and function. Advanced spectroscopic methods continue to unravel the intricacies of photophysical behavior, paving the way for more efficient and versatile materials. However, challenges such as stability under environmental stressors, quantum yield optimization, and cost-effective scalability remain significant. Addressing these limitations through interdisciplinary research will unlock new possibilities in areas like flexible electronics, bioimaging, and energy harvesting. By embracing these advancements, the transformative potential of photoluminescent materials can be fully harnessed to meet the demands of future technologies.

References

1. Kumar, M., Kumar, P.: Applications of white light emitting materials, pp. 127–139 (2024). https://doi.org/10.1007/978-981-97-6744-1_6
2. Li, K., Ren, T.-B., Huan, S., Yuan, L., Zhang, X.-B.: Progress and perspective of solid-state organic fluorophores for biomedical applications. J. Am. Chem. Soc. **143**(50), 21143–21160 (2021). https://doi.org/10.1021/jacs.1c10925
3. Wang, Y., Omoniyi, A.O., Zhang, M., Yang, M., Li, T., Li, D., Zhang, J.: Photoreversible shape memory polyurethane films prepared using demulsification-induced fast solidification for multilevel information encryption application. ACS Appl. Polym. Mater. **6**(10), 5788–5802 (2024). https://doi.org/10.1021/acsapm.4c00444
4. Wang, A., Hou, Y.L., Kang, F., Lyu, F., Xiong, Y., Chen, W.C., Li, Y.Y.: Rare earth-free composites of carbon dots/metal-organic frameworks as white light emitting phosphors. J. Mater. Chem. C **7**(8), 2207–2211 (2019). https://doi.org/10.1039/c8tc04171g

5. Cui, S., Wang, B., Zan, Y., Shen, Z., Liu, S., Fang, W., Chen, L.: Colorful, time-dependent carbon dot-based afterglow with ultralong lifetime. Chem. Eng. J., **431**, (2022). https://doi.org/10.1016/j.cej.2021.133373
6. Lastusaari, M., Laamanen, T., Malkamäki, M., Eskola, K.O., Kotlov, A., Carlson, S., Hölsä, J.: The Bologna stone: history's first persistent luminescent material. Eur. J. Mineral. **24**(5), 885–890 (2012). https://doi.org/10.1127/0935-1221/2012/0024-2224
7. Pathak, P.K., Kurchania, R.: Synthesis and thermoluminescence properties of SrAl2O4 (EU) phosphor irradiated with cobalt-60, 6MV and 16MV photon beams. Radiat. Phys. Chem. **117**, 48–53 (2015). https://doi.org/10.1016/j.radphyschem.2015.07.009
8. Wan, M., Jiang, X., Nie, J., Cao, Q., Zheng, W., Dong, X., Zhou, W.: Phosphor powders-incorporated polylactic acid polymeric composite used as 3D printing filaments with green luminescence properties. J. Appl. Polym. Sci., **137**(18), (2020). https://doi.org/10.1002/app.48644
9. Rafiq, Q., Khan, M.T., Hayat, S.S., Azam, S., Rahman, A.U., Elansary, H.O., Shan, M.: Adsorption and solar light activity of noble metal adatoms (Au and Zn) on Fe(111) surface: a first-principles study. Phys. Chem. Chem. Phys. **26**(24), 17118–17131 (2024). https://doi.org/10.1039/D3CP04504H
10. Chan, N.N.M.Y., Idris, A., Abidin, Z.H.Z., Tajuddin, H.A., Abdullah, Z.: Correction: White light employing luminescent engineered large (mega) Stokes shift molecules: A review. RSC Advances, **11**(29), 17646–17647 (2021). https://doi.org/10.1039/D1RA90109E
11. Yao, J., Yang, M., Duan, Y.: Chemistry, biology, and medicine of fluorescent nanomaterials and related systems: new insights into biosensing, bioimaging, genomics, diagnostics, and therapy. Chem. Rev. **114**(12), 6130–6178 (2014). https://doi.org/10.1021/cr200359p
12. Gao, R., Kodaimati, M.S., Yan, D.: Recent advances in persistent luminescence based on molecular hybrid materials. Chem. Soc. Rev. **50**(9), 5564–5589 (2021). https://doi.org/10.1039/D0CS01463J
13. Wagner, A.M., Knipe, J.M., Orive, G., Peppas, N.A.: Quantum dots in biomedical applications. Acta Biomater. **94**, 44–63 (2019). https://doi.org/10.1016/j.actbio.2019.05.022
14. Dong, H., Du, S.-R., Zheng, X.-Y., Lyu, G.-M., Sun, L.-D., Li, L.-D., Yan, C.-H.: Lanthanide nanoparticles: From design toward bioimaging and therapy. Chem. Rev. **115**(19), 10725–10815 (2015). https://doi.org/10.1021/acs.chemrev.5b00091
15. Yi, Z., Luo, Z., Qin, X., Chen, Q., Liu, X.: Lanthanide-activated nanoparticles: A toolbox for bioimaging, therapeutics, and neuromodulation. Acc. Chem. Res. **53**(11), 2692–2704 (2020). https://doi.org/10.1021/acs.accounts.0c00513
16. Zhang, J., Lin, Y., Zhou, H., He, H., Ma, J.-J., Luo, M.-Y., Pang, D.-W.: Cell membrane-camouflaged NIR II fluorescent Ag2 Te quantum dots-based nanobioprobes for enhanced in vivo homotypic tumor imaging. Adv. Healthcare Mater. **8**(14), 1900341 (2019). https://doi.org/10.1002/adhm.201900341
17. Liu, Y., Li, Y., Koo, S., Sun, Y., Liu, Y., Liu, X., Hong, X.: Versatile types of inorganic/organic NIR-IIa/IIb fluorophores: From strategic design toward molecular imaging and theranostics. Chem. Rev. **122**(1), 209–268 (2022). https://doi.org/10.1021/acs.chemrev.1c00553
18. Xiang, C., Wu, L., Lu, Z., Li, M., Wen, Y., Yang, Y., Qian, L.: High efficiency and stability of ink-jet printed quantum dot light emitting diodes. Nat. Commun. **11**(1), 1646 (2020). https://doi.org/10.1038/s41467-020-15481-9
19. Lu, H., Carroll, G.M., Neale, N.R., Beard, M.C.: Infrared quantum dots: Progress, challenges, and opportunities. ACS Nano, **13**(2), acsnano.8b09815 (2019). https://doi.org/10.1021/acsnano.8b09815
20. Chinnathambi, S., Shirahata, N.: Recent advances on fluorescent biomarkers of near-infrared quantum dots for in vitro and in vivo imaging. Sci. Technol. Adv. Mater. **20**(1), 337–355 (2019). https://doi.org/10.1080/14686996.2019.1590731
21. Kosaka, N., Ogawa, M., Sato, N., Choyke, P.L., Kobayashi, H.: In vivo real-time, multicolor, quantum dot lymphatic imaging. J. Investig. Dermatol. **129**(12), 2818–2822 (2009). https://doi.org/10.1038/jid.2009.161

22. Dong, Y., Chen, C., Zheng, X., Gao, L., Cui, Z., Yang, H., Li, C.M.: One-step and high yield simultaneous preparation of single- and multi-layer graphene quantum dots from CX-72 carbon black. J. Mater. Chem. **22**(18), 8764 (2012). https://doi.org/10.1039/c2jm30658a
23. Deng, D., Chen, Y., Cao, J., Tian, J., Qian, Z., Achilefu, S., Gu, Y.: High-quality CuInS2/ZnS quantum dots for in vitro and in vivo bioimaging. Chem. Mater. **24**(15), 3029–3037 (2012). https://doi.org/10.1021/cm3015594
24. Badıllı, U., Mollarasouli, F., Bakirhan, N.K., Ozkan, Y., Ozkan, S.A.: Role of quantum dots in pharmaceutical and biomedical analysis, and its application in drug delivery. TrAC, Trends Anal. Chem. **131**, 116013 (2020). https://doi.org/10.1016/j.trac.2020.116013
25. Muthusankar, G., Devi, R.K., Gopu, G.: Nitrogen-doped carbon quantum dots embedded Co3O4 with multiwall carbon nanotubes: An efficient probe for the simultaneous determination of anticancer and antibiotic drugs. Biosens. Bioelectron. **150**, 111947 (2020). https://doi.org/10.1016/j.bios.2019.111947
26. Yang, Y., Liu, Q., Liu, Y., Cui, J., Liu, H., Wang, P., Dong, Y.: A novel label-free electrochemical immunosensor based on functionalized nitrogen-doped graphene quantum dots for carcinoembryonic antigen detection. Biosens. Bioelectron. **90**, 31–38 (2017). https://doi.org/10.1016/j.bios.2016.11.029
27. Elmizadeh, H., Faridbod, F., Soleimani, M., Ganjali, M.R., Bardajee, G.R.: Fluorescent apta-nanobiosensors for fast and sensitive detection of digoxin in biological fluids using rGQDs: Comparison of two approaches for immobilization of aptamer. Sens. Actuators, B Chem. **302**, 127133 (2020). https://doi.org/10.1016/j.snb.2019.127133
28. Rafiee, F., Tajfar, N., Mohammadnejad, M.: The synthesis and efficiency investigation of a boronic acid-modified magnetic chitosan quantum dot nanocomposite in the detection of Cu2+ ions. Int. J. Biol. Macromol. **189**, 477–482 (2021). https://doi.org/10.1016/j.ijbiomac.2021.08.158
29. Bao, W., Ma, H., Wang, N., He, Z.: PH-sensitive carbon quantum dots−doxorubicin nanoparticles for tumor cellular targeted drug delivery. Polym. Adv. Technol. **30**(11), 2664–2673 (2019). https://doi.org/10.1002/pat.4696
30. Liu, L., Jiang, H., Dong, J., Zhang, W., Dang, G., Yang, M., Dong, L.: PEGylated MoS2 quantum dots for traceable and pH-responsive chemotherapeutic drug delivery. Colloids Surf., B **185**, 110590 (2020). https://doi.org/10.1016/j.colsurfb.2019.110590
31. Javanbakht, S., Namazi, H.: Doxorubicin loaded carboxymethyl cellulose/graphene quantum dot nanocomposite hydrogel films as a potential anticancer drug delivery system. Mater. Sci. Eng., C **87**, 50–59 (2018). https://doi.org/10.1016/j.msec.2018.02.010
32. Chen, A.A.: Quantum dots to monitor RNAi delivery and improve gene silencing. Nucleic Acids Res. **33**(22), e190–e190 (2005). https://doi.org/10.1093/nar/gni188
33. Xu, D., Li, L., Chu, C., Zhang, X., Liu, G.: Advances and perspectives in near-infrared fluorescent organic probes for surgical oncology. WIREs Nanomed. Nanobiotechnol. **12**(5), e1635 (2020). https://doi.org/10.1002/wnan.1635
34. Zhu, H., Li, W., Ai, S., Wan, Y., Lin, W.: Novel activated NIR-II fluorescence/Ratio photoacoustic probe for dual-modality accurate imaging of palladium ions overload in mouse liver. J. Hazard. Mater. **470**, 134275 (2024). https://doi.org/10.1016/j.jhazmat.2024.134275
35. Xia, B., Ren, F., Ma, X., Yang, Z.-C., Jiang, Z.-L., Fang, W.-W., Li, Z.: Preparation of NIR-II polymer nanoprobe through twisted intramolecular charge transfer and förster resonance energy transfer of NIR-I dye. Adv. Healthcare Mater. **13**(22), 2400760 (2024). https://doi.org/10.1002/adhm.202400760
36. Li, B., Wang, W., Zhao, L., Wu, Y., Li, X., Yan, D., Liao, Y.: Photothermal therapy of tuberculosis using targeting pre-activated macrophage membrane-coated nanoparticles. Nat. Nanotechnol. **19**(6), 834–845 (2024). https://doi.org/10.1038/s41565-024-01618-0
37. Tian, R., Ma, H., Yang, Q., Wan, H., Zhu, S., Chandra, S., Chen, X.: Rational design of a super-contrast NIR-II fluorophore affords high-performance NIR-II molecular imaging guided microsurgery. Chem. Sci. **10**(1), 326–332 (2019). https://doi.org/10.1039/C8SC03751E

38. Naleway, J.J., Fox, C.M.J., Robinhold, D., Terpetschnig, E., Olson, N.A., Haugland, R.P.: Synthesis and use of new fluorogenic precipitating substrates. Tetrahedron Lett. **35**(46), 8569–8572 (1994). https://doi.org/10.1016/S0040-4039(00)78438-3
39. Shi, H., Kwok, R.T.K., Liu, J., Xing, B., Tang, B.Z., Liu, B.: Real-time monitoring of cell apoptosis and drug screening using fluorescent light-up probe with aggregation-induced emission characteristics. J. Am. Chem. Soc. **134**(43), 17972–17981 (2012). https://doi.org/10.1021/ja3064588
40. Chen, Y., Pei, P., Lei, Z., Zhang, X., Yin, D., Zhang, F.: A promising NIR-II fluorescent sensor for peptide-mediated long-term monitoring of kidney dysfunction. Angew. Chem. **133**(29), 15943–15949 (2021). https://doi.org/10.1002/ange.202103071
41. Qin, Z., Ren, T.-B., Zhou, H., Zhang, X., He, L., Li, Z., Yuan, L.: NIRII-HDs: A versatile platform for developing activatable NIR-II fluorogenic probes for reliable in vivo analyte sensing. Angew. Chem. Int. Ed. **61**(19), e202201541 (2022). https://doi.org/10.1002/anie.202201541
42. Xue, X., Zhao, Y., Dai, L., Zhang, X., Hao, X., Zhang, C., Liang, X.: Spatiotemporal drug release visualized through a drug delivery system with tunable aggregation-induced emission. Adv. Mater. **26**(5), 712–717 (2014). https://doi.org/10.1002/adma.201302365
43. Kim, K.Y., Jin, H., Park, J., Jung, S.H., Lee, J.H., Park, H., Jung, J.H.: Mitochondria-targeting self-assembled nanoparticles derived from triphenylphosphonium-conjugated cyanostilbene enable site-specific imaging and anticancer drug delivery. Nano Res. **11**(2), 1082–1098 (2018). https://doi.org/10.1007/s12274-017-1728-7
44. Lunardi, C.N., Gomes, A.J., Palepu, S., Galwaduge, P.T., Hillman, E.M.C.: PLGA nano/microparticles loaded with cresyl violet as a tracer for drug delivery: Characterization and in-situ hyperspectral fluorescence and 2-photon localization. Mater. Sci. Eng., C **70**, 505–511 (2017). https://doi.org/10.1016/j.msec.2016.09.020
45. Bao, G., Wen, S., Lin, G., Yuan, J., Lin, J., Wong, K.-L., Jin, D.: Learning from lanthanide complexes: The development of dye-lanthanide nanoparticles and their biomedical applications. Coord. Chem. Rev. **429**, 213642 (2021). https://doi.org/10.1016/j.ccr.2020.213642
46. Mejía-Méndez, J.L., Navarro-López, D.E., Sanchez-Martinez, A., Ceballos-Sanchez, O., Garcia-Amezquita, L.E., Tiwari, N., López-Mena, E.R.: Lanthanide-doped ZnO nanoparticles: Unraveling their role in cytotoxicity, antioxidant capacity, and nanotoxicology. Antioxidants **13**(2), 213 (2024). https://doi.org/10.3390/antiox13020213
47. Ahmad, M.Y., Yue, H., Tegafaw, T., Liu, S., Ho, S.L., Lee, G.H., Chang, Y.: Functionalized lanthanide oxide nanoparticles for tumor targeting, medical imaging, and therapy. Pharmaceutics **13**(11), 1890 (2021). https://doi.org/10.3390/pharmaceutics13111890
48. Naczynski, D.J., Sun, C., Türkcan, S., Jenkins, C., Koh, A.L., Ikeda, D., Xing, L.: X-ray-induced shortwave infrared biomedical imaging using rare-earth nanoprobes. Nano Lett. **15**(1), 96–102 (2015). https://doi.org/10.1021/nl504123r
49. Yi, Z., Luo, Z., Barth, N.D., Meng, X., Liu, H., Bu, W., Liu, X.: In vivo tumor visualization through MRI off-on switching of NaGdF4–$CaCO_3$ nanoconjugates. Adv. Mater. **31**(37), 1901851 (2019). https://doi.org/10.1002/adma.201901851
50. Jethva, P., Momin, M., Khan, T., Omri, A.: Lanthanide-doped upconversion luminescent nanoparticles—evolving role in bioimaging, biosensing, and drug delivery. Materials **15**(7), 2374 (2022). https://doi.org/10.3390/ma15072374
51. Wei, R., Wei, Z., Sun, L., Zhang, J.Z., Liu, J., Ge, X., Shi, L.: Nile red derivative-modified nanostructure for upconversion luminescence sensing and intracellular detection of Fe3+ and MR imaging. ACS Appl. Mater. Interfaces. **8**(1), 400–410 (2016). https://doi.org/10.1021/acsami.5b09132
52. Liu, Y., Chen, M., Cao, T., Sun, Y., Li, C., Liu, Q., Li, F.: A cyanine-modified nanosystem for in vivo upconversion luminescence bioimaging of methylmercury. J. Am. Chem. Soc. **135**(26), 9869–9876 (2013). https://doi.org/10.1021/ja403798m
53. Ancel, L., Gateau, C., Lebrun, C., Delangle, P.: DNA sensing by a Eu-binding peptide containing a proflavine unit. Inorg. Chem. **52**(2), 552–554 (2013). https://doi.org/10.1021/ic302456q

54. Yang, L., Zhang, K., Bi, S., Zhu, J.-J.: Dual-acceptor-based upconversion luminescence nanosensor with enhanced quenching efficiency for in situ imaging and quantification of MicroRNA in living cells. ACS Appl. Mater. Interfaces. **11**(42), 38459–38466 (2019). https://doi.org/10.1021/acsami.9b12254
55. Pershagen, E., Nordholm, J., Borbas, K.E.: Luminescent lanthanide complexes with analyte-triggered antenna formation. J. Am. Chem. Soc. **134**(24), 9832–9835 (2012). https://doi.org/10.1021/ja3004045
56. Xu, M., Zou, X., Su, Q., Yuan, W., Cao, C., Wang, Q., Li, F.: Ratiometric nanothermometer in vivo based on triplet sensitized upconversion. Nat. Commun. **9**(1), 2698 (2018). https://doi.org/10.1038/s41467-018-05160-1
57. Liu, J., Liu, Y., Bu, W., Bu, J., Sun, Y., Du, J., Shi, J.: Ultrasensitive nanosensors based on upconversion nanoparticles for selective hypoxia imaging in vivo upon near-infrared excitation. J. Am. Chem. Soc. **136**(27), 9701–9709 (2014). https://doi.org/10.1021/ja5042989
58. del Barrio, M., de Marcos, S., Cebolla, V., Heiland, J., Wilhelm, S., Hirsch, T., Galbán, J.: Enzyme-induced modulation of the emission of upconverting nanoparticles: Towards a new sensing scheme for glucose. Biosens. Bioelectron. **59**, 14–20 (2014). https://doi.org/10.1016/j.bios.2014.02.076
59. Chen, Z., Chen, H., Hu, H., Yu, M., Li, F., Zhang, Q., Huang, C.: Versatile synthesis strategy for carboxylic acid−functionalized upconverting nanophosphors as biological labels. J. Am. Chem. Soc. **130**(10), 3023–3029 (2008). https://doi.org/10.1021/ja076151k
60. Zhou, F., Noor, M.O., Krull, U.J.: Luminescence resonance energy transfer-based nucleic acid hybridization assay on cellulose paper with upconverting phosphor as donors. Anal. Chem. **86**(5), 2719–2726 (2014). https://doi.org/10.1021/ac404129t
61. Zhang, C., Yuan, Y., Zhang, S., Wang, Y., Liu, Z.: Biosensing platform based on fluorescence resonance energy transfer from upconverting nanocrystals to graphene oxide. Angew. Chem. Int. Ed. **50**(30), 6851–6854 (2011). https://doi.org/10.1002/anie.201100769
62. Navya, P.N., Kaphle, A., Srinivas, S.P., Bhargava, S.K., Rotello, V.M., Daima, H.K.: Current trends and challenges in cancer management and therapy using designer nanomaterials. Nano Convergence **6**(1), 23 (2019). https://doi.org/10.1186/s40580-019-0193-2
63. Zhang, Y., Zhang, Y., Song, G., He, Y., Zhang, X., Liu, Y., Ju, H.: A DNA–azobenzene nanopump fueled by upconversion luminescence for controllable intracellular drug release. Angew. Chem. **131**(50), 18375–18379 (2019). https://doi.org/10.1002/ange.201909870
64. Zhu, X., Li, J., Qiu, X., Liu, Y., Feng, W., Li, F.: Upconversion nanocomposite for programming combination cancer therapy by precise control of microscopic temperature. Nat. Commun. **9**(1), 2176 (2018). https://doi.org/10.1038/s41467-018-04571-4
65. Zhang, P., Hou, Y., Zeng, J., Li, Y., Wang, Z., Zhu, R., Gao, M.: Coordinatively unsaturated Fe3+ based activatable probes for enhanced MRI and therapy of tumors. Angew. Chem. Int. Ed. **58**(32), 11088–11096 (2019). https://doi.org/10.1002/anie.201904880
66. Wei, D., Yu, Y., Huang, Y., Jiang, Y., Zhao, Y., Nie, Z., Xiao, H.: A Near-infrared-II polymer with tandem fluorophores demonstrates superior biodegradability for simultaneous drug tracking and treatment efficacy feedback. ACS Nano **15**(3), 5428–5438 (2021). https://doi.org/10.1021/acsnano.1c00076
67. Kucherenko, M.G.: The role of spatial correlations in diffusion-controlled luminescent reactions. Chem. Phys. **179**(3), 279–286 (1994). https://doi.org/10.1016/0301-0104(94)87007-1
68. Umberger, J.Q., LaMer, V.K.: The kinetics of diffusion controlled molecular and ionic reactions in solution as determined by measurements of the quenching of fluorescence. J. Am. Chem. Soc. **67**(7), 1099–1109 (1945). https://doi.org/10.1021/ja01223a023
69. Hua, Y., Yu, J.S.: Synthesis and luminescent properties of near-UV excited NaLa(MoO4)2:Er3+ phosphors for multifunctional applications. J. Alloy. Compd. **811**, 152050 (2019). https://doi.org/10.1016/j.jallcom.2019.152050
70. Ayachi, F., Saidi, K., Chaabani, W., Dammak, M.: Synthesis and luminescence properties of Er3+ doped and Er3+–Yb3+ codoped phosphovanadate YP0.5V0.5O4 phosphors. J. Lumin., **240**, 118451 (2021). https://doi.org/10.1016/j.jlumin.2021.118451

71. Devi, H.J., Loitongbam, R.S., Singh, W.R.: Luminescence switching in Ce3+ ion sensitized YPO4:Tb3+ through Redox reaction. Mater. Res. Bull. **92**, 74–84 (2017). https://doi.org/10.1016/j.materresbull.2017.03.056
72. Kitsuda, M., Fujihara, S.: Quantitative luminescence switching in CePO4: Tb by redox reactions. J. Phys. Chem. C **115**(17), 8808–8815 (2011). https://doi.org/10.1021/jp201406y
73. Yan, Y., Shang, M., Huang, S., Wang, Y., Sun, Y., Dang, P., Lin, J.: Photoluminescence properties of AScSi2O6:Cr3+(A = Na and Li) phosphors with high efficiency and thermal stability for near-infrared phosphor-converted light-emitting diode light sources. ACS Appl. Mater. Interfaces. **14**(6), 8179–8190 (2022). https://doi.org/10.1021/acsami.1c23940
74. Chen, Y., Wu, H., Li, Y., Hu, Y.: Luminescence characteristics of ultra-broadband near-infrared emission Li3Mg2SbO6:Cr3+ phosphors and their applications in light-emitting diodes. J. Lumin. **264**, 120189 (2023). https://doi.org/10.1016/j.jlumin.2023.120189
75. Sun, Y., Zhou, X., Lun, Z., Han, K., Xiong, P., Xia, Z.: Amorphous to crystalline phase transformation enables tunable persistent luminescence for multi-mode optical information storage. Adv. Funct. Mater., 2406336, (2024). https://doi.org/10.1002/adfm.202406336
76. Vishwakarma, P.K., Rai, S.B., Bahadur, A.: Enhanced green up/down-conversion emissions through phase transformation in Ho3+/Yb3+ co-doped Y2O3:ZrO2 phosphors in presence of Na+ ions. Opt. Mater. **139**, 113814 (2023). https://doi.org/10.1016/j.optmat.2023.113814
77. Ali, N., Sahare, P.D., Kachere, A.R., Kakade, P.M., Mandlik, N.T., Dhole, S.D.: Luminescence and dosimetric characteristics of microcrystalline SrB4O7:Eu3+ synthesized by solid state diffusion method. J. Radioanal. Nucl. Chem. **330**(3), 1397–1408 (2021). https://doi.org/10.1007/s10967-021-07965-9
78. Altunal, V., Guckan, V., Ozdemir, A., Can, N., Yegingil, Z.: Luminescence characteristics of Al-and Ca-doped BeO obtained via a sol-gel method. J. Phys. Chem. Solids **131**, 230–242 (2019). https://doi.org/10.1016/j.jpcs.2019.04.003
79. Parashar, M., Shukla, V.K., Singh, R.: Metal oxides nanoparticles via sol–gel method: a review on synthesis, characterization and applications. J. Mater. Sci.: Mater. Electron. **31**(5), 3729–3749 (2020). https://doi.org/10.1007/s10854-020-02994-8
80. Kati, M., Gökçe, S., Keskin, Türemiş, M., Çetin, A., Kibar, R.: Luminescence characteristics and kinetic parameters of LiBaPO4: Tb3+, Dy3+ phosphors synthesized by sol-gel method. J. Lumin., **266**, 120312 (2024). https://doi.org/10.1016/j.jlumin.2023.120312
81. Gökçe, S., Keskin, İ.Ç., Katı, M.İ., Kibar, R., Çetin, A., Arslanlar, Y.T.: Kinetic parameters and luminescence properties of rare earth (Tb, Nd) doped and transition metal (Mn) doped/co-doped YAlO3 prepared via sol-gel method. J. Lumin.,**261**, 119883 (2023). https://doi.org/10.1016/j.jlumin.2023.119883
82. Verma, A., Sharma, R., Bisen, D.P., Brahme, N., Thakkar, K., Tigga, S., Chandrakar, P.: Luminescence investigation of CaY2Al4SiO12:Dy3+ phosphor synthesized by sol–gel method. Luminescence **38**(5), 576–584 (2023). https://doi.org/10.1002/bio.4485
83. Morey, G.W., Niggli, P.: The hydrothermal formation of silicates, A review. J. Am. Chem. Soc. **35**(9), 1086–1130 (1913). https://doi.org/10.1021/ja02198a600
84. Yoshimura, M., Suda, H.: Hydrothermal processing of hydroxyapatite: past, present, and future. In: Hydroxyapatite and related materials, pp. 45–72. CRC press, (2017)
85. Yang, G., Park, S.-J.: Conventional and microwave hydrothermal synthesis and application of functional materials: A review. Materials **12**(7), 1177 (2019). https://doi.org/10.3390/ma12071177
86. Yang, G., Park, S.J.: Author response to comment on: Conventional and microwave hydrothermal synthesis and application of functional materials: A review. Materials **12**(21), 1177 (2019). https://doi.org/10.3390/ma12213640
87. Piticescu, R.R., Monty, C., Taloi, D., Motoc, A., Axinte, S.: Hydrothermal synthesis of zirconia nanomaterials. J. Eur. Ceram. Soc. **21**(10–11), 2057–2060 (2001). https://doi.org/10.1016/S0955-2219(01)00171-6
88. Feng, S., Xu, R.: New materials in hydrothermal synthesis. Acc. Chem. Res. **34**(3), 239–247 (2001). https://doi.org/10.1021/ar0000105

89. Qi, P., Cong, Y., Yu, L., Ge, X., Hao, C., Wang, F., He, L.: Research on the progress of Ce3+,Tb3+ co-activated phosphate luminescent materials prepared by hydrothermal method. In: Journal of physics: Conference series, vol. 2430, p. 12018 (2023). https://doi.org/10.1088/1742-6596/2430/1/012018
90. Cao, C., Yang, H.K., Chung, J.W., Moon, B.K., Choi, B.C., Jeong, J.H., Kim, K.H.: Hydrothermal synthesis and enhanced photoluminescence of Tb3+ in Ce3+/Tb3+ doped KGdF4 nanocrystals. J. Mater. Chem. **21**(28), 10342–10347 (2011). https://doi.org/10.1039/c1jm10832h
91. Cao, C., Xie, A., Noh, H.M., Jeong, J.H.: Ce3+/Tb3+ non-/single-/co-doped K-Lu-F materials: Synthesis, optical properties, and energy transfer. Luminescence **31**(5), 1063–1068 (2016). https://doi.org/10.1002/bio.3072
92. Etafo, N.O.: Advancements of lanthanide-doped phosphors in solid-state lighting applications. Curr. Phys., **01**, (2024). https://doi.org/10.2174/0127723348280880240115054806
93. Al-Madhagi, H., Yazbik, V., Abdelwahed, W., Alchab, L.: Magnetite nanoparticle co-precipitation synthesis, characterization, and applications: mini review. BioNanoScience **13**(2), 853–859 (2023). https://doi.org/10.1007/s12668-023-01113-1
94. Mehrabi, M., Zahedifar, M., Sadeghi, E.: Luminescence properties of pure $CaSO_4$ nanoparticles produced by co-precipitation method. Jns **4**(4), 425–431 (2014). https://doi.org/10.7508/jns.2014.04.004
95. Chauhan, A., Kataria, S., Busko, D., Cardona, F.A., Turshatov, A., Richards, B.S.: Elucidating the role of metal-ion co-doping towards boosting upconversion luminescence in gadolinium vanadate. J. Mater. Chem. C **9**(46), 16709–16720 (2021). https://doi.org/10.1039/d1tc03205d
96. Fang, M., Yang, J., Li, Z.: Light emission of organic luminogens: Generation, mechanism and application. Prog. Mater Sci. **125**, 100914 (2022). https://doi.org/10.1016/j.pmatsci.2021.100914
97. Yang, J., Fang, M., Li, Z.: Organic luminescent materials: The concentration on aggregates from aggregation-induced emission. Aggregate **1**(1), 6–18 (2020). https://doi.org/10.1002/agt2.2
98. Meng, L., Jiang, S., Song, M., Yan, F., Zhang, W., Xu, B., Tian, W.: TICT-Based near-infrared ratiometric organic fluorescent thermometer for intracellular temperature sensing. ACS Appl. Mater. Interfaces. **12**(24), 26842–26851 (2020). https://doi.org/10.1021/acsami.0c03714
99. Zhou, Z., Yang, J., Yang, B., Han, Y., Zhu, L., Xue, X.-S., Zhu, F.: Photoredox nickel-catalysed stille cross-coupling reactions. Angew. Chem. Int. Ed. **62**(52), e202314832 (2023). https://doi.org/10.1002/anie.202314832
100. Bellomo, C., Chaari, M., Cabrera-González, J., Blangetti, M., Lombardi, C., Deagostino, A., Prandi, C.: Carborane-BODIPY dyads: New photoluminescent materials through an efficient heck coupling. Chem. Eur. J. **24**(58), 15622–15630 (2018). https://doi.org/10.1002/chem.201802901
101. Yamaguchi, E., Karin, O., Itoh, A.: Direct arylation reaction of heteroarenes mediated by photoinduced electron transfer. J. Photochem. Photobiol. **16**, 100183 (2023). https://doi.org/10.1016/j.jpap.2023.100183
102. Zani, L., Dessì, A., Franchi, D., Calamante, M., Reginato, G., Mordini, A.: Transition metal-catalyzed cross-coupling methodologies for the engineering of small molecules with applications in organic electronics and photovoltaics. Coord. Chem. Rev. **392**, 177–236 (2019). https://doi.org/10.1016/j.ccr.2019.04.007
103. Yang, R., Jess, A.D., Fai, C., Hages, C.J.: Low-temperature, solution-based synthesis of luminescent chalcogenide perovskite BaZrS3 nanoparticles. J. Am. Chem. Soc. **144**(35), 15928–15931 (2022). https://doi.org/10.1021/jacs.2c06168
104. Sun, L., Zou, Y., Liang, Z., Yu, J., Xu, R.: A one-pot synthetic strategy via tandem Suzuki-Heck reactions for the construction of luminescent microporous organic polymers. Polym. Chem. **5**(2), 471–478 (2014). https://doi.org/10.1039/c3py00980g
105. Zangade, S., Patil, P.: A review on solvent-free methods in organic synthesis. Curr. Org. Chem. **23**(21), 2295–2318 (2020). https://doi.org/10.2174/1385272823666191016165532

106. Choy, W.C.H., Chan, W.K., Yuan, Y.: Recent advances in transition metal complexes and light-management engineering in organic optoelectronic devices. Adv. Mater. **26**(31), 5368–5399 (2014). https://doi.org/10.1002/adma.201306133
107. Papaspyrides, C.D., Vouyiouka, S.N.: Solid state polymerization, vol. 236). Wiley Online Library, (2009). https://doi.org/10.1002/9780470451830
108. Wegner, G.: Solid-state polymerization mechanisms. Pure Appl. Chem. **49**(4), 443–454 (1977). https://doi.org/10.1351/pac197749040443
109. Takacs, L.: Self-sustaining reactions induced by ball milling. Prog. Mater Sci. **47**(4), 355–414 (2002). https://doi.org/10.1016/S0079-6425(01)00002-0
110. Szczesniak, B., Borysiuk, S., Choma, J., Jaroniec, M.: Mechanochemical synthesis of highly porous materials. Mater. Horiz. **7**(6), 1457–1473 (2020). https://doi.org/10.1039/d0mh00081g
111. Penczner, S.H., Kumar, P., Patel, M., Bouchard, L.S., Iacopino, D., Patel, R.: Innovations in mechanochemical synthesis: Luminescent materials and their applications. Mater. Today Chem. **39**, 102177 (2024). https://doi.org/10.1016/j.mtchem.2024.102177
112. Amado-Briseño, M.Á., Hernández-Ortíz, O.J., Rodríguez, M.A.V., Ayala, K.A., del Pozo Melero, G., Herrero, B.R., Vázquez-García, R.A.: Mechanosynthesis of 2,2′-((1E,1′E)-(2,5-bis(octyloxy)-1,4-phenylene)bis(ethene-2,1-diyl))bis(6-bromoquinoline): Optical, electroluminescence, electrical, electrochemical, and morphological studies. J. Mater. Sci.: Mater. Electron. **33**(1), 126–138 (2022). https://doi.org/10.1007/s10854-021-07271-w
113. Ma, X., Lim, G.K., Harris, K.D.M., Apperley, D.C., Horton, P.N., Hursthouse, M.B., James, S.L.: Efficient, scalable, and solvent-free mechanochemical synthesis of the OLED material Alq3 (q = 8-hydroxyquinolinate). Cryst. Growth Des. **12**(12), 5869–5872 (2012). https://doi.org/10.1021/cg301291w
114. Martín-Palma, R.J., Lakhtakia, A.: Vapor-deposition techniques. In: Engineered biomimicry, pp. 383–398. Elsevier, (2013). https://doi.org/10.1016/B978-0-12-415995-2.00015-5
115. Harsha, K.S.: Principles of vapor deposition of thin films. Elsevier, Principles of vapor deposition of thin films (2006). https://doi.org/10.1016/B978-0-08-044699-8.X5000-1
116. Biswas, S., Shalev, O., Shtein, M.: Thin-film growth and patterning techniques for small molecular organic compounds used in optoelectronic device applications. Annu. Rev. Chem. Biomol. Eng. **4**(1), 289–317 (2013). https://doi.org/10.1146/annurev-chembioeng-061312-103356
117. Jiang, Y., He, S., Qiu, L., Zhao, Y., Qi, Y.: Perovskite solar cells by vapor deposition based and assisted methods. Appl. Phys. Rev., **9**(2), (2022). https://doi.org/10.1063/5.0085221
118. Crowell, J.E.: Chemical methods of thin film deposition: Chemical vapor deposition, atomic layer deposition, and related technologies. J. Vac. Sci. Technol., A: Vac., Surf. Films **21**(5), S88–S95 (2003). https://doi.org/10.1116/1.1600451
119. Matsumoto, S., Ito, A.: Chemical vapor deposition route to transparent thick films of Eu 3+ -doped HfO_2 and Lu_2O_3 for luminescent phosphors. Opt. Mater. Express **10**(4), 899 (2020). https://doi.org/10.1364/ome.386425
120. Sun, L., Yuan, G., Gao, L., Yang, J., Chhowalla, M., Gharahcheshmeh, M.H., Liu, Z.: Chemical vapour deposition. Nat. Rev. Methods Prim **1**(1), 5 (2021). https://doi.org/10.1038/s43586-020-00005-y
121. Mattox, D.M.: Handbook of Physical Vapor Deposition (PVD) processing, pp. 1–945. (2007). https://doi.org/10.1016/c2009-0-18800-1
122. Singh, J., Wolfe, D.E.: Nanostructured component fabrication by electron beam-physical vapor deposition. J. Mater. Eng. Perform. **14**(4), 448–459 (2005). https://doi.org/10.1361/105994905X56223
123. Fernandes, J.D., Alessio, P., Silva, M.R.M., Aroca, R.F., De Souza, A.E., Constantino, C.J.L.: Physical vapor deposited films of a perylene derivative: Supramolecular arrangement and thermal stability. Mater. Res. **20**(4), 882–890 (2017). https://doi.org/10.1590/1980-5373-MR-2016-0692
124. He, J., Li, F., Long, Y., Song, Y., Wei, L., Liang, X., Kang, K.: PVD preparation and spectral study of organic electroluminescent material 8-hydroxyquinoline lithium. Results in Optics **15**, 100628 (2024). https://doi.org/10.1016/j.rio.2024.100628

125. Lunt, R.R., Lassiter, B.E., Benziger, J.B., Forrest, S.R.: Organic vapor phase deposition for the growth of large area organic electronic devices. Appl. Phys. Lett., **95**(23), (2009). https://doi.org/10.1063/1.3271797
126. Qu, B., Ding, K., Sun, K., Hou, S., Morris, S., Shtein, M., Forrest, S.R.: Fast organic vapor phase deposition of thin films in light-emitting diodes. ACS Nano **14**(10), 14157–14163 (2020). https://doi.org/10.1021/acsnano.0c07017
127. Kreis, J., Schwambera, M., Keiper, D., Gersdorff, M., Long, M., Heuken, M.: Organic Vapor Phase Deposition (OVPD) for efficient OLED manufacturing: the specific advantages and possibilities of carrier-gas enhanced vapor phase deposition for the manufacturing of organic thin film devices. In: Organic light emitting materials and devices XVI, vol. 8476, p. 84761L, (2012). https://doi.org/10.1117/12.930502
128. Burrows, P.E., Forrest, S.R., Sapochak, L.S., Schwartz, J., Fenter, P., Buma, T., Forrest, J.L.: Organic vapor phase deposition: a new method for the growth of organic thin films with large optical non-linearities. J. Cryst. Growth **156**(1–2), 91–98 (1995). https://doi.org/10.1016/0022-0248(95)00310-X
129. Nicole, L., Laberty-Robert, C., Rozes, L., Sanchez, C.: Hybrid materials science: A promised land for the integrative design of multifunctional materials. Nanoscale **6**(12), 6267–6292 (2014). https://doi.org/10.1039/c4nr01788a
130. Richardson, J.J., Cui, J., Björnmalm, M., Braunger, J.A., Ejima, H., Caruso, F.: Innovation in layer-by-layer assembly. Chem. Rev. **116**(23), 14828–14867 (2016). https://doi.org/10.1021/acs.chemrev.6b00627
131. Srivastava, S., Kotov, N.A.: Layer-by-layer (LBL) assembly with semiconductor nanoparticles and nanowires. Semiconductor Nanocrystal Quantum Dots: Synthesis, Assembly, Spectroscopy and Applications **41**(12), 197–216 (2008). https://doi.org/10.1007/978-3-211-75237-1_7
132. Liu, N., Li, S., Chen, L., Zheng, W.: A promising temperature sensor based on all-quantum-dot multilayer via layer-by-layer self-assembled method. Opt. Mater. **108**, 110460 (2020). https://doi.org/10.1016/j.optmat.2020.110460
133. Li, F., Klepzig, L.F., Keppler, N., Behrens, P., Bigall, N.C., Menzel, H., Lauth, J.: Layer-by-layer deposition of 2D CdSe/CdS nanoplatelets and polymers for photoluminescent composite materials. Langmuir **38**(37), 11149–11159 (2022). https://doi.org/10.1021/acs.langmuir.2c00455
134. Phillips, J.M., Coltrin, M.E., Crawford, M.H., Fischer, A.J., Krames, M.R., Mueller-Mach, R., Tsao, J.Y.: Research challenges to ultra-efficient inorganic solid-state lighting. Laser Photonics Rev. **1**(4), 307–333 (2007). https://doi.org/10.1002/lpor.200710019
135. Blasse, G., Bril, A.: A new phosphor for flying-spot cathode-ray tubes for color television: Yellow-emitting Y3Al5O12-Ce3+. Appl. Phys. Lett. **11**(2), 53–55 (1967). https://doi.org/10.1063/1.1755025
136. Rai, P., Song, M.K., Song, H.M., Kim, J.H., Kim, Y.S., Lee, I.H., Yu, Y.T.: Synthesis, growth mechanism and photoluminescence of monodispersed cubic shape Ce doped YAG nanophosphor. Ceram. Int. **38**(1), 235–242 (2012). https://doi.org/10.1016/j.ceramint.2011.06.057
137. Sato, Y., Kuwahara, H., Kato, H., Kobayashi, M., Masaki, T., Kakihana, M.: Large redshifts in emission and excitation from Eu2+-Activated Sr2SiO4 and Ba2SiO4 phosphors induced by controlling Eu2+ occupancy on the basis on crystal-site engineering. Opt. Photonics J. **5**(11), 326–333 (2015). https://doi.org/10.4236/opj.2015.511031
138. Pardha Saradhi, M., Varadaraju, U.V.: Photoluminescence studies on Eu2+-activated Li 2SrSiO4-A potential orange-yellow phosphor for solid-state lighting. Chem. Mater. **18**(22), 5267–5272 (2006). https://doi.org/10.1021/cm061362u
139. Baginskiy, I., Liu, R.S., Wang, C.L., Lin, R.T., Yao, Y.J.: Temperature dependent emission of strontium-barium Orthosilicate (Sr 2–x Ba x)SiO4: Eu 2+ phosphors for high-power white light-emitting diodes. J. Electrochem. Soc. **158**(10), P118–P121 (2011). https://doi.org/10.1149/1.3625282

140. Höppe, H.A., Lutz, H., Morys, P., Schnick, W., Seilmeier, A.: Luminescence in Eu2+-doped Ba2Si5N8: Fluorescence, thermoluminescence, and upconversion. J. Phys. Chem. Solids **61**(12), 2001–2006 (2000). https://doi.org/10.1016/S0022-3697(00)00194-3
141. Pust, P., Weiler, V., Hecht, C., Tücks, A., Wochnik, A.S., Henß, A.-K., Schnick, W.: Narrow-band red-emitting Sr[LiAl3N4]:Eu2+ as a next-generation LED-phosphor material. Nat. Mater. **13**(9), 891–896 (2014). https://doi.org/10.1038/nmat4012
142. Zhu, H., Lin, C.C., Luo, W., Shu, S., Liu, Z., Liu, Y., Chen, X.: Highly efficient non-rare-earth red emitting phosphor for warm white light-emitting diodes. Nat. Commun., **5**, (2014). https://doi.org/10.1038/ncomms5312
143. Frayret, J., Castetbon, A., Trouve, G., Potin-Gautier, M.: Solubility of (NH4)2SiF6, K2SiF6 and Na2SiF6 in acidic solutions. Chem. Phys. Lett. **427**(4–6), 356–364 (2006). https://doi.org/10.1016/j.cplett.2006.06.044
144. Matsuzawa, T., Aoki, Y., Takeuchi, N., Murayama, Y.: A new long phosphorescent phosphor with high brightness, SrAl2 O 4: Eu2 +, Dy3 +. J. Electrochem. Soc. **143**(8), 2670–2673 (1996). https://doi.org/10.1149/1.1837067
145. Meyer, J., Tappe, F.: Photoluminescent materials for solid-state lighting: State of the art and future challenges. Adv. Opt. Mater. **3**(4), 424–430 (2015). https://doi.org/10.1002/adom.201400511
146. Zhao, X., Wang, X., Chen, B., Meng, Q., Di, W., Ren, G., Yang, Y.: Novel Eu3+-doped red-emitting phosphor Gd2Mo3O9 for white-light-emitting-diodes (WLEDs) application. J. Alloy. Compd. **433**(1–2), 352–355 (2007). https://doi.org/10.1016/j.jallcom.2006.06.096
147. Lv, W., Jia, Y., Zhao, Q., Jiao, M., Shao, B., Lü, W., You, H.: Crystal structure and luminescence properties of Ca8Mg3Al2Si7O28: Eu2+ for WLEDs. Adv. Opt. Mater. **2**(2), 183–188 (2014). https://doi.org/10.1002/adom.201300448
148. Gou, J., Wang, J., Yu, B., Duan, D., Ye, S., Liu, S.: Li doping effect on the photoluminescence behaviors of KSrPO4:Dy3+ phosphors for WLED light. Mater. Res. Bull. **64**, 364–369 (2015). https://doi.org/10.1016/j.materresbull.2015.01.005
149. Lei, W., Luo, Z., He, Y., Liu, S., Zhang, P., Liang, H., Lu, A.: Preparation and broadband white emission of Ce3+-doped transparent glass-ceramics containing ZnO nanocrystals for WLEDs applications. J. Alloy. Compd., 875. https://doi.org/10.1016/j.jallcom.2021.159979
150. Ling, S., Xiong, F.B., Yang, W.B., Lin, H.F., Zhu, W.Z.: Novel Sm3+/Eu3+ co-doped Sr7Sb2O12 red-emitting phosphor for white LED. Inorg. Chem. Commun. **150**, 110365 (2023). https://doi.org/10.1016/j.inoche.2022.110365
151. Naik, R., Prashantha, S.C., Nagabhushana, H., Nagaswarupa, H.P., Anantharaju, K.S., Sharma, S.C., Girish, K.M.: Mg_2SiO_4:Tb3+ nanophosphor: Auto ignition route and near UV excited photoluminescence properties for WLEDs. J. Alloy. Compd. **617**, 69–75 (2014). https://doi.org/10.1016/j.jallcom.2014.07.100
152. Bawanthade, B.P., Mistry, A.A., Ugemuge, N., Chaudari, I.S., Dhoble, S.J.: Synthesis and study of optical properties of a Gd3+-doped $NaYF_4$ phosphor for phototherapy lamp application. Lumin., **39**(4). https://doi.org/10.1002/bio.4736
153. Raghu Raman, T., Ratnakaram, Y.C., Deva Prasad Raju, B.: Synthesis and spectroscopic investigations on Pr3+-doped LiPbB5O9 phosphor: A blue converting red phosphor for white LEDs. Optik, **225**, (2021). https://doi.org/10.1016/j.ijleo.2020.165758
154. Yuan, J., Feng, G., Dong, J., Lei, S., Hu, W.: Dual-functional porous MOFs with hierarchical guest encapsulation for room-temperature phosphorescence and white-light-emission. Nanoscale **13**(29), 12466–12474 (2021). https://doi.org/10.1039/d1nr03006j
155. Won, Y.H., Cho, O., Kim, T., Chung, D.Y., Kim, T., Chung, H., Jang, E.: Highly efficient and stable InP/ZnSe/ZnS quantum dot light-emitting diodes. Nature **575**(7784), 634–638 (2019). https://doi.org/10.1038/s41586-019-1771-5
156. Yuan, T., Yuan, F., Li, X., Li, Y., Fan, L., Yang, S.: Fluorescence-phosphorescence dual emissive carbon nitride quantum dots show 25% white emission efficiency enabling single-component WLEDs. Chem. Sci. **10**(42), 9801–9806 (2019). https://doi.org/10.1039/c9sc03492g

157. Guo, M.C., Zhong, W. Di, Wu, T., Han, W. Da, Gao, X.S., Ren, X.M.: Two Bi-MOFs with pyridylmulticarboxylate ligands showing distinct crystal structures and phosphorescence properties. J. Solid State Chem., **309**, (2022). https://doi.org/10.1016/j.jssc.2022.123005
158. Long, Z.Q., Wu, Y.L., Zheng, Y., Shi, R.H., Lu, D.F.: Room-temperature phosphorescence of a calcium-based metal-organic framework. Mater. Lett., 357. https://doi.org/10.1016/j.matlet.2023.135753
159. Liu, H., Ye, W., Mu, Y., Ma, H., Lv, A., Han, S., Huang, W.: Highly efficient blue phosphorescence from pillar-layer MOFs by ligand functionalization. Adv. Mater., **34**(5), (2022). https://doi.org/10.1002/adma.202107612
160. Wang, J., Song, B., Tang, J., Hu, G., Wang, J., Cui, M., He, Y.: Multi-modal anti-counterfeiting and encryption enabled through silicon-based materials featuring pH-responsive fluorescence and room-temperature phosphorescence. Nano Res. **13**(6), 1614–1619 (2020). https://doi.org/10.1007/s12274-020-2781-1
161. Le, T.H., Choi, Y., Kim, S., Lee, U., Heo, E., Lee, H., Yoon, H.: Highly elastic and >200% reversibly stretchable down-conversion white light-emitting diodes based on quantum dot gel emitters. Adv. Opt. Mater., **8**(7), (2020). https://doi.org/10.1002/adom.201901972
162. Sun, X., Wang, Y., Yang, J., Li, D., Wang, C.Z., Zhou, S., Zhou, J.: Rapid synthesis of rare-earth-element-free yellow-emissive carbon quantum ring-based crystals in a large scale for white light-emitting diodes. ACS Sustain. Chem. Eng. **10**(3), 1195–1204 (2022). https://doi.org/10.1021/acssuschemeng.1c06657
163. Meng, T., Wang, Z., Yuan, T., Li, X., Li, Y., Zhang, Y., Fan, L.: Gram-scale synthesis of highly efficient rare-earth-element-free red/green/blue solid-state bandgap fluorescent carbon quantum rings for white light-emitting diodes. Angew. Chemie—International Ed. **60**(30), 16343–16348 (2021). https://doi.org/10.1002/anie.202103361
164. Hu, J., Lei, M., Yan, L., Chen, L., Yang, Y., Zheng, J., Xu, B.: Carbon dot-based afterglow composite with tunable room temperature phosphorescence and thermally activated delayed fluorescence and their anti-counterfeiting and encryption application. Chem. Eng. J., **489**, (2024). https://doi.org/10.1016/j.cej.2024.151245
165. Pan, G., Bai, X., Xu, W., Chen, X., Zhou, D., Zhu, J., Song, H.: Impurity ions codoped cesium lead halide perovskite nanocrystals with bright white light emission toward ultraviolet-white light-emitting diode. ACS Appl. Mater. Interfaces. **10**(45), 39040–39048 (2018). https://doi.org/10.1021/acsami.8b14275
166. Moon, B.J., Kim, S.J., Lee, S., Lee, A., Lee, H., Lee, D.S., Lee, S.H.: Rare-earth-element-ytterbium-substituted lead-free inorganic perovskite nanocrystals for optoelectronic applications. Adv. Mater., **31**(33), (2019). https://doi.org/10.1002/adma.201901716
167. Wang, Y., Gao, H., Yang, J., Fang, M., Ding, D., Tang, B.Z., Li, Z.: High performance of simple organic phosphorescence host–guest materials and their application in time-resolved bioimaging. Adv. Mater., **33**(18), (2021). https://doi.org/10.1002/adma.202007811
168. Krishnan, R., Nair, G.B., Menon, S.G., Erasmus, L., Swart, H.C.: Synthesis of Tm2WO6:Er3+ upconversion phosphor for high-contrast imaging of latent-fingerprints. J. Alloy. Compd., 878, (2021). https://doi.org/10.1016/j.jallcom.2021.160386
169. Wei, J.H., Liao, J.F., Zhou, L., Luo, J. Bin, Wang, X.D., Kuang, D.B.: Indium-antimony-halide single crystals for high-efficiency white-light emission and anti-counterfeiting. Sci. Adv., **7**(34), (2021). https://doi.org/10.1126/sciadv.abg3989
170. Abdelhameed, M.M., Attia, Y.A., Abdelrahman, M.S., Khattab, T.A.: Photochromic and fluorescent ink using photoluminescent strontium aluminate pigment and screen printing towards anticounterfeiting documents. Luminescence **36**(4), 865–874 (2021). https://doi.org/10.1002/bio.3987
171. He, Y., Zhang, L.M., Chen, Y.M., Sun, L., Hu, C., Wang, M.X., Zhang, Q.Q.: Biocompatible photoluminescent silk fibers with stability and durability. ACS Biomater. Sci. Eng. **5**(5), 2657–2668 (2019). https://doi.org/10.1021/acsbiomaterials.9b00200
172. Cho, H., Kim, Y., Wolf, C., Lee, H., Lee, T.: Improving the stability of metal halide perovskite materials and light-emitting diodes. Adv. Mater. **30**(42), 1704587 (2018). https://doi.org/10.1002/adma.201704587

173. Zhang, H., Zhang, H., Pan, A., Yang, B., He, L., Wu, Y.: Rare earth-free luminescent materials for wLEDs: Recent progress and perspectives. Adv. Mater. Technol. **6**(1), 2000648 (2021). https://doi.org/10.1002/admt.202000648
174. Wei, Y., Cheng, Z., Lin, J.: An overview on enhancing the stability of lead halide perovskite quantum dots and their applications in phosphor-converted LEDs. Chem. Soc. Rev. **48**(1), 310–350 (2019). https://doi.org/10.1039/C8CS00740C
175. Omoniyi, A.O., Wang, Y., Yang, S., Liu, J., Zhang, J., Su, Z.: High-security information encryption strategy based on optical functional materials: A review on materials design, problems, multiple coding, and beyond. Mater. Today Commun. **36**, 106508 (2023). https://doi.org/10.1016/j.mtcomm.2023.106508
176. Christé, S., Esteves da Silva, J.C.G., Pinto da Silva, L.: Evaluation of the environmental impact and efficiency of N-doping strategies in the synthesis of carbon dots. Materials **13**(3), 504 (2020). https://doi.org/10.3390/ma13030504
177. Johny, A., Pinto da Silva, L., Pereira, C.M., Esteves da Silva, J.C.G.: Sustainability assessment of highly fluorescent carbon dots derived from eucalyptus leaves. Environments **11**(1), 6 (2024). https://doi.org/10.3390/environments11010006
178. Panigrahi, K., Nag, A.: Challenges and strategies to design phosphors for future white light emitting diodes. J. Phys. Chem. C **126**(20), 8553–8564 (2022). https://doi.org/10.1021/acs.jpcc.2c01679
179. Neacsu, I.A., Stoica, A.E., Vasile, B.S., Andronescu, E.: Luminescent hydroxyapatite doped with rare earth elements for biomedical applications. Nanomaterials **9**(2), 239 (2019). https://doi.org/10.3390/nano9020239
180. Krishnan, R., Shibu, S.N., Poelman, D., Badyal, A.K., Kunti, A.K., Swart, H.C., Menon, S.G.: Recent advances in microwave synthesis for photoluminescence and photocatalysis. Mater. Today Commun. **32**, 103890 (2022). https://doi.org/10.1016/j.mtcomm.2022.103890
181. Wang, J., Ma, Q., Wang, Y., Shen, H., Yuan, Q.: Recent progress in biomedical applications of persistent luminescence nanoparticles. Nanoscale **9**(19), 6204–6218 (2017). https://doi.org/10.1039/C7NR01488K
182. Abdollahi, A., Roghani-Mamaqani, H., Razavi, B., Salami-Kalajahi, M.: Photoluminescent and chromic nanomaterials for anticounterfeiting technologies: Recent advances and future challenges. ACS Nano **14**(11), 14417–14492 (2020). https://doi.org/10.1021/acsnano.0c07289
183. Chimene, D., Alge, D.L., Gaharwar, A.K.: Two-dimensional nanomaterials for biomedical applications: Emerging trends and future prospects. Adv. Mater. **27**(45), 7261–7284 (2015). https://doi.org/10.1002/adma.201502422

Biocompatible Materials for Light Emitters

Saheed Abiola Raheem and Olayinka Oderinde

Abstract Biocompatible materials are explicitly designed to collaborate with biological systems, serving a wide range of applications, without causing damage to the host-tissue. To date, biocompatible materials have attracted remarkable attention in display, drug delivery, and lighting devices due to their numerous merits, involving cytotoxicity, biocompatibility, and flexibility. As light emitters, biocompatible materials emit corresponding light to the photon energy when current circulates through it. This chapter highlights the recent developments in the synthesis and functionalization of biocompatible materials for light-emitting applications.

1 Introduction

Light emitting and display technology are crucial to developing the information and technology industries. Amid the global energy crisis affecting everyday life, the demand for low-energy, eco-friendly light emitters has risen, positioning them as promising candidates for next-generation display applications. Light emitters with low energy consumption and minimal toxicity are specifically appealing for advancing display technology [1, 2]. Hence, there is a growing demand for materials that combine high energy efficiency with minimal or no damage to biological systems [3]. Biocompatible materials perform a particular function without unintended effects and do not bring about inflammatory reactions. These materials are safe, interact with biological systems, and do not cause any damaging effects on the body. Thus, materials with the properties as mentioned above are known to be biocompatible. Biocompatible materials find wide applications in drug delivery, gene therapy, electronics, etc. [4–6]. Strategies for improving the biocompatibility of biomaterials and

S. A. Raheem (✉)
Department of Applied and Environmental Chemistry, University of Szeged, Rerrich Béla tér 1, Szeged H-6720, Hungary
e-mail: saheedabiola9@gmail.com

O. Oderinde
Department of Chemistry, Faculty of Natural and Applied Sciences, Lead City University, Ibadan, Nigeria

© The Author(s), under exclusive license to Springer Nature Switzerland AG 2025

N. O. Etafo (ed.), *Tailored Light Emitters For Biomedical Applications*, Engineering Materials, https://doi.org/10.1007/978-3-031-88731-4_3

examples of biocompatible materials as light emitters for biomedical applications will be discussed in the sub-sections below.

2 Strategies for Biocompatibility

Light-emitting biomaterials may increase the risk of infection when implanted into biological systems because of their associated intrinsic risk. However, it is on record that biomaterials' biological responses are notably affected by surface properties (such as elasticity, topography, charge, surface free energy, etc.) [7]. Thus, certain techniques are used to enhance the biological properties and the biocompatibility of such biomaterials, thereby reducing related infections [8, 9]. In this chapter, we will highlight surface modification and polymer encapsulation as forms of biocompatibility procedures.

2.1 Surface Modification

This process involves modifying the surface properties of biomaterials to increase their biocompatibility for improved stability. Surface modification involves various intricacies, varying from the incorporation of a single functional group to a more difficult multi-step reaction. These modifications can be achieved through processes such as hydrolysis, aminolysis, oxidation, and plasma treatment [10, 11]. For instance, del Olmo et al. coated chitosan-based hydrogel on (α+β) titanium alloy (Ti_6Al_4V) via hydrolysis and aminolysis to increase the biocompatibility of the Ti_6Al_4V. When evaluated, the modified Ti_6Al_4V exceptionally boosts cell proliferation and displays a remarkable cell-repelling and contact-killing potential [12]. Similarly, Li et al. constructed macro/micro/nano three-layer structures on titanium via a two-step micro-arc oxidation method. The modification is assumed to enhance the adhesion of osteoblasts to implants [13].

In another related study, Bax et al. coated tropoelastin on polyurethane co-polymer by plasma ion immersion implantation to improve the biocompatibility of the latter. When tested, the modified polyurethane co-polymer shows improved human dermal fibroblast and human umbilical vein endothelial cell adhesion [14].

2.2 Polymer Encapsulation

Polymer encapsulation involves the modification of the biomaterials with an additional polymer layer to make them hydrophilic and increase their biocompatibility. To date, silk has been developed into different forms via surface morphology control. For instance, Lawrence and co-researchers incorporated haemoglobin and enzyme peroxidase into silk to create nanopatterning for biocompatibility. The modification leads to excellent optical quality and biological uses [15]. In another study carried out by Losi et al., a modified poly(ether)urethane/polydimethylsiloxane/fibrin-based scaffold displayed enhanced granulation tissue formation and maturity [16]. Through polymer encapsulation, Lin et al. prepared dextran-modified bacterial cellulose hydrogel that possesses high water content and is rigid. When tested, the modified bacterial cellulose hydrogel displays improved cell proliferation with no cytotoxicity, unlike pure bacterial cellulose hydrogel. It also shows promise for quick healing in in vivo wound healing tests [17].

Based on the aforementioned studies, we can conclude that both surface modification and polymer encapsulation have improved the biocompatibility of biomaterials by tackling the complications that are associated with simple biomaterials.

3 Examples of Biocompatible Materials

In the following subsections, we will highlight a few examples of biocompatible materials for biomedical applications, namely silica nanoparticles, polymeric micelles, and carbon nanomaterials.

3.1 Silica Nanoparticles

To date, silica-based nanoparticles have received significant attention as superior biocompatible materials because of their adaptable properties. Studies have shown that silica nanoparticle properties such as morphology and nanostructures do have a remarkable effect on the therapeutic efficacy of drugs and side effects [18–20]. To show the biocompatibility of silica nanoparticles in biological systems, Li et al. prepared cisplatin and cholorin e6-conjugated silica nanoparticles for use a cancer therapy. When applied as infrared light irradiation in mice for in vivo chemo-photodynamic therapy, it successfully represses the tumour growth. The performance observed in tumours is shown (Fig. 1a and b) with a drastic reduction in their weight after the treatment [21]. Similarly, Amin et al. reported the preparation of mesoporous silica nanoparticles coated with Poly (D, L-lactide-co-glycolide) for photodynamic therapy (PDT) of curcumin. During hemocompatibility assay, it decreases haemolytic effects that are connected with silanol and erythrocytes interaction [22]. In other related work by Lalegül-Ülker et al., silica-coated iron oxide/polyaniline nanocomposites were prepared through chemical oxidative polymerization. It is concluded that the prepared silica nanocomposites show great potential for use in controlled drug delivery and tissue engineering [23].

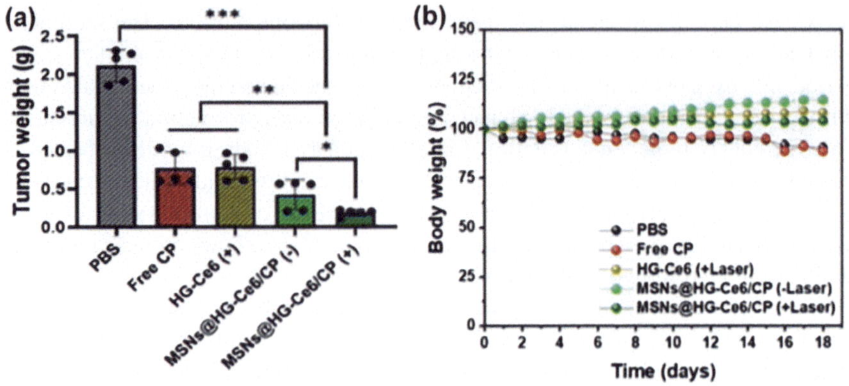

Fig. 1 **a** Tumour treatment after treatment, and **b** Body weight of the mice after treatment. Reproduced under the permission of Li et al. [21]

3.2 Polymeric Micelles

Polymeric micelles are co-polymers produced through the self-assembly of amphiphilic molecules in aqueous solutions. Polymeric micelles have attracted attention over the years for use as specific drug and protein delivery, it is also commonly used in brain-specific delivery. These applications are made possible because of their nano-size and steric stabilization which make them easily infiltrate the blood-brain barrier and reach the brain's parenchyma [24]. In a study carried out by Li et al. fluorinated amphiphilic polymers were synthesized via living cationic polymerization. Due to the aforementioned unique properties, it is assumed to be a promising anti-cancer drug carrier [25]. In another study carried out by Dule et al., Cysteine-based amphiphilic peptide polymer was synthesized via a thiol-mediated radical polymerization process. The as-prepared sample is cytotoxic and was applied to probe the critical aggregation concentration of the Chinese Hamster Ovary cells [26]. By coating polymeric micelles on mesoporous silica nanoparticles, Xu et al. prepared a multifunctional nanocarrier. When evaluated, the polymeric micelles-coated silica nanoparticles display a remarkable fluorescence, unlike the pure silica nanoparticle, demonstrating its use in drug delivery systems [27].

3.3 Carbon Nanomaterials

Carbon nanomaterials consist of members of the carbon family that have attracted extensive attraction and found applications in the biomedical field. The members consist of carbon nanotubes (CNT), carbon nanofiber (CNF), carbon sheets (CS), graphene, graphene oxide (GO), and fullerenes [28]. By employing hazard-free and simple methods of preparation, Chen et al. synthesized red-emitting carbon dots

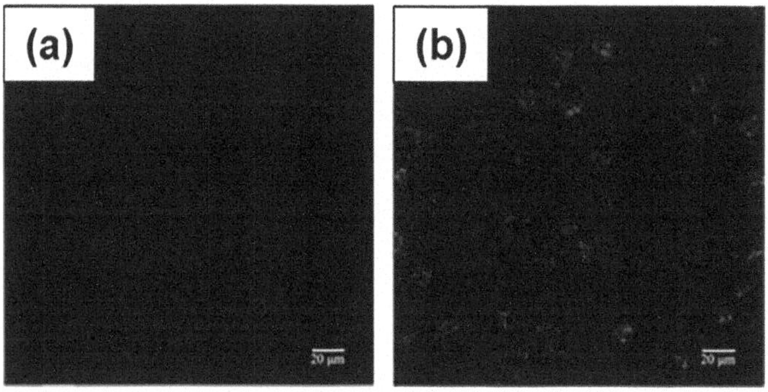

Fig. 2 **a** A549 cells without rCDs **b** A549 cells with rCDs. Reproduced under the permission of Chen et al. [29]

(rCDs) via hydrothermal procedure. When tested for cytotoxicity and acute toxicity *in vitro* and *in vivo*, the rCDs show great biocompatibility and minimal toxicity. These qualities position them as a potential candidate for bioimaging, where rCDs serve as the fluorescent probe in A549 cells, zebrafish and mice. For instance, when compared against the control in A549 cells, rCDs display bright red fluorescence (Fig. 2) [29]. In a similar work on carbon dots, Sun et al. prepared nitrogen-doped carbon dots via a solvothermal method with urea as the nitrogen source. CDs demonstrated impressive imaging depths when used for probing mesenchyme (a subtype of triple-negative breast cancer cell line) [30]. In another study carried out by Yuan et al., graphene quantum dots were synthesized and combined with prepared gold nanoclusters to develop paper-based analytical devices. When employed in immunoassay, these devices demonstrated swift and numerous pathogen detection in resource-limited zones, enabling prompt diagnosis of bacterial infections [31].

Various properties of biomaterials, ranging from biological, chemical, mechanical, and optical characteristics play an important role in their application in biomedical, as highlighted by the representatives listed (Table 1).

Table 1 Different biocompatible for biomedical applications and their properties

Biocompatible material	Irradiation parameter	Irradiation effect	Quantum yield	Refs. (%)
Dextran/bacterial cellulose hydrogel	Absorbance 450 nm		–	[18]
PLGA/mesoporous silica nanoparticles	PDT-457 nm 220.2 W/m^2	–	–	[22]
Thiolate/ nanoclusters	460/490 nm	–	1.5	[32]
N, F-doped carbon Dots	428 nm	Effective against *Escherichia coli* & *Staphylococcus aureus*	52.2	[33]
Graphene films	812 nm 0.15 W/m^2	Kills ~ 99 % planktonic bacteria	–	[34]
Carbon dots	365 nm	–	20.5	[35]

4 Conclusion

In this chapter, up-to-date studies on biocompatible materials for light-emitters have been highlighted. Biocompatible materials are promising candidate for fluorescence because of their unique properties that can be modified for enhanced performance. By focusing on the specific modifications, these materials are poised revolutionize lightning display technology and spearhead advancement in biomedical research. For light-emitting applications, the modification process should be highly efficient and hazard-free to reduce any negative impacts on biological systems.

References

1. Salehi, A., Fu, X., Shin, D.H., So, F.: Recent advances in OLED optical design. Wiley-VCH Verlag, (2019). https://doi.org/10.1002/adfm.201808803
2. Mei, W., et al.: High-resolution, full-color quantum dot light-emitting diode display fabricated via photolithography approach. Nano Res. **13**(9), 2485–2491 (2020). https://doi.org/10.1007/s12274-020-2883-9
3. Hsiang, E.L., Yang, Z., Yang, Q., Lan, Y.F., Wu, S.T.: Prospects and challenges of mini-LED, OLED, and micro-LED displays. J. Soc. Inf. Disp. **29**(6), 446–465 (2021). https://doi.org/10.1002/jsid.1058
4. Hasanin, M.S.: Cellulose-based biomaterials: Chemistry and biomedical applications. John Wiley and Sons Inc., (2022). https://doi.org/10.1002/star.202200060
5. Lingait, D., et al.: A review on versatile applications of biomaterial/polycationic chitosan: An insight into the structure-property relationship. Elsevier B.V., (2024). https://doi.org/10.1016/j.ijbiomac.2023.128676
6. Zimmermann, J., Porcarelli, L., Rödlmeier, T., Sanchez-Sanchez, A., Mecerreyes, D., Hernandez-Sosa, G.: Fully printed light-emitting electrochemical cells utilizing biocompatible materials. Adv. Funct. Mater. **28**(24), (2018). https://doi.org/10.1002/adfm.201705795

7. Hernandez, J.L., et al.: Effect of tissue microenvironment on fibrous capsule formation to biomaterial-coated implants. Biomaterials, **273**, (2021). https://doi.org/10.1016/j.biomaterials.2021.120806
8. Benčina, M., Resnik, M., Starič, P., Junkar, I.: Use of plasma technologies for antibacterial surface properties of metals. Molecules, **26**(5), (2021). https://doi.org/10.3390/molecules26051418
9. Chen, S.T., Wu, C.Y., Chen, H.Y.: Enhanced growth activities of stem cell spheroids based on a durable and chemically defined surface modification coating. ACS Appl. Mater. Interfaces **10**(38), 31882–31891 (2018). https://doi.org/10.1021/acsami.8b09103
10. Chouirfa, H., Bouloussa, H., Migonney, V., Falentin-Daudré, C.: Review of titanium surface modification techniques and coatings for antibacterial applications. Acta Materialia Inc., (2019). https://doi.org/10.1016/j.actbio.2018.10.036
11. Roh, S., Jang, Y., Yoo, J., Seong, H.: Surface modification strategies for biomedical applications: enhancing cell–biomaterial interfaces and biochip performances. SpringerOpen, (2023). https://doi.org/10.1007/s13206-023-00104-4
12. Andrade del Olmo, J., et al.: Multifunctional antibacterial chitosan-based hydrogel coatings on Ti6Al4V biomaterial for biomedical implant applications. Int. J. Biol. Macromol. **231**, (2023). https://doi.org/10.1016/j.ijbiomac.2023.123328
13. Li, Y., Wang, W., Duan, J., Qi, M.: A super-hydrophilic coating with a macro/micro/nano triple hierarchical structure on titanium by two-step micro-arc oxidation treatment for biomedical applications. Surf. Coatings Technol. **311**, 1–9 (2017). https://doi.org/10.1016/j.surfcoat.2016.12.065
14. Bax, D.V., Kondyurin, A., Waterhouse, A., McKenzie, D.R., Weiss, A.S., Bilek, M.M.M.: Surface plasma modification and tropoelastin coating of a polyurethane co-polymer for enhanced cell attachment and reduced thrombogenicity. Biomaterials **35**(25), 6797–6809 (2014). https://doi.org/10.1016/j.biomaterials.2014.04.082
15. Lawrence, B.D., Cronin-Golomb, M., Georgakoudi, I., Kaplan, D.L., Omenetto, F.G.: Bioactive silk protein biomaterial systems for optical devices. Biomacromolecules **9**(4), 1214–1220 (2008). https://doi.org/10.1021/bm701235f
16. Losi, P., et al.: Fibrin-based scaffold incorporating VEGF- and bFGF-loaded nanoparticles stimulates wound healing in diabetic mice. Acta Biomater. **9**(8), 7814–7821 (2013). https://doi.org/10.1016/j.actbio.2013.04.019
17. Lin, S.P., Kung, H.N., Tsai, Y.S., Tseng, T.N., Di Hsu, K., Cheng, K.C.: Novel dextran modified bacterial cellulose hydrogel accelerating cutaneous wound healing. Cellulose **24**(11), 4927–4937 (2017). https://doi.org/10.1007/s10570-017-1448-x
18. Li, L., Liu, T., Fu, C., Tan, L., Meng, X., Liu, H.: Biodistribution, excretion, and toxicity of mesoporous silica nanoparticles after oral administration depend on their shape. Nanomedicine Nanotechnol., Biol. Med. **11**(8), 1915–1924 (2015). https://doi.org/10.1016/j.nano.2015.07.004
19. Wang, X., et al.: Hollow structure improved anti-cancer immunity of mesoporous silica nanospheres in vivo. Small **12**(26), 3510–3515 (2016). https://doi.org/10.1002/smll.201600677
20. Yang, Y., Zhang, M., Song, H., Yu, C.: Silica-based nanoparticles for biomedical applications: from nanocarriers to biomodulators. Acc. Chem. Res. **53**(8), 1545–1556 (2020). https://doi.org/10.1021/acs.accounts.0c00280
21. Li, Y., et al.: Integrated and hyaluronic acid-coated mesoporous silica nanoparticles conjugated with cisplatin and chlorin e6 for combined chemo and photodynamic cancer therapy. Eur. Polym. J. **220**, (2024). https://doi.org/10.1016/j.eurpolymj.2024.113426
22. Umair Amin, M., et al.: Enhanced photodynamic therapy of curcumin using biodegradable PLGA coated mesoporous silica nanoparticles. Eur. J. Pharm. Biopharm. **204**, (2024). https://doi.org/10.1016/j.ejpb.2024.114503
23. Lalegül-Ülker, Ö., Elçin, Y.M.: Magnetic and electrically conductive silica-coated iron oxide/polyaniline nanocomposites for biomedical applications. Mater. Sci. Eng. C. **119**, (2021). https://doi.org/10.1016/j.msec.2020.111600

24. Kaur, J., et al.: Advances in designing of polymeric micelles for biomedical application in brain related diseases. Elsevier Ireland Ltd. https://doi.org/10.1016/j.cbi.2022.109960
25. Wei, B.X., Cui, Y.T., Ma, S.C., Liu, H.H., Bai, Y.P.: Synthesis of stimulus-responsive ABC triblock fluorinated polyether amphiphilic polymer and application as low toxicity smart drug carrier. Eur. Polym. J. **175**, (2022). https://doi.org/10.1016/j.eurpolymj.2022.111389
26. Dule, M., Biswas, M., Biswas, Y., Mandal, K., Jana, N.R., Mandal, T.K.: Cysteine-based amphiphilic peptide-polymer conjugates via thiol-mediated radical polymerization: Synthesis, self-assembly, RNA polyplexation and N-terminus fluorescent labeling for cell imaging. Polymer (Guildf) **112**, 125–135 (2017). https://doi.org/10.1016/j.polymer.2017.01.083
27. Xu, X., et al.: Polymeric micelle-coated mesoporous silica nanoparticle for enhanced fluorescent imaging and pH-responsive drug delivery. Chem. Eng. J. **279**, 851–860 (2015). https://doi.org/10.1016/j.cej.2015.05.085
28. Las-Casas, B., et al.: The emergence of hybrid cellulose nanomaterials as promising biomaterials. Int. J. Biol. Macromol. **250**, (2023). https://doi.org/10.1016/j.ijbiomac.2023.126007
29. Chen, J., Li, T., Lin, C., Hou, Y., Cheng, S., Gao, B.: Green synthesis of red-emitting carbon dots for bioimaging, sensing, and antibacterial applications. Spectrochim. Acta—Part A Mol. Biomol. Spectrosc. **328**, (2025). https://doi.org/10.1016/j.saa.2024.125458
30. Sun, Z., et al.: A yellow-emitting nitrogen-doped carbon dots for sensing of vitamin B12 and their cell-imaging. Dye. Pigment. **176**, (2020). https://doi.org/10.1016/j.dyepig.2020.108227
31. Yuan, H., et al.: Detection of pathogens using graphene quantum dots and gold nanoclusters on paper-based analytical devices. Sensors Actuators B Chem. **363**, (2022). https://doi.org/10.1016/j.snb.2022.131824
32. Ramadurai, M., Rajendran, G., Bama, T.S., Prabhu, P., Kathiravan, K.: Biocompatible thiolate protected copper nanoclusters for an efficient imaging of lung cancer cells. J Photochem. Photobiol. B Biol. **205**, (2020). https://doi.org/10.1016/j.jphotobiol.2020.111845
33. Hua, J., Hua, P., Qin, K.: Highly fluorescent N, F co-doped carbon dots with tunable light emission for multicolor bio-labeling and antibacterial applications. J. Hazard. Mater, **459**, (2023). https://doi.org/10.1016/j.jhazmat.2023.132331
34. Henriques, P.C., et al.: Graphene films irradiated with safe low-power NIR-emitting diodes kill multidrug resistant bacteria. Carbon N. Y. **180**, 10–21 (2021). https://doi.org/10.1016/j.carbon.2021.04.085
35. Wang, H.J., Hou, W.Y., Yu, T.T., Chen, H.L., Zhang, Q.Q.: Facile microwave synthesis of carbon dots powder with enhanced solid-state fluorescence and its applications in rapid fingerprints detection and white-light-emitting diodes. Dye. Pigment. **170**, (2019). https://doi.org/10.1016/j.dyepig.2019.107623

Applications in Diagnostics

Targeted Drug Delivery with Photoluminescent Emitters: Applications in Diagnostic

Abayomi Bamisaye, Nelson Oshogwue Etafo, Muyideen Olaitan Bamidele, and Olaolu Samuel Awobifa

Abstract Targeted drug delivery has been transformed by photoluminescent emitters, enabling combined therapeutic and diagnostic (theranostic) applications. These systems use materials like quantum dots, carbon dots, and rare-earth nanoparticles to achieve precise targeting, reduced side effects, and real-time imaging. Passive and active mechanisms guide the drug to specific sites, minimizing off-target effects. Innovations in materials that respond to stimuli, like those affected by pH or redox changes, allow controlled drug release in environments like tumor microenvironments. Advanced encapsulation improves drug stability, loading capacity, and responsiveness to triggers. Light-triggered delivery systems use near-infrared or visible light for precise, non-invasive drug activation, while photodynamic therapy integrates treatment and imaging for better cancer care. Biocompatible and biodegradable materials are prioritized to ensure safety and minimize toxicity. Surface modifications, such as PEGylation and ligand attachment, enhance targeting accuracy and extend circulation time. Stability issues, including sensitivity to the environment and limited shelf life, are addressed through improved encapsulation techniques. Pharmacokinetic and pharmacodynamic studies optimize drug distribution, circulation, and toxicity reduction. Photoluminescent systems enable real-time monitoring, dose adjustments, and tracking therapeutic progress. Despite challenges in scalability, cost, and regulatory approvals, these systems represent a breakthrough in personalized medicine, combining precision, diagnostics, and treatment.

A. Bamisaye (✉) · M. O. Bamidele
Department of Chemistry, Faculty of Natural and Applied Sciences, Lead City University, Ibadan, Oyo State, Nigeria
e-mail: abayomibamisaye@gmail.com; bamisaye.olusegun@lcu.edu.ng

N. O. Etafo
Carolina Universidad, Saltillo, Coahuila, Mexico

M. O. Bamidele
Department of Food Research, School of Chemistry, Universidad Autonoma de Coahuila, Saltillo Coahuila, Mexico

O. S. Awobifa
Facultad de Ciencias Químicas, Universidad Autónoma de Coahuila, Saltillo, Coahuila, México

© The Author(s), under exclusive license to Springer Nature Switzerland AG 2025
N. O. Etafo (ed.), *Tailored Light Emitters For Biomedical Applications*, Engineering Materials, https://doi.org/10.1007/978-3-031-88731-4_4

Keywords Photoluminescent emitters · Targeted drug delivery · Real-time imaging · Stimuli-responsive materials · Theranostic

1 Introduction

The demand for effective and personalized therapeutic solutions has significantly advanced the field of targeted drug delivery. These systems enhance therapeutic characteristic of bioactive materials or drug by minimizing adverse effects through precise delivery to targeted sites [1]. Recently, the integration of photoluminescent materials has introduced a diagnostic capability that allows real-time imaging, tracking, and monitoring within biological environments [2]. This theranostic approach, which combines therapeutic and diagnostic functionalities, paves new avenues for personalized medicine [3]. Photoluminescent substances, examples include quantum dots, carbon dots, and nanoparticles with embedded rare-earth elements offer unique optical properties that are ideal for theranostic applications. For example, quantum dots exhibit tunable emission spectra, high brightness, and photostability, enabling prolonged imaging without signal loss [4]. Carbon dots, noted for their excellent compatibility with biological tissues and a low risk of causing harm, are particularly suitable in vivo studies [5]. These materials may be coupled with therapeutic agents, directing moieties of ligands, or biofunctional molecules to form multifunctional nanostructures that selectively target diseased cells, thus improving treatment precision and providing clinicians with real-time feedback for optimized patient outcomes [6]. Several recent studies have highlighted these innovations. Hussain et al. [7] developed naturally occurring carbon dots (PACDs) with antioxidant properties, biocompatibility, and colloidal stability using a one-step thermal coupling procedure. PACDs exhibit prolonged release patterns and pH-sensitive drug release, rendering them advantageous for controlled drug delivery in acidic disease environments. Similarly, Parsaeifar et al. [8] prepared carbon quantum dots/45S5 nanohybrids that demonstrated in vitro luminescent emissions and rapid doxorubicin release, suggesting their potential for bioactive applications in bone fillers and implant coatings. Other studies have explored novel nanomaterials' such as B-doped carbon dots [9] and mesoporous silica hybrids [10], which exhibit high drug encapsulation efficiency, pH-sensitive release, and strong optical absorption for cancer theranostics. Photoluminescent emitters also serve as biomarkers, which can be used to monitor physiological states, disease indicators, and facilitate personalized treatment planning [11]. Certain photoluminescent materials provide controlled drug release mechanisms triggered with release triggered by pH or temperature changes, minimizing side effects and safeguarding tissues in good conditions [12, 13]. Additionally, multiplexed imaging capabilities support the simultaneous visualization of multiple biomarkers, which are crucial for complex conditions, such as cancer [14]. Despite these promising developments, photoluminescent drug delivery systems face challenges in their clinical translation to adopt this novel approach, the following should be ensured; biocompatibility, minimizing toxicity, maintaining stability in physiological environments, and probable scalable production [15]. Additionally, some photoluminescent materials may generate reactive oxygen species (ROS) when illuminated by light, potentially compromising cellular potential [16].

This review offers an in-depth analysis of photoluminescent emitters for targeted drug delivery emphasizing their diagnostic and theranostic capabilities. We examined the photoluminescence mechanisms in drug delivery, discussed recent innovations in targeting and ligand design, and highlighted advancements in in vivo imaging and tracking. Finally, we address clinical translation challenges and suggest strategies to bridge laboratory research and practical applications, with the aim of fostering further research to bring these technologies closer to clinical use in personalized medicine.

2 Design Consideration for Drug Delivery Systems

Designing these therapeutic delivery transport systems entails focusing on specific delivery, enhanced diagnostic capabilities, and the integration of photoluminescent emitters. All these points involve a blend of biomedical engineering, materials science, pharmacology, and optical diagnostics. This section provides an insight into certain factors that warrant careful examination in fabricating the drug delivery system as shown in the section, thus.

2.1 Photoluminescent Emitters in Diagnostics

Luminophores emitting in the 650–1350 nm range (the therapeutic window) are advantageous for imaging applications. This spectral region minimizes absorption by biological matter, enabling deeper tissue penetration and improved image quality in both in vitro and in vivo settings [17]. While organic dyes are frequently employed, inorganic red/NIR emitters offer distinct advantages. These include ruthenium complexes, rare-earth compounds, quantum dots, and molybdenum/tungsten octahedral cluster complexes. They not only exhibit strong emission within the expected red/near-infrared (NIR) wavelength range but also possess unique functionalities. These functionalities encompass upconversion luminescence, photoactivation effects, and the capacity to photosensitize singlet oxygen generation. However, a significant limitation of these inorganic emitters is their inherent instability in aqueous environments within a functional body condition. This instability persists even when there are no further alterations, despite their exceptional functional potential. Silica encapsulation has emerged as a prominent and effective strategy to address this limitation. Silica is readily available, biocompatible, and non-toxic [17]. Furthermore, Li et al. reported that photoluminescence (PL) imaging has emerged as a key instrument for surgical navigation, therapeutic assessment, and illness diagnosis.

The design of nanoprobes with optimal efficiency for in vivo imaging and seamless personalized medicine is still a significant challenge. Nonetheless, growing interest is now towards the sub-10 nm ultra-small nanoprobes for in vivo photoluminescence imaging. These nanoprobes have gained attention because of their superior imaging signal-to-noise ratio, promising potential for clinical applications, and efficient clearance from the body [18]. In the same view Li et al., also assert that the creation of fluorescent probes has drawn much attention in recent years. Modern biological applications greatly benefit from the non-invasive, safe, images in real time of living objects with enhanced spectrum resolution possible by fluorescence signaling. In vitro and in vivo fluorescence sensing and imaging are characterized by several fundamental photophysical mechanisms, including Förster Resonance Energy Transfer (FRET), Aggregation-Induced Emission (AIE), Photoinduced Electron Transfer (PET), Excited-State Intramolecular Proton Transfer (ESIPT), Intramolecular Charge Transfer (ICT), and Twisted Intramolecular Charge Transfer (TICT) [18].

2.2 *Brightness and Quantum Yield*

Abdellatif et al. highlighted that quantum dots (QDs), which are semiconductor-based nanomaterials, have diverse applications spanning biomedical fields such as drug delivery, live imaging, and medical diagnostics, as well as non-medical areas like solar cell technology. Despite their potential, the clinical utility of QDs remains underappreciated [19]. Tools that allow for more precise cancer targeting and enhanced tumor visibility will be necessary to increase the efficacy of cancer treatment. Because they can be used as both diagnostics and treatments, theranostics holds promise for improving cancer care; nevertheless, tissue-associated light absorption and scattering frequently limit their diagnostic value. The synthesis of CuInSe2@ZnS; Mn quantum dots (QDs) with inherent multifunctionality are powerful tumor ablation agents and allow precise localization of tiny metastases. Abdellatif et al developed biocompatible quantum dots (QDs) exhibiting remarkable near-infrared (NIR)-II fluorescence efficiency of up to 31.2%, exceptional contrast in magnetic resonance imaging (MRI), and selective accumulation in 4T1 breast cancer tumors [19]. This was accomplished by controlling the growth kinetics of a ZnS shell around a biocompatible CuInSe2 core, incorporating manganese doping, and applying folic acid functionalization. These nanoprobes' MRI-enabled contrast is adequate for promptly detecting minor lung metastases, which is crucial for stopping the spread and recurrence of cancer. Additionally, the excitation of tumor-localized QDs with NIR light induces heat and radical generation via non-radiative recombination pathways, effectively destroying cancer cells and stimulating an anticancer immune response. This approach eradicates tumors and prevents their regrowth in

80% of treated mice, while simultaneously enabling tumor visualization through fluorescence emitted via radiative recombination pathways [20]. Despite their protein-like size, exceptional photostability, and long-term biosafety in vivo, photoluminescent graphene quantum dots (GQDs), which have been regarded as highly suitable for bioimaging, have yet to achieve certain critical and unique in vivo bioimaging applications. The NP-GQD-PEG nanocomposite was synthesized by embedding graphene quantum dots (GQDs) within a poly (ethylene glycol) (PEG) layer of PEGylated nanoparticles using a bottom-up molecular approach. In vivo evaluations reveal that these embedded GQDs achieve 7–8 times greater tumor accumulation and sustain over four times longer blood circulation compared to standard GQDs. This multifunctional NPs-GQDs-PEG nanocomposite provides targeted, multimodal molecular imaging for specific tumor types both in vitro and in vivo, with straightforward modifications to enhance specificity [21].

2.3 *Photostability*

Photostability is essential in targeted drugs delivery systems that make use of light emitting materials. These polymers enable precise monitoring of drug carriers in the body. Excellent photostability ensures long-term brightness while preventing damage from prolonged light exposure. This increases medication delivery effectiveness and dependability, allowing for the development of more complex and least intrusive therapies. Jiang et al. reported an approach to enhance the characteristics of conventional fluorophores based on the dyes' photostability, brightness, and Stokes shift which are the key factors in the fidelity and use of super-resolution fluorescence imaging. Conventional rhodamines can be modified to include a quinoxaline motif with a finely tuned electron density. This leads to the development of novel dyes featuring a vibrational structure and suppressed twisted intramolecular charge transfer (TICT), which collectively enhance brightness, photostability, and the Stokes shift. YL578, a new fluorophore produced from Rhodamine B, has twice the brightness and Stokes shift of its parent molecule. YL578-based probes exhibit improved photostability in STED microscopy, outperforming carbocyanine-based standards (CPY-Halo and 580CP-Halo) by three times. This method provides a versatile framework for developing a novel category of vibrant, photostable luminescent probes with prolonged Stokes shifts (up to 136 nm), which are suitable for improved biosensing and bioimaging applications [22]. Researchers may benefit more from biological imaging if fluorescent labels with higher bleaching resistance are used [23].

2.4 *Biocompatibility and Non-toxicity*

The report given by Umezawa & Soga showed that some research is being done on using polymers to enclose bioactive compounds and nanomaterials to minimize their interactions with organs and biomolecules outside the target areas, hence controlling their toxicity and beneficial effects [24]. This idea is well-recognized as nanoparticle-based medication delivery systems. RNA vaccines exemplify an innovative approach by encapsulating highly fragile RNA within lipid nanoparticles, ensuring stable delivery of RNA to immune cells. It is anticipated that these approaches will be successful in creating low-toxicity nanoscale materials. Umezawa and Soga [24] investigated the effectiveness of hybrid nanomaterials (HNMs), combining inorganic and organic components, for photodynamic therapy (PDT) targeting deep tissue lesions. In this regard, HNM synthesized was used as biodegradable polymer nanoparticles to enclose UCL-NPs, rose bengal (RB), and a PDT dye. By combining (1) PDT dyes with (2) Near-infrared (NIR) light-activated upconversion luminescent nanoparticles (UCL-NPs) excited dyes. When encapsulated in highly transparent biological tissues (HNMs), the nanoparticles maintained their luminescence while significantly reducing the toxicity of the dye (RB).

Furthermore, Guo et al. also reported that semiconducting polymer nanoparticles, often known as Pdots, have numerous biomedical applications, including biomolecular probes, tumor imaging, and treatment. Despite their potential, the physiological effects and biocompatibility of Pdots in vitro and in vivo have not been extensively investigated [25]. This study systematically evaluated the biological impacts of Pdots with diverse surface alterations, addressing the critical concern of their interactions with biological systems. Investigations revealed how Pdots interact with organisms at both cellular and animal levels. The functional usefulness is enhanced, when various groups such as thiol, carboxyl, and amino were introduced onto the Pdots' surfaces, resulting in Pdots@SH, Pdots@COOH, and Pdots@NH2. According to extracellular research, the physicochemical characteristics of Pdots were not significantly impacted by the configuration of the sulfhydryl, carboxyl, or amino groups; however, the stability of Pdots was somewhat affected by the amino modification. Because of their instability in solution, Pdots@NH_2 increased cytotoxicity and decreased cellular absorption capability at the cellular level. At the in vivo level, Pdots@SH and Pdots@COOH demonstrated enhanced blood flow and rapid detoxification compared to Pdots@NH2. The study shows that the mice's blood indices and histological lesions in the major tissues and organs were not significantly impacted by the four types of Pdots.

2.5 Pharmacokinetics and Pharmacodynamics (Biodistribution)

A magnetic field from the outside increases the desired biodistribution of nanoparticles, such as in malignant tumors. Therefore, understanding these nanoparticles' biodistribution is crucial for medical purposes. Nowak-Jary and Machnicka reported that magnetic iron oxide nanoparticles, such as magnetite and maghemite, are being thoroughly researched because of their many potential uses in the biological and medical sciences. By focusing on an external magnetic field, their special qualities like their nanometric size, huge specific surface area, and super-paramagnetism allow them to be utilized in internal radiotherapy and targeted drug administration. They also work well for radiolabelling, hyperthermia, and magnetic resonance imaging (MRI). Properly designed nanoparticles can effectively target specific tissues and organs [26]. mRNA molecules are frequently delivered using lipid nanoparticles (LNPs). Nevertheless, little is known about the metric relationships between transgene expression dynamics, biodistribution, and the pharmacokinetics (PK) of the nanoparticle carrier. LNPs of various sizes were made with mRNAs expressing the firefly luciferase gene. Liquid chromatography with tandem mass spectrometry or fluorescence bioimaging was used to assess the biodistributions of injected LNPs in mice [27]. Furthermore, enzyme activity assays and bioluminescence imaging were used to measure the amounts of luciferase expression [28]. Some intramuscularly injected LNPs, particularly those of smaller size, were shown to circulate throughout the body, accumulating in the liver and spleen. Biomolecules in locally injected LNPs, such as mRNAs, can move to various organs and tissues via systemic circulation. The LNP biodistribution and pharmacokinetics (PK) have an impact on gene expression levels, as do the injection method and particle size [27]. He et al. [29] described nanoassemblies that respond to reactive oxygen species (ROS) and can reduce in size. These structures are formed through several host–guest interactions between β-cyclodextrin (β-CD)-attached discoidal recombinant high-density lipoprotein (NP3ST) and hyaluronic acid-ferrocene (HA-Fc) conjugates. The pharmacokinetics and distribution of the nanoparticles in mice are shown in Fig. 1a–h.

2.6 *Stability and Shelf Life (Environmental Sensitivity)*

According to He et al. [30], environmental sensitivity is crucial for photoluminescent materials. Encapsulation methods, including the use of zeolitic imidazole framework-8 (ZIF-8), can greatly improve nitrogen-doped graphene quantum dots' photo–, thermal–, pH–, and storage stability. Time–temperature indicators could benefit from persistent luminous materials, which have superior environmental stability and recyclability [31]. Photo- and thermal-sensitivity are common in therapeutic protein formulations, according to a survey of approved biotechnology-derived pharmaceutical products; liquid formulations and specific container types exhibit more pronounced sensitivity [32]. Smart magnetic composites that are triple responsive to temperature, pH, and UV light have been created for effective phosphopeptide enrichment. These composites exhibit high sensitivity, selectivity, and reusability in a variety of biological samples [33].

Moreover, the fabrication of drug delivery systems requires attention to compatibility with the body, precise targeting, and controlled drug release. Important factors include the composition of characteristics of the drug, the needed distribution pattern, and the method of delivery (e.g., oral, skin application, injection). Some of the

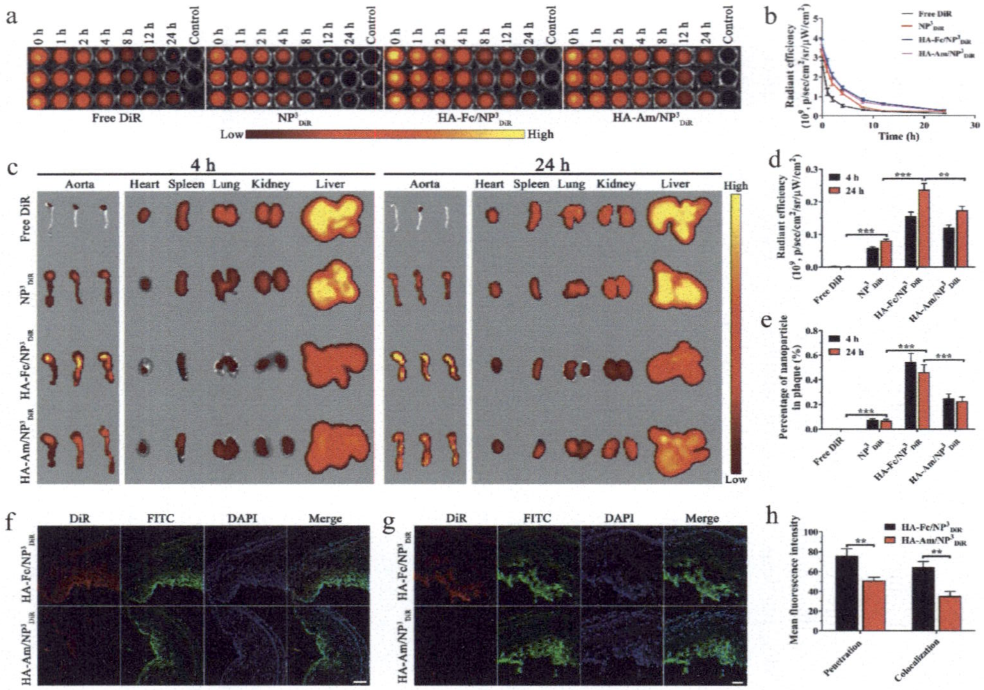

Fig. 1 Pharmacokinetic and distribution of nanoparticles in mice. **a** Ex vivo images, and **b** quantified DiR fluorescence intensities of whole blood collected from wild-type C57BL/6 mice at fixed time points measured by IVIS spectrum system (n = 3); **c** Ex vivo images of the aortas and main organs in atherosclerotic mice imaged by IVIS spectrum system, **d** quantified fluorescence intensities in the aortas and **e** the percentage of nanoparticle in plaque (n = 3). Immunofluorescence analysis of **f** the penetration ability of DiR-labeled nanoparticles (Red)across the CD31-labeled plaque tissues (Green), and **g** the colocalization of DiR-labeled nanoparticles (Red) and CD68-labeled cells (Green) imaged by CLSM, **h** quantification of DiR fluorescence intensity in the aortic root sections

other factors that determines the fabrication of drug delivery system, decryption, and advantage and disadvantage of each methods is summarized in Table 1. The materials should be safe, harmless, able to naturally degrade, ensuring stability, and easy use. These are essential for effective therapy outcome for patient.

Table 1 Showing design consideration for drug delivery systems

Design consideration	Description	Advantages	Disadvantages	References
Targeting mechanisms	Mechanisms to direct the drug to specific tissues (passive, active, stimuli-responsive)	Promotes medication concentration at a particular site Reduces general adverse effects	Complexity of design Potential off-target effects if targeting is not precise	[34, 35]
Material selection	Choosing biocompatible and biodegradable materials	Reduced toxicity and immune reaction Biodegradable materials minimize accumulation	Limited material options that balance biocompatibility, biodegradability, and functionality	[36–38]
Photo-luminescent emitters	Materials that emit light for real-time tracking and diagnostic imaging	Allows simultaneous therapy and diagnostics Enables real-time tracking of the delivery of drugs	Possible toxicity (e.g., some quantum dots) Limited penetration with some emission wavelengths	[17, 39, 40]
Encapsulation and drug loading	Techniques to protect and control release of drugs	Controlled release optimizes therapeutic effects Reduces premature degradation of the drug	Potential for low drug loading Complex preparation may increase costs	[41–43]
Optical properties for imaging	Using NIR or other suitable wavelengths for deeper tissue imaging	Enables tracking in vivo NIR wavelengths allow deeper tissue penetration Multiplexing capabilities	Emission may decrease over time (photobleaching) Imaging equipment required	[44–46]

(continued)

Table 1 (continued)

Design consideration	Description	Advantages	Disadvantages	References
Surface modification and functionalization	Adding ligands, antibodies, PEG, etc., to enhance targeting, circulation, and cellular uptake	Enhances specificity to target cells Extends circulation time Reduces immune detection (PEGylation)	Additional steps in the synthesis Potential immune response to ligands and modification agents	[47–49]
Pharmacokinetics and pharmacodynamics	Controlling drug distribution, half-life, and toxicity	Increases therapeutic effect and reduces toxicity Improved control over drug release and clearance	Variability in patient responses Toxicity from certain materials (e.g., inorganic nanoparticles)	[50–52]
Stability and shelf life	Ensuring the system remains stable during storage and transport	Extended shelf life and stability Reduced risk of degradation during administration	Sensitive to environmental factors (e.g., temperature, light) Packaging requirements for stability	[53–55]
Theranostic capability	Combining therapeutic and diagnostic functions in one system	Reduces need for multiple treatments Real-time feedback on therapeutic efficacy	Complexity of integration Higher production costs and regulatory challenges	[53, 56–58]

3 Light-Triggered Drug Release Mechanism

According to the 2024 report by the National Cancer Institute, 14, 910 children and adolescents (0–19 years) are estimated to contract cancer resulting in 1,590 mortalities with the expected new cancer cases will be expected to 29.9 million by 2040 [59]. The challenges for the drug method of administration as a delivery system for the therapy are bioavailability, instability, and toxicity [60]. Light-activated drug release systems provide an advanced method for drug delivery, allowing accurate oversight over both the duration and site of therapeutic release [61]. These systems harness illumination to activate the release of enclosed drugs, offering a non-invasive and precisely targeted treatment method at designated times and sites within the body [62]. Table 2 shows the superior properties of the light-activated drug delivery devices better than the conventional drug delivery system. This customized delivery strategy has tremendous potential to enhance therapeutic efficacy while minimizing the negative effects often associated with traditional drug administration methods [63]. There are several advantages attributed to light-triggered drug release system, these include:

- **Precision and Control**: Light can be precisely focused to certain specific tissues or cells, minimizing off-target effects. Agiba et al. [61] noted that these systems are capable of responding to different light wavelengths, such as UV, visible, and near-infrared, based on the specific photosensitive elements and the composition of the nanocarriers. Gao et al. stated that Lipid nanoparticles (LNPs) are now recognized as an acceptable medium for targeted distribution, employing passive and active targeting techniques, as well as stimuli-responsive mechanisms for controlled release [74].

Table 2 The comparative study of the traditional and light-triggered delivery system

Feature	Traditional drug delivery system	Light-triggered delivery system	References
Drug release mechanism	Based on physical or chemical processes like diffusion, dissolution, or enzymatic degradation	It is triggered by exposure to specific wavelengths of light, leading to a controlled release of the drug	[62, 64]
Timing of drug release	Predetermined and often occurs over a prolonged period	Can be precisely controlled by applying light at specific times and durations	[65, 66]
Spatial control	Limited spatial control over drug release	Offers precise spatial control by focusing light on specific target areas	[66]
Side effects	Can lead to systemic side effects due to widespread drug distribution	Reduces systemic side effects by targeting drug release to specific sites	[67, 68]
Patient compliance	Requires strict adherence to dosing schedules	Offers flexibility and patient convenience, as drug release can be triggered on demand	[69, 70]
Complexity	Relatively simpler in design and formulation	Requires more complex formulations and delivery systems, often involving light-sensitive materials	[71, 72]
Applications	Widely used for various therapeutic applications, including oral, intravenous, and topical delivery	Primarily used for targeted drug delivery, particularly in cancer therapy and ophthalmology	[66, 73]

- **Non-Invasive**: Light-based triggers are non-invasive, avoiding the need for surgical procedures or injections. Shamsipur et al. highlighted that several phototriggered structures, such as o-nitrobenzyl, coumarinyl, and anthracenyl, have been created to improve the regulated release of medicinal substances [75]. Singh et al. [76] indicated that systems based on ESIPT, AIE, and AIE + ESIPT enable successful and tailored administration of medicines and gaseous compounds, with low cytotoxicity and real-time monitoring. Jiang et al. stated that mechanoluminescent nano transducers activated by focused ultrasound have been developed to overcome light attenuation in deep tissues, allowing noninvasive light delivery to deep-seated structures with submillimeter resolution and millisecond response times [77].
- **Temporal and Spatial Control**: Drug release can be initiated and terminated at specific times by controlling light exposure. Light-triggered liposomes enable on-demand drug release, improving therapy and minimizing side effects [61]. A study developed by Jung et al. highlighted a mitochondria-targeting prodrug that releases mechlorethamine upon light activation, with the process monitored through fluorescence signals [67]. Moreso, irradiation can be directed on certain locations within the body, which is known as spatial control. This is also crucial for targeted drug delivery. These systems utilize photoresponsive polymers and nanocarriers that release drugs upon light exposure [78]. Light-responsive liposomes have emerged as promising nanocarriers, capable of releasing drugs when activated at various light wavelengths, from UV to near-infrared [61].
- **Remote Activation**: Light-triggered systems can be remotely activated, allowing for flexible and personalized treatment. Polymeric nanoparticles are versatile carriers that can incorporate various medications and mitigate challenges in traditional retinal drug delivery [79]. Light-responsive nanosystems have been developed to penetrate deeper tissues using near-infrared light, ultrasound, or X-ray excitation [80]. These systems have showed potential in the fight against cancer, as light activation can elicit apoptotic alterations in cancer cells [81].

3.1 Photothermal Therapy (PTT)

Photothermal therapy (PTT) is a non-invasive form of cancer therapy that uses radiation-absorbing substances to generate heat upon the contact with light, resulting in the selective destruction of tumor cells [82]. PTT, which uses near-infrared (NIR) light to target tumors, absorbs deep tissue with minimal injury to healthy tissue [83]. Malekzadeh et al. stated that PTT is accomplished by introducing nanoparticles into the tumor, which absorb near-infrared (NIR) light and transform it into heat. NIR light's capacity to penetrate extensively into tissues makes it particularly effective for targeting tumors located deep within the body [84]. This involves 3 main processes: light absorption, heat generation, and cell death.

Hu et al. reported an innovative approach might inspire new strategies for overcoming thermoresistance and enhancing tumour therapy. Because Conventional photothermal therapy (PTT) often requires hyperthermia (>50°C), which can harm normal tissues. Mild-temperature PTT, while less toxic, is limited by cancer cell thermoresistance. To overcome this challenge, they created a nanocarrier that delivers nitric oxide (NO) and the photothermal agent DCTBT for mild-temperature PTT using NIR-II AIE. Intracellular NO release and DCTBT-induced ROS generation upon 808 nm laser irradiation synergistically produce peroxynitrite ($ONOO^-$), which inhibits heat shock proteins (HSPs) and enhances cancer cell sensitivity to mild-temperature PTT. The efficacy of $ONOO^-$-potentiated mild-temperature PTT was validated in subcutaneous and orthotopic hepatocellular carcinoma (HCC) models [85].

Liao et al. developed small-sized Ti3C2Tx MXene nanosheets loaded with (–)-epigallocatechin gallate (EGCG) to enhance the efficacy of near-infrared (NIR) light-based photothermal therapy (PTT), an attractive alternative to chemotherapy known for its simplicity and minimal side effects, while also addressing the challenges posed by inflammation and heat shock protein (HSP) overexpression that can reduce its effectiveness. These nanosheets exhibit high photothermal conversion efficiency, excellent drug delivery capability, and potent antioxidant properties. EGCG, released in acidic tumor microenvironments, inhibits HSP expression and reduces inflammation. In vitro and in vivo studies demonstrated enhanced tumor ablation and reduced inflammation with MXene@EGCG, offering a novel approach for cancer therapy [86].

Moreover, Jia et al. developed a novel injectable hydrogel system composed of CoSnSx, L-arginine, chitosan (CTS), and carboxymethyl cellulose (CMC) designed for sonodynamic and dual-gas enhanced photothermal therapy (PTT). Since PTT activates the immune system and near-infrared lasers have limited tissue penetration, single PTT treatments are often insufficient. CoSnSx, with its hollow structure, generates a significant amount of singlet oxygen (1O2) under ultrasonic (US) irradiation and produces H2S gas in acidic conditions, thereby offering sonodynamic and gas therapeutic effects. Moreover, in both in vitro and in vivo studies, this multifunctional injectable hydrogel system demonstrated exceptional therapeutic outcomes through sonodynamic and dual-gas treatment-enhanced PTT. Under 808 nm laser irradiation, CoSnSx exhibited excellent photothermal conversion efficiency (48.24%). L-arginine, a nitric oxide (NO) a precursor, was incorporated into the hydrogel to enable controlled NO release during US/laser irradiation, thereby enhancing the PTT response. This innovative injectable hydrogel technology offers a promising strategy to enhance PTT effectiveness [87].

3.1.1 Mechanism of Photothermal Therapy (PTT)

The mechanism of photothermal therapy involves three main processes which include, light absoprtion, heat generation and cell death. This is shown in Fig. 2.

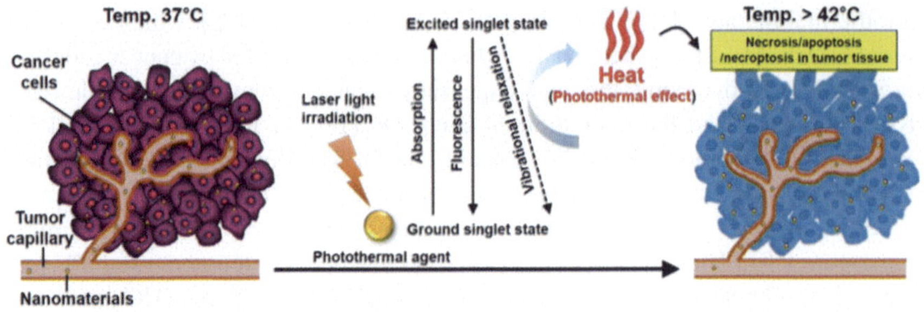

Fig. 2 The mechanism reaction of photothermal therapy (PTT) [88]

- **Light Absorption**: Nanoparticles, often synthesized from precious metals like gold or semiconductor materials, are injected into the tumor. These nanoparticles efficiently absorb near-infrared (NIR) radiation that can penetrate deeply into body parts while causing minimal harm. Kurokawa et al. [89] reported that gold nanoparticles (AuNPs) can be engineered to absorb near-infrared (NIR) light, enabling deep tissue penetration without causing damage. This property, combined with their potential for cancer-specific accumulation, makes AuNPs promising candidates for cancer therapy. To enhance their cancer-targeting ability, they synthesized Au-HpD, a porphyrin-conjugated gold compound. Their results demonstrate that Au-HpD aggregates predominantly in cancer cells as opposed to normal cells. When cancer cells treated with Au-HpD were exposed to 870 nm laser irradiation, they exhibited significant cell death, characterized by structural alterations, such as nuclear disintegration. In contrast, normal cells were unaffected by this treatment. These results indicate that using Au-HpD in combination with NIR laser irradiation could be an effective approach for selective destruction of cancer cells.
- **Heat Generation**: When the nanoparticles absorb light, they quickly release the energy as heat through vibrational relaxation, raising the temperature within the tumor microenvironment. According to the report of Thirumurugan et al. [90], Photothermal therapy (PTT) is a minimally invasive cancer treatment. It employs nanoparticles (NPs) to convert near-infrared (NIR) light into heat, resulting in the destruction of cancer cells. NPs deliver photothermal agents (PTAs) to the tumor microenvironment (TME), where they absorb NIR light and generate heat. This localized hyperthermia damages cancer cells. NPs, with their ability to target the TME and enhance drug delivery, significantly improve PTT's effectiveness.
- **Cell Death**: The increased temperature disrupts cellular structures, denatures proteins, and triggers cell death, effectively destroying the tumor cells.

Lukácsi et al. [91] reported a study on PTT, its molecular, cellular, and immunological effects of hyperthermia, a cancer treatment involving elevated tumor temperatures ($\geq$39 °C), this shows promise as an adjuvant therapy. The molecular and cellular effects include DNA repair inhibition, cell cycle arrest and apoptosis, and heat shock protein modulation. The immunological effects results in mild systemic hyperthermia

(39–41°C) activates immune cells, mimicking fever. All these is followed by an intense heat (>50 °C) with the potential to release tumor antigens, thereby enhancing immune responses. Immunotherapy synergy results where hyperthermia, particularly when combined with photothermal nanoparticles, can modulate the immunity and improve the therapeutic value of immune checkpoint inhibitors. The clinical outcomes demonstrate that hyperthermia is a economic viable and acceptable adjunctive treatment, especially when combined with immunotherapy. Thereby providing valuable insights for selecting patient-specific treatments and guiding future research.

3.2 Photodynamic Therapy

Photodynamic therapy (PDT) has gained attention due to its targeted curative strategy for applications in cancer, antimicrobial treatments, and other localized diseases. PDT selectively destroys diseased cells while preserving healthy tissues by using photosensitizers that are activated upon light exposure [92]. Recent advances in the integration of photoluminescent materials with PDT have enhanced treatment precision by enabling dual functionality as both therapeutic and visualization agents [45, 93]. This theranostic approach supports the real-time visualization of personalized treatment planning and monitoring by clinicians, thereby advancing precision and personalized medicine [94, 95]. In a recent study by Zhou et al. [96], a two-photon activation technique for the TiO_2-curcumin-sofast (TCS) complex was developed to enhance the generation and penetration depth of reactive oxygen species (ROS), surpassing traditional curcumin (CUR). TCS exhibited a 6–sevenfold increase in ROS production, showing significant phototoxicity and induction of apoptosis in HeLa and T24 cancer cell lines. Simulated deep-tissue trials using pig skin further supported TCS's potential of TCS for treating cancers and deep-seated lesions. Wang et al. [97] synthesized a hyaluronic acid-carbon dot (HA-CD) composite via hydrothermal methods, integrating cisplatin (DDP) for dual chemotherapeutic and PDT functionality. This composite, through ROS generation, effectively inhibited tumor growth in vivo, underscoring its potential for combined chemotherapy and PDT in oral squamous cell carcinoma (OSCC) treatment. Chen et al. [98] introduced Hcy-I, a near-infrared mitochondrial-targeted photosensitizer with enhanced singlet oxygen generation due to iodine atom inclusion, which increases spin–orbit coupling and intersystem crossing. This mitochondrial targeting, validated in vitro, induces apoptosis by disrupting membrane potential, illustrating a promising avenue for integrating cancer diagnostics and therapeutics. Shi et al. [99] developed a graphene oxide-based DNA nanodevice (DND) for fluorescence signal amplification and PDT in tumor cells. The DND Y-type DNA structures amplify Ce6 fluorescence and ROS release, inducing cell apoptosis with high specificity for miRNA-21, indicating their utility in early cancer diagnosis and timely treatment. Tong et al. [100] synthesized two organic porphyrin-based molecules, ONP and SNP, with modified photophysical properties for enhanced PDT and photothermal effects. Their acceptor–donor–acceptor architecture improved intersystem crossing and ROS generation, displaying biocompatibility and cytotoxicity in Hepa1-6 cells, offering a synergistic approach to photodynamic and photothermal therapy.

3.2.1 Mechanisms of Action in PDT

In PDT, a photosensitizing agent is administered and selectively accumulates in diseased tissues, guided by mechanisms such as ligand-receptor interactions or nanoparticle-based delivery systems [101, 102]. When stimulated to light of the appropriate wavelength, the photosensitizer gets excited and transmits energy to surrounding molecular oxygen, which triggers the formation of ROS, such as singlet oxygen and free radicals, as illustrated in Fig. 3 [103]. These reactive oxygen species (ROS) cause oxidative harm to cellular structures, including lipids, proteins, and DNA, eventually resulting in cell death [104]. In tumors, ROS-induced cell damage disrupts the vasculature and activates immune responses, thereby enhancing the therapeutic effect [105]. Incorporating photoluminescent emitters in PDT has further improved both precision and efficacy [106]. Photoluminescent materials, such as quantum dots, carbon dots, and conjugated polymers emit light when activated, enabling dual functions for treatment and real-time imaging. This approach facilitates precise localization of the treatment area, allows real-time dosage adjustments, and optimizes therapeutic outcomes [107]. Unlike traditional photosensitizers, photoluminescent emitters can be engineered for specific emission and absorption spectra, which enhances their compatibility with diverse tissue optical properties and improves imaging clarity by minimizing interference from tissue autofluorescence [108]. New studies centres on the use of advanced PDT. Xiong et al. [109] developed Apt-LPR, a light-activated PDT/RNAi synergy enhancer. This system combines miR-34a and photosensitizers within cationic liposomes to form a "Liposome-Aptamer-Target" interface, reducing cytotoxicity, enhancing DNase

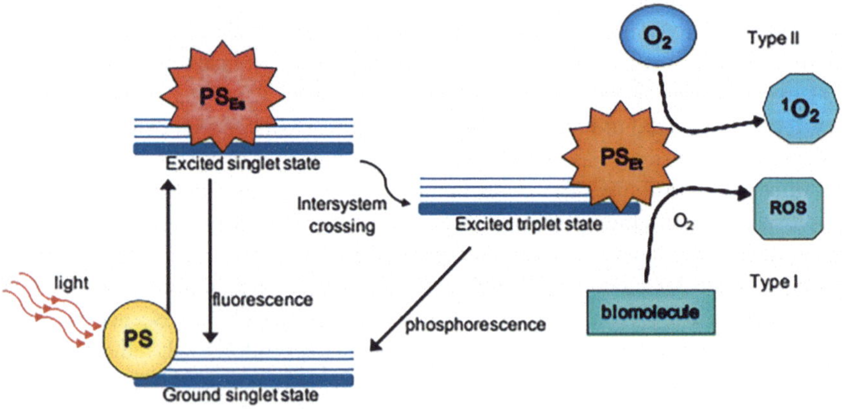

Fig. 3 Mechanisms of action in photodynamic therapy [112]

resistance, and preserving selective targeting for drug delivery. Apt-LPR effectively stimulated antitumor immunity and suppressed tumor growth in mouse models, while zebrafish models demonstrated its photo-controlled drug release and tumor-targeting precision. Chen et al. [110] synthesized PyCF3SiPc, a photosensitizer enhanced with a DSPE-mPEG2000 nanocarrier for targeted visualization of lipid droplets. In vitro studies revealed that DSPE@PyCF3SiPc selectively accumulated in lipid droplets and exhibited phototoxic effects against MCF-7 breast cancer cells, demonstrating its potential for precise therapeutic action and real-time tracking. Oliveira et al. [111] synthesized various palladium (II) and platinum (II) complexes with thiosemicarbazones derived from thiophene to evaluate their cytotoxic properties. Among these, $PdCH_3$ showed significant cytotoxicity against A549 and A2780cis cancer cell lines by inducing apoptosis and inhibiting colony formation. This study emphasizes the utility of Pd-based complexes as tailored cytotoxic treatments to certain cancer types.

Quantum dots (QDs) offer unique advantages, like high photostability, adjustable emission spectra, and high light absorption [113]. Unlike traditional organic photosensitizers, QDs can be engineered to specific wavelengths, optimizing ROS production, and boosting phototoxicity against targeted cells [114]. Their surfaces can be modified with targeting ligands, antibodies, or peptides to boost their ability to selectively target sick parts. This considerably broadens the therapeutic potential of PDT [115]. Carbon dots (CDs) are another promising option on account of their low toxicity, tissue compatibility, and ease of synthetic feasibility from sustainable carbon sources, including biowastes [116]. These properties make CDs cost effective and versatile. Their efficient ROS generation and customizable surface chemistry allows conjugation with targeting agents, enhancing their therapeutic potential [117]. CDs also exhibit high aqueous solubility, supporting their targeted accumulation in diseased tissues [118]. Conjugated polymer nanoparticles (CPNs) are structurally flexible alternatives to inorganic particles with tunable light absorption properties and high ROS generation efficiency [119]. Lin et al. [120] created a scanty X-ray activated phosphor, $Ca_2P_2O_7{:}Pr^{3+}$, exhibiting exceptional afterglow luminescence over a wide range, highlighting its promise as a red phosphor for LEDs and a potent agent for PDT. Additionally, [121] created Mito CPs-p, a mitochondrial-targeting, pH-responsive nanozyme that combines platinum with pH-responsive porphyrin polymers, significantly increasing ROS production and therapeutic efficacy in the tumor environment. In a further study, [122] engineered Bi2Se3 nanosheets modified with thiolated ultrasmall gold nanoclusters (AuNCs), enhancing both photothermal and photocatalytic capabilities for combined photothermal/photodynamic therapy in tumors. These nanosheets present an innovative approach for theranostic applications by integrating therapeutic action with imaging functionality. Further studies by, [122] have investigated cyclometalated Ir (III) complexes and Ru (II) polypyridyl derivatives. These compounds, containing thiazolyl-β-carboline ligands, demonstrate exceptional photostability when exposed to blue light and show strong anticancer effects. In particular, the Ir (III) complexes demonstrated high cytotoxicity, which was further enhanced by blue-light activation. These complexes demonstrate the potential of multifunctional nanoplatforms that combine drug delivery, imaging, and photodynamic effects in a single system.

3.2.2 Advances in Targeting and Selectivity of PDT

A significant challenge in PDT is the targeted collection of photosensitizers in diseased tissues to avoid off-target ROS production [123]. To enhance targeting precision, photosensitizers can be conjugated with ligands like folic acid, antibodies, or aptamers that targetedly bind to receptors overexpressed on cancer cells or pathogens [124, 125]. Nanoparticle carriers, including liposomes and micelles, further increase the bioavailability and provide controlled target area for a release [126]. Stimuli-responsive delivery systems, which activate photosensitizers under specific conditions (e.g., acidic pH or enzyme presence characteristic of tumor environments), have also been shown to significantly improve PDT precision by restricting their activation to diseased tissues [127, 128]. Dual-targeting strategies that use two ligands to bind distinct receptors on target cells add an extra level of specificity. By recognizing multiple cell surface markers, these dual-targeted photosensitizers reduce non-specific accumulation and enhance the therapeutic index for complex conditions, such as cancer [129]. Recent studies have highlighted these advancements. For instance, [130] developed a series of iridium (III) complexes, with IrC8 demonstrating high potential for image-guided PDT by enabling dual-photon emissions and increased phototoxicity. Similarly, [131] created a COF-based nanosatellite designed for tumor-targeted chemoimmunotherapy. This system, coated with mannose-modified gold nanoparticles and doxorubicin, promotes immunogenic cell death and antigen exposure, allowing targeted delivery and sustained immune activation, which suppresses tumor growth and metastasis. Another innovative approach by [132] aimed to address tumor hypoxia by incorporating perfluorohexane into TPASIC-PFH@PLGA nanoparticles. By reversing hypoxic conditions, these nanoparticles enhance phototherapeutic effectiveness and improve antitumor outcomes. Zheng et al. [133] explored calreticulin (CALR)-targeted therapies for cancer by developing a nanobody that binds to the immunogenic cell death marker calreticulin. When combined with indocyanine green, this CALR-targeting nanobody enables near-infrared imaging-guided photothermal therapy. This strategy modulates the tumor microenvironment and boosts antitumor immunity by inhibiting the CD47-SIRPα pathway, thereby enhancing safety and treatment precision. Overall, these advanced targeting strategies enable more precise localization, allow dose reduction, minimize side effects, and increase the therapeutic safety of PDT.

3.2.3 Theranostic Potential and Real-Time Monitoring in PDT

The theranostic capabilities of photoluminescent emitters in PDT provide both therapeutic and diagnostic benefits, enabling real-time imaging along with targeted treatment [134]. These emitters allow clinicians to track photosensitizer distribution in diseased tissues and confirm precise localization prior to light activation, reducing unintended ROS exposure in healthy areas [80, 135]. Continuous visualization during therapy further enables adaptive dosing adjustments and optimizes treatment efficacy in real-time [136]. Post-treatment imaging offers valuable insights into therapeutic success and disease progression, which are critical in managing cancer, and real-time response data can guide subsequent treatments and improve patient outcomes [137, 138]. This combination of diagnostic feedback and treatment precision marks the photoluminescent-enhanced PDT as a significant advancement in precision medicine. Recent progress in photoluminescent materials has further refined PDT's accuracy, efficiency, and safety of PDT for various applications, including oncology and antimicrobial therapy. For example, Fan et al. [139] stated a versatile nanoplatform for cancer therapy was developed by combining aPD-L1 with gadolinium-doped near-infrared carbon dots. This platform amplifies immunogenic cell death and enhances the efficacy of immune checkpoint blockade therapy Additionally, Kim et al. [140] improved coumarin-based fluorescent probes by integrating a protonatable lysosome-targeting group with bovine serum albumin nanoparticles, which enhanced ROS production, induced lysosomal dysfunction, and promoted cancer cell apoptosis. Other innovative approaches include that of Xu et al. [141], who developed a water-soluble molecule (DTPAP-TBZ-I@BSA) for self-reporting PDT, achieving an 84% tumor inhibition rate in vivo through enhanced fluorescence and ROS generation. Shi et al. [142] synthesized a mitochondria-targeted photosensitizer, TSPy-SS-P, capable of selective hydrogen sulfide (H_2S) detection and efficient tumor ablation via both type I and type II PDT. Feng et al. [143] created a mitochondria-specific photosensitizer, TPA-NH_2-B, utilizing peroxynitrite (ONOO–) as a recognition group, which showed increased ROS production and improved electron transfer efficiency, effectively suppressing tumor growth. Despite ongoing challenges in biocompatibility and targeted delivery, advances in material science, nanotechnology, and biomedical engineering continue to propel PDT toward safer, more effective, and personalized clinical applications.

3.3 *Stimuli-Responsive Release (e.g. pH, Redox)*

Drugs and bioactive materials can be controlled and precisely released at specified site. Stimuli-responsive drug delivery systems achieve controlled release of bioactive materials by responding to specific environmental cues. This method improves treatment efficacy and real-time diagnostic monitoring, making it particularly useful for targeted drug administration using photoluminescent emitters. Several examples of stimuli, such as pH and redox triggers employed in these systems are presented in this section.

3.3.1 pH-Responsive Release

pH-responsive drug delivery systems exploit acidic cellular environments, characteristic of tumors, to improve therapeutic outcomes and reduce systemic side effects [144]. These systems rely on pH-sensitive polymers that undergo changes in solubility, conformation, surface activity, and hydrophilicity owing to their self-assembling properties when exposed to specific pH levels. These polymers are suitable for delivering diverse biomolecules, ranging from small molecules to antibodies. Tewari et al. [145], enabling targeted delivery across diverse physiological pH ranges from the acidic nucleus to the alkaline cytoplasm and from highly acidic stomach juices to mildly alkaline plasma [146]. Considering the patient's physiological and pathological conditions, non-invasive drug delivery routes such as the oral, ocular, nasal, pulmonary, transdermal, and rectal pathways are being explored for the administration of small molecules, monoclonal antibodies, and recombinant proteins. Singh and Nayak highlighted that these polymers can be fabricated into various structures, including metallic nanoparticles, liposomes, dendrimers, and micelles, which serve as drug reservoirs for controlled and sustained release [147]. Another innovative approach involves nanoconjugates incorporating β-cyclodextrin, quantum dots, and folic acid as targeting agents for pH-dependent drug release, offering enhanced selectivity for cancer cells over healthy cells [148]. Several pH-responsive systems have been developed, including.

- **Micelles**: pH-sensitive polymeric micelles have shown promise as cancer treatment medication delivery vehicles. In acidic tumor settings, these micelles could encapsulate hydrophobic medications and release them. pH-responsive micelles with adjustable drug release profiles have been made using a variety of polymers, including mPEG-pH-PCL and PEG-b-PVP [149, 150]. Hyaluronic acid-modified polyhistidine (HA-PHis) and folic acid-modified Pluronic (PF127-FA), characterized by $1H$ NMR, were utilized to construct HPPF micelles. The optimal mixing ratio of HA-PHis to PF127-FA was determined to be 8:2, based on variations in particle size and zeta potential. Compared to HA-PHis and PF127-FA individually, HPPF micelles exhibited enhanced stability due to their higher zeta potential and lower critical micelle concentration. The micelles demonstrated pH sensitivity, as drug release significantly increased from 45 to 90% with a decrease in pH, attributed to the protonation of PHis [151]. Furthermore, fatty acid-grafted chitosan-based micelles show sensitivity to both pH and temperature, enabling extended drug circulation and targeted tumor growth [152].
- **Hydrogels**: Vegad et al. and Wu et al. stated that the recent studies have focused on pH-responsive hydrogels for controlled drug delivery. These hydrogels, capable of swelling or shrinking in response to pH changes, allow for site-specific drug release. The pH-responsive qualities of several non-cellulosic biopolymers, including chitosan and alginate, have been investigated and following Fickian diffusion, a dual-cross-linked PEI/PVA hydrogel showed enhanced drug release in acidic environments [153, 154].

3.3.2 Mechanism of pH Sensitivity

Photosensitizers for drug delivery exploit pH gradients between healthy and diseased tissues. Designed for stability at physiological pH, these agents undergo structural changes in response to pH shifts, enabling controlled drug release. This pH-sensitive mechanism enhances therapeutic precision by minimizing off-target effects and improving drug efficacy. Various types of drug delivery systems are pH sensitive, with different mechanisms, these include:

- **Polymer-Based Systems**: Singh and Nayak reported that systems based on polymers have shown great promise as a vehicle for drug delivery because they provide tailored and responsive release mechanisms. When the pH of the environment varies, pH-responsive polymers, such as poly (β-amino esters) and poly (acrylic acid), can change their characteristics, allowing for regulated medication release under physiological situations [147]. Additionally, engineered polymer structures like nanoparticles, liposomes, dendrimers, and micelles serve as promising drug reservoirs for controlled release. Key challenges in this field include material selection, efficient drug loading, stability, consistent data generation, and regulatory approval. Hydrogels, with their high-water content and responsiveness to stimuli like pH and temperature, are particularly promising for controlled drug delivery [147, 155].
- **Hydrophobic-Hydrophilic Transitions**: Leng et al. reported that pH-sensitive materials have been investigated recently for targeted medication administration, especially in treating cancer. In acidic medium, these materials change from hydrophobic to hydrophilic, allowing for the regulated drug sustained release. Numerous strategies have been studied, including the protonation of polymeric nanoparticles, pH-sensitive connections between carriers and pharmaceuticals, and the release of polymers that shield drug-loaded nanoparticles [156]. More than 60% of drugs in developed by pharmaceutical sector recorded a decrease in therapeutic efficacy, and this problem is associated with hydrophobicity resulting to poor availability. There is a method used to show a significant and continuous number of released payloads while permitting their controlled release under favourable conditions. This approach utilizes polymer nanofibers conjugated with solubilizers via responsive linkages to encapsulate payloads. Thioether ester linkages within these fibers degrade in mildly acidic conditions, releasing hydrotropes and kosmotropes, which in turn triggers the release of model payloads, such as drugs and dyes [157].
- **Protonation of Functional Groups**: A recent study explored the use of functionalized nanoparticles and smart nanogels for targeted cancer drug delivery. These systems leverage pH-responsive release mechanisms, incorporating functional groups like amines and carboxylic acids [158, 159]. Carbon nanotubes functionalized with folic acid have been investigated as pH-controlled fluorouracil carriers, showing improved drug release in low pH conditions [160]. The pH sensitivity and biodegradability of polyacrylic acid (PAA) have made it a useful polymer for directed drug delivery systems [161].

3.3.3 Applications of pH Responsive Material in Drug Delivery with Photoluminescent Emitters in Diagnostics and Cancer Therapy

The Warburg effect leads tumor cells to produce lactate and hydrogen ions (H+), resulting in an acidic tumor microenvironment (TME) that can be exploited for customized tumor therapy. pH-responsive nanocarriers have recently gained much attention in nanotechnology because of their advancements. They show controlled release profiles of therapeutic reagents and targeted accumulation within tumor locations under acidic tumor settings, allowing for precision tumor therapy as reported by Bhattacharya et al. and Chen et al. [162, 163]. Since less than 1% of systemically administered nanoparticles build up in tumors, several innovative strategies have been developed to target and administer the treatment in or close to tumors. One such strategy relies on the tumor's endosomes and extracellular matrix having an acidic pH. Greater specificity is made possible by the extracellular tumor matrix's gradient, which has an average pH of 6.8, which allows pH-responsive particles to aggregate. Nanoparticles undergo additional exposure to lower pHs after being taken up by tumor cells; in late endosomes, their pH reaches 5. Macromolecular drug delivery systems have utilized pH-sensitive targeting for efficient chemotherapy and combined chemo-nucleic acid therapies like keratin protein or polymeric nanoparticles, leveraging the acidic conditions present in tumors [156]. In diagnostics, stimuli-responsive polymers coupled with photluminiscent emmiter hold promise for the regulated release of therapeutic and diagnostic chemicals, enhanced stability during circulation, and targeted administration [164]. The diverse pH environments within the body, including bodily fluids and cellular organelles, and the pH fluctuations observed in various diseases, have driven the development of pH-responsive polymeric nanocarriers. For instance, the tumor's acidic extracellular environment can be used to promote targeted delivery.

Given that most nanocarriers are internalized through endocytosis, leading to a pH reduction from 6.5 in the endosome to 5.0 in the lysosome, pH-sensitive groups have been designed to enhance cargo release during cellular uptake [164]. Although swarming magnetic micro/nanorobots show promise in healthcare, but their chemical sensing capabilities within local microenvironments are currently limited. This study introduces swarming magnetic photonic crystal microrobots (PC-bots) that can detect pH changes, autonomously control drug release, and provide real-time visual pH feedback. These PC-bots comprise pH-responsive hydrogel microspheres encapsulating 1D periodic arrays of Fe_3O_4 nanoparticles [165].

3.3.4 Redox-Responsive Release

Glutathione (GSH) gradient-based redox-responsive drug delivery devices have been studied recently for targeted cancer treatment. Selective drug release are used by researchers for creating nanocarriers that react to increased GSH levels in tumor cells [166, 167]. Chemotherapy and photodynamic therapy were combined to create a biodegradable covalent organic framework that would release 5-fluorouracil in response to GSH, resulting in a synergistic tumor treatment [167]. Figure 4 shows the stimuli initiate the release of drugs. Furthermore, Sastre et al. reported that the pancreatic redox homeostasis is crucial for normal function and is maintained by various regulatory systems [168]. The study further highlighted that an imbalance in this system results in oxidative stress, a critical component influencing progress of various pancreatic diseases. Additionally, it revealed that chronic pancreatitis is associated with oxidative damage driven by NADPH oxidase and CYP2E1, which contributes to fibrosis and inflammation [169]. Pancreatic cancer development is driven by oxidative stress induced by mutant KRAS, which promotes cell proliferation and transformation. In diabetes, oxidative stress contributes to β-cell dysfunction and apoptosis [170, 171]. Understanding the role of redox signaling in these diseases may provide novel therapeutic targets.

In a novel study, Ji et al. developed disulfide bond-bridged prodrug self-assembled nanoparticles (DSSS NPs) to target and treat ALI because acute lung injury (ALI) is a serious condition caused by excessive inflammation, often progressing to acute respiratory distress syndrome (ARDS). Current therapeutic options for acute lung injury (ALI) remain limited. DSSS nanoparticles, formulated from dexamethasone (Dex) and stearic acid (SA), exhibited a remarkably high drug loading capacity (37.75% Dex), far exceeding that of traditional nanomedicines (typically less than 10%). These nanoparticles enabled targeted drug release in inflamed lung tissues and responsive release within the inflammatory microenvironment. In a mouse model of LPS-induced ALI, DSSS NPs effectively reduced pro-inflammatory cytokines and

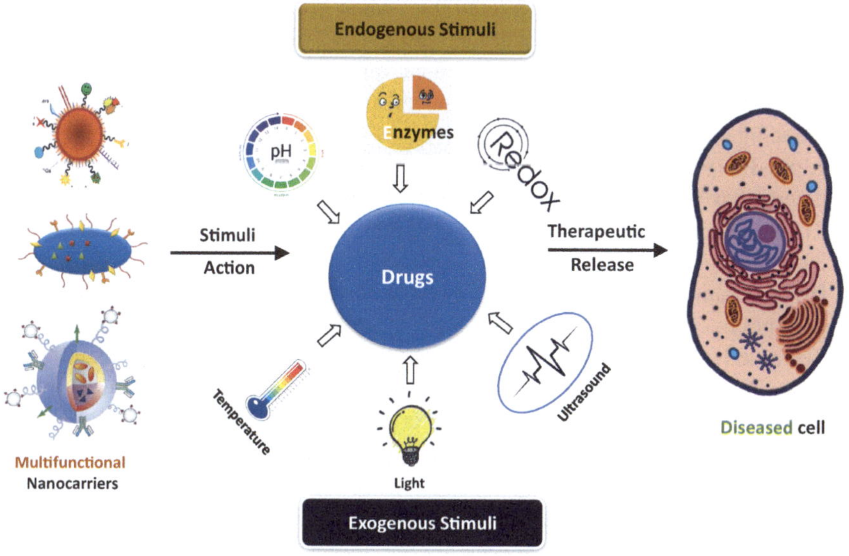

Fig. 4 The release of drugs in response to stimuli

mitigated tissue damage. These findings indicate that DSSS NPs hold significant promise as a therapeutic approach for ALI [172].

3.3.5 Other Stimuli-Responsive Mechanisms

Although redox and pH stimuli are the most employed, photoluminescent drug delivery systems can also incorporate other stimuli for improved control and diagnostic potential.

- **Temperature-Responsive Systems**: Poly(N-isopropylacrylamide) (PNIPAAm)-based temperature-responsive drug delivery systems have received a lot of attention because of their capacity to release medicines in reaction to temperature changes. With a lower critical solution temperature (LCST) of roughly 32 °C, which is similar to physiological temperature, PNIPAAm is suited for biomedical applications. PNIPAAm-based nanocarriers and hydrogels provide for controlled and prolonged medication release by reducing fast drug release and increasing delivery efficiency. Moreover, multi-stimuli-responsive drug delivery vehicles can be created by combining these temperature-responsive systems with pH-responsive components [173, 174].
- **Enzyme-Responsive Systems**: Guo et al. and Zhang et al. said that targeted cancer therapy has shown promise using enzyme-responsive drug delivery systems, especially those that target matrix metalloproteinases (MMPs). Numerous tumor micro-environments overexpress MMPs, particularly MMP-2, which are essential for tumor growth and metastasis [175, 176]. While the studies by the groups of Wei and Zong also demonstrated that, when liposomes or other nanocarriers encounter high MMP levels in tumor tissues, they can react to enzymes and release their payload. By providing better medication targeting, increased tumor penetration, and controlled release, these devices may boost therapeutic efficacy while reducing adverse effects [177, 178].
- **Light-Responsive Systems**: Particularly in treating cancer, light-responsive devices have shown great promise as instruments for targeted medication delivery. These devices use a range of light wavelengths, such as visible, ultraviolet, and near-infrared, to initiate the controlled release of medicinal substances [61]. Commonly used as light-responsive drug delivery vehicles, liposomes, and polymer-based nanocarriers provide improved therapeutic efficacy and decreased systemic toxicity [61, 179]. Additionally, novel technologies utilizing aggregation-induced emission (AIE) and excited-state intramolecular proton transfer (ESIPT) were studied for the creation of light-activated drug delivery devices and bioactive molecule donors [76].

4 In Vivo Imaging and Tracking of Drug Carriers

Using light-emitting markers to track drug carriers in living organisms has revolutionized drug delivery research, providing insights into how drugs are distributed, released, and targeted to specific regions within the body. Materials that emit light, such as near-infrared (NIR) dyes, quantum dots, and upconversion nanoparticles (UCNPs), are commonly employed due to their stable and intense signals, with the ability to emit in the NIR spectrum, which is optimal for tissue penetration and clear signal detection. NIR imaging enables deep tissue visualization with reduced background fluorescence, crucial for tracking drug carriers (liposomes, nanoparticles, micelles). These carriers are labeled with luminescent markers and monitored in vivo using techniques like fluorescence microscopy, PET, or photoacoustic imaging, allowing researchers to observe their distribution and drug release within the body. The intensity and positioning of the signals enable real-time tracking of carrier movement and assessment of their distribution and transit within the body.

Quantum dots and NIR dyes are popular choices for tracking because of their adjustable light properties and strong NIR emission. UCNPs, which contain rare-earth elements like ytterbium and erbium, offer an alternative approach by converting lower-energy NIR light into visible light, allowing tracking with less energy and reducing potential damage. The main benefit of using these light-emitting markers in drug carrier tracking is that they are non-invasive, enabling continuous observation without harming the subject. This feature is essential for refining drug formulations and delivery strategies on the go, supporting personalized medicine by enabling precise control over where and how much drug is delivered. Additionally, tracking with photoluminescent markers helps evaluate the effectiveness and safety of new drug delivery systems, leading to quicker and more dependable preclinical testing.

4.1 In Vivo Imaging

Luminescence imaging has become an essential tool in biomedical research, offering valuable insights into the structure of diseased tissues, signaling pathways, and cellular interactions. It is increasingly being adopted for diagnostic purposes and image-guided surgery. Imaging in the near-infrared (NIR) range (700–1,700 nm) is particularly advantageous as NIR light interacts less with tissue through scattering and absorption compared to visible light, enabling deeper penetration and reduced interference from natural body fluorescence, which enhances image clarity and contrast. Although preclinical studies have shown promising results, only a limited number of NIR fluorophores have been approved for clinical use. This review explores the main engineering challenges that must be overcome for NIR luminescence imaging to become a widespread clinical tool, including improving probe designs to enhance imaging contrast, reducing natural tissue fluorescence, and increasing the probes' ability to target specific areas in the body. Chen et al. presented research on NIR luminescence for high-contrast in vivo biomedical imaging [180]. NIR fluorophores offer distinct advantages over conventional dyes emitting at shorter wavelengths. As a result, NIR fluorophores are widely used in fluorescence and photoacoustic imaging, as well as photodynamic and photothermal therapies. However, non-targeted NIR fluorescence-emitting organic molecules lack specificity for tumors, potentially causing harm to healthy tissues and leading to significant side effects. Therefore, developing NIR fluorophore-based compounds that specifically target tumors has become a key focus in medicinal chemistry. Recent efforts have led to the development of various tumor-targeted NIR fluorophore-based imaging and therapeutic agents. This review highlights research conducted between 2012 and 2021, particularly focusing on studies involving cancer-selective strategies for designing small organic dye-based NIR imaging and therapeutic agents [181].

Saeboe et al. [182] studies introduced highly red-emitting InP QDs with tunable near-infrared (NIR) photoluminescence (PL) and multiplexing capabilities within the first optical tissue window, synthesized without harmful substances. By employing an inverted ZnSe/InP/ZnS core/shell/shell heterostructure, we overcome the 'growth bottleneck' in InP QD synthesis and shift their emission deeper into the NIR. The InP shell thickness controls the emission peak, ranging from 515 to 845 nm. The high absorptivity of InP enables efficient excitation across UV, visible, and NIR wavelengths. These QDs expand the tunable emission range of InP-based nanostructures, addressing a key synthetic limitation for NIR imaging applications. We demonstrate the potential of these NIR-emitting InP particles for in vivo imaging through multiplexed lymph node imaging in a mouse model. Figure 5 illustrates a typical example and images of photoluminescent emitters for in vivo imaging.

Ren et al. [185] demonstrates the potential of SWIR-emitting probes to monitor the efficacy of a polymer-coated NaErF4/NaYF4 nanoparticle-based cancer vaccine in vivo. By imaging vaccine distribution and immune cell infiltration in mice, they observed rapid lymphatic drainage and subsequent tumor regression. The presence of antigen-specific CD8 + T cells within the tumor microenvironment, visualized using NIR-emitting probes and light-sheet microscopy, correlated with successful tumor eradication. These findings highlight the value of infrared imaging for optimizing nanoparticle-based cancer immunotherapy. Swamy et al. [186] investigated biocompatible, water-soluble cyanine dyes emitting in the short-wave infrared (SWIR) region for in vivo multiplexed molecular imaging. By leveraging the advantages of SWIR imaging, including deeper tissue penetration and reduced autofluorescence, the study developed ICG-based dyes (ICG-C9 and ICG-C11) with emission wavelengths of 922 nm and 1010 nm. These dyes were successfully applied for three-color SWIR fluorescence imaging of breast tumors in live mice, targeting surface receptors and blood vessels. Furthermore, two-color imaging was utilized to monitor tumor cell death using ICG-conjugated Kadcyla and annexin V-linked dyes. Long-term imaging over 38 days demonstrated tumor shrinkage, highlighting the potential of SWIR-emitting cyanine probes for in vivo molecular imaging applications.

Zhong et al. [184] worked on in vivo deep brain multiphoton fluorescence imaging that spanned the NIR-I, NIR-II, and NIR-IV optical windows. This approach utilized

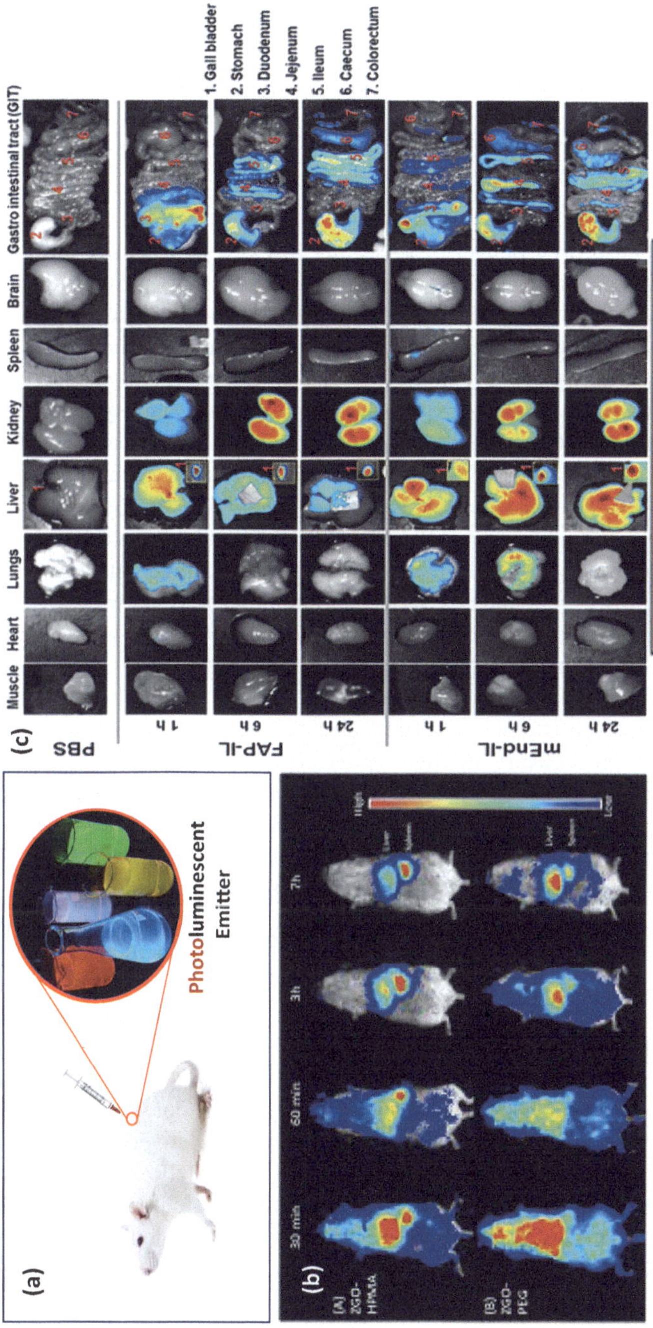

Fig. 5 Showing the application of photoresponsive emitters in in vivo imaging **a**: Injecting Wistar rat with Photoresponive emitters; **b**: In vivo biodistribution of coated ZGO-HPMA and ZGO-PEG in in healthy mice [183] and **c**: Representative scaled NIRF images of mouse organs illustrating the distribution of liposomal fluorescence at various time intervals after injection [184]

ICG as a label to enable deep brain imaging using a custom-built multiphoton microscope. The study demonstrated the ability to image deep into the mouse brain at depths of 950 μm (NIR-I) and 850 μm (NIR-II), verifying the promise of multi-optical window multiphoton microscopy (MPM) for deep brain imaging.

4.2 Tracking of Drug Carriers

The biggest challenge in drug delivery for treating diseases is primarily the low bioavailability of the molecules involved. However, nanotechnology provides a way to overcome these issues by using various approaches. Adding fluorescent probes to nanosystems can be a helpful strategy to track the paths taken by nanocarriers in the body and enhance targeting precision. Using fluorescence to label nanocarrier surfaces or encapsulating fluorophore molecules transforms these nanosystems into light probes that are valuable in diagnostics and theranostics. Moreover, photoluminescent (PL) metal nanoclusters (NCs) have gained substantial attention owing to their remarkable physical and chemical characteristics, high biocompatibility, and vast range of potential applications [187]. In addition, sustained-release carriers exhibiting strong luminescence hold great potential for integrating imaging with the delivery of bioactive compounds. A variety of luminescent systems have been reported in the literature, such as metal nanoclusters, nanoparticles, luminescent polymers [188], and nanoemulsions [189, 190].

Lai et al. present a gel-forming clusteroluminogenic polymer with adjustable emission properties that functions as a sustained-release carrier, allowing for real-time tracking during the delivery of bioactive agents [188]. They describe the synthesis and characteristics of CT, a highly tunable, non-conjugated polymer with inherent luminescence. The emission of CT can be fine-tuned based on the excitation wavelength, enabling optical imaging across a wide range of wavelengths. This study marks the first proof-of-concept to successfully integrate clusterization-triggered emission into carrier design, merging imaging capabilities with bioactive agent delivery. In the context of cancer treatment, their findings demonstrate that CT not only enhances the in vivo antitumor effectiveness but also facilitates real-time tracking of its location and gelation through intrinsic blue fluorescence. With its excellent biocompatibility, CT holds substantial promise for self-illuminating therapies aimed at cancer treatment.

Ding et al. explored X-ray-activated dual near-infrared and short-wave infrared persistent luminescence imaging for prolonged tracking of drug delivery [191]. Both short-wave infrared (SWIR: 900–1700 nm) and near-infrared (NIR: 650–900 nm) luminescence offer reduced optical scattering and improved signal-to-noise ratios in deep tissues, which makes them increasingly valuable in biomedicine. In this study, they developed mesoporous silica-coated Yb-doped magnesium germanate nanoparticles (mMGOs) that demonstrate exceptional dual NIR and SWIR persistent luminescence upon X-ray irradiation by adjusting the valence of rare-earth ions. These nanoparticles also feature high cargo capacity and controlled release in tumor regions. Both in vitro and in vivo experiments revealed that mMGOs can be reactivated multiple times for rechargeable persistent luminescence imaging, enabling effective monitoring of cargo delivery in mice. Additionally, the drug release profile led to significant tumor growth inhibition. The X-ray-excited dual NIR and SWIR persistent luminescence imaging not only facilitated rechargeable imaging of deep tumors but also enabled long-term tracking with notable tumor suppression.

Rahal et al. describe the preparation of carbon quantum dots via a one-step microwave-assisted synthesis for detecting the antibiotic Minocycline [192]. A linear correlation was established between the photoluminescence quenching of CQDs and Minocycline concentrations ranging from 0.28 to 30.39 μM. UV–vis and PL spectroscopy revealed that the photoluminescence reduction was due to the inner filter effect. Selectivity studies were conducted to evaluate the impact of various compounds on Minocycline detection. Additionally, Minocycline was loaded onto chitosan-grafted-oligomeric lactic acid microspheres as a drug carrier. CQDs were utilized to assess the loading capacity, encapsulation efficiency, and cumulative drug release of the Minocycline-loaded microspheres. The optimal samples demonstrated a loading capacity of 14.1–26.344% and encapsulation efficiency of 34.48–64.37%. The CHS-g-OLA2 sample showed reduced burst release, with 50% cumulative drug release occurring within four days. Mathematical modeling suggested that the CHS-g-OLA2 sample followed the Higuchi kinetic model for drug release from a swellable matrix via diffusion.

Nisar et al. developed a photoinduced electron transfer-based glutathione-sensing theranostic nanoprodrug for real-time drug release monitoring and cancer treatment [193]. The glutathione-responsive nanoprodrug, featuring a high drug-loading content of 59.4 wt% and an average size of 46 nm, consists of the anticancer drug paclitaxel linked to a fluorescent imaging probe with a high fluorescence quantum yield. The fluorescence allows for efficient self-tracking and sensitive glutathione sensing. In the presence of high glutathione levels in cancer cells, the disulphide bond is cleaved, releasing the drug and fluorescence-off imaging probe. This change in fluorescence enables the drug release process to be monitored. The nanoprodrugs exhibited high cytotoxicity against various cancer cells, especially A549 and HEK-293 cells, showing superior therapeutic effects compared to free paclitaxel, offering a new strategy for precision cancer therapy.

Wang et al. [194] synthesized near-infrared-emitting persistent luminescence nanoparticles loaded in mesoporous silica nanoparticles (mZGC), with macrophages as cellular carriers to enhance the targeted delivery of theranostic agents to tumor sites. This system improves the signal-to-noise ratio by reducing interference from short-lived autofluorescence during in situ excitation, and using macrophages as carriers significantly boosts targeting efficiency in cancer treatment. Additionally, the photothermal properties of ICG@mZGC were assessed, demonstrating excellent photothermal performance with a photothermal conversion efficiency of 23.29%.

In a study focusing on water-soluble photoluminescent (PL) metal nanoclusters (NCs), Qiao et al. [187] developed ultrabright and stable PL Au/Ag nanoclusters for efficient drug delivery to cancer cells, achieving a PL quantum yield (QY) of 73% and exceptional photostability through heteroatom doping and surface rigidization.

These Au/Ag NCs maintain over 61% QY across varying pH levels and ionic conditions, showing substantial resistance to photobleaching. Spectroscopic analyses, both steady-state and time-resolved, reveal that silver doping enhances the photostability and electronic structure of the Au/Ag NCs, resulting in an improved PL QY. In vitro studies demonstrate that the Au/Ag NCs have high drug-loading capacity and pH-triggered release capability for doxorubicin (DOX), which can be tracked via PL intensity and lifetime changes. Imaging-guided experiments in cancer cells show efficient delivery and release of DOX in the nucleus, with preferential accumulation in the nucleolus. In vivo tests reveal a tumor suppression rate of 90.2% in mice, highlighting Au/Ag NCs as an efficient mechanism for bioimaging and visual medication delivery in biomedical settings.

5 Challenges and Future Directions

5.1 Challenges

While light-triggered drug release mechanisms offer enhanced precision, control, and therapeutic potential, ongoing research focuses on overcoming current challenges and exploring innovative strategies to fully realize their clinical applications These are:

- **Light Penetration**: Deep tissue penetration of light remains a challenge, limiting the applicability of light-triggered systems in certain clinical settings. This limited penetration could be due to 3 main factors: (i) Limited Reach: Even with longer wavelengths, the depth of light penetration is still relatively shallow, often reaching only a few millimeters. This limits the ability to target deeper tissues or organs. (ii) Scattering Effects: As light travels through tissue, it undergoes scattering, which can further reduce its intensity and directionality. This makes it difficult to precisely deliver light to specific target areas. (iii) Tissue Heterogeneity: Different tissues have varying optical properties, which can further complicate light penetration. For example, highly pigmented organs like the liver or skin rich in melanin can absorb more light, reducing penetration.
- **Light Source Development**: Developing efficient and safe light sources for clinical use is an ongoing area of research. This involves several key areas of focus which include Developing light sources that consume less energy, reducing operational costs and environmental impact, and maximizing the amount of visible light produced per unit of energy input, ensuring optimal illumination with minimal energy waste. Ensuring that the light sources operate within safe limits to prevent damage to the eyes, particularly during prolonged exposure. Avoid the emission of harmful radiation or substances that could potentially harm patients or medical staff. Designing light sources that dissipate Heat proficiently to avoid scorching and ensure peak efficiency.

- **Phototoxicity**: Phototoxicity refers to the harmful effects caused by the interaction of light with certain substances, leading to cellular damage and tissue injury. Careful consideration must be given to the potential phototoxic effects of light and photosensitive agents. phototoxicity can arise from two main sources.
- **Light Source**: The wavelength of light used to activate the drug release mechanism plays a significant role in phototoxicity. Shorter wavelengths, such as UV light, are more energetic and have a higher potential for causing cellular damage. Longer wavelengths, like near-infrared (NIR) light, are generally considered safer because they have lower energy and deeper penetration into tissue. The intensity of light exposure is another critical factor. Excessive light exposure can lead to phototoxic reactions, even with longer wavelengths. Therefore, precisely regulating light exposure is crucial to minimizing the risk of phototoxicity. (ii) Photosensitive Agents: Photosensitizers are chemicals that absorb light energy and move it to oxygen molecules, generating reactive oxygen species (ROS). While ROS are essential for certain biological processes, excessive ROS production can damage cellular components, leading to cell death eventually phototoxicity. In addition some drugs themselves may be photosensitive, meaning they can undergo photochemical reactions upon light exposure, generating toxic byproducts.
- **Complex Delivery Systems**: Light-triggered medication delivery devices provide a precise and non-invasive way to control drug release. These devices use light to offer tailored therapy while minimizing negative effects. However, designing complex light-triggered systems that integrate multiple functionalities and respond to various stimuli presents significant challenges. Designing complex light-triggered systems that integrate multiple functionalities and respond to various stimuli is a significant challenge. (i) Precise Light Control: Ensuring light delivery to precise target areas throughout the body may prove difficult, especially for deep-tissue applications. The precise timing of light exposure is crucial to regulate drug release kinetics. The intensity of light must be carefully controlled to avoid unintended side effects and ensure optimal drug release. (ii) Multifunctional Integration: Integrating multiple therapeutic agents into a single delivery system requires careful design to prevent interactions and ensure simultaneous or sequential release. Additionally, integrating diagnostic and therapeutic capabilities into a single platform enables continuous tracking of drug distribution and treatment efficacy. (iii) Stimuli-Responsive Materials: Developing materials that react to various stimuli, including light, pH, temperature, or redox potential, enables precise regulation of drug release within intricate biological settings. The materials used in light-triggered systems must be biocompatible and biodegradable to minimize adverse effects.

5.2 *Future Directions*

The Ongoing research on light-triggered drug delivery aims to improve the following key challenges.

- **Light Penetration**: The system of light-triggered drug delivery has a future that lies in developing devices that can deliver drugs to deeper tissues with greater precision and control. Improving light penetration in light-triggered drug delivery systems is a key area of research such as NIR light penetrates deeper tissues than visible or UV light. Developing systems that respond to NIR light would allow for more precise drug delivery to deeper tissues. Upconversion nanoparticles transform lower-energy NIR light to higher-energy visible light, allowing for deeper tissue invasion while retaining light-sensitive drug carriers. Photoacoustic imaging techniques can monitor light penetration and drug release in real-time, allowing for treatment optimization. Combining light-triggered drug delivery with other modalities, such as ultrasound or magnetic fields, could further enhance tissue penetration and drug release.
- **Light Source Development**: Investigating novel light source technologies, especially organic light-emitting diodes (OLEDs) and quantum dot light-emitting diodes (QLEDs), for possible clinical purposes. Developing adaptive lighting systems that can adjust the light output based on the specific needs of the patient and the clinical procedure to produce personalized lighting. Combining light sources with other medical technologies, such as imaging systems and robotic devices, to create integrated solutions for advanced clinical applications.
- **Phototoxicity**: To mitigate phototoxicity in light-triggered drug delivery systems, researchers and clinicians must consider the following: Prioritize longer wavelengths like NIR light, which has lower energy and deeper tissue penetration, and optimize light intensity and exposure duration to minimize potential harm. Select photosensitizers with high selectivity for target tissues and minimal off-target effects and consider the potential for generating ROS and their impact on surrounding tissues. Develop formulations that minimize the release of photosensitive drugs in the absence of light and incorporate protective agents or antioxidants to scavenge excess ROS. Rigorous preclinical studies to assess phototoxicity potential, and careful monitoring of patients during clinical trials to identify and manage any adverse effects.
- **Innovative Light-Triggered Therapeutics**: These include (i) Advanced light delivery systems with unique properties such as precise targeting, deep tissue penetration, spatial and temporal control e.g. fiber optics, upconversion particles. (ii) Multifunctional nanomaterials with distinctive qualities include light responsiveness, drug absorption capacity, directed administration, and regulated discharge. e.g. polymer-based system, lipid-based system, and inorganic particles. (iii) Stimuli-Responsive Hydrogels with the unique properties of light sensitivity, drug encapsulation, controlled release, biocompatibility and biodegradability e.g. light sensitive hydrogels, multi-stimuli response hydrogels.

6 Conclusion

Integrating light-emitting materials into drug delivery systems has revolutionized modern medicine, offering dual benefits in diagnosis and treatment. These systems connect design strategies, material choices, and drug behavior to improve precision and effectiveness. Materials like quantum dots, carbon dots, and rare-earth-doped nanoparticles enable non-invasive imaging, real-time tracking, and targeted delivery through passive and active mechanisms. Functional modifications, such as molecule attachment or PEG coating, enhance targeting accuracy, biocompatibility, and circulation time while reducing toxicity. Advances in drug encapsulation have improved loading capacity, stability, and release mechanisms responsive to conditions like pH, redox states, and temperature. Light-triggered release and photodynamic therapy offer precise spatial and temporal control, further enhancing treatment outcomes. Theranostics, which combines therapy and diagnosis in a single system, is particularly transformational since it allows for simultaneous treatment and monitoring. However, challenges such as improving stability, extending shelf life, and ensuring scalability must be overcome for clinical applications.

Despite obstacles like production scalability and regulatory hurdles, light-emitting material-based drug delivery represents a significant leap in precision medicine, offering personalized treatment strategies, real-time feedback, and reduced side effects.

References

1. Zhao, K., Zeng, Z., He, Y., Zhao, R., Niu, J., Sun, H., et al.: Recent advances in targeted therapy for inflammatory vascular diseases. J. Control. Release **372**, 730–50 (2024). https://doi.org/10.1016/j.jconrel.2024.06.063
2. Fang, X., Wang, X., Ding, B.: Applications of luminescent metal-organic frameworks as pioneering biosensors for biological and chemical detection. Chin. Chem. Lett., 110453, (2024). https://doi.org/10.1016/j.cclet.2024.110453
3. Dhoundiyal, S., Srivastava, S., Kumar, S., Singh, G., Ashique, S., Pal, R., et al.: Radiopharmaceuticals: navigating the frontier of precision medicine and therapeutic innovation. Eur. J. Med. Res. **29**, 26 (2024). https://doi.org/10.1186/s40001-023-01627-0
4. Liu, M., Liang, J., Vetrone, F.: Toward accurate photoluminescence nanothermometry using rare-earth doped nanoparticles for biomedical applications. Acc. Chem. Res. **57**, 2653–64 (2024). https://doi.org/10.1021/acs.accounts.4c00342
5. Farshidfar, N., Fooladi, S., Nematollahi, M.H., Iravani, S.: Carbon dots with tissue engineering and regenerative medicine applications. RSC Adv. **13**, 14517–29 (2023). https://doi.org/10.1039/D3RA02336B
6. Al Ragib, A., Al Amin, A., Alanazi, Y.M., Kormoker, T., Uddin, M., Siddique, M.D.A.B., et al.: Multifunctional carbon dots in nanomaterial surface modification: a descriptive review. Carbon Res. **2**, 37 (2023). https://doi.org/10.1007/s44246-023-00069-x
7. Hussain, A., Alajmi, M.F., Ganguly, S.: Pentetic acid derived dual purpose fluorescent carbon dots for pH responsive drug delivery and antioxidant proficiency. Diam. Relat. Mater. **145**, 111101 (2024). https://doi.org/10.1016/j.diamond.2024.111101

8. Parsaeifar, N., Salimi, E., Molaei, M.J.: Preparation and characterization of fluorescent CQDs/45S5 bioactive nanohybrids as bone targeted drug carriers. Ceram Int. **50**, 41315–41326 (2024). https://doi.org/10.1016/j.ceramint.2024.07.443
9. Wibrianto, A., Putri, F.S.D., Nisa, U.K., Mahyahani, N., Sugito, S.F.A., Wardana, A.P., et al.: Strategic assessment of boron-enriched carbon dots/naproxen: diagnostic, toxicity, and in vivo therapeutic evaluation. Mol. Pharm. **21**, 801–12 (2024). https://doi.org/10.1021/acs.molpharmaceut.3c00919
10. de Lara Andrade, J., Gonçalves de Oliveira, A., Augusto Moreira, C., Scanferla, C.E., Lima, S.M., da Cunha Andrade, L.H., et al.: Multifunctional nanoplatforms based on alumina-coated mesoporous silica with potential for cancer theranostics applications. Microporous Mesoporous Mater. **382**, 113373 (2025). https://doi.org/10.1016/j.micromeso.2024.113373
11. Khondakar, K.R., Tripathi, D., Mazumdar, H., Ahuja, K., Kaushik, A.: Tailored MXenes and graphene as efficient telemedicine platforms for personalized health wellness. Mater Adv **5**, 4091–111 (2024). https://doi.org/10.1039/D4MA00234B
12. Agiba, A.M., Elsayyad, N., ElShagea, H.N., Metwalli, M.A., Mahmoudsalehi, A.O., Beigi-Boroujeni, S., et al.: Advances in light-responsive smart multifunctional nanofibers: implications for targeted drug delivery and cancer therapy. Pharmaceutics **16**, 1017 (2024). https://doi.org/10.3390/pharmaceutics16081017
13. Luobin, L., Wanxin, H., Yingxin, G., Qinzhou, Z., Zefeng, L., Danyang, W., et al.: Nanomedicine-induced programmed cell death in cancer therapy: mechanisms and perspectives. Cell Death Discov **10**, 386 (2024). https://doi.org/10.1038/s41420-024-02121-0
14. Das, S., Mazumdar, H., Khondakar, K.R., Kaushik, A.: Machine learning integrated graphene oxide-based diagnostics, drug delivery, analytical approaches to empower cancer diagnosis. BMEMat (2024). https://doi.org/10.1002/bmm2.12117
15. Tong, J., Wang, Z., Zhang, J., Gao, R., Liu, X., Liao, Y., et al.: Advanced applications of nanomaterials in atherosclerosis diagnosis and treatment: Challenges and future prospects. ACS Appl. Mater. Inter. **16**, 58072–99 (2024). https://doi.org/10.1021/acsami.4c13607
16. Kargar, E., Meshkini, A.: Improved photocatalytic disinfection performance of graphitic carbon nitride through hybridization with humic acid /zinc peroxide: A synergistic generation of antimicrobial reactive oxygen species. J Photochem Photobiol A Chem. **452**, 115577 (2024). https://doi.org/10.1016/j.jphotochem.2024.115577
17. Vorotnikov, Y.A., Vorotnikova, N.A., Shestopalov, M.A.: Silica-based materials containing inorganic Red/NIR emitters and their application in biomedicine. Materials **16**, 5869 (2023). https://doi.org/10.3390/ma16175869
18. Li, S., Wei, J., Yao, Q., Song, X., Xie, J., Yang, H.: Emerging ultrasmall luminescent nanoprobes for *in vivo* bioimaging. Chem. Soc. Rev. **52**, 1672–96 (2023). https://doi.org/10.1039/D2CS00497F
19. Abdellatif, A.A., Younis, M.A., Alsharidah, M., Al Rugaie, O., Tawfeek, H.M.: Biomedical applications of quantum dots: Overview, challenges, and clinical potential. Int. J. Nanomedicine **17**, 1951–70 (2022). https://doi.org/10.2147/IJN.S357980
20. Li, Y., Zhang, P., Tang, W., McHugh, K.J., Kershaw, S.V., Jiao, M., et al.: Bright, magnetic NIR-II quantum dot probe for sensitive dual-modality imaging and intensive combination therapy of cancer. ACS Nano **16**, 8076–94 (2022). https://doi.org/10.1021/acsnano.2c01153
21. Yan, H., Wang, Q., Wang, J., Shang, W., Xiong, Z., Zhao, L., et al.: Planted graphene quantum dots for targeted, enhanced tumor imaging and long-term visualization of local pharmacokinetics. Adv. Mater. **35**, (2023). https://doi.org/10.1002/adma.202210809
22. Jiang, G., Ren, T.-B., D'Este, E., Xiong, M., Xiong, B., Johnsson, K., et al.: A synergistic strategy to develop photostable and bright dyes with long Stokes shift for nanoscopy. Nat. Commun. **13**, 2264 (2022). https://doi.org/10.1038/s41467-022-29547-3
23. Remmel, A.: How to keep the lights on: the mission to make more photostable fluorophores. Nature. **630**, 258–60 (2024). https://doi.org/10.1038/d41586-024-01591-7
24. Umezawa, M., Soga, K.: 134 hybrid nanostructures using polymers to reduce the toxicity of inorganic luminescent nanomaterials and organic dyes. Ann Work Expo Health. **67**, i98–i98 (2023). https://doi.org/10.1093/annweh/wxac087.241

25. Guo, W., Chen, M., Yang, Y., Ge, G., Tang, L., He, S., et al.: Biocompatibility and biological effects of surface-modified conjugated polymer nanoparticles. Molecules **28**, 2034 (2023). https://doi.org/10.3390/molecules28052034
26. Nowak-Jary, J., Machnicka, B.: In vivo biodistribution and clearance of magnetic iron oxide nanoparticles for medical applications. Int. J. Nanomedicine **18**, 4067–100 (2023). https://doi.org/10.2147/IJN.S415063
27. Di, J., Du, Z., Wu, K., Jin, S., Wang, X., Li, T., et al.: Biodistribution and non-linear gene expression of mRNA LNPs affected by delivery route and particle size. Pharm. Res. **39**, 105–14 (2022). https://doi.org/10.1007/s11095-022-03166-5
28. Gibbons, A.E., Luker, K.E., Luker, G.D.: Dual reporter bioluminescence imaging with nanoluc and firefly luciferase, pp. 41–50 (2018). https://doi.org/10.1007/978-1-4939-7860-1_4
29. He, J., Zhang, W., Zhou, X., Xu, F., Zou, J., Zhang, Q., et al.: Reactive oxygen species (ROS)-responsive size-reducible nanoassemblies for deeper atherosclerotic plaque penetration and enhanced macrophage-targeted drug delivery. Bioact Mater. **19**, 115–126 (2023). https://doi.org/10.1016/j.bioactmat.2022.03.041
30. Balakrishnan, T., Ang, W.L., Mahmoudi, E.: Enhancing photoluminescence stability of blue emissive nitrogen doped graphene quantum dots by encapsulating inside zeolitic imidazole framework-8. J. Solid State Chem. **328**, 124343 (2023). https://doi.org/10.1016/j.jssc.2023.124343
31. Song, Y., Du, J., Yang, R., Lin, C., Chen, W., Wu, Z., et al.: Recyclable time–temperature indicator enabled by light storage in particles. Adv. Opt. Mater. **11**, (2023). https://doi.org/10.1002/adom.202202654
32. Kim, J.J., Pritts, J.D., Ngo, M., Estoll, C.R., Rao, V.A.: Trends in light and temperature sensitivity recommendations among licensed biotechnology drug products. Pharm. Res. **40**, 1491–505 (2023). https://doi.org/10.1007/s11095-023-03494-0
33. Zhao, Y., Xu, W., Zheng, H., Jia, Q.: Light, pH, and temperature triple-responsive magnetic composites for highly efficient phosphopeptide enrichment. Anal. Chem. **95**, 9043–51 (2023). https://doi.org/10.1021/acs.analchem.3c01330
34. Abdelkawi, A., Slim, A., Zinoune, Z., Pathak, Y.: Surface modification of metallic nanoparticles for targeting drugs. Coatings **13**, 1660 (2023). https://doi.org/10.3390/coatings13091660
35. Bhaladhare, S., Bhattacharjee, S.: Chemical, physical, and biological stimuli-responsive nanogels for biomedical applications (mechanisms, concepts, and advancements): A review. Int. J. Biol. Macromol. **226**, 535–53 (2023). https://doi.org/10.1016/j.ijbiomac.2022.12.076
36. Oleksy, M., Dynarowicz, K., Aebisher, D.: Advances in biodegradable polymers and biomaterials for medical applications—a review. Molecules **28**, 6213 (2023). https://doi.org/10.3390/molecules28176213
37. Faheed, N.K.: Advantages of natural fiber composites for biomedical applications: a review of recent advances. Emergent Mater **7**, 63–75 (2024). https://doi.org/10.1007/s42247-023-00620-x
38. Kong, L., Heydari, Z., Lami, G.H., Saberi, A., Baltatu, M.S., Vizureanu, P.: A comprehensive review of the current research status of biodegradable zinc alloys and composites for biomedical applications. Materials **16**, 4797 (2023). https://doi.org/10.3390/ma16134797
39. Kumara, B.N., Kalimuthu, P., Prasad, K.S.: Synthesis, properties and potential applications of photoluminescent carbon nanoparticles: A review. Anal. Chim. Acta **1268**, 341430 (2023). https://doi.org/10.1016/j.aca.2023.341430
40. Li, C., Huang, J., Yuan, L., Xie, W., Ying, Y., Li, C., et al.: Recent progress of emitting long-wavelength carbon dots and their merits for visualization tracking, target delivery and theranostics. Theranostics **13**, 3064–102 (2023). https://doi.org/10.7150/thno.80579
41. Sivadasan, D., Sultan, M.H., Alqahtani, S.S., Javed, S.: Cubosomes in drug delivery—a comprehensive review on its structural components. Prep. Tech. Ther. Applications. Biomed. **11**, 1114 (2023). https://doi.org/10.3390/biomedicines11041114
42. Shi, M., McHugh, K.J.: Strategies for overcoming protein and peptide instability in biodegradable drug delivery systems. Adv. Drug Deliv. Rev. **199**, 114904 (2023). https://doi.org/10.1016/j.addr.2023.114904

43. Lai, J., Azad, A.K., Sulaiman, W.M.A.W., Kumarasamy, V., Subramaniyan, V., Alshehade, S.A.: Alginate-based encapsulation fabrication technique for drug delivery: An updated review of particle type, formulation technique, pharmaceutical ingredient, and targeted delivery system. Pharmaceutics **16**, 370 (2024). https://doi.org/10.3390/pharmaceutics16030370
44. Yang, Y., Jiang, Q., Zhang, F.: Nanocrystals for deep-tissue *in vivo* luminescence imaging in the near-infrared region. Chem. Rev. **124**, 554–628 (2024). https://doi.org/10.1021/acs.chemrev.3c00506
45. Li, C., Pang, Y., Xu, Y., Lu, M., Tu, L., Li, Q., et al.: Near-infrared metal agents assisting precision medicine: from strategic design to bioimaging and therapeutic applications. Chem. Soc. Rev. **52**, 4392–442 (2023). https://doi.org/10.1039/D3CS00227F
46. Ren, F., Li, T., Yao, T., Chen, G., Li, C., Wang, Q.: Near-infrared-II fluorophores for in vivo multichannel biosensing. Chemosensors **11**, 433 (2023). https://doi.org/10.3390/chemosensors11080433
47. Ju, Y., Kim, C.-J., Caruso, F.: Functional ligand-enabled particle assembly for bio-nano interactions. Acc. Chem. Res. **56**, 1826–37 (2023). https://doi.org/10.1021/acs.accounts.3c00172
48. Huang, P., Wang, C., Deng, H., Zhou, Y., Chen, X.: Surface engineering of nanoparticles toward cancer theranostics. Acc. Chem. Res. **56**, 1766–79 (2023). https://doi.org/10.1021/acs.accounts.3c00122
49. Singh, R., Srinivas, S.P., Kumawat, M., Daima, H.K.: Ligand-based surface engineering of nanomaterials: Trends, challenges, and biomedical perspectives. OpenNano **15**, 100194 (2024). https://doi.org/10.1016/j.onano.2023.100194
50. Yuan, L., Chen, Q., Riviere, J.E., Lin, Z.: Pharmacokinetics and tumor delivery of nanoparticles. J Drug Deliv Sci Technol **83**, 104404 (2023). https://doi.org/10.1016/j.jddst.2023.104404
51. Feliu, N., Parak, W.J.: Developing future nanomedicines. Science **2024**(384), 385–6 (1979). https://doi.org/10.1126/science.abq3711
52. Niroumand, U., Firouzabadi, N., Goshtasbi, G., Hassani, B., Ghasemiyeh, P., Mohammadi-Samani, S.: The effect of size, morphology and surface properties of mesoporous silica nanoparticles on pharmacokinetic aspects and potential toxicity concerns. Front Mater. **10**, (2023). https://doi.org/10.3389/fmats.2023.1189463
53. Furness, M.S., Cai, H., Chandramouli, S., Chelliah, M., Chen, X.H., Ghosh, D., et al.: Modeling Approaches to Reimagine Stability (MARS) for enabling earlier access to critical drugs for patients with unmet medical needs. AAPS PharmSciTech. **24**, 35 (2023). https://doi.org/10.1208/s12249-022-02498-0
54. Reinhart, A.-G., Osterwald, A., Ringler, P., Leiser, Y., Lauer, M.E., Martin, R.E., et al.: Investigations into mRNA lipid nanoparticles shelf-life stability under nonfrozen conditions. Mol. Pharm. **20**, 6492–503 (2023). https://doi.org/10.1021/acs.molpharmaceut.3c00956
55. Reichard, J.F., Phelps, S.E., Lehnhardt, K.R., Young, M., Easter, B.D.: The effect of long-term spaceflight on drug potency and the risk of medication failure. NPJ Microgravity **9**, 35 (2023). https://doi.org/10.1038/s41526-023-00271-6
56. Bauri, S., Tripathi, S., Choudhury, A.M., Mandal, S.S., Raj, H., Maiti, P.: Nanomaterials as theranostic agents for cancer therapy. ACS Appl Nano Mater **6**, 21462–95 (2023). https://doi.org/10.1021/acsanm.3c04235
57. Hosseini, S.M., Mohammadnejad, J., Salamat, S., Beiram Zadeh, Z., Tanhaei, M., Ramakrishna, S.: Theranostic polymeric nanoparticles as a new approach in cancer therapy and diagnosis: A review. Mater Today Chem **29**, 101400 (2023). https://doi.org/10.1016/j.mtchem.2023.101400
58. Pratihar, S., Bhagavath, K.K., Govindaraju, T.: Small molecules and conjugates as theranostic agents. RSC Chem Biol **4**, 826–49 (2023). https://doi.org/10.1039/D3CB00073G
59. National Cancer Institute.: Cancer Statistics. US Department of Health and Human Services, National Institute of Health, USA (2024)
60. Lorscheider, M., Gaudin, A., Nakhlé, J., Veiman, K.-L., Richard, J., Chassaing, C.: Challenges and opportunities in the delivery of cancer therapeutics: Update on recent progress. Ther. Deliv. **12**, 55–76 (2021). https://doi.org/10.4155/tde-2020-0079

61. Agiba, A.M., Arreola-Ramírez, J.L., Carbajal, V., Segura-Medina, P.: Light-responsive and dual-targeting liposomes: From mechanisms to targeting strategies. Molecules **29**, 636 (2024). https://doi.org/10.3390/molecules29030636
62. Salkho, N.M., Awad, N.S., Pitt, W.G., Husseini, G.A.: Photo-induced drug release from polymeric micelles and liposomes: phototriggering mechanisms in drug delivery systems. Polymers (Basel) **14**, 1286 (2022). https://doi.org/10.3390/polym14071286
63. Yuan, S., Yao, B., Yang, G., Lei, H.: Light-driven multi-core/shell microdroplets as a targeted drug delivery system. Adv. Funct. Mater. **34**, (2024). https://doi.org/10.1002/adfm.202401905
64. Al Ragib, A., Chakma, R., Dewan, K., Islam, T., Kormoker, T., Idris, A.M.: Current advanced drug delivery systems: Challenges and potentialities. J Drug Deliv Sci Technol **76**, 103727 (2022). https://doi.org/10.1016/j.jddst.2022.103727
65. Magill, E., Demartis, S., Gavini, E., Permana, A.D., Thakur, R.R.S., Adrianto, M.F., et al.: Solid implantable devices for sustained drug delivery. Adv. Drug Deliv. Rev. **199**, 114950 (2023). https://doi.org/10.1016/j.addr.2023.114950
66. Tao, Y., Chan, H.F., Shi, B., Li, M., Leong, K.W.: Light: A magical tool for controlled drug delivery. Adv Funct Mater. **30**, (2020). https://doi.org/10.1002/adfm.202005029
67. Jung, Y.L., Yang, Y.J., Shil, A., Sarkar, S., Ahn, K.H.: Anticancer prodrug capable of mitochondria-targeting, light-triggered release, and fluorescence monitoring. ACS Appl. Bio Mater. **7**, 3991–6 (2024). https://doi.org/10.1021/acsabm.4c00342
68. Losada-Barreiro, S., Celik, S., Sezgin-Bayindir, Z., Bravo-Fernández, S., Bravo-Díaz, C.: Carrier systems for advanced drug delivery: Improving drug solubility/bioavailability and administration routes. Pharmaceutics **16**, 852 (2024). https://doi.org/10.3390/pharmaceutics16070852
69. Pokharel, M., Park, K.: Light mediated drug delivery systems: A review. J. Drug Target. **30**, 368–80 (2022). https://doi.org/10.1080/1061186X.2021.2005610
70. James, A., Palanisamy, M., Radhakrishnan, A., Khanam, J.: Contemporary technologies in chronopharmaceutic drug delivery system. J Pharm Res Int. 35–57 (2022). https://doi.org/10.9734/jpri/2022/v34i35A36161
71. Rapp, T.L., DeForest, C.A.: Targeting drug delivery with light: A highly focused approach. Adv. Drug Deliv. Rev. **171**, 94–107 (2021). https://doi.org/10.1016/j.addr.2021.01.009
72. Jain, S., Kirar, M., Bindeliya, M., Sen, L., Soni, M., Shan, M., et al.: Novel drug delivery systems: An overview. Asian J. Dent. Health Sci. **2**, 33–39 (2022). https://doi.org/10.22270/ajdhs.v2i1.14
73. Benson, H.A.E., Roberts, M.S.: Challenges and innovations of controlled drug delivery. Fundamentals of Drug Delivery, Wiley, pp. 1–14 (2021). https://doi.org/10.1002/9781119769644.ch1
74. Gao, P.: Advancements in lipid nanoparticle technologies for precision targeting in therapeutic delivery. Precis Nanomed. **7**, (2024). https://doi.org/10.33218/001c.121633
75. Shamsipur, M., Ghavidast, A., Pashabadi, A.: Phototriggered structures: Latest advances in biomedical applications. Acta Pharm Sin B **13**, 2844–76 (2023). https://doi.org/10.1016/j.apsb.2023.04.005
76. Singh, A.K., Nair, A.V., Shah, S.K.S., Ray, S., Singh, N.D.P.: ESIPT–, AIE–, and AIE + ESIPT-based light-activated drug delivery systems and bioactive donors for targeted disease treatment. J Med. Chem. **66**, 3732–3745 (2023). https://doi.org/10.1021/acs.jmedchem.2c01466
77. Jiang, S., Wu, X., Yang, F., Rommelfanger, N.J., Hong, G.: Activation of mechanoluminescent nanotransducers by focused ultrasound enables light delivery to deep-seated tissue in vivo. Nat. Protoc. **18**, 3787–820 (2023). https://doi.org/10.1038/s41596-023-00895-8
78. Aundhia, C., Parmar, G., Talele, C., Kardani, S., Maheshwari, R.: Light-responsive polymers: Developments in drug delivery systems. Curr Org Chem. **28**, 1179–1189 (2024). https://doi.org/10.2174/0113852728307241240430055059
79. Guidi, L., Cascone, M.G., Rosellini, E.: Light-responsive polymeric nanoparticles for retinal drug delivery: Design cues, challenges and future perspectives. Heliyon **10**, e26616 (2024). https://doi.org/10.1016/j.heliyon.2024.e26616

80. Tsang, C.Y., Zhang, Y.: Nanomaterials for light-mediated therapeutics in deep tissue. Chem. Soc. Rev. **53**, 2898–931 (2024). https://doi.org/10.1039/D3CS00862B
81. Kapoor, D., Maheshwari, N., Bag, A., Sharma, M.C., Prajapati, B., Maheshwari, R.: Polymer mediated light responsive therapeutics delivery system to treat cancer. Eur. Polym. J. **210**, 112923 (2024). https://doi.org/10.1016/j.eurpolymj.2024.112923
82. Chen, J., Ning, C., Zhou, Z., Yu, P., Zhu, Y., Tan, G., et al.: Nanomaterials as photothermal therapeutic agents. Prog. Mater. Sci. **99**, 1–26 (2019). https://doi.org/10.1016/j.pmatsci.2018.07.005
83. Beniwal, N., Verma, A., Putta, C.L., Rengan, A.K.: Recent trends in bio-nanomaterials and non-invasive combinatorial approaches of photothermal therapy against cancer. Nanotheranostics **8**, 219–38 (2024). https://doi.org/10.7150/ntno.91356
84. Malekzadeh, R., Mortezazadeh, T., Abdulsahib, W.K., Babaye Abdollahi, B., Hamblin, M.R., Mansoori, B., et al.: Nanoarchitecture-based photothermal ablation of cancer: A systematic review. Environ Res. **236**, 116526 (2023). https://doi.org/10.1016/j.envres.2023.116526
85. Hu, H., Li, D., Dai, W., Jin, Q., Wang, D., Ji, J., et al.: A NIR-II AIEgen-based supramolecular nanodot for peroxynitrite-potentiated mild-temperature photothermal therapy of hepatocellular carcinoma. Adv Funct Mater. **33**, (2023). https://doi.org/10.1002/adfm.202213134
86. Liao, T., Chen, Z., Kuang, Y., Ren, Z., Yu, W., Rao, W., et al.: Small-size Ti3C2Tx MXene nanosheets coated with metal-polyphenol nanodots for enhanced cancer photothermal therapy and anti-inflammation. Acta Biomater. **159**, 312–23 (2023). https://doi.org/10.1016/j.actbio.2023.01.049
87. Jia, L., Wang, Y., Hu, T., Yang, C., Lin, H., Zhang, F., et al.: Boosting the tumor photothermal therapy with hollow CoSnSx-based injectable hydrogel via the sonodynamic and dual-gas therapy. Chem. Eng. J. **469**, 143969 (2023). https://doi.org/10.1016/j.cej.2023.143969
88. Han, H.S., Choi, K.Y.: Advances in nanomaterial-mediated photothermal cancer therapies: Toward clinical applications. Biomedicines **9**, 305 (2021). https://doi.org/10.3390/biomedicines9030305
89. Kurokawa, H., Taninaka, A., Yoshitomi, T., Shigekawa, H., Matsui, H.: Near-infrared light irradiation of porphyrin-modified gold nanoparticles promotes cancer-cell-specific cytotoxicity. Molecules **27**, 1238 (2022). https://doi.org/10.3390/molecules27041238
90. Thirumurugan, S., Ramanathan, S., Muthiah, K.S., Lin, Y.-C., Hsiao, M., Dhawan, U., et al.: Inorganic nanoparticles for photothermal treatment of cancer. J Mater Chem B **12**, 3569–93 (2024). https://doi.org/10.1039/D3TB02797J
91. Lukácsi, S., Munkácsy, G., Győrffy, B.: Harnessing hyperthermia: Molecular, cellular, and immunological insights for enhanced anticancer therapies. Integr. Cancer. Ther. **23**, (2024). https://doi.org/10.1177/15347354241242094
92. Kazemi, K.S., Kazemi, P., Mivehchi, H., Nasiri, K., Eshagh Hoseini, S.S., Nejati, S.T., et al.: Photodynamic therapy: A novel approach for head and neck cancer treatment with focusing on oral cavity. Biol Proced Online **26**, 25 (2024). https://doi.org/10.1186/s12575-024-00252-3
93. Wang, Y., Yin, X.-B.: Persistent luminescence materials for imaging and therapeutic applications. Coord. Chem. Rev. **522**, 216192 (2025). https://doi.org/10.1016/j.ccr.2024.216192
94. Marques, L., Costa, B., Pereira, M., Silva, A., Santos, J., Saldanha, L., et al.: Advancing precision medicine: a review of innovative in silico approaches for drug development. Clinical pharmacology and personalized healthcare. Pharmaceutics **16**, 332 (2024). https://doi.org/10.3390/pharmaceutics16030332
95. Suhag, D., Kaushik, S., Taxak, V.B.: Theranostics: Combining diagnosis and therapy, pp. 271–95 (2024). https://doi.org/10.1007/978-981-97-4818-1_10
96. Zhou, Y., Xie, Y., Zhang, J., Li, Y., Fan, Y., Wang, H., et al.: PEGylate engineering for preparing water-soluble deep/near-infrared red type I/II photosensitizer and its efficient photodynamic therapy of cancer cells. J. Mol. Struct. **1321**, 139956 (2025). https://doi.org/10.1016/j.molstruc.2024.139956

97. Wang, Y., Du, M., Wang, J., Bai, Z., Cui, C., Tong, J., et al.: Carbon dots-cisplatin nano drug delivery system induces the death of oral tongue squamous cell under self-targeting chemical/photodynamic combined therapy. Colloids Surf A Physicochem Eng Asp **704**, 135511 (2025). https://doi.org/10.1016/j.colsurfa.2024.135511
98. Chen, W., Sun, J., Xiao, H., Zhu, Z., Xing, J., Zhang, Y., et al.: Near-infrared hemicyanine photosensitizer for targeted mitochondrial viscosity imaging and efficient photodynamic therapy. Spectrochim Acta A Mol Biomol Spectrosc **325**, 125049 (2025). https://doi.org/10.1016/j.saa.2024.125049
99. Shi, M., He, Y., Li, Y., Fan, M., Huang, H., Zhong, X., et al.: A self-powered theranostic DNA nanodevice for amplification of both intracellular microRNA imaging and photodynamic therapy. Spectrochim Acta A Mol Biomol Spectrosc. **324**, 124987 (2025). https://doi.org/10.1016/j.saa.2024.124987
100. Tong, S., Cheng, Y., Liu, H., Pang, Y., Lin, X., Hu, Z., et al.: Thionation of conjugated porphyrin with enhanced photodynamic and photothermal effects for cancer therapy. J Photochem Photobiol A Chem **459**, 116085 (2025). https://doi.org/10.1016/j.jphotochem.2024.116085
101. Alizadeh Nobari, S., Doustvandi, M.A., Yaghoubi, S.M., Shahriar Oskouei, S.S., Alizadeh, E., Afrashteh Nour, M., et al.: Emerging trends in quantum dot-based photosensitizers for enhanced photodynamic therapy in cancer treatment. J. Pharm. Investig. (2024). https://doi.org/10.1007/s40005-024-00698-3
102. Truong, T.T., Mondal, S., Doan, V.H.M., Tak, S., Choi, J., Oh, H., et al.: Precision-engineered metal and metal-oxide nanoparticles for biomedical imaging and healthcare applications. Adv. Colloid Interface Sci. **332**, 103263 (2024). https://doi.org/10.1016/j.cis.2024.103263
103. Bastos, E.L., Quina, F.H., Baptista, M.S.: Endogenous photosensitizers in human skin. Chem. Rev. **123**, 9720–85 (2023). https://doi.org/10.1021/acs.chemrev.2c00787
104. Wang, B., Wang, Y., Zhang, J., Hu, C., Jiang, J., Li, Y., et al.: ROS-induced lipid peroxidation modulates cell death outcome: mechanisms behind apoptosis, autophagy, and ferroptosis. Arch. Toxicol. **97**, 1439–51 (2023). https://doi.org/10.1007/s00204-023-03476-6
105. Lin, J., Li, D., Li, C., Zhuang, Z., Chu, C., Ostrikov, K., et al.: A review on reactive oxygen species (ROS)-inducing nanoparticles activated by uni- or multi-modal dynamic treatment for oncotherapy. Nanoscale. **15**, 11813–11833. https://doi.org/10.1039/D3NR01735D
106. Cui, X., Li, X., Peng, C., Qiu, Y., Shi, Y., Liu, Y., et al.: Beyond external light: On-spot light generation or light delivery for highly penetrated photodynamic therapy. ACS Nano **17**, 20776–803 (2023). https://doi.org/10.1021/acsnano.3c05619
107. Pathak, R., Punetha, V.D., Bhatt, S., Punetha, M.: Multifunctional role of carbon dot-based polymer nanocomposites in biomedical applications: a review. J. Mater. Sci. **58**, 6419–43 (2023). https://doi.org/10.1007/s10853-023-08408-4
108. Wang, F., Zhong, Y., Bruns, O., Liang, Y., Dai, H.: In vivo NIR-II fluorescence imaging for biology and medicine. Nat. Photonics **18**, 535–47 (2024). https://doi.org/10.1038/s41566-024-01391-5
109. Xiong, H., Song, Z., Wang, T., Huang, K., Yu, F., Sun, W., et al.: Photoswitchable dynamics and RNAi synergist with tailored interface and controlled release reprogramming tumor immunosuppressive niche. Biomaterials **312**, 122712 (2025). https://doi.org/10.1016/j.biomaterials.2024.122712
110. Chen, X., Chen, G., Dong, S., Qiu, L., Qiu, R., Han, X., et al.: Trifluoromethyl-pyrrolidone phthalocyanine nanoparticles for targeted lipid droplet imaging and in vitro photodynamic therapy in breast cancer cells. Spectrochim Acta A Mol Biomol Spectrosc **325**, 125012 (2025). https://doi.org/10.1016/j.saa.2024.125012
111. Oliveira, G.P., Lima, M.A., Pereira, G.B.S., Costa, A.R., Batista, A.A., Forim, M.R., et al.: Palladium(II) and platinum(II) thiophene-based thiosemicarbazones: Synthesis, properties, and anticancer studies. J. Mol. Struct. **1322**, 140306 (2025). https://doi.org/10.1016/j.molstruc.2024.140306
112. Calixto, G., Bernegossi, J., De Freitas, L., Fontana, C., Chorilli, M.: Nanotechnology-based drug delivery systems for photodynamic therapy of cancer: A review. Molecules **21**, 342 (2016). https://doi.org/10.3390/molecules21030342

113. Chen, S., Zu, B., Wu, L.: Optical applications of $CuInSe_2$ colloidal quantum dots. ACS Omega. **9**, 43288–301 (2024). https://doi.org/10.1021/acsomega.4c03802
114. Karami, M., Aghabarari, B.: The advancement of molybdenum disulfide quantum dots nanoparticles as nanocarrier for drug delivery systems: Cutting-edge in dual therapeutic roles. J. Mol. Struct. **1318**, 139149 (2024). https://doi.org/10.1016/j.molstruc.2024.139149
115. Pandey, T., Pandey, V.: Advancements in increasing efficiency of hydrogen sulfide in therapeutics: Strategies for targeted delivery as prodrugs. Nitric Oxide **152**, 1–10 (2024). https://doi.org/10.1016/j.niox.2024.09.001
116. Soni, H., Bhattu, M., SD, P., Kaur, M., Verma, M., Singh, J.: Recent advances in waste-derived carbon dots and their nanocomposites for environmental remediation and biological applications. Environ Res. **251**, 118560 (2024). https://doi.org/10.1016/j.envres.2024.118560
117. Guo, W., Song, X., Liu, J., Liu, W., Chu, X., Lei, Z.: Quantum dots as a potential multifunctional material for the enhancement of clinical diagnosis strategies and cancer treatments. Nanomaterials **14**, 1088 (2024). https://doi.org/10.3390/nano14131088
118. Shang, S., Li, X., Wang, H., Zhou, Y., Pang, K., Li, P., et al.: Targeted therapy of kidney disease with nanoparticle drug delivery materials. Bioact Mater **37**, 206–21 (2024). https://doi.org/10.1016/j.bioactmat.2024.03.014
119. Shen, Q., Song, G., Lin, H., Bai, H., Huang, Y., Lv, F., et al.: Sensing, imaging, and therapeutic strategies endowing by conjugate polymers for precision medicine. Adv. Mater. **36**, (2024). https://doi.org/10.1002/adma.202310032
120. Lin, T., Fu, X., Liu, Z., Chen, N., Zhang, J., Liu, R., et al.: X-ray induced long afterglow luminescence from UVC to red region in Ca2P2O7:Pr3+. J. Rare Earths (2024). https://doi.org/10.1016/j.jre.2024.08.012
121. Huang, B., Xie, J., Wang, P., Tian, J., Zhang, W.: Nanozyme-catalyzed oxygen self-supplying mitochondria-targeting nanoplatform for precise photodynamic therapy. Next Materials **5**, 100230 (2024). https://doi.org/10.1016/j.nxmate.2024.100230
122. Li, C., Fang, X., Zeng, Q., Zeng, L., Zhang, B., Nie, G.: Ultra small gold nanoclusters supported on two-dimensional bismuth selenium nanosheets for synergistic photothermal and photodynamic tumor therapy. RSC Adv. **14**, 24335–44 (2024). https://doi.org/10.1039/D4RA03142C
123. Zhang, Q., Luo, Q., Liu, Z., Sun, M., Dong, X.: Nano-ROS-generating approaches to cancer dynamic therapy: Lessons from nanoparticles. Chem. Eng. J. **457**, 141225 (2023). https://doi.org/10.1016/j.cej.2022.141225
124. Akpa, P.A., Peter, I.E., Onwuka, A.M., Obi, B.C., Akunne, M.O., Nworu, C.S., et al.: Nanotheranostics: Platforms, current applications, and mechanisms of targeting in breast and prostate cancers. J. Nanotheranostics **4**, 346–83 (2023). https://doi.org/10.3390/jnt4030016
125. Bandyopadhyay, A., Das, T., Nandy, S., Sahib, S., Preetam, S., Gopalakrishnan, A.V., et al.: Ligand-based active targeting strategies for cancer theranostics. Naunyn Schmiedebergs Arch. Pharmacol. **396**, 3417–41 (2023). https://doi.org/10.1007/s00210-023-02612-4
126. Munir, M., Zaman, M., Waqar, M.A., Khan, M.A., Alvi, M.N.: Solid lipid nanoparticles: A versatile approach for controlled release and targeted drug delivery. J. Liposome Res. **34**, 335–48 (2024). https://doi.org/10.1080/08982104.2023.2268711
127. Wei, D., Sun, Y., Zhu, H., Fu, Q.: Stimuli-responsive polymer-based nanosystems for cancer theranostics. ACS Nano **17**, 23223–61 (2023). https://doi.org/10.1021/acsnano.3c06019
128. Zhao, H., Li, Y., Chen, J., Zhang, J., Yang, Q., Cui, J., et al.: Environmental stimulus-responsive mesoporous silica nanoparticles as anticancer drug delivery platforms. Colloids Surf. B Biointerfaces **234**, 113758 (2024). https://doi.org/10.1016/j.colsurfb.2024.113758
129. Sultana, N., David, A.E.: Improving cancer targeting: A study on the effect of dual-ligand density on targeting of cells having differential expression of target biomarkers. Int. J. Mol. Sci. **24**, 13048 (2023). https://doi.org/10.3390/ijms241713048
130. Shao, T., Feng, Z., Shen, Y., Chen, D., Xiang, P., Zhang, Q., et al.: Fine-tuning the side-chain length of iridium(III) complexes for enhanced photophysical properties in cancer theranostics. J. Inorg. Biochem. **262**, 112760 (2025). https://doi.org/10.1016/j.jinorgbio.2024.112760

131. Lin, D., Lv, W., Qian, M., Jiang, G., Lin, X., Gantulga, D., et al.: Engineering cell membrane-camouflaged COF-based nanosatellite for enhanced tumor-targeted photothermal chemoimmunotherapy. Biomaterials **314**, 122869 (2025). https://doi.org/10.1016/j.biomaterials.2024.122869
132. Zhang, L., Yu, Y., Ding, K., Ji, C., Zhang, D., Liang, P., et al.: Tumor microenvironment ameliorative and adaptive nanoparticles with photothermal-to-photodynamic switch for cancer phototherapy. Biomaterials **313**, 122771 (2025). https://doi.org/10.1016/j.biomaterials.2024.122771
133. Zheng, L., Wang, H., Zhong, X., Jia, L., Shi, G., Bai, C., et al.: Reprogramming tumor microenvironment with precise photothermal therapy by calreticulin nanobody-engineered probiotics. Biomaterials **314**, 122809 (2025). https://doi.org/10.1016/j.biomaterials.2024.122809
134. Teng, M., Liang, X., Liu, H., Li, Z., Gao, X., Zhang, C., et al.: Cerenkov radiation shining a light for cancer theranostics. Nano Today **55**, 102174 (2024). https://doi.org/10.1016/j.nantod.2024.102174
135. Strobl, M.A.R., Gallaher, J., Robertson-Tessi, M., West, J., Anderson, A.R.A.: Treatment of evolving cancers will require dynamic decision support. Ann. Oncol. **34**, 867–84 (2023). https://doi.org/10.1016/j.annonc.2023.08.008
136. Liu, B., Zhou, H., Tan, L., Siu, K.T.H., Guan, X.-Y.: Exploring treatment options in cancer: Tumor treatment strategies. Signal Transduct. Target. Ther. **9**, 175 (2024). https://doi.org/10.1038/s41392-024-01856-7
137. Zhong, N.-N., Wang, H.-Q., Huang, X.-Y., Li, Z.-Z., Cao, L.-M., Huo, F.-Y., et al.: Enhancing head and neck tumor management with artificial intelligence: Integration and perspectives. Semin. Cancer Biol. **95**, 52–74 (2023). https://doi.org/10.1016/j.semcancer.2023.07.002
138. Hussain, M.M., Khan, W.U., Ahmed, F., Wei, Y., Xiong, H.: Recent developments of Red/NIR carbon dots in biosensing, bioimaging, and tumor theranostics. Chem. Eng. J. **465**, 143010 (2023). https://doi.org/10.1016/j.cej.2023.143010
139. Fan, Y., Zhang, R., Shi, J., Tian, F., Zhang, Y., Zhang, L., et al.: Mild near-infrared laser-triggered photo-immunotherapy potentiates immune checkpoint blockade via an all-in-one theranostic nanoplatform. J. Colloid Interface Sci. **678**, 1088–103 (2025). https://doi.org/10.1016/j.jcis.2024.09.020
140. Kim, G., Han, J., Nguyen, V.K.T., Lee, S., Min, S., Park, S., et al.: Two strategies of enhancing the therapeutic potential of a coumarin probe: Integration of a protonatable moiety and BSA-based nanoparticle formation. Dyes Pigm. **232**, 112475 (2025). https://doi.org/10.1016/j.dyepig.2024.112475
141. Xu, Y., Zhang, J., Wang, Z., Zhang, P., Zhang, Z., Yang, Z., et al.: Water-soluble AIE photosensitizer in short-wave infrared region for albumin-enhanced and self-reporting phototheranostics. Biomaterials **314**, 122847 (2025). https://doi.org/10.1016/j.biomaterials.2024.122847
142. Shi, J., Liang, M., Qiu, Y., Zhang, J., Wang, S., Fang, H., et al.: Two-pronged strategy: A mitochondria targeting AIE photosensitizer for hydrogen sulfide detection and type I and type II photodynamic therapy. Talanta **282**, 127074 (2025). https://doi.org/10.1016/j.talanta.2024.127074
143. Feng, B., Zhong, L., Yang, Y., Qu, W., Wang, Y., Wang, K., et al.: ONOO-regulating ICT of mitochondria-targeted photosensitizers to enhance type-I photochemical reactions. Sens Actuators B Chem **423**, 136810 (2025). https://doi.org/10.1016/j.snb.2024.136810
144. Verkhovskii, R., Ivanov, A., Lengert, E., Tulyakova, K., Shilyagina, N., Ermakov, A.: Current principles, challenges, and new metrics in pH-responsive drug delivery systems for systemic cancer therapy. Pharmaceutics **15**, 1566 (2023). https://doi.org/10.3390/pharmaceutics15051566
145. Tewari, A.K., Upadhyay, S.C., Kumar, M., Pathak, K., Kaushik, D., Verma, R., et al.: Insights on development aspects of polymeric nanocarriers: The translation from bench to clinic. Polymers (Basel) **14**, 3545 (2022). https://doi.org/10.3390/polym14173545
146. Singh, J., Nayak, P.: PH-responsive polymers for drug delivery: Trends and opportunities. J. Polym. Sci. **61**, 2828–50 (2023). https://doi.org/10.1002/pol.20230403

147. Singh, J., Nayak, P.: <scp>pH</scp> -responsive polymers for drug delivery: Trends and opportunities. J. Polym. Sci. **61**, 2828–50 (2023). https://doi.org/10.1002/pol.20230403
148. Pilch, J., Potęga, A., Kowalczyk, A., Kasprzak, A., Kowalik, P., Bujak, P., et al.: PH-responsive drug delivery nanoplatforms as smart carriers of unsymmetrical bisacridines for targeted cancer therapy. Pharmaceutics **15**, 201 (2023). https://doi.org/10.3390/pharmaceutics15010201
149. Jo, M.J., Shin, H.J., Yoon, M.S., Kim, S.Y., Jin, C.E., Park, C.-W., et al.: Evaluation of pH-sensitive polymeric micelles using citraconic amide bonds for the co-delivery of paclitaxel, etoposide, and rapamycin. Pharmaceutics **15**, 154 (2023). https://doi.org/10.3390/pharmaceutics15010154
150. Brewer, K., Bai, F., Blencowe, A.: PH-responsive poly(ethylene glycol)-b-poly(2-vinylpyridine) micelles for the triggered release of therapeutics. Pharmaceutics **15**, 977 (2023). https://doi.org/10.3390/pharmaceutics15030977
151. Yang, D., Li, Z., Zhang, Y., Chen, X., Liu, M., Yang, C.: Design of dual-targeted pH-sensitive hybrid polymer micelles for breast cancer treatment: Three birds with one stone. Pharmaceutics **15**, 1580 (2023). https://doi.org/10.3390/pharmaceutics15061580
152. Zlotnikov, I.D., Streltsov, D.A., Ezhov, A.A., Kudryashova, E.V.: Smart pH- and temperature-sensitive micelles based on chitosan grafted with fatty acids to increase the efficiency and selectivity of doxorubicin and its adjuvant regarding the tumor cells. Pharmaceutics **15**, 1135 (2023). https://doi.org/10.3390/pharmaceutics15041135
153. Vegad, U., Patel, M., Khunt, D., Zupančič, O., Chauhan, S., Paudel, A.: pH stimuli-responsive hydrogels from non-cellulosic biopolymers for drug delivery. Front. Bioeng Biotechnol. **11**, (2023). https://doi.org/10.3389/fbioe.2023.1270364
154. Wu, Y., Li, Y., Han, R., Long, Z., Si, P., Zhang, D.: Dual-cross-linked PEI/PVA hydrogel for pH-responsive drug delivery. Biomacromol **24**, 5364–70 (2023). https://doi.org/10.1021/acs.biomac.3c00824
155. Thang, N.H., Chien, T.B., Cuong, D.X.: Polymer-based hydrogels applied in drug delivery: An overview. Gels **9**, 523 (2023). https://doi.org/10.3390/gels9070523
156. Leng, Q., Imtiyaz, Z., Woodle, M.C., Mixson, A.J.: Delivery of chemotherapy agents and nucleic acids with pH-dependent nanoparticles. Pharmaceutics **15**, 1482 (2023). https://doi.org/10.3390/pharmaceutics15051482
157. Kongkatigumjorn, N., Crespy, D.: Cascade release of payloads from polymer nanofibers with conjugated hydrotropes and kosmotropes. Macromolecules **57**, 3502–14 (2024). https://doi.org/10.1021/acs.macromol.4c00526
158. Yu, J., Liu, Y., Zhang, Y., Ran, R., Kong, Z., Zhao, D., et al.: Smart nanogels for cancer treatment from the perspective of functional groups. Front. Bioeng Biotechnol. **11**, (2024). https://doi.org/10.3389/fbioe.2023.1329311
159. Santhamoorthy, M., Ramkumar, V., Thirupathi, K., Gnanasekaran, L., Karuppannan, V., Phan, T.T.V., et al.: L-lysine functionalized mesoporous silica hybrid nanoparticles for pH-responsive delivery of curcumin. Pharmaceutics **15**, 1631 (2023). https://doi.org/10.3390/pharmaceutics15061631
160. Yahyavi, M., Badalkhani-Khamseh, F., Hadipour, N.L.: Folic acid functionalized carbon nanotubes as pH controlled carriers of fluorouracil: Molecular dynamics simulations. J. Mol. Liq. **377**, 121393 (2023). https://doi.org/10.1016/j.molliq.2023.121393
161. Pourmadadi, M., Farokh, A., Rahmani, E., Eshaghi, M.M., Aslani, A., Rahdar, A., et al.: Polyacrylic acid mediated targeted drug delivery nano-systems: A review. J Drug Deliv Sci Technol **80**, 104169 (2023). https://doi.org/10.1016/j.jddst.2023.104169
162. Chen, Z., Wang, X., Zhao, N., Chen, H., Guo, G.: Advancements in pH-responsive nanocarriers: enhancing drug delivery for tumor therapy. Expert Opin. Drug Deliv. **20**, 1623–42 (2023). https://doi.org/10.1080/17425247.2023.2292678
163. Bhattacharya, S., Prajapati, B.G., Singh, S.: A critical review on the dissemination of PH and stimuli-responsive polymeric nanoparticular systems to improve drug delivery in cancer therapy. Crit. Rev. Oncol. Hematol. **185**, 103961 (2023). https://doi.org/10.1016/j.critrevonc.2023.103961

164. Khan, R.U., Shao, J., Liao, J.-Y., Qian, L.: PH-triggered cancer-targeting polymers: From extracellular accumulation to intracellular release. Nano Res. **16**, 5155–68 (2023). https://doi.org/10.1007/s12274-022-5252-z
165. Yu, Z., Li, L., Mou, F., Yu, S., Zhang, D., Yang, M., et al.: Swarming magnetic photonic-crystal microrobots with on-the-fly visual <scp>pH</scp> detection and self-regulated drug delivery. Info. Mat. **5**, (2023). https://doi.org/10.1002/inf2.12464
166. Yang, S., Xie, J., Wang, D., Tian, S., Di, Y., Yan, L.: A dual-responsive polyurethane nanocarrier for drug release triggered by intracellular GSH and NQO1 enzyme. Polym. Chem. **15**, 2513–27 (2024). https://doi.org/10.1039/D4PY00320A
167. Tang, X., Wen, Y., Zhang, Z., Zhu, J., Song, X., Li, J.: Rationally designed multifunctional nanoparticles as GSH-responsive anticancer drug delivery systems based on host-guest polymers derived from dextran and β-cyclodextrin. Carbohydr. Polym. **320**, 121207 (2023). https://doi.org/10.1016/j.carbpol.2023.121207
168. Sastre, J., Pérez, S., Sabater, L., Rius-Pérez, S.: Redox signalling in the pancreas in health and disease. Physiol. Rev. (2024). https://doi.org/10.1152/physrev.00044.2023
169. Lai, W., Zhang, J., Sun, J., Min, T., Bai, Y., He, J., et al.: Oxidative stress in alcoholic liver disease, focusing on proteins, nucleic acids, and lipids: A review. Int. J. Biol. Macromol. **278**, 134809 (2024). https://doi.org/10.1016/J.IJBIOMAC.2024.134809
170. Yavuz, O., Dincel, G.C., Yildirim, S., El-Ashram, S., Al-Olayan, E.: Impact of apoptosis and oxidative stress on pancreatic beta cell pathophysiology in streptozotocin-induced Type 1 diabetes mellitus. Tissue Cell **91**, 102552 (2024). https://doi.org/10.1016/J.TICE.2024.102552
171. Eguchi, N., Vaziri, N.D., Dafoe, D.C., Ichii, H.: The role of oxidative stress in pancreatic β cell dysfunction in diabetes. Int. J. Mol. Sci. **22**, 1509 (2021). https://doi.org/10.3390/IJMS22041509
172. Ji, M., Liu, H., Wei, M., Shi, D., Gou, J., Yin, T., et al.: Redox-sensitive disulfide-bridged self-assembled nanoparticles of dexamethasone with high drug loading for acute lung injury therapy. Int. J. Pharm. **664**, 124600 (2024). https://doi.org/10.1016/j.ijpharm.2024.124600
173. Shaibie, N.A., Ramli, N.A., Mohammad Faizal, N.D.F., Srichana, T., Mohd Amin M.C.I.: Poly (*N*isopropylacrylamide)-based polymers: recent overview for the development of temperature-responsive drug delivery and biomedical applications. Macromol Chem Phys. **224**, (2023). https://doi.org/10.1002/macp.202300157
174. Thirupathi, K., Santhamoorthy, M., Radhakrishnan, S., Ulagesan, S., Nam, T.-J., Phan, T.T.V., et al.: Thermosensitive polymer-modified mesoporous silica for pH and temperature-responsive drug delivery. Pharmaceutics **15**, 795 (2023). https://doi.org/10.3390/pharmaceutics15030795
175. Zhang, C., Jiang, G., Gao, X.: Matrix metalloproteinase-responsive drug delivery systems. Bioconjug. Chem. **34**, 1349–65 (2023). https://doi.org/10.1021/acs.bioconjchem.3c00266
176. Guo, F., Du, Y., Wang, Y., Wang, M., Wang, L., Yu, N., et al.: Targeted drug delivery systems for matrix metalloproteinase-responsive anoparticles in tumor cells: A review. Int. J. Biol. Macromol. **257**, 128658 (2024). https://doi.org/10.1016/j.ijbiomac.2023.128658
177. Zong, L., Xu, H., Zhang, H., Tu, Z., Zhang, X., Wang, S., et al.: A review of matrix metalloproteinase-2-sensitive nanoparticles as a novel drug delivery for tumor therapy. Int. J. Biol. Macromol. **262**, 130043 (2024). https://doi.org/10.1016/j.ijbiomac.2024.130043
178. Wei, Y., Lv, J., Zhu, S., Wang, S., Su, J., Xu, C.: Enzyme-responsive liposomes for controlled drug release. Drug Discov. Today **29**, 104014 (2024). https://doi.org/10.1016/j.drudis.2024.104014

179. Brion, A., Chaud, J., Klimezak, M., Bolze, F., Ohlmann, L., Léonard, J., et al.: Photoactivatable liposomes for blue to deep red light-activated surface drug release: Application to controlled delivery of the antitumoral drug melphalan. Bioconjug. Chem. **34**, 1304–15 (2023). https://doi.org/10.1021/acs.bioconjchem.3c00197
180. Chen, Y., Wang, S., Zhang, F.: Near-infrared luminescence high-contrast in vivo biomedical imaging. Nat. Rev. Bioeng. **1**, 60–78 (2023). https://doi.org/10.1038/s44222-022-00002-8
181. Li, H., Kim, Y., Jung, H., Hyun, J.Y., Shin, I.: Near-infrared (NIR) fluorescence-emitting small organic molecules for cancer imaging and therapy. Chem. Soc. Rev. **51**, 8957–9008 (2022). https://doi.org/10.1039/D2CS00722C
182. Saeboe, A.M., Nikiforov, A.Y., Toufanian, R., Kays, J.C., Chern, M., Casas, J.P., et al.: Extending the near-infrared emission range of indium phosphide quantum dots for multiplexed in vivo imaging. Nano Lett. **21**, 3271–9 (2021). https://doi.org/10.1021/ACS.NANOLETT.1C00600/SUPPL_FILE/NL1C00600_SI_001.PDF
183. Liu, J., Kotrchová, L., Lécuyer, T., Corvis, Y., Seguin, J., Mignet, N., et al.: Coating persistent luminescence nanoparticles with hydrophilic polymers for in vivo imaging. Front. Chem. **8**, (2020). https://doi.org/10.3389/fchem.2020.584114
184. Tansi, F.L., Rüger, R., Kollmeier, A.M., Böhm, C., Kontermann, R.E., Teichgraeber, U.K., et al.: A fast and effective determination of the biodistribution and subcellular localization of fluorescent immunoliposomes in freshly excised animal organs. BMC Biotechnol. **17**, 8 (2017). https://doi.org/10.1186/s12896-017-0327-8
185. Ren, F., Wang, F., Baghdasaryan, A., Li, Y., Liu, H., Hsu, R., et al.: Shortwave-infrared-light-emitting probes for the in vivo tracking of cancer vaccines and the elicited immune responses. Nat. Biomed. Eng. **8**, 726–39 (2024). https://doi.org/10.1038/s41551-023-01083-5
186. Swamy, M.M.M., Murai, Y., Monde, K., Tsuboi, S., Swamy, A.K., Jin, T.: Biocompatible and Water-Soluble Shortwave-Infrared (SWIR)-emitting cyanine-based fluorescent probes for in vivo multiplexed molecular imaging. ACS Appl. Mater. Interfaces **16**, 17253–66 (2024). https://doi.org/10.1021/acsami.4c01000
187. Qiao, L., Fu, Z., Li, B., Liu, Z., Cai, L., Pan, Y., et al.: Heteroatom doping promoted ultrabright and ultrastable photoluminescence of water-soluble Au/Ag nanoclusters for visual and efficient drug delivery to cancer cells. ACS Appl. Mater. Interfaces. **16**, 34510–23 (2024). https://doi.org/10.1021/ACSAMI.4C04303/SUPPL_FILE/AM4C04303_SI_001.PDF
188. Lai, W.F., Huang, E.M., Wong, W.T.: A gel-forming clusteroluminogenic polymer with tunable emission behavior as a sustained-release carrier enabling real-time tracking during bioactive agent delivery. Appl. Mater. Today **21**, 100876 (2020). https://doi.org/10.1016/J.APMT.2020.100876
189. Bamisaye, A., Adegoke, K.A., Alli, Y.A., Bamidele, M.O., Idowu, M.A., Ogunjinmi, O.E.: Recent advances in nanoemulsion for sustainable development of farm-to-fork systems. J. Clean. Prod. **429**. https://doi.org/10.1016/j.jclepro.2023.139226
190. Bamisaye, A., Eromosele, C.O., Dare, E.O., Akinloye, O.A., Idowu, M.A., Ighodaro, O.M., et al.: Fabrication, characterization, antimicrobial, toxicity and potential drug-delivery studies of PEGylated Sesamum indicum oil based nanoemulsion system. Beni. Suef. Univ J. Basic. Appl. Sci. **12**. https://doi.org/10.1186/s43088-023-00371-y
191. Ding, D., Li, S., Xu, H., Zhu, L., Meng, S., Liu, J., et al.: X-ray-activated simultaneous near-infrared and short-wave infrared persistent luminescence imaging for long-term tracking of drug delivery. ACS Appl. Mater. Interfaces **13**, 16166–72 (2021). https://doi.org/10.1021/acsami.1c02372
192. Rahal, M., Atassi, Y., Alghoraibi, I.: Quenching photoluminescence of carbon quantum dots for detecting and tracking the release of minocycline. J Photochem Photobiol A Chem **412**, 113257 (2021). https://doi.org/10.1016/J.JPHOTOCHEM.2021.113257
193. Nisar, S., Starosta, E., Elayyan, M., Regmi, A., Sui, B.: Photoinduced electron transfer-based glutathione-sensing theranostic nanoprodrug with self-tracking and real-time drug release monitoring for cancer treatment. ACS Appl. Mater. Interfaces **16**, 6859–67 (2024). https://doi.org/10.1021/acsami.3c16585

194. Wang, H., Zhang, J., Zheng, B., Yang, Z., Sun, J., Liu, X., et al.: Near infrared-emitting persistent luminescence nanoparticles@macrophages as cell-based carriers for precise imaging-guided cancer cell ablation. New J. Chem. **48**, 9052–61 (2024). https://doi.org/10.1039/D3NJ02936K

Photoluminescence for Biosensing and Diagnostics

Chiamaka Linda Mgbechidinma, Samuel Ukpong Okon, Omoremime Elizabeth Dania, Fatai Oladipupo Oladoyinbo, Chibueze Anslem Mgbechidimma, Olayinka Oderinde, Isaac Sewanu Bankole, and Olubunmi Ayoni Ogundiran

Abstract Photoluminescence-based biosensors, such as Fluorescence Resonance Energy Transfer (FRET) and chemiluminescence assays, have revolutionized biosensing and diagnostics. Their unique mechanisms, coupled with advancements in fluorescent materials and detection technologies, continue to expand their applications, offering unparalleled precision and sensitivity in detecting biological and chemical targets. This chapter provides comprehensive details on photoluminescence

C. L. Mgbechidinma
School of Life Sciences, Centre for Cell and Development Biology and State Key Laboratory of Agrobiotechnology, The Chinese University of Hong Kong, Shatin, New Territories, Hong Kong, China

Department of Microbiology, University of Ibadan, Ibadan, Oyo State 200243, Nigeria

S. U. Okon
Suzhou Industrial Technological Research Institute of Zhejiang University, Suzhou 215163, China

Department of Marine Science, Akwa Ibom State University, Mkpat Enin, P.M.B. 1167, Nigeria

O. E. Dania
Department of Biochemistry, College of Science and Technology, Covenant University, PMB 1023, Ota, Ogun State, Nigeria

F. O. Oladoyinbo
Department of Chemistry, College of Physical Sciences, Federal University of Agriculture, Abeokuta, P.M.B. 2240, Abeokuta, Nigeria

C. A. Mgbechidimma
Department of Computer Science, University of Ibadan, Ibadan, Nigeria

O. Oderinde (✉)
Department of Chemistry, Faculty of Natural and Applied Sciences, Lead City University, Ibadan, Nigeria
e-mail: yinkaoderinde@yahoo.com; oderinde.olayinka@lcu.edu.ng

I. S. Bankole
Department of Science Laboratory Technology, Ogun State Institute of Technology, Igbesa, Ogun State, Nigeria

O. A. Ogundiran
Department of Chemical Sciences, Faculty of Sciences, Taraba State University, Jalingo, Nigeria

© The Author(s), under exclusive license to Springer Nature Switzerland AG 2025
N. O. Etafo (ed.), *Tailored Light Emitters For Biomedical Applications*, Engineering Materials, https://doi.org/10.1007/978-3-031-88731-4_5

for biosensing and diagnostics, biosensors utilizing photoluminescent emitters, and the in vitro and in vivo diagnostic applications for disease biomarker detection and imaging of cellular processes.

Keywords Biomarker detection · Cellular imaging · Chemiluminescence assays · Fluorescence Resonance Energy Transfer (FRET) · Medical diagnostics · Photoluminescence biosensor

1 Introduction

Urbanization, industrialization, and the increasing population have escalated factors threatening human health, with the unpredictable occurrence of epidemic and pandemic diseases currently being important issues of public concern. Polymerase chain reaction (PCR) and enzyme-linked immunosorbent assay (ELISA) are known serological diagnostic testing methods for these diseases, especially the most recent severe acute respiratory syndrome coronavirus (SARS-CoV-2), otherwise known as COVID-19 [1]. However, they are less attractive due to their complexity, high cost, and the need for large equipment space and skilled labor. Therefore, there is a need for rapid detection of pathogens and their human mechanistic invasion. Through improving techniques, researchers are continually proving the impeccable benefits of the synergy of synthetic chemistry and material sciences to advancing the health sector, even beyond Sustainable Development Goal 3 (SDG 3) on good health and well-being [2]. Incorporating optimized novel materials has proven effective recently, with a significant focus on engineering luminescence technologies for real-time surveillance and diagnostic testing. These techniques are instrumental in identifying the root causes of disease in patients, monitoring treatment efficacy, and screening potential diseases in asymptomatic but high-risk populations.

Luminescence involves the absorption of energy and its subsequent emission of light. Luminescent substances can either fluoresce (fast nanosecond time scale) or phosphoresce (slower, longer time scales of hours or days) [3]. Photoluminescence, the emission of light upon photon absorption, is a fundamental principle in diverse applications, notably biosensing and diagnostics. Photoluminescence-based biosensors offer high sensitivity, specificity, and versatility, making them indispensable tools in modern healthcare and biological research. These sensors often exploit molecular interactions to generate measurable photoluminescence signals indicative of specific analyte presence or concentration [4, 5]. In addition to the biosensor and diagnostic functions, photoluminescence is also well used in various fields, such as catalysis, lubrication, and the manufacture of optoelectronic devices. Experimental photoluminescence studies have and are still exploring steady-state photoluminescence (excitation spectra), time-resolved photoluminescence (light sources and photon counting), photoluminescence quantum yields (absolute and relative), and variable-temperature photoluminescence. Known classes of photoluminescent compounds are conjugated organic compounds (polycyclic aromatic hydrocarbons and laser dyes), transition metal coordination compounds (cyclometalated iridium complexes), coordination complexes with *d–d* transitions (Cr(III)), lanthanide compounds, nanomaterials and extended solids (quantum dots, solid-state phosphors, and carbon dots).

Most photoluminescence emitters are simple, rapid, affordable, and user-friendly, making them desirable for manufacturing point-of-care (POC) diagnostic testing tools. For instance, carbon dots, which are ultra-small in size, have excellent catalytic performance and outstanding biocompatibility, are environmentally friendly, and have low toxicity [6]. Carbon dots (CDs) have abundant surface groups that confer excellent long-term dispersibility and water solubility. They can be synthesized from many carbon-based materials, including graphene oxide, graphite, glucose, organic acids, carbon nanotubes, coal, grass, petroleum coke, as well as domestic waste; hence, highly fluorescent carbon quantum dots have been reported to have been greenly-synthesized for biomedical applications [7]. The photoluminescence mechanisms of CDs depend on their synthesis mode, ultimately affecting their applications. These mechanisms are divided into surface state, carbon core state, molecule state, and the synergistic effect of all the states. The synergistic effect mechanism is because none of the earlier three mechanisms can fully explain the photoluminescence ability of some CDs, as seen in multi-emission CDs [8]. Doping enhances the quantum yield and intrinsic properties of CDs' photoluminescence, translating to its possible biological applications. Doping can be single-atom or dual-atom doping, and the main doping agents include N, O, P, and B. The selection of doping agents/dopants is important and depends on the proposed applications [9].

Medically, diagnostic instruments must possess characteristic properties, including rapidity, high sensitivity, cost-effectiveness, specificity, and ease of implementation (Fig. 1c). Owing to these characteristics, they are widely explored as biosensors. In designing biosensors for SARS-CoV-2, significant attention is given to the S-protein (sticking out from the surface of viral particles and allows attachment/entry into host cells) and the N-protein (located within the SARS-CoV-2 virus and involved in RNA synthesis and translation with high concentration and immunogenicity in patient serum) [10]. This highlights the importance of understanding pathogen physiology to create biosensors with target biorecognition elements for specific organelles, antibodies, proteins, nucleic acids, and other biomolecules. In this case, signal transmission systems incorporated in the photoluminescence biosensors for diagnostics can be optical (spectrophotometric analysis) or electrochemical. Biosensors from both combinations include zinc oxide ZnO nanostructures—with high surface and room temperature photoluminescence and the novel ZnO tetrapods (ZnO-Ts) nanostructures [10]. Both have photoluminescence properties that can be used as biosensor transducers (Fig. 1a), revealing advances in the photoluminescence technological buildup by incorporating optical methods with nanotechnology and electrochemical techniques. Therefore, in this chapter, we herein present a comprehensive review of biosensors and photoluminescent emitters in biosensors, the major types, their fundamental working principles, and diagnostic applications for in vitro and in vivo examinations, especially for fluorescence resonance energy transfer (FRET) and chemiluminescence assays (Fig. 1b).

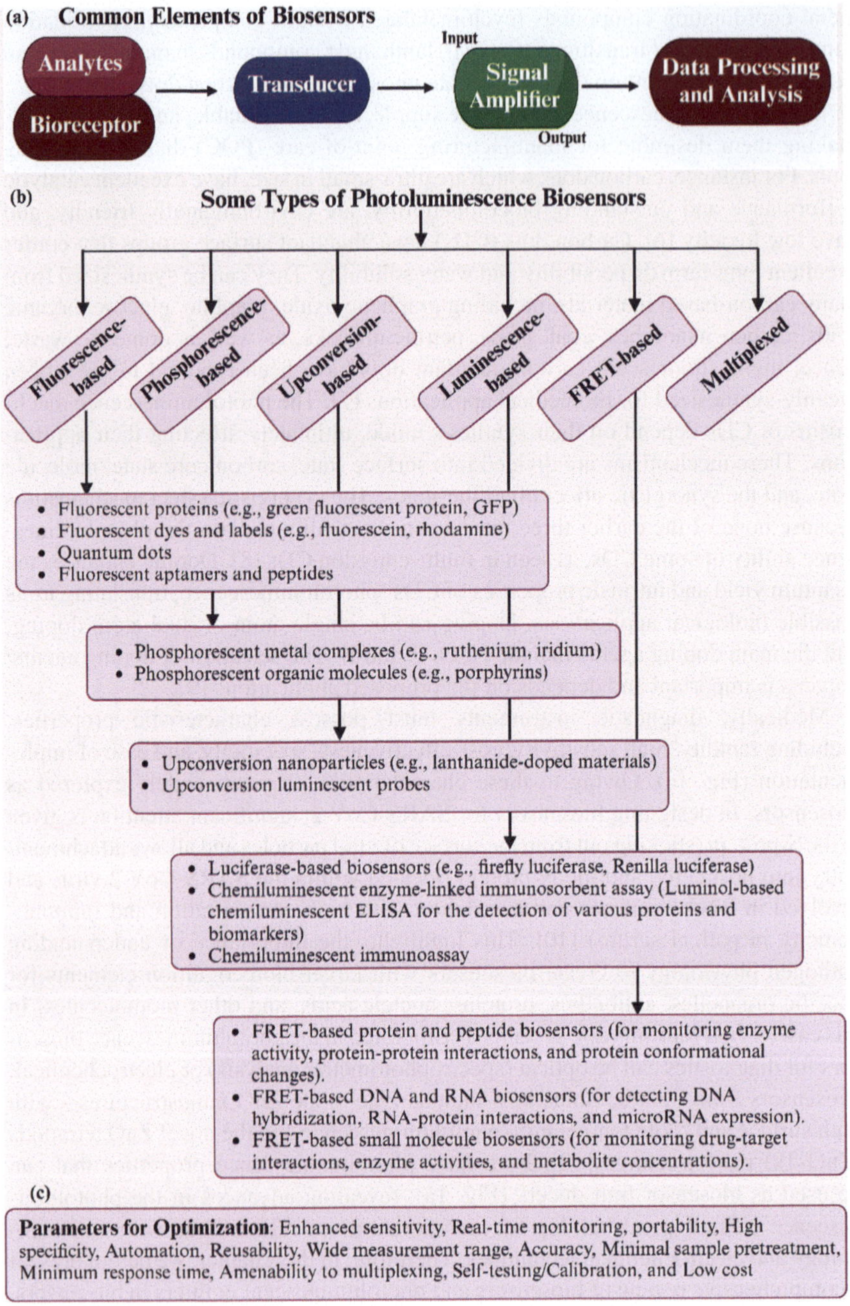

Fig. 1 The operation principle of biosensors shows the common elements (**a**), types of photoluminescent biosensors and their examples (**b**), and the specific properties that can be optimized (**c**)

2 Biosensors Utilizing Photoluminescent Emitters

A biosensor is a device that identifies variations in a biological analyte and employs a transducer to transform these variations into an electrical signal (Fig. 1a) [11, 12]. They are important instruments in medical diagnostics, environmental assessment, and food safety [13–15]. The biological recognition element, including enzymes, antibodies, DNA, or cells, engages with the target analyte, while the transducer transforms this contact into a noticeable signal [16]. Photoluminescence refers to light emission from matter following photon absorption, wherein the excited state experiences relaxation processes before photon reradiation. The observation of photoluminescence at specific energies signifies the population of the state linked to that transition energy [17]. Optical transducers that employ photoluminescent materials are esteemed for their exceptional sensitivity, fast response, and non-invasive sensing abilities.

Photoluminescence is categorized into two primary types: fluorescence, characterized by the fast emission of light following stimulation (within nanoseconds), and phosphorescence, which involves a delayed emission ranging from milliseconds to minutes [17]. Photoluminescent materials, including organic dyes, quantum dots, and rare-earth elements, are especially advantageous in optical biosensors because they generate quantifiable optical signals in reaction to biological interactions. The optical biosensors quantify chemiluminescence, absorban-ce, and fluorescence characteristics [13].

2.1 Types of Photoluminescent Emitters Used in Biosensors

Photoluminescent emitters employed in biosensors are classified into various types, each providing specific advantages regarding sensitivity, stability, and spectrum properties.

i. **Organic dyes**, including fluorescein, rhodamine, and cyanine, are typical fluorescent substances extensively used in biosensors due to their high quantum yield and capacity for conjugation with biological molecules for specific analyte detection [18]. Nonetheless, their effectiveness is frequently undermined by photobleaching, a phenomenon in which their fluorescence intensity decreases with extended light exposure, rendering them less appropriate for sustained applications.
ii. **Quantum dots (QDs)** are semiconductor nanoparticles characterized by their ultrasmall size, generally ranging from 1 to 10 nm, commonly reported as carbon, graphene, and graphdiyne quantum dots [19]. They present notable advantages, including size-tunable fluorescence, exceptional brightness, and a strong resistance to photobleaching. The combination of these properties and

Table 1 Types of photoluminescent emitters used in biosensors

Emitter type	Characteristics	Examples
Organic dyes	High quantum yield, easy conjugation with biomolecules, prone to photobleaching	Fluorescein, rhodamine
Quantum Dots (QDs)	Size-tunable emission, high photostability, narrow emission spectra	CdSe, PbS QDs
Rare-earth-doped materials	Long-lived luminescence, highly resistant to photobleaching, useful for time-resolved assays	Europium (Eu^{3+})-and terbium (Tb^{3+})-doped nanoparticles

their broad absorption and narrow emission spectra make QDs ideal for multiplexed biosensing, enabling the simultaneous detection of several analytes with a mono-light source [20, 21].

iii. **Rare-earth elements** have received considerable interest as fluorescent labeling reagents for microsecond time-resolved fluorescence bioassays owing to their distinctive spectroscopic properties, such as large Stokes shift, extended fluorescence lifetimes, and sharp emission bands at longer wavelengths [22]. Materials doped with rare-earth elements, including europium- and terbium-based nanoparticles, demonstrate prolonged luminescence and outstanding photostability [22]. The value of these materials is especially pronounced in time-resolved fluorescence assays, as their delayed emission capability minimizes background interference, thereby enhancing their suitability for sensitive biosensing applications (see Table 1).

2.2 Working Principles of Biosensors with Photoluminescent Emitters

Photoluminescent biosensors transform biological interactions into optical signals, with the detection technique predominantly dependent on alterations in photoluminescent characteristics, including intensity, wavelength variations, or fluorescence lifetime in reaction to the target analyte. The interaction between the photoluminescent emitter and either the recognition element or the ambient environment prompts alterations. Multiple essential sensing techniques are employed in photoluminescent biosensors. **Förster Resonance Energy Transfer (FRET)** is a quantum mechanical process wherein energy from an excited donor is non-radiatively conveyed to a ground state acceptor at a less than 10 nm proximity [23]. This distance is why FRET is frequently used biologically to investigate molecular interactions that typically occur in close proximity. FRET has been extensively adopted in many fluorescent applications, such as medical diagnostics, optical imaging, DNA analysis, and other sensing capabilities [24]. **Quenching-based biosensors** detect analytes by reducing the fluorescence intensity of the emitter through its interaction with a quencher, a technique especially efficient for detecting tiny molecules such as glucose or metal ions. In contrast, **turn-on fluorescence biosensors** depend on activating a previously quenched emitter upon analyte binding, resulting in a recovered fluorescence signal by providing excellent sensitivity due to minimal background noise. Finally, **ratiometric fluorescence biosensors** quantify substances by assessing the variation in the ratio of fluorescence intensities at two distinct wavelengths [25], thereby enhancing detection accuracy and stability by reducing the impact of environmental variables such as pH or light fluctuations. Figure 1a shows the generic working principles of biosensors with photoluminescent emitters.

2.3 Applications for Photoluminescent Biosensors

Photoluminescent biosensors have various applications in multiple fields, such as medical diagnostics, drug discovery, food safety, and environmental monitoring [10, 26]. In medical diagnostics, these biosensors are employed to identify illnesses, biomarkers, and infections with great sensitivity. Quantum dot (QD)-based immunoassays can identify prostate-specific antigen (PSA), a biomarker for prostate cancer, facilitating early and accurate detection. In environmental monitoring, photoluminescent biosensors are essential for identifying contaminants such as heavy metals and pesticides in water and air. QD-based sensors, designed for mercury (Hg^{2+}) and cadmium (Cd^{2+}) ions detection, offer efficient and sensitive techniques for monitoring these hazardous materials. In the food industry, these biosensors serve to detect foodborne pathogens such as *Escherichia coli* and *Salmonella*, facilitating prompt identification and prevention of contamination. Overall, photoluminescent biosensors play an important function in drug discovery, being used in high-throughput screening to observe molecular interactions, enzyme activities, and cellular responses [10]. Their exceptional photostability and ability to multiplex render them especially advantageous for monitoring several drug targets simultaneously.

3 Two Major Primary Mechanisms Employed in Photoluminescent Biosensors

3.1 Fluorescence Resonance Energy Transfer (FRET)

Fluorescence resonance energy transfer (FRET), which depends on the energy transfer between acceptor and donor molecules, is an effective method for observing biomolecular interactions at the nanoscale. The FRET-based aptasensor is highly promising owing to its immediate responsiveness and practical quantification [26, 27]. FRET, as a photophysical process, exhibits exceptional sensitivity to the distance between the donor and acceptor, generally within 1–10 nm of the non-radiative energy transfer, rendering it a suitable technique for investigating molecular interactions, conformational alterations, and precise spatial correlations [28]. Efficient energy transfer requires that the donor and acceptor are in close proximity and that the donor's emission spectrum substantially overlaps with the acceptor's absorption spectrum. Thus, this mechanism is highly reliant on relative orientation and distance. Significantly, energy is conveyed directly through space, avoiding photon emission through dipole–dipole interactions. The efficiency of energy transfer (E) relies on the distance (r) separating the acceptor and donor and can be articulated by the subsequent equation:

$$E = \frac{R_0^6}{R_0^6 + r^6}$$

where:

E is the FRET efficiency,

r is the distance between the donor and acceptor fluorophores,

R_0 is the Förster distance, the distance at which the efficiency of energy transfer is 50%.

The Förster distance (R_0) is an important parameter in FRET studies since it dictates the sensitivity of energy transfer between donor and acceptor molecules. Förster distance (R_0), the intermolecular distance at which 50% of the maximum potential energy transfer occurs is an important parameter for all types of resonance energy transfer (RET). It offers a method for determining the range of distances measurable by any RET probe pair [29]. R_0 is affected by multiple parameters, such as the donor's quantum yield, the refractive index of the surrounding medium, and the degree of overlap between the donor's emission spectrum and the acceptor's absorption spectrum. The Förster distance for most FRET couples generally ranges from 2 to 6 nm, serving as an essential parameter for evaluating molecule closeness and interaction efficacy. The formula for determining R_0 is:

$$R_0^6 = \frac{8.79 \times 10^{-25} \cdot \kappa^2 \cdot \Phi_D \cdot n^{-4} \cdot J(\lambda)}{L}$$

where:

κ^2 is the orientation factor between the donor and acceptor dipoles,

Φ_D is the donor's quantum yield,

n is the medium's refractive index,

$J(\lambda)$ is the spectral overlap integral, which quantifies the overlap between donor emission and acceptor absorption,

L is the Avogadro constant.

$$E = 1 - \frac{F_D}{F_{D0}}$$

where:

F_D is the fluorescence intensity of the donor in the presence of the acceptor,

F_{D0} is the fluorescence intensity of the donor in the absence of the acceptor.

FRET can also be used to estimate distances using the relationship between FRET efficiency and distance:

$$r = R_0 \left(\frac{1 - E}{E} \right)^{\frac{1}{6}}$$

This enables researchers to precisely quantify molecular distances within the 1–10 nm range, which is especially advantageous for investigating protein–protein interactions, conformational alterations, and macromolecular assemblies.

3.1.1 Application of Fluorescence Resonance Energy Transfer (FRET)

FRET has extensive biological research applications, rendering it an indispensable instrument for examining molecular interactions and dynamic processes. A common use involves examining protein–protein interactions, wherein proteins are tagged with donors and acceptor fluorophores to assess their closeness and deduce potential connections. This has been used in examining interactions among signaling proteins, enzymes, and their substrates, as well as receptors and their ligands. FRET is essential for observing conformational alterations in biomolecules such as proteins and nucleic acids. By positioning fluorophores at designated sites, researchers may monitor distance variations that transpire during structural alterations, providing immediate insights into the dynamic behavior of these molecules. FRET is employed in nucleic acid research to investigate nucleic acid (DNA and RNA) structural conformation and folding, yielding insights into their secondary and tertiary structures and their interactions with other molecules.

Furthermore, FRET-based biosensors have been developed to identify diverse biological and chemical substances. These biosensors function by detecting FRET signals induced by conformational alterations or interactions that position fluorophores in close proximity. They have also been used to observe cellular activities such as calcium ion concentration, pH variations, and enzyme activity. A significant application of FRET-based biosensors lies in nucleic acid hybridization assays, where FRET signals indicate successful complementary DNA or RNA strand binding.

Moreover, nanotechnology advancements have enabled the integration of quantum dots as FRET donors, offering superior photostability and tunable emission properties compared to traditional organic dyes [5]. Furthermore, FRET is extensively employed in microscopy, especially with fluorescence microscopy methods like confocal and total internal reflection fluorescence (TIRF) imaging. FRET microscopy facilitates high spatial and temporal resolution observation of molecular interactions in living cells, enabling researchers to examine dynamic processes within subcellular compartments in real time [4]. These biosensors often incorporate genetically encoded fluorescent proteins or synthetic dyes as donor–acceptor pairs.

Notwithstanding its extensive application and adaptability, FRET has several limitations that necessitate careful consideration in experimental design. One major challenge is the careful selection of donor and acceptor fluorophore pairings to guarantee adequate spectrum overlap while reducing interference from autofluorescence. Moreover, FRET's sensitivity to the orientation and distance between fluorophores implies that structural alterations or environmental variables can influence the accuracy of results. Also, the photobleaching of fluorophores over time presents a challenge, potentially compromising the reliability of long-term measurements. When optimized by careful fluorophore selection and regulated experimental conditions, FRET continues to be an effective method for investigating molecular interactions and dynamics at nanometer-scale distances. Its capacity to deliver real-time, in situ measurements renders it indispensable for various biological and biochemical applications, providing profound insights into the principles governing molecular processes in living cells and complicated molecular systems [4]. Table 2 shows the common donor–acceptor pairs used in FRET experiments, their excitation and emission wavelengths, and their Förster distances.

3.2 Chemiluminescence Assays—Biosensors Utilizing Photoluminescent Emitters

Chemiluminescence assays are highly sensitive analytical methods that quantify light emission resulting from a chemical process. Chemiluminescence offers excellent analytical performance, attributed to its independence from external light sources, absence of background interference, and remarkable sensitivity and selectivity [30]. In recent times, chemiluminescence assays have been extensively employed as innovative quantification methods in disease diagnosis microbiological safety, food and drug analysis, pollutant detection, etc. due to their simplicity, high sensitivity, and specificity. In contrast to fluorescence, which necessitates external light to stimulate molecules, chemiluminescence occurs directly from the process, wherein specific molecules emit energy as photons while transitioning to a lower energy state. Chemiluminescence is based on the oxidation of a luminophore, a light-emitting molecule, during a chemical reaction [31, 32]. Common luminophores (light-emitting molecules) include luminol, acridinium esters, and peroxyoxalates,

Table 2 Comparison of FRET and chemiluminescence assays

Features	FRET	Chemiluminescence
Excitation source	Needed	Not needed
Sensitivity	High	Very high
Spatial resolution	Excellent	Limited
Temporal resolution	High	Moderate
Photobleaching/phototoxicity	Significant	Minimal
Background interference	Moderate	Low
Materials	(a) Quantum Dots (QDs) (b) Fluorescent Tagged Proteins (XFP): (i) CFP (Cyan Donor Fluorophore); YFP (Yellow Acceptor Fluorophore); 433 nm Donor Excitation; 527 nm Acceptor Emission; 5.0 nm Förster Distance (ii) GFP (Green Donor Fluorophore); RFP (Red Acceptor Fluorophore); 488 nm Donor Excitation; 607 nm Acceptor Emission; 4.8 nm Förster Distance (iii) Alexa Fluor 488 (Donor Fluorophore); Alexa Fluor 555 (Acceptor Fluorophore); 490 nm Donor Excitation; 565 nm Acceptor Emission; 6.0 nm Förster Distance	Luminol, Cypridina luciferin, 2-methyl-6-phenyl-3,7-dihydroimidazo[1,2-α]pyrazin-3-one (CLA), Oxalate, Dioxetane, 1,2-Dioxetane, etc.
Key process	(a) Excitation of the donor fluorophore, promoting electrons from the ground state to an excited state by absorbing light energy at a specific wavelength, such as a laser (b) Non-radiative energy transfer to nearby acceptor fluorophore from the excited donor fluorophore through dipole–dipole interactions in a highly distance dependent manner (c) Acceptor fluorophore, upon receiving the donor energy, becomes excited and subsequently emits light at a longer wavelength (lower energy) than the donor's emission. The acceptor fluorescence can then be detected and measured	(a) Formation of high-energy intermediates such as 1,2-dioxetane, 1,2-dioxetanone, and 1,2-dioxetanedione, which release sufficient energy to produce visible light (ranging from 40 to 70 kcal/mol) (b) Decomposition of these high-energy intermediates and chemiexcitation to an excited state (c) Emission of light from the excited state
Applications	Protein localization and interactions, live-cell imaging and dynamics	Clinical diagnostics, gene tracking and ROS detection

which react with specific analytes or enzymatic products and release light upon oxidation products [33]. The produced light's intensity is directly proportional to the reactants' concentration, facilitating quantitative measurement with equipment like luminometers.

The general reaction can be summarized as:

$$\text{Oxidant} + \text{Luminophore} \rightarrow \text{Excited-state intermediate} \rightarrow \text{Light emission} + \text{Stable product}$$

3.2.1 Types of Chemiluminescence Assays

Chemiluminescence assays are recognized for their sensitive signals, minimal background interference, and extensive applicability in research and clinical settings [34, 35]. They exist in various forms, each characterized by distinct mechanisms for producing light through chemical reactions. In **direct chemiluminescence assays**, the luminous response arises directly from the pertinent chemical interaction, exemplified by luminol reacting with hydrogen peroxide in biological samples, where the light intensity correlates with the concentration of hydrogen peroxide [32]. **Enzyme-linked chemiluminescence assays (ECLAs)** employ enzymes such as horseradish peroxidase (HRP) or alkaline phosphatase to facilitate a luminous reaction. In these assays, typically employed in immunoassays, an antibody or antigen is conjugated to an enzyme, and following binding to the target molecule, a chemiluminescent substrate is injected, with the enzyme facilitating light production. ECLAs often cover procedures including antigen or antibody immobilization, analyte binding, introduction of enzyme-labeled antibodies, and light detection using plate readers [36]. **Electrochemiluminescence (ECL) assays** integrate electrochemical methods with chemiluminescence, wherein light is produced by species stimulated through oxidation or reduction at an electrode interface. ECL assays, recognized for their elevated sensitivity and little background signal, are extensively employed in diagnostic applications, exemplified by the Roche Elecsys® system for detecting biomarkers, including hormones and tumor markers. Enhanced chemiluminescence applies specialized enhancers, such as *p*-iodophenol and luminol, to augment light intensity and duration, facilitating the identification of minimal concentrations of proteins or antibodies in complex biological samples. This method is especially beneficial in applications like Western blotting and ELISAs.

3.2.2 Applications for Chemiluminescence Assays

Chemiluminescence assays possess widespread applications in diverse disciplines due to their exceptional sensitivity and specificity. Immunoassays, as detailed by [30], are frequently employed in techniques such as enzyme-linked immunosorbent assays (ELISAs), western blotting, and radioimmunoassays, rendering them optimal for diagnostic applications, especially in the detection of hormones, medicines, and biomarkers associated with infectious diseases. Chemiluminescence immunoassay integrates chemiluminescence with immunoassay methodologies commonly employed in clinical diagnostics and biomolecule detection, showcasing its applicability in food safety assessments, such as mycotoxin, heavy metal and drug residue analysis [37, 38]. Chemiluminescent immunoassays (CLIA) are extensively used for the quantitative detection of biomarkers. In CLIA, antibodies conjugated with chemiluminescent labels emit light upon binding to the target analyte. The intensity of the emitted light, directly proportional to the concentration of analyte, is measured using a luminometer [33, 39–41]. Another noteworthy application of chemiluminescence is in oxidative stress measurement, where reactive oxygen species (ROS) interact with chemiluminescent probes to produce light. This approach is widely used in research exploring the role of oxidative stress in various diseases [42]. Chemiluminescent assays are essential **in nucleic acid** detection within molecular biology, particularly in hybridization techniques such as Southern and Northern blotting, where DNA or RNA probes hybridize with target sequences, and chemiluminescence facilitates the detection and quantification of specific nucleic acids. **In genetic research** [43], chemiluminescent reporter gene assays, including luciferase-based assays, are employed to investigate gene expression, with light emission directly correlating to the transcriptional activity of the gene of interest, while **in environmental monitoring and food safety testing** [44] chemiluminescence assays have been used to monitor and identify pollutants, pathogens or hazardous chemicals in food such as pesticides, heavy metals, and toxins.

3.2.3 Advantages and Limitations of Chemiluminescence Assays

Chemiluminescence assays have numerous substantial benefits, rendering them extremely effective for detecting and quantifying various analytes. They are recognized for their exceptional sensitivity, enabling the detection of minimal analyte concentrations owing to the elevated quantum efficiency of the light-emitting processes. These assays have an extensive dynamic range, facilitating precise measurement of both low and high concentrations. In contrast to fluorescence-based tests, chemiluminescence exhibits little background noise as it does not necessitate external light sources for excitation, hence improving the signal-to-noise ratio. Chemiluminescent reactions occur rapidly, generally within seconds to minutes, rendering them suitable for rapid analysis. Moreover, numerous chemiluminescence experiments are more affordable, requiring fewer components than fluorescence-based techniques. However, there are limitations, such as signal attenuation in specific reactions, necessitating precise timing for detection, and potential interference from compounds in complex biological samples, resulting in false positives or negatives. The high cost of equipment, including luminometers, may also be a factor for smaller laboratories. Notwithstanding these problems, chemiluminescence assays are effective in fields including molecular biology, clinical diagnostics, and environmental monitoring. Their continuous advancement, especially in reagent chemistry and detection technologies, expands their capabilities and applications, as shown in Table 2.

4 In Vitro and in Vivo Diagnostic Applications

Photoluminescence-applied sensors are used to detect biomarkers, toxins, and adulterations because of their high sensitivity, cost-effectiveness, stability, and biocompatibility. Photoluminescence is a dynamic part of sensing acquired due to surface passivation and functionalization of the CDs and graphene QDs [45, 46]. The sensing mechanism of photoluminescence carbon dots and graphene quantum dots is based on quenching or fluorescence enhancement [47, 48].

Numerous red/NIR emitting CDs can monitor and visualize Cr^{6+} and Fe^{3+} in living cells and also analyze intracellular temperature [49]. An in vitro diagnostic application of photoluminescence uses orange-emissive carbon dots immobilized in medical cotton cloth to monitor wound pH due to its pH-sensitive fluorescence, thereby acting as a pH sensor. Monitoring wound pH can be used in identifying nonhealing wounds and detecting early infections, as the orange CDs can respond distinctly to changes in pH, giving pH-sensitive fluorescence over the pH range of 5 to 9. This is indicative of CDs fluorescence colour variation in pH, thus giving precise measurements. Apart from the portable nature of CD pH sensors, CDs coated cloths are gaining increasing attention as they are resistant to blood contamination influence and long-term storage [50].

Another way photoluminescence is used in point-of-care diagnostics involves the formation of quantum dot-biomolecule hybrids, i.e., quantum dots conjugated to aptamers, antibodies, etc. These probes are employed in in vitro bioassays and biosensors [51]. An advantage of quantum dots over organic dyes is the ability to simultaneously determine different biomolecules using a single excitation wavelength in addition to their size-controlled luminescence [7]. Advances in the bioconjugation of quantum dots have resulted in their application in the monitoring of molecular surface dynamics of membrane-associated molecules, detection of tumor biomarkers, molecular interactions quantification at subcellular and cellular levels, and cell motility measurement [7, 19, 47, 48].

As biomarkers, they are functional indicators of the biological processes occurring in living systems that show either normal physiological or pathological states [2, 29, 34]. Photoluminescence offers a clearer approach to detecting inflammatory biomarkers such as C-reactive protein (CRP) and glycoprotein procalcitonin (PCT). C-reactive protein is an important biomarker of infection, inflammation, obesity, and cardiovascular diseases, and it can be measured in the blood. The standard clinical assays do not have sufficient sensitivity for low levels of CRP, which is believed to have participated in the acute myocardial infarction- and coronary heart disease development needed for the prediction of cardiovascular diseases [52], while in the case of PCT, it is essential for the diagnosis of sepsis [53] since viral infections do not cause an elevation in PCT levels neither do autoimmune diseases. Using long-lived emissive nanoparticles provides a sensitive time selection-based analytical method because they have a luminescence lifetime of 10^{-4} to 10^{2} s, which lowers the fluorescent background while improving analysis accuracy [54].

Chemiluminescence assays, leveraging light emission from chemical reactions, are powerful tools for detecting and quantifying analytes with exceptional sensitivity [55, 56]. By eliminating the need for external excitation sources, chemiluminescence minimizes background noise and enhances signal-to-noise ratios, making it highly suitable for both in vitro and in vivo diagnostics. This section highlights two major applications: disease biomarker detection and imaging of cellular processes.

4.1 Disease Biomarker Detection

The sensitive and selective identification of biomarkers is important in diagnosing disease progression, organ dysfunction and estimating disease state. Biomarkers are found in body fluids such as plasma, saliva, and urine, as well as in different body tissues. The construction of fluorogenic biosensors has enabled the successful detection of multiple analytes. Various disease biomarkers can now be detected simultaneously in homogenous solutions or cells, resulting in accurate diagnosis [1, 57]. For example, three tumor suppressor genes-p16, p21, and p53 can be detected simultaneously using a multicolour graphene oxide probe. It was observed that a selective increase in fluorescence was recorded on the interaction of the graphene oxide/multi-DNA sensor and a given tumor suppressor gene without any interference from none-selected genes, as carbon dots are also widely explored in drug (gene, vaccine, and antiviral) delivery [57]. Also, carbohydrate interactions with proteins are common in pathological processes; the efficient identification and analysis of these interactions could serve as an avenue for diagnosing such diseases and devising treatment modalities [1, 2, 58]. Biosensors are devised with two glycoligands having different fluorophores conjugated to graphene oxide, whereby the presence of the glycoligand receptors resulted in the restoration of fluorescence similar to the "turn on fluorescence sensors" [59].

Chemiluminescence-based assays [5, 39, 41] are widely used for detecting disease biomarkers in clinical diagnostics due to their high sensitivity and specificity (Fig. 2). These assays are commonly employed in immunoassays, where chemiluminescent probes are conjugated to antibodies or other recognition molecules. A chemical reaction is triggered upon binding to the target analyte, resulting in light emission directly proportional to the analyte concentration [41]. A notable example is the detection of cardiac troponin, a myocardial infarction biomarker. Chemiluminescent immunoassays (CLIAs) offer superior performance in quantifying troponin levels, enabling rapid and accurate diagnosis of heart attacks. Similarly, CLIAs are widely used to measure levels of hormones, cytokines, and infectious disease markers [40]. Recent advancements in chemiluminescence technology, such as nanoparticle-based probes and novel luminophores, offer enhanced stability, brightness, and tunability.

These innovations expand the range of detectable biomarkers and improve assay performance in complex biological matrices [41, 55].

microRNAs (miRNAs) regulate gene expression by interacting with proteins or altering epigenetic pathways. A malfunction in miRNAs expression has been associated with human diseases like cancer [19]. Label-free fluorescent probe based on a G-quadruplex/thioflavin T (ThT) complex can be used to generate the signal output for miRNA detection. While G-quadruplex structure is formed by the combination of the catalytic hairpin assembly (CHA), DNAzyme-based cycling, and primer exchange reaction (PER) amplification process for enhanced sensitivity, the fluorescence signal enhancement results from the binding of G-quadruplex to ThT. Thus, G-quadruplex/ThT complex produces photoluminescence signal transduction mechanism that is measured and correlated with the concentration of the target miRNAs such as miRNA-21 in cellular extracts [60]. Glucose monitoring is essential in managing diabetes, a metabolic disorder of public health concern. The development of non-invasive blood glucose monitoring nanotechnology is highly desired. A nanosensor for continuous fluorescent sensing of glucose with biocompatibility photostable fluorophores made of nanodiamond boronic hydrogel system was designed by Zhang and team members [42]. Hyperbilirubinemia can occur in both children and adults, with the potential to result in jaundice, hepatitis, brain injury, or death. Also, low levels are associated with iron deficiencies and cardiovascular diseases. One method developed for accurately quantifying bilirubin involves using L-cysteine stabilized copper nanocluster (L-cys-CuNC). The interaction between bilirubin, biliverdin, and L-cys-CuNCs results in fluorescence quenching [61]. B-type natriuretic peptides are used

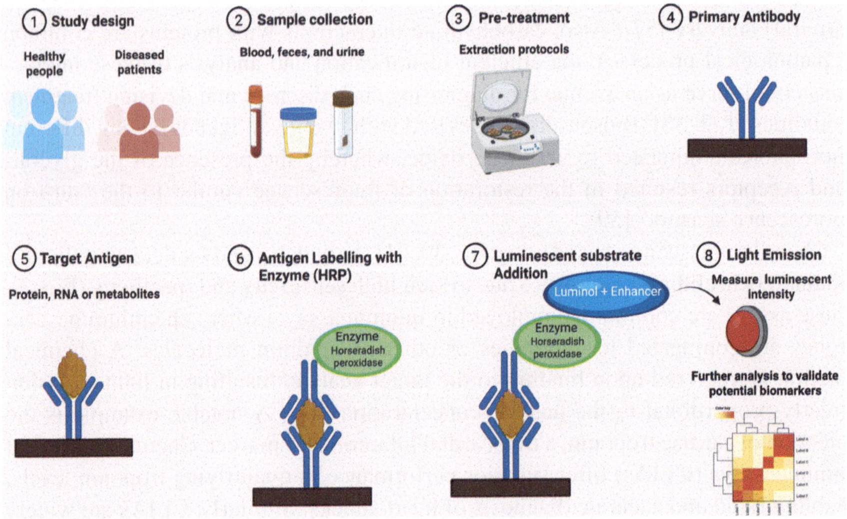

Fig. 2 A systematic illustration of the exploration of chemiluminescence enzyme immunoassay in detecting biomarkers from diseased patients in an antibody-conjugated system. The figure was created using BioRender

for diagnosing/prognoses of acute myocardial infarction and are released from the heart [62]. With the aid of core technology and probe technique made up of upconversion nanoparticles lateral flow strips (UCNPs-LFS), B-type natriuretic peptide and suppression of tumorigenicity two (2) were measured concurrently.

For multiplexed cancer detection, antibody-conjugated single-band up-conversion nanoparticles (UCNPs), which have multiple colouration were fabricated to surmount the ineffectiveness of conventional biochemical techniques. These UCNPs produce photoluminescence through tissue-transparent near-infrared irradiation. This was used to detect the expression of typical breast cancer biomarkers: progesterone- and estrogen receptor, and the human epidermal growth factor receptor 2 in cells and tissue samples [1, 2, 29, 34, 57, 58]. The burgeoning of multiplexed photoluminescent sensors to multiple biomarkers in homologous solutions, identifying a specific cell in a mixture of cells, or imaging multiple biomarkers of a single cell or pathogen is now possible [63].

4.2 *Imaging of Cellular Processes*

Optical imaging provided by photoluminescent probes is a powerful tool in the biomedical field for the early detection, screening, and treatment of diseases [10, 58]. Targeting specific molecules in vitro and in vivo serves as a means of identifying events happening at the molecular level within cells or tissues. Photoluminescent CDs are used for bioimaging due to their solubility, photo- and thermal stability, low toxicity, tunable photoluminescence, and biocompatibility [27, 47, 58]. The first set of carbon dots utilized in bioimaging encountered the problem of low image quality due to spin–orbit coupling effects. The higher-grade carbon dots recently synthesized have red/NIR emissions with excellent photostability, larger penetration depth, and the avoidance of background fluorescence [47, 57]. CDs and graphene QDs are applied in biosensing and diagnostics because CDs have active components like H, N, C, and O on their surfaces and exhibit tunable bright fluorescence properties across the visible range. Graphene QDs, though having tunable photoluminescence properties, are also biocompatible with high photostability [19].

The first recorded use of photoluminescence in bioimaging was achieved in 2006 by labeling the *Escherichia coli* cells using PEG1500N-passivated CDs; however recent studies reveal the probing polarity and pH sensitivity of CDs in *E. coli* intracellular domain through time-resolved fluorescence analyses [64]. Wavelength-tunable luminescent CDs with cross-linker glutaraldehyde linked to yellow luminescent CDs can be used to study HeLa cells in relation to several diseases such as cervix cancer [59], breast cancer [19], and cervical cancer [60]. These CDs have high-quality nucleolus imaging capacity in fixed and living cells, providing a means for the possible delivery of drugs to the nucleus specifically and for cancer therapy. N-doped CDs, when synthesized from pyrrolic nitrogen concentrated in the mitochondria, serve as good mitochondria imaging molecules [65]. In addition, N-doped CDs with two-photon excitation at 800 nm can be used in imaging the human breast cancer cells when femtosecond pulsed laser is applied or through the precise and swift ablation process [66]. Under a fluorescence microscope in a temperature-dependent manner, the carbon dots imaged the cell membranes and cytoplasm without entering the nucleus. N, Se-carbon dots have free radical scavenging ability and, therefore, could protect cells from oxidative stress in a structure-properties relationship giving good signals during bioimaging [67]. Also, the in vivo imaging of nude mice administered carbon dots (CDs) aqueous solution through intravenous injection showed biocompatibility and excellent imaging at different time points [68]. Notably, FRET as shown in Fig. 3 is widely explored method in cellular imaging.

Chemiluminescence is a valuable tool for imaging cellular processes, particularly in live cells and animal models [55]. Its high sensitivity and minimal background interference enable real-time visualization of biochemical reactions and cellular activities. Unlike fluorescence imaging, which requires external illumination, chemiluminescence avoids photobleaching and phototoxicity, making it ideal for longitudinal studies [41]. One prominent application is the monitoring of reactive oxygen species (ROS) and other oxidative stress markers [69]. Chemiluminescent probes, such as luminol or coelenterazine, react with ROS to emit light, providing insights into

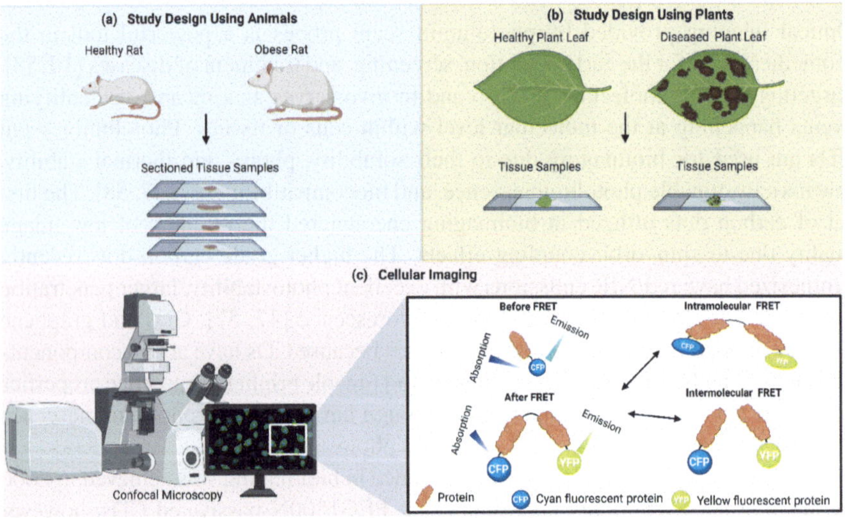

Fig. 3 Systematic illustration of FRET application. **a** The study was designed using a healthy or obese rat to understand the protein interactions that trigger the phenotypic change. **b** The study design used healthy and diseased plant leaves to deduce the protein interaction or conformational changes resulting in black spot formation in diseased leaves. **c** Cellular imaging of FRET mostly requires the use of confocal microscopes such as STELLARIS confocal microscope platform by Leica, ZEISS LSM 900 confocal, and recently MINIFLUX microscopy in observing the CFP (donor) and YFP (acceptor) absorption and emission spectra. Overlap between the emission and absorption of CFP and YFP leads to efficient FRET interaction. This interaction can be used to deduce intramolecular FRET or intermolecular FRET. The figure was created using BioRender

oxidative stress-related diseases. Additionally, genetically encoded chemiluminescent reporters, like NanoLuc luciferase, allow for the non-invasive tracking of gene expression and protein–protein interactions in vivo. Chemiluminescence assays serve as versatile tools in disease biomarker detection and imaging of cellular processes. With continuous advancements in probe design and detection systems, these assays hold significant promise for improving diagnostic precision and broadening the scope of biomedical research.

5 Challenges and Future Perspectives

While photoluminescent biosensors offer numerous benefits, several challenges must be overcome to realize their full potential. High and persistent emission efficiencies in carbon quantum dots and desirable longevity have yet to be achieved, which is important for applications requiring long-term safety. Although the literature presents some evidence indicating that carbon quantum dots demonstrate high photostability over extended periods of UV exposure, numerous studies have also documented their photobleaching behavior. Given that quantum dots and rare-earth-based emitters demonstrate better photostability, additional investigations are necessary to improve their long-term performance. The biocompatibility of functionalized carbon quantum dots is a significant concern for their application in live cells, tissues, and animals, posing a possible limitation for medical therapy trials. A further problem pertains to the complication and expense associated with fabricating photoluminescent materials such as quantum dots and rare-earth nanoparticles, which require meticulous synthesis and functionalization methods and can be excessively costly. Future research may concentrate on developing more biocompatible and stable photoluminescent materials, enhancing detection sensitivity via innovative transduction processes, and expanding the scope of applications, especially in personalized medicine and point-of-care diagnostics. Advancements in materials science, bioconjugation, and nanomaterial synthesis indicate that next-generation photoluminescent biosensors will be increasingly sensitive, durable, and adaptable, hence expanding opportunities in healthcare, environmental monitoring, food safety, and other fields.

6 Conclusion

This chapter has discussed in-depth the advances and applications of several photoluminescent biosensors, focusing on medical diagnostics. The combination of nanotechnology, albeit new surface modification techniques and improved materials, has considerably increased these sensors' specificity and sensitivity. These advancements are critical for detecting very low biomarker concentrations required for disease diagnosis and monitoring. The chapter also emphasizes the importance of designing and implementing biosensors that use low-cost, novel materials with high surface area, variable porosity, and chemical activity to detect analytes efficiently while diffusing them quickly. Such properties are especially useful in biomedical applications and wearable sensors, where biomarker detection must be rapid and accurate. Although photoluminescent biosensors have demonstrated remarkable potential in medical diagnostics; however, incorporating innovative materials into biosensor design can increase signal transduction, which is critical for detecting low-concentration analytes, hence increasing sensor reliability and efficiency. Advances in functional nanomaterial sciences have created new biosensor synthesis and fabrication opportunities, resulting in more effective diagnostic tools. Notably, photoluminescent biosensors' capacity to detect specific biomarkers in vivo and in vitro with high precision and sensitivity renders them highly valuable in the early detection of diseases like cancer and cardiovascular diseases, just to mention a few. The early identification revealed by these sensors enables timely intervention, potentially enhancing patient outcomes and lowering healthcare expenditures. Nonetheless, further studies are needed to overcome obstacles in applying photoluminescent biosensors, such as sensor material stability, reproducibility of results, and sensor integration into user-friendly devices.

Disclosure of Funding Sources Not applicable.

Financial Disclosure The authors have no sources of funding or other financial disclosures concerning the manuscript.

Declaration of Competing Interest The authors declare that there are no conflicts of interest.

References

1. Bakhshipour, F., Zibaei, M., Rokni, M.B., Miahipour, A., Firoozeh, F., Beheshti, M., et al.: Comparative evaluation of real-time PCR and ELISA for the detection of human fascioliasis. Sci. Rep. **14**, 3865 (2024). https://doi.org/10.1038/s41598-024-54602-y
2. Elbasiony, A.M., Alharthi, S., Mohamady Ghobashy, M., Boraie, W.E., Attia, M.S., Madani, M., et al.: Development and application of novel biosensors for enhanced detection in medical diagnostics. Microchem. J. **207**, 111938 (2024). https://doi.org/10.1016/j.microc.2024.111938
3. Chiatti, C., Fabiani, C., Bondi, R., Zampini, G., Latterini, L., Pisello, A.L.: Controlled combination of phosphorescent and fluorescent materials to exploit energy-saving potential in the built environment. Energy **275**, 127333 (2023). https://doi.org/10.1016/j.energy.2023.127333
4. Neema, P.M., Tomy, A.M., Cyriac, J.: Chemical sensor platforms based on fluorescence resonance energy transfer (FRET) and 2D materials. TrAC-Trends Anal. Chem. **124**, 115797 (2020). https://doi.org/10.1016/j.trac.2019.115797
5. Choi, J.H., Ha, T., Shin, M., Lee, S.N., Choi, J.W.: Nanomaterial-based fluorescence resonance energy transfer (FRET) and metal-enhanced fluorescence (MEF) to detect nucleic acid in cancer diagnosis. Biomedicines **9** (2021). https://doi.org/10.3390/biomedicines9080928
6. Kaurav, H., Verma, D., Bansal, A., Kapoor, D.N., Sheth, S.: Progress in drug delivery and diagnostic applications of carbon dots: a systematic review. Front. Chem. **11** (2023). https://doi.org/10.3389/fchem.2023.1227843
7. Praseetha, P.K., Litany, R.I.J., Alharbi, H.M., Khojah, A.A., Akash, S., Bourhia, M., et al.: Green synthesis of highly fluorescent carbon quantum dots from almond resin for advanced theranostics in biomedical applications. Sci. Rep. **14**, 24435 (2024). https://doi.org/10.1038/s41598-024-75333-0

8. He, C., Xu, P., Zhang, X., Long, W.: The synthetic strategies, photoluminescence mechanisms and promising applications of carbon dots: current state and future perspective. Carbon N Y **186**, 91–127 (2022). https://doi.org/10.1016/j.carbon.2021.10.002
9. Miao, S., Liang, K., Zhu, J., Yang, B., Zhao, D., Kong, B.: Hetero-atom-doped carbon dots: doping strategies, properties and applications. Nano Today **33**, 100879 (2020). https://doi.org/10.1016/j.nantod.2020.100879
10. Viter, R., Tepliakova, I., Drobysh, M., Zbolotnii, V., Rackauskas, S., Ramanavicius, S., et al.: Photoluminescence-based biosensor for the detection of antibodies against SARS-CoV-2 virus proteins by ZnO tetrapod structure integrated within microfluidic system. Sci. Total. Environ. **939** (2024). https://doi.org/10.1016/j.scitotenv.2024.173333
11. Wang, Y., Liu, K., Zhang, M., Xu, T., Du, H., Pang, B., et al.: Sustainable polysaccharide-based materials for intelligent packaging. Carbohydr. Polym. **313**, 120851 (2023). https://doi.org/10.1016/j.carbpol.2023.120851
12. Jain, U., Saxena, K., Hooda, V., Balayan, S., Singh, A.P., Tikadar, M., et al.: Emerging vistas on pesticides detection based on electrochemical biosensors—an update. Food Chem. **371**, 131126 (2022). https://doi.org/10.1016/j.foodchem.2021.131126
13. Sagar Shrikrishna, N., Sharma, R., Sahoo, J., Kaushik, A., Gandhi, S.: Navigating the landscape of optical biosensors. Chem. Eng. J. **490** (2024). https://doi.org/10.1016/j.cej.2024.151661
14. Salinas, R.A., Martínez Tolibia, S.E., Galdámez-Martínez, A., Romero, J.E., García-Barrera, L.J., Orduña, A., et al.: Real-time nanoscale bacterial detection utilizing a 1DZnO optical nanobiosensor. Adv. Nanobiomed. Res. (2024). https://doi.org/10.1002/anbr.202400013
15. Li, H., Hu, Y., Zhang, Y., Zhang, H., Yao, D., Lin, Y., et al.: Metal halide perovskite nanocrystals-intermediated hydrogel for boosting the biosensing performance. Adv. Mater. **36**, 2409090 (2024). https://doi.org/10.1002/adma.202409090
16. Viter, R., Tepliakova, I., Drobysh, M., Zbolotnii, V., Rackauskas, S., Ramanavicius, S., et al.: Photoluminescence-based biosensor for the detection of antibodies against SARS-CoV-2 virus proteins by ZnO tetrapod structure integrated within microfluidic system. Sci. Total. Environ. **939**, 173333 (2024). https://doi.org/10.1016/j.scitotenv.2024.173333
17. Park, K., Kim, H., Jung, G.W., Gwon, S.Y., Kim, D.H.: Photoluminescence and energy transfer of $Lu_3Al_5O_{12}:Ce^{3+}$, Pr^{3+} phosphors. Ceram. Int. **48**, 5312–5320 (2022). https://doi.org/10.1016/j.ceramint.2021.11.074
18. Floris, F., Figus, C., Quochi, F., Marabelli, F.: Enhanced photoluminescence of organic dyes embedded in sol-gel organosilane thin films. Opt. Mater. (Amst) **156**, 115912 (2024). https://doi.org/10.1016/j.optmat.2024.115912
19. Bahari, D., Babamiri, B., Salimi, A., Rashidi, A.: Graphdiyne/graphene quantum dots for development of FRET ratiometric fluorescent assay toward sensitive detection of miRNA in human serum and bioimaging of living cancer cells. J. Lumin. **239**, 118371 (2021). https://doi.org/10.1016/j.jlumin.2021.118371
20. Zhang, L., Yang, X., Yin, Z., Sun, L.: A review on carbon quantum dots: synthesis, photoluminescence mechanisms and applications. Luminescence **37**, 1612–1638 (2022). https://doi.org/10.1002/bio.4351
21. Zhang, H., Zhang, H.: Special issue: rare earth luminescent materials. Light Sci. Appl. **11**, 260 (2022). https://doi.org/10.1038/s41377-022-00956-9
22. Zhang, H., Zhang, H.: Rare earth luminescent materials. Light Sci. Appl. **11**, 260 (2022). https://doi.org/10.1038/s41377-022-00956-9
23. Li, Y., Qian, M., Cheng, Y., Qiu, X.: Robust visualization of membrane protein by aptamer mediated proximity ligation assay and Förster resonance energy transfer. Colloids Surf. B Biointerfaces **248**, 114486 (2025). https://doi.org/10.1016/j.colsurfb.2024.114486
24. Roy, L., Mukherjee, D., Singh, S., Banerjee, A., Bhattacharyya, N., Halder, A., et al.: Picosecond resolved Förster resonance energy transfer (FRET) differentiates self-assembled biological macromolecules in aqueous medium. Chem. Phys. Impact **4** (2022). https://doi.org/10.1016/j.chphi.2022.100081
25. Han, Y., An, J., Fang, J., Zhang, J., Liu, Y.: Novel hydrogel pillar array based ratiometric multicolor fluorescence biosensor for visual detection of alkaline phosphatase activity. Spectrochim. Acta A Mol. Biomol. Spectrosc. **319** (2024). https://doi.org/10.1016/j.saa.2024.124542.

26. Jain, S., Nehra, M., Kumar, R., Dilbaghi, N., Kim, K.H., Kumar, S.: Development of a FRET aptasensor based on MoS2-doped Zn-MOF as luminophore for selective detection of cadmium in aqueous solutions. Microchim. Acta **191**, 324 (2024). https://doi.org/10.1007/s00604-024-06382-5
27. Chen, J., Zhang, Y., Wang, X., Li, F., Wu, S., Wang, W., et al.: A FRET based ultrasensitive fluorescent aptasensor for 6′-sialyllactose detection. Anal. Biochem. **688**, 115462 (2024). https://doi.org/10.1016/j.ab.2024.115462
28. Ryan, L.S., Gerberich, J., Haris, U., Nguyen, D., Mason, R.P., Lippert, A.R.: Ratiometric pH imaging using a 1,2-dioxetane chemiluminescence resonance energy transfer sensor in live animals. ACS Sens. **5**, 2925–2932 (2020). https://doi.org/10.1021/acssensors.0c01393
29. Weihs, F., Anderson, A., Trowell, S., Caron, K.: Resonance energy transfer-based biosensors for point-of-need diagnosis—progress and perspectives. Sensors (Switzerland) **21**, 1–18 (2021). https://doi.org/10.3390/s21020660
30. Rink, S., Duerkop, A., Jacobi von Wangelin, A., Seidel, M., Baeumner, A.J.: Next generation luminol derivative as powerful benchmark probe for chemiluminescence assays. Anal. Chim. Acta **1188** (2021). https://doi.org/10.1016/j.aca.2021.339161.
31. Jiang, Y., Yang, X., Li, S., Qiao, Y., Zhou, Y., Li, Y.: Chemiluminescence initiated by nebulization of oxidant- and catalyst-free aqueous luminol solutions. Chem. Eng. J. **481**, 148753 (2024). https://doi.org/10.1016/j.cej.2024.148753
32. Tzani, M.A., Gioftsidou, D.K., Kallitsakis, M.G., Pliatsios, N.V., Kalogiouri, N.P., Angaridis, P.A., et al.: Direct and indirect chemiluminescence: reactions, mechanisms and challenges. Molecules **26**, 7664 (2021). https://doi.org/10.3390/molecules26247664
33. Nirala, N.R., Harel, Y., Lellouche, J.P., Shtenberg, G.: Ultrasensitive haptoglobin biomarker detection based on amplified chemiluminescence of magnetite nanoparticles. J. Nanobiotechnol. **18**, 1–10 (2020). https://doi.org/10.1186/s12951-019-0569-9
34. Tannenberg, R., Paul, M., Röder, B., Gande, S.L., Sreeramulu, S., Saxena, K., et al.: Chemiluminescence biosensor for the determination of cardiac troponin I (cTnI). Biosensors (Basel) 13 (2023). https://doi.org/10.3390/bios13040455
35. Roda, B., Deo, S.K., O'Connor, G., Moraskie, M., Giordani, S., Marassi, V., et al.: Shining light on biosensors: chemiluminescence and bioluminescence in enabling technologies. TrAC-Trends Anal. Chem. **180**, 117975 (2024). https://doi.org/10.1016/j.trac.2024.117975
36. Abbasi, R., Hu, X., Zhang, A., Dummer, I., Wachsmann-Hogiu, S.: Optical image sensors for smart analytical chemiluminescence biosensors. Bioengineering **11**, 912 (2024). https://doi.org/10.3390/bioengineering11090912
37. Dai, L., Lou, Y., Liu, L., Wei, Q., Ma, H.: Gold nanoclusters-incorporated nanogels as hybrid nanozymes for sensitive chemiluminescence immunoassays. Biomed. Anal. **1**, 280–286 (2024). https://doi.org/10.1016/j.bioana.2024.11.001
38. Liu, H., Shi, Y., Ye, J., Ni, B., Xuan, Z., Li, F., et al.: An automated magnetic beads-based chemiluminescence immunoassay system for simultaneous quantification of multi-mycotoxins in agricultural products. Sens. Actuators B Chem. **420** (2024). https://doi.org/10.1016/j.snb.2024.136424
39. Zhao, L.Z., Fu, Y.Z., Ren, S.W., Cao, J.T., Liu, Y.M.: A novel chemiluminescence imaging immunosensor for prostate specific antigen detection based on a multiple signal amplification strategy. Biosens. Bioelectron. **171**, 112729 (2021). https://doi.org/10.1016/j.bios.2020.112729
40. Xiao, Q., Xu, C.: Research progress on chemiluminescence immunoassay combined with novel technologies. TrAC-Trends Anal. Chem. **124**, 115780 (2020). https://doi.org/10.1016/j.trac.2019.115780
41. Abbasi, R., Hu, X., Zhang, A., Dummer, I., Wachsmann-Hogiu, S.: Optical image sensors for smart analytical chemiluminescence biosensors. Bioengineering **11**, 912 (2024)
42. Zhang, Y., Zhang, Z., Wu, M., Zhang, R.: Advances and perspectives of responsive probes for measuring γ-glutamyl transpeptidase. ACS Meas. Sci. Au **4**, 54–75 (2024). https://doi.org/10.1021/acsmeasuresciau.3c00045
43. Mao, F., Yang, X., He, Z., Sun, Z., Zhang, S., Liu, X.: Mimotope peptides for nanobodies: a nontoxic alternative to ochratoxin A and its application in chemiluminescence immunoassays

for analysis of pepper samples. Food Chem. **465** (2025). https://doi.org/10.1016/j.foodchem.2024.142061
44. Su, D., Han, J., Chen, L., Zhu, S., Jiang, Y., Wang, Z.: Fabrication of dextran-grafted magnetic polymer microspheres with low nonspecific protein adsorption as carriers for chemiluminescence immunoassays. Colloids Surf. A Physicochem. Eng. Asp. **694** (2024). https://doi.org/10.1016/j.colsurfa.2024.134115
45. Sharma, V., Tiwari, P., Kaur, N., Mobin, S.M.: Optical nanosensors based on fluorescent carbon dots for the detection of water contaminants: a review. Environ. Chem. Lett. **19**, 3229–3241 (2021). https://doi.org/10.1007/s10311-021-01241-8
46. Ji, C., Zhou, Y., Leblanc, R.M., Peng, Z.: Recent developments of carbon dots in biosensing: a review. ACS Sens. **5**, 2724–2741 (2020). https://doi.org/10.1021/acssensors.0c01556
47. Kong, J., Wei, Y., Zhou, F., Shi, L., Zhao, S., Wan, M., et al.: Carbon quantum dots: properties, preparation, and applications. Molecules **29**, 2002 (2024). https://doi.org/10.3390/molecules29092002
48. Rahal, M., Atassi, Y., Alghoraibi, I.: Quenching photoluminescence of Carbon Quantum Dots for detecting and tracking the release of Minocycline. J. Photochem. Photobiol. A Chem. **412**, 113257 (2021). https://doi.org/10.1016/j.jphotochem.2021.113257
49. Xu, Y., Yang, Y., Lin, S., Xiao, L.: Red-emitting carbon nanodot-based wide-range responsive nanothermometer for intracellular temperature sensing. Anal. Chem. **92**, 15632–15638 (2020). https://doi.org/10.1021/acs.analchem.0c03912
50. Liu, J., Li, R., Yang, B.: Carbon dots: a new type of carbon-based nanomaterial with wide applications. ACS Cent. Sci. **6**, 2179–2195 (2020). https://doi.org/10.1021/acscentsci.0c01306
51. Díaz-González, M., de la Escosura-Muñiz, A., Fernandez-Argüelles, M.T., García Alonso, F.J., Costa-Fernandez, J.M.: Quantum dot bioconjugates for diagnostic applications. Top. Curr. Chem. **378** (2020). https://doi.org/10.1007/s41061-020-0296-6
52. Kokorina, A.A., Ponomaryova, T.S., Goryacheva, I.Y.: Photoluminescence-based immunochemical methods for determination of C-reactive protein and procalcitonin. Talanta **224** (2021). https://doi.org/10.1016/j.talanta.2020.121837
53. Shao, X.Y., Wang, C.R., Xie, C.M., Wang, X.G., Liang, R.L., Xu, W.W.: Rapid and sensitive lateral flow immunoassay method for procalcitonin (PCT) based on time-resolved immunochromatography. Sensors **17**, 480 (2017). https://doi.org/10.3390/S17030480
54. Zhang, K.Y., Yu, Q., Wei, H., Liu, S., Zhao, Q., Huang, W.: Long-lived emissive probes for time-resolved photoluminescence bioimaging and biosensing. Chem. Rev. **118**, 1770–1839 (2018). https://doi.org/10.1021/ACS.CHEMREV.7B00425/SUPPL_FILE/CR7B00425_SI_001.PDF
55. Yang, M., Huang, J., Fan, J., Du, J., Pu, K., Peng, X.: Chemiluminescence for bioimaging and therapeutics: recent advances and challenges. Chem. Soc. Rev. **49**, 6800–6815 (2020). https://doi.org/10.1039/D0CS00348D
56. Wang, C., Wang, T., Zhang, M., Li, N., Fan, M., Cui, X.: Chemiluminescence molecular sensor for endogenous HOCl in vivo. Sens. Actuators B Chem. **339**, 129927 (2021). https://doi.org/10.1016/j.snb.2021.129927
57. Kaurav, H., Verma, D., Bansal, A., Kapoor, D.N., Sheth, S.: Progress in drug delivery and diagnostic applications of carbon dots: a systematic review. Front. Chem. **11**, 1227843 (2023). https://doi.org/10.3389/fchem.2023.1227843
58. Lv, C.C., Han, J.P., Zhao, G., Xie, F., Mo, H.L., Yang, X.K., et al.: Atomically precise Au_4Cu_4-alkynyl clusters with bright photoluminescence for hydroxyl radical detection and arthritis diagnosis. Sens. Actuators B. Chem. **426**, 137029 (2025). https://doi.org/10.1016/j.snb.2024.137029
59. Ou, F., Lin, Z., Li, L., Tang, Y., Zhang, Z.: Turn on fluorescence sensor for specific detection of glycoligand-receptor recognitions based graphene oxide nanocomposite. Results Chem. **3**, 100140 (2021). https://doi.org/10.1016/j.rechem.2021.100140
60. Wang, H., Sun, Y.: Sensitive and label-free fluorescent microRNA detection via catalytic DNAzyme assembly initiated primer exchange reaction. Results Chem. **13** (2025). https://doi.org/10.1016/j.rechem.2024.101967

61. Anand, S.K., Mathew, M.R., Kumar, K.G.: A simple and cost effective turn off fluorescence sensor for biliverdin and bilirubin based on L-cysteine modulated copper nanoclusters. J. Fluoresc. **30**, 63–70 (2020). https://doi.org/10.1007/S10895-019-02470-5/METRICS
62. Dobrzycka, M., Kołakowski, A., Stefanowicz, M., Matulewicz, N., Nikołajuk, A., Karczewska-Kupczewska, M.: Inverse regulation of serum osteoprotegerin and B-type natriuretic peptide concentrations by free fatty acids elevation in young healthy humans. Nutrients **14** (2022). https://doi.org/10.3390/NU14040837
63. Ding, L., Zhong, Z., Chen, C., Liu, B., Chen, Z., Zhang, L., et al.: Advances in multiplexed photoelectrochemical sensors for multiple components. Chem. Eng. J. **505** (2025). https://doi.org/10.1016/j.cej.2025.159319
64. Yahav, G., Pawar, S., Lipovsky, A., Gupta, A., Gedanken, A., Duadi, H., et al.: Probing polarity and pH sensitivity of carbon dots in escherichia coli through time-resolved fluorescence analyses. Nanomaterials **13** (2023). https://doi.org/10.3390/nano13142068
65. Wang, H., Zhang, M., Wei, K., Zhao, Y., Nie, H., Ma, Y., et al.: Pyrrolic nitrogen dominated the carbon dot mimic oxidase activity. Carbon N Y **179**, 692–700 (2021). https://doi.org/10.1016/J.CARBON.2021.04.061
66. Li, D., Huang, K., She, J., Cai, Y., Liu, B., Wei, Z., et al.: Two-photon fluorescence-guided precise photothermal therapy located in a single cancer cell utilizing bifunctional N-doped carbon quantum dots. J. Colloid Interface Sci. **662**, 719–726 (2024). https://doi.org/10.1016/j.jcis.2024.02.114
67. Innocenzi, P., Stagi, L.: Carbon dots as oxidant-antioxidant nanomaterials, understanding the structure-properties relationship. A critical review. Nano Today 50 (2023). https://doi.org/10.1016/j.nantod.2023.101837
68. Sun, Y., Zheng, S., Liu, L., Kong, Y., Zhang, A., Xu, K., et al.: The cost-effective preparation of green fluorescent carbon dots for bioimaging and enhanced intracellular drug delivery. Nanoscale Res. Lett. **15**, 1–9 (2020). https://doi.org/10.1186/S11671-020-3288-0/FIGURES/6
69. Mostafa, I.M., Abdussalam, A., Zholudov, Y.T., Snizhko, D.V., Zhang, W., Hosseini, M., et al.: Recent applications and future perspectives of chemiluminescent and bioluminescent imaging technologies. Chem. Biomed. Imaging **1**, 297–314 (2023). https://doi.org/10.1021/cbmi.2c00002

Light-Emitting Materials for Point-of-Care Diagnostics

Sreedeep Dey

Abstract Light-emitting materials encompass organic fluorescent compounds, semiconductor nanocrystals like quantum dots (QDs), perovskite-based light emitting diodes, etc. These rapid, accurate, and easy-to-access materials reshape point-of-care (POC) diagnostics. With their astonishing optical qualities, they improve the sensitivity and specificity of devices that monitor glucose levels, detect pathogens, and are used as wearable health systems. Glucose-detecting Fluorescence-based microneedles and immunoarray chips for insulin and glycated hemoglobin testing are some of the mentioned devices, demonstrating precision and clinical relevance. Water-based nanoparticle production and biodegradable polymer integration are some of the mentioned eco-friendly methods through which sustainability could be achieved. Here it has been shown that QD-modified biosensors, self-healing electroluminescent devices, and Artificial Intelligence (AI)-enhanced imaging systems potentially improve diagnostic performance. It has been anticipated that continuous health monitoring can be performed with wearable systems equipped with light-emitting sensors. As a result, early disease detection and individualized care can be obtained. Integrated photonic systems use plasmonic photothermal processes. DNA can be rapidly amplified with plasmonic photothermal polymerase chain reaction. AI-driven frameworks increase signal interpretation. It also boosts self-diagnostic capabilities. Future research should focus on multiplexed sensing. Biodegradability should be improved, and AI should be utilized for predictive healthcare. These potentials will be able to close technological gaps. Diagnostic accessibility should be increased in resource-constrained countries. Light-emitting materials are merging material science, nanotechnology, and healthcare systems and breaking through global healthcare solutions.

Keywords Light-emitting materials · Point-of-care diagnostics · Quantum dots · Biosensors · Sustainability · Wearable devices · Artificial intelligence

S. Dey (✉)
Department of Chemical Engineering, University of Calcutta, 92 A. P. C. Road, Kolkata 700009, West Bengal, India
e-mail: sreedeepdey04@gmail.com

© The Author(s), under exclusive license to Springer Nature Switzerland AG 2025
N. O. Etafo (ed.), *Tailored Light Emitters For Biomedical Applications*, Engineering Materials, https://doi.org/10.1007/978-3-031-88731-4_6

1 Introduction

Clinical testing is a vital component in accurately detecting infectious diseases and other medical disorders. The traditional model for such testing is to collect a test sample from the patient at a physician's clinic and then analyze it in a lab. Lubin et al. [1] reviewed that this method provides a high level of test accuracy, but the findings can take several days and may necessitate multiple patient visits [1]. POC Testing is a type of testing that uses technology to perform analyses at the point of service rather than in a traditional clinical laboratory setting. According to Luppa et al. [2], most POC testing systems can be utilized in any environment that has received a CLIA certificate of waiver from the Centers for Medicare and Medicaid Services [2]. POC testing can be found in one's doctor's clinic, a pharmacy, a long-term care facility, and, more recently, in licensed drive-through locations and workplaces. Chan et al. [3] mentioned that POC testing can offer results in minutes, allowing for faster decisions about patient care and expanding testing to communities and people who do not have easy access to healthcare [3].

Unfortunately, laboratories in India are generally located in larger towns or cities, particularly high-end laboratories that can provide inquiry reports promptly. With such a referral system, the sample will have to travel considerable distances, and sample integrity is frequently questioned. So, when one considers the breadth and width of our country, we have a large people base to serve, as well as a large region to cover. Engel et al. [4] reviewed that a large proportion of our population resides in Tier 2 and Tier 3 cities and towns, as well as villages. It is practically impossible for healthcare providers to establish a referral laboratory in every small town and village. As a result, having a POC strategy would be ideal because they would be able to provide a test closer to the patient while also receiving the information promptly. POC testing provides a speedy result, which one may act on right away and possibly even transfer the patient to the appropriate center. As a result, POC testing plays an important strategic role in countries such as India and developing nations [4]. Many tests performed at the point of care may not be directly interpretable by the patient. Even interpretations can be difficult at times, which is where a POC coordinator can help. The POC coordinator will eventually assist one in bridging the gap between what is performed at the point of care and the skills required to interpret that specific POC testing so that one can provide the correct results to the patient. Drancourt et al. [5] emphasized that there have been a few situations that researchers have encountered recently where one connected this POC gadget that they were utilizing at the patient site to somewhere in the country, and the interpretation came from a subject matter expert somewhere else in the country. So, a very coordinated effort from the POC coordinator is required, and that is the primary responsibility of the POC person [5].

POC diagnostics have increased the ability to identify a variety of medical diseases. Holtgrewe et al. [6] mentioned that the primary advantage of this approach is the significant reduction in turnaround time. The COVID-19 pandemic has escalated the POC diagnostics industry, leading to increasing rivalry among companies

[6]. According to Shang et al. [7], this has resulted in the development of gadgets that provide faster and more reliable virus detection. Diabetes, HIV, and *H. Pylori* infection are some diseases that are frequently checked with POC diagnostic devices [7].

According to Global Data, the POC diagnostics market is anticipated to be valued at over 72 billion US dollars by 2027 [8]. The high prevalence of infectious diseases, together with investment in new product development, will drive market expansion. POC diagnostic products allow for quick medical decisions because diseases can be diagnosed at an early stage. This corresponds to an earlier commencement of treatment and thus better health outcomes for patients. POC diagnostics also play an important role in providing health care in remote locations.

Integrating light-emitting materials into POC platforms leverages superior optical properties. Their enhanced sensitivity and specificity allow real-time monitoring. Light-emitting materials encompass QDs, perovskites, and hybrid organic–inorganic systems. Hu et al. [9] mentioned that these materials have some distinct properties. Tunable emission spectra, high quantum yields, and photostability make them ideal candidates for detecting biomarkers, infections, and physiological changes precisely [9]. Tao et al. [10] added that apart from clinical diagnostics, we can adapt these materials to wearable health monitoring systems [10]. Investigation of Zhang [11] shows that we can use them for environmental monitoring and delivering drugs [11]. Zhu et al. [12] worthily elaborated the discussion mentioning that there is an ongoing global demand for efficient diagnostic systems. This demand has fueled the need for sustainable light-emitting technologies. Environmental issues can be addressed globally with environmentally friendly, water-based synthesis methods. Biodegradable polymers and non-toxic QDs are some potent alternatives [12]. Diagnostic capabilities increase by integrating AI. As per the study of Bajwa et al. [13], AI allows for data-driven insights and develops predictive healthcare [13]. A thorough overview of light-emitting materials recently being used in POC diagnostics has been discussed in this chapter. The focus has been on their applications in monitoring glucose levels, detecting infectious diseases, and wearable appliances. Some of the most recent advancements in material synthesis processes, engineering of devices, and AI-enhanced diagnostics have also been investigated. The emphasis is on how they resolve global health inequities, particularly in low-resource countries. In those countries, healthcare delivery gaps can be filled with POC diagnostics. In this chapter, the convergence of material science, nanotechnology, and medical diagnostics has highlighted the potential of light-emitting materials altering global healthcare systems. Major problems and future approaches have also been outlined. These insights lay the groundwork for long-term and equitable advances in diagnostic technologies.

2 Overview of Point-of-Care Diagnostics

2.1 How Point-of-Care Diagnostics Evaluated: From Strips to Smart Systems?

POC testing has grown dramatically in recent years, owing primarily to the use of new technology. Nayak et al. [14] reported that the development of POCT products has occurred in roughly four stages. (1) The initial generation of qualitative testing consisted of test strips and paper. (2) The second generation of the semi-quantitative is the colorimetric swatch card or semi-quantitative instrument reading. (3) Manual operation represents the third generation of full quantitative systems. (4) The fourth generation of technology platforms includes automation, information technology, and intelligence [14].

2.2 Bridging Science and Technology with the Foundations of POCT

The fundamental principles of POC testing technologies can be generally classified into four steps. (1) In the classic procedure, liquid reagents are infiltrated into absorbent materials such as filter paper and microporous membranes before being integrated into dry reagent blocks. Then, they are adhered to hard substrates to generate various types of diagnostic reagent strips. (2) Miniaturization of traditional analytical instruments and simplification of operational procedures. The POCT diagnostic device becomes portable and palm-sized. (3) Integration of the preceding two into a cohesive system. (4) Use of biosensing technology, which employs biosensors to detect the object to be measured.

2.3 Classification of POCT Technologies

According to Luppa et al. [2], there are seven categories of POC testing technology. (1) *Visual observation:* Simple color development is based on direct observation. This is a semi-quantitative analysis method. (2) *Enzyme labeling*: This is an immune response. (3) *Immunodiafiltration and immunochromatography:* This is an immune reaction. (4) *Biosensor:* It detects enzymes and antibodies using optical and electrical technologies. (5) *Electrochemical detection:* This technique takes advantage of electronic probes' sensitivity to certain chemical compounds. (6) *Spectrophotometric analysis:* Spectrophotometric analysis uses optical absorbance. (7) *Biochip:* This device uses protein interactions [2].

3 Categories of Light-Emitting Materials in POC

Optical biosensors are applied in POC diagnostics. Light-emitting materials are at the core of those biosensors. We can divide these materials into various categories. Each category is equipped with distinct qualities. These distinct qualities make them suitable for different purposes. Organic Light-Emitting Diodes (OLEDs), QDs, Rare-Earth Doped Materials, and Upconversion Nanoparticles are some of the major categories. Perovskite nanocrystals, classic fluorescent dyes, and proteins are some additional examples of emerging materials used in POC diagnosis.

3.1 OLEDs in Point-of-Care Systems

OLEDs are flexible materials. They are distinguished for achieving impressive brightness with customizable emission spectra and being energetically efficient. With these properties, OLEDs become an attractive choice for small and versatile diagnostic equipment. They provide precise and customized light emission. It is useful for developing portable and wearable POC diagnostic systems. Katchman et al. [15] successfully detected IgG antibodies to several viral antigens in patient serum samples using commercial flat panel OLED display technology and protein microarray technology. Human IgG detection limits were found to be 10 pg/mL [15].

3.2 Quantum Dots: Precisely Diagnosing Multiplexed Point-of-Care

QDs have size-dependent optical characteristics. Their absorption spectra are broad. These qualities make them suitable for very sensitive and multiplexed detection. They can simultaneously detect multiple biomarkers accurately. They cause minimal interference. They are helpful in the detection of infectious diseases in POC systems. However, typical AuNPs-LFIAs are moderately sensitive; therefore quick detection remains a hurdle. QDs-based LFIA has been evaluated for very sensitive, quick detection of infectious diseases. Qassimet et al. in 2009 discussed the basics of LFIA and ways for using QDs to increase sensitivity [16].

3.3 Rare-Earth Doped Materials for POC

Rare earth elements like lanthanides have distinct photophysical properties. Their luminescence lifetimes are longer. The emission spectra are characterized by narrow, sharp bands due to inner-shell electronic transitions (*f*-*f* transitions) that are relatively insensitive to the surrounding environment. Jethva et al. [17] elaborated that they are ideally fit for time-resolved fluorescence methods. Light emission occurs in specific spectral regions. As a result, background noise gets reduced and detection sensitivity increases [17].

3.4 Upconversion Nanoparticles for POC

UCNPs are unique. They transform low-energy photons (like near-infrared light) into high-energy photons (like visible light) by a process called upconversion luminescence. This characteristic makes them relevant in deep tissue imaging and high-sensitivity detection in POC systems. However, the study by Wu et al. [18] shows that these potent UCNP-based systems have some constraints. The Quantum yields are sometimes inadequate. Absorption cross-sections are short. These constraints demand future development for their performance improvement in real-world diagnostic purposes [18].

3.5 Perovskite Nanocrystals as the Next-Generation Fluorescence for Precision Diagnostics

Perovskite nanocrystals (Pe-NCs) show high photoluminescence quantum yield and tunable emission features. These features grow the interest in utilizing them for next-generation diagnostic tools. As their photoluminescence spectra are narrower than typical fluorophores, they fit ideally for sensitive diagnostic procedures. The Perovskite Nanocrystal Fluorescence-Linked Immunosorbent Assay is a breakthrough in POC diagnostics. It is a quantitative fluorescence-based approach which is used in food safety and clinical diagnostics. The fluorescent probes (perovskite antibodies) have been developed by Dong et al. [19] via electrostatic adsorption with a narrow full width at half-maximum (18 nm), setting the groundwork for future research into multi-target detection [19].

3.6 Traditional Fluorescent Dyes and Proteins in Modern Diagnostics in POC

Fluorescent dyes and proteins are regarded as traditional approaches. Still, they seem essential in POC biosensing applications. They are versatile in labeling and producing signals. For example, diabetic foot ulcer (DFU) is a significant diabetes consequence, and fluorescent materials have provided novel diagnostic treatments for DFUs. Traditional approaches are focused on examining visual wounds. Whereas a fluorescent pH-sensing bandage, which is an improved molecular diagnostic tool, monitors wounds faster and more accurately, improving patient outcomes. In a fluorescent dye screen, Al-Hawat et al. [20] identified pyranine as the lead chemical because of its pH-sensing characteristics in the clinically important pH range of 6–9. This pH-sensing diagnostic wound dressing was evaluated on mice's full-thickness dorsal wounds, and it demonstrated a linear fluorescence response ($R^2 = 0.9909$) to clinically relevant pH levels [20].

4 Mechanisms of Detection of Light-Emitting Materials in POC

Recent studies have demonstrated that light-emitting materials play an important role in POC diagnostics. They offer a range of detection modalities that are highly sensitive, specific, and fast. These materials interact with biomolecules and environmental variables. They provide localized bio information and insights that reflect status of patient health and stage of occuring disease. Therefore, these materials are important players in biosensing systems. The primary mechanisms for detecting POCs with light-emitting materials are discussed below.

4.1 Fluorescence-Based Detection for POC

Being technologically simple and providing rapid response, fluorescence-based detection has become a popular biosensing technique in POC. Fluorescent probes precisely target organelles and specific biochemical variables by detecting changes in biomolecular quantities or microenvironments. This tailored detection emphasizes the roles of analytes in normal and pathological situations and improves diagnosis accuracy. Zhu et al. [21] have expanded the diversity by creating organelle-specific responsive probes that can detect changes even in biomolecular levels (reactive oxygen species, fluoride ion, hydrogen sulfide, zinc cation, thiol-containing amino acids, and cyclooxygenase-2) as well as the microenvironment (viscosity, polarity, pH) [21].

4.2 Luminescence Resonance Energy Transfer (LRET) for POC

LRET transfers energy from a source molecule (such as a light-emitting substance) to an acceptor molecule. This method is especially useful for label-free or weakly labeled detection. Upconversion nanoparticles (UCNPs) have remarkable luminescent characteristics. They are commonly used as donors in LRET-based biosensors. Being larger in size, proteins (also known as macromolecules) and antibodies hurdle protein detection. A recent study by Chen et al. [22] has addressed this constraint in their study. The researchers have developed a magnetic UCNP-based LRET biosensor. It detects SARS-CoV-2 spike proteins. This technique used antibody-functionalized UCNPs and magnetic gold nanoparticles. Therefore, donor–acceptor coupling lengths were adjusted to provide ultrasensitive and extremely selective detection. Their findings revealed that this platform reversibly reduced the coupling distance between UCNPs and MGNs, increasing the LRET signal by a factor of ten, from 20.6 pg/mL without magnetic modulation to 2.1 pg/mL with magnetic modulation within 1 h [22].

4.3 Colorimetric and Electrochemical Transduction in POC

For providing data, sometimes, biosensors have to rely on transduction mechanisms. Electrochemical tests and colorimetric lateral flow immunoassays (LFIs) are two prevalent approaches. Findings from study of Weihs et al. [23] report that despite fulfilling basic diagnostic requirements, they demand significant modification for detecting broader biomarkers. Being known for quantitative and diverse capabilities, Förster Resonance Energy Transfer (FRET)–based biosensors appear as a viable alternative. FRET-based systems accurately quantify biomolecular interactions. Therefore, they are widely employed for research purposes [23].

4.4 Chemiluminescence in POC

Chemiluminescence may be referred to as light emission from chemical reactions without external excitation. This process has a high signal-to-noise ratio. This property makes it excellent for POC diagnostics. A chemiluminescent immunoassay for pepsinogen I (PGI) was performed by Liu et al. [24] where a fully automated, compact apparatus was utilized. This assay was designed for community health check-ups. The detection limit of 0.048 ng/mL was proven outstanding compared to other available POC diagnostic devices. A wide detection range of 0–200 ng/mL indicated its potentiality for large-scale stomach cancer screening, specifically in resource-limited situations [24].

4.5 *Electrochemiluminescence (ECL) in POC*

ECL is a combination of the advantages of electrochemical and luminescent methods. ECL is highly sensitive and detects faster. It is highly potential for proof-of-concept applications. However, developing portable and precise ECL devices for on-site testing is still a matter of challenge. There are some recent improvements in ECL technology. Ying et al. [25] investigated that, making small devices and utilizing novel sensing components can overcome these limits. Such advancements have to be practically applicable for accelerating the commercialization of ECL-based diagnostic instruments [25].

5 Fabrication and Integration of Light-Emitting Materials in POC Devices

For developing POC devices using light-emitting materials, fabrication techniques have to be advanced in terms of their engineering. Moreover, these devices have to be designed in such ways that they could be integrated seamlessly. This section discusses what are the promising fabrication techniques and integration strategies being practiced in recent years. Additionally, related difficulties and advancements have also been focused on. These techniques and strategies have been shown in Fig. 1.

Thin Films and Nanoparticles in POC: High-quality thin films and nanoparticles are applied for POC applications. These thin films and nanoparticles can be created by a number of fabrication technologies applied for POC applications.

Spin-Coating, Vapor Deposition, and Inkjet Printing in POC: Among several up-and-coming methods, spin-coating, vapor deposition, and inkjet printing are commonly used ones. They deposit homogeneous layers of light-emitting materials like OLEDs and QDs onto substrates.

Inkjet-Printed Quantum Dot LEDs in POC: Inkjet printing is a promising method. This method has been found to produce quantum dot light-emitting diodes (QLEDs). However, inkjet-printed QLEDs are less efficient and stable compared to spin-coated QLEDs. A pressure-assisted thermal annealing (PTA) method was devised by Wei et al. [26] for enhancing inkjet-printed CdZnSe/CdZnS/ZnS QD films to solve this issue. This approach was able to improve packing order. It reduced surface roughness. Photoluminescence and electrical characteristics were remarkably increased. Ultimately, a high-performance film was reproduced. Inkjet-printed red and green CdZnSe-based QLEDs reached a record high external quantum efficiency (EQE) of 23.08% with an amazing operating lifetime (T_{50}) of up to 343,342 h@100 cd m^{-2}, and a record EQE of 22.43% with T_{50} exceeding 1,500,463 h@100 cd m^{-2} [26].

Nanoparticle Synthesis in POC: Sol–Gel, Hydrothermal, and Hot Injection Methods are the fabrication method for developing nanoparticles. Sol–gel synthesis,

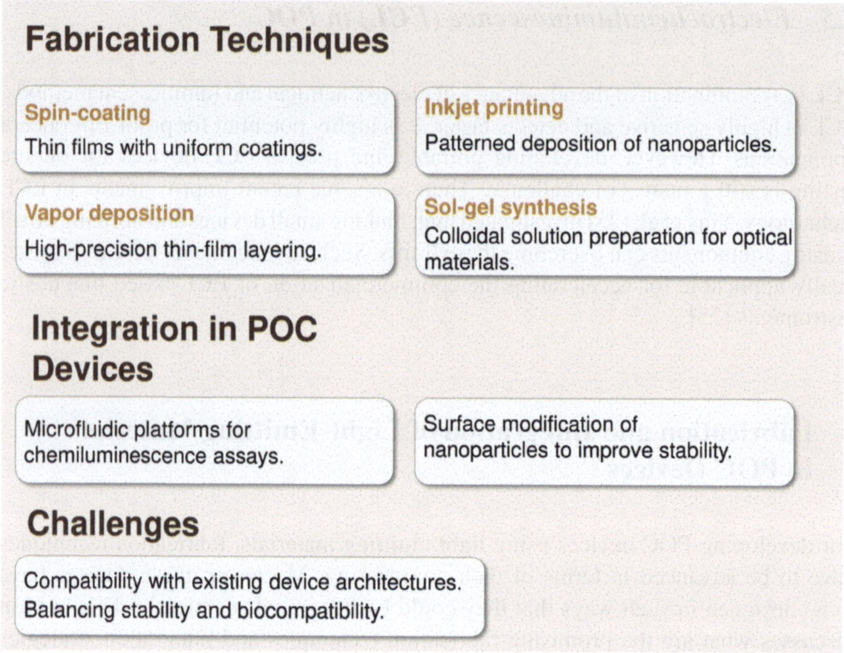

Fig. 1 Fabrication techniques and integration strategies of light-emitting materials in POC devices

hydrothermal methods, and hot injection are preferably used for creating QDs, upconversion nanoparticles (UCNPs), and perovskite nanocrystals.

Tailoring Surface Properties in POC: Surface changes after synthesis make nanoparticles more stable and biocompatible for biological purposes. Zhang et al. [27] previously reviewed that Cadmium-based QDs show broader UV excitation. Their emission spectra are narrower. They show intense photoluminescence and are highly photostable. These properties make them utilizable for sensors, bioimaging, and electroluminescent operators [27].

Microfluidic Platforms in POC: Incorporation of light-emitting materials onto microfluidic platforms for lab-on-chip applications is a substantial barrier. Energy sources are required for driving light emissions. Storti et al. [28] demonstrated that Chemiluminescence (CL) is an innovative approach. It needs no external energy sources. CL-based systems are considerably increasing their utility as they provide complete geometric flexibility and three-dimensional positioning of light-emitting materials [28].

Photolithography and Soft Lithography in POC: Photolithography and soft lithography are frequently used for creating microchannels within microfluidic devices. Optimal interaction between light-emitting materials and biological samples can be ensured with those materials.

Advanced Microfabrication in POC: With these microfabrication techniques, we can accurately manipulate fluid at the microscale. This property makes them critical for diagnostic applications. Recent research by Ravi et al. [29] has created sophisticated, multicellular channels. They are useful for studying tumor microenvironments (TMEs) and cellular interactions [29].

Laser micromachining, 3D printing, and electron beam lithography are some sophisticated techniques enabling high-resolution features on microfluidic substrates. These methods construct complex device geometries and functional components. This broadens microfluidics to be used in diagnosis, discovering drugs, and performing biomedical research.

Integration of Chemiluminescence in POC: Trautmann et al. [30] have shown the production and characterization of a chemiluminescent light source that is fully integrated on a microfluidic platform using the direct writing technique known as Femtosecond Laser Micromachining [30].

6 Applications of Light-Emitting Materials in POC Diagnostics

The key players in POC diagnostics—light-emitting materials—have a wide range of medical applications, from detecting infectious diseases to identifying cancer biomarkers. With subsequent focus on current developments and potential significance, this section identifies their use in diagnostic tools. Figure 2 shows some of the notable applications.

6.1 Infectious Disease Diagnostics in POC

From the COVID-19 pandemic, we have understood why rapid, sensitive diagnostic tools are needed. Having outstanding optical qualities, QDs have been used in lateral flow immunoassays (LFAs). They improve detection sensitivity for SARS-CoV-2 antigens. Traditional LFAs were cost-effective and portable. However, they could not detect low (undetectable) viral loads. The first use of QDs in bioimaging occurred in 1998.

Quantum Dots in Lateral Flow Immunoassays in POC: Mousavi et al. [31] reported that, this restriction was overcome by QD-based LFAs. Viral antigen detection performance was improved, and a small sample size was required. With nanotechnology, diagnostics of infectious diseases have been improved. This technology has utilized nanoparticles (NPs) as drug carriers and vaccine delivery systems [31].

Single-Virus Tracking Systems in POC: These materials (QDs) can increase bioavailability, maintain specificity, and trigger developed immunogenic responses.

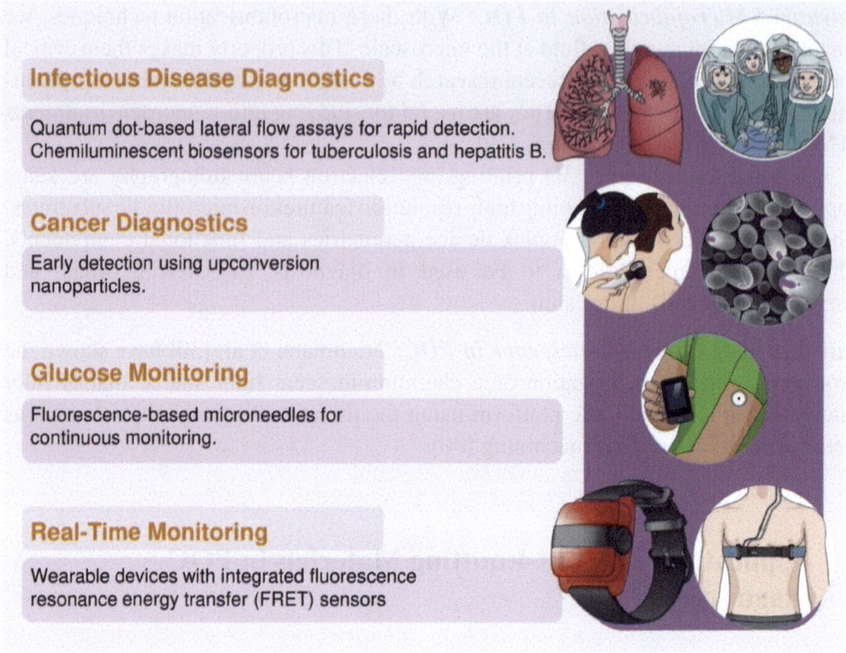

Fig. 2 Applications of light-emitting materials in POC diagnostics

For example, using QDs in single-virus tracking (SVT) systems permit real-time monitoring of viral interactions in living cells. From this system, crucial insights into infection mechanisms can be gained. Liu et al. [32] highlighted that, the QSVT approach has generated amazing results in determining the mechanisms underlying viral entrance, trafficking, and egress. The protocol requires 1–2 weeks from the development of viruses and cellular specimens to image collection, with 1 day for image processing and data analysis [32].

6.2 Chemiluminescent and Paper-Based Biosensors in POC

Electrogenerated Chemiluminescence (ECL) in POC: Electrogenerated chemiluminescence (ECL) is a notable chemiluminescent (CL) biosensor that is becoming popular for being exceptionally sensitive and convenient. Study by Ge et al. [33] shows that there are low-cost paper substrates that detect CL. These substrates make the construction process of lab-on-paper devices easier. These devices can be used for detecting infectious agents. As one of the novel solutions, smartphones are being used as analyzers, enabling quantitative, on-site detection of bacterial pathogens [33].

FLASH Biosensor in POC: FLASH (Fast, Luminescent, and Affordable Sensor of Hip1) is a type of CL biosensor. Babin et al. [34] considered that it is a promising choice for diagnostic purposes in resource-limited environments and is able to detect diseases like tuberculosis (TB). Similarly, chemiluminescent techniques can detect hepatitis B virus (HBV) DNA. They exhibit higher sensitivity than nested PCR. Therefore we can consider them as scalable alternatives for monitoring blood safety. CL and ECL offer superior performance while maintaining the simplicity, cheap cost, multifunctionality, versatility, flexibility, and disposability of μ-PADS [34].

Peroxidase-Like Chemiluminescent Systems in POC: A CL system with long, persistent, and intensive intensity was introduced by Chen et al. [35] based on the peroxidase-like property of 4-mercaptophenylboronic acid (MPBA)-functionalized CuSe nanoprobes (CuSeNPs@MPBA) [35].

6.3 Cancer Biomarker Detection in POC

Detecting cancer in early stages is important as it increases the chances of successful treatment. Central to this effort are light-emitting materials like rare-earth-doped nanoparticles and upconversion nanoparticles (UCNPs). These nanoparticles exhibit minimal background interference. They are exceptionally specific. Physicians recommend them for detecting circulating tumor cells (CTCs) and other biomarkers. UCNPs have unique optical and chemical properties. They are applicable in bioimaging, biosensing, and theranostic applications. Li et al. [36] suggested that identifying CTCs in blood samples is regarded as a vital step in the diagnosis process of early-stage cancers. Time-resolved fluorescence assays using UCNPs have been proven excellent for this purpose. UCNP-based platforms are a leap forward in cancer diagnostics. However, there are high demands for advanced research that can enhance the detection efficiency of UCNP-based platforms [36].

6.4 Emerging Applications and Future Directions of POC

Light-emitting materials are being investigated to be used for novel purposes. They are being used in photochemical processes and theranostics. In these ways, diagnostic and therapeutic abilities can be combined on a single platform. To realize their full potential, further refinements are important in every stage of synthesis, stability, and performance.

6.4.1 Innovations in Continuous Glucose Monitoring (CGM) Sensors in POC

Advancements in CGM Technology in POC

Continuous glucose monitoring (CGM) is transforming diabetes management. This system tracks blood glucose levels in real-time, interprets the trend analysis, and provides alerts for hypoglycemia. As a result, diabetes treatments become safer and more efficient, cases of hypoglycemic episodes are reduced, and glycemic fluctuation decreases. With real-time glucose monitoring modifications in insulin dosage can be precisely performed, which results in better patient outcomes.

mbNIR Sensors and Shallow Dense Neural Networks in POC: Over the last two decades, CGM technology has significantly been advanced. Cutting-edge sensors are being used to improve precision and deliver a better user experience. For example, a multiple photonic band near-infrared (mbNIR) sensor was combined with personalized medical features (PMF) in shallow dense neural networks (SDNN). This system performed exceptionally well for classifying diabetes on the basis of fasting glucose levels. The accuracy and specificity were 97.8% and 98.7%, respectively.

Non-Invasive Blood Glucose Monitoring in POC: The model developed by Srichan et al. [37] for non-invasive real-time blood glucose monitoring showed a $\pm$15% inaccuracy with a 95% confidence interval and a detection limit of 60–400 mg/dL when verified with the standard hexokinase enzymatic method for glucose level determination [37].

Glucose-Responsive Fluorescence-Based Microneedle Systems in POC: The discovery of glucose-responsive fluorescence-based microneedle systems is a crucial breakthrough in CGM technology. These devices deliver continuous glucose monitoring. As these devices show lesser invasiveness, the incidents of pain, wounds, and irritation in the skin can be minimized.

Wearable and Implantable Monitoring Solutions in POC: When microneedle CGM systems were combined by Sang et al. [38] with mobile applications and portable devices, it drastically changed the concepts of wearable and implantable monitoring solutions [38].

Biomarker Detection for Diabetes in POC

Key biomarkers like insulin and glycated hemoglobin (HbA1c) can be monitored through advanced immunoarray chips. These chips have been found to incorporate magnetite nanoparticles. Those nanoparticles are coated with QDs. The coating makes them able to immobilize aptamers. A study by Singh et al. [39] examined that their detection limits are 4 pM for insulin and 1% for HbA1c. Fluorescence imaging has confirmed the successful outcome of surface plasmon microarray technology. As this technology deals with molecular binding interactions, we can accurately diagnose which biomarker can be utilized for diabetes management. Surface plasmon kinetic study revealed binding constants of 0.24 (±0.08) nM and 37 (±3) μM for insulin and HbA1c on immobilized monoclonal antibodies [39].

Quantum Dot Nanoparticles in Glucose Sensing in POC

As QDs exhibit superior optical qualities, they are increasingly being used in glucose monitoring. A noteworthy study was performed by Ripoll et al. [40] where, CdSe/ZnS QDs have been coupled with aminophenylboronic acid (APBA) and demonstrated promising results as glucose nanosensors. Their photoluminescence durations are longer. This property improves selectivity as it reduces possible interference that comes from cell autofluorescence. As a result, it becomes an accurate sensing solution. The nanosensors were successfully used for the detection of glucose in MDA-MB-231 cells using FLIM [40].

6.4.2 Emerging Diagnostic Techniques in POC

Nowadays, glucose monitoring and therapeutic drug monitoring (TDM) are being revolutionized by advancements in optical and photonic techniques. A successfully established study by Son et al. [41] reveals that Plasmonic photothermal polymerase chain reaction (PCR) techniques utilize ultrafast light-to-heat conversion. Rapid thermal cycling results in amplified DNA in less than five minutes. With the help of fluorescence resonance energy transfer (FRET), the sensitivity and specificity of diagnostic procedures get increased as biological activities can be monitored in real time. Oligonucleotides having a DNA backbone and one or more chromophore tags have numerous applications as FRET probes [41].

6.4.3 Wearable and Integrated Optical Devices in POC

Fluorescence, luminescence, and colorimetry-based Wearable optical sensors are being used in medical diagnosis, like drug monitoring and maintaining cardiovascular health. These sensors provide continuous health monitoring and light-based therapies that form a versatile platform for integrated diagnostics and treatment.

6.4.4 Cerenkov Luminescence Imaging (CLI) in POC

CLI is a new alternative to nuclear imaging modalities. Being cost-effective and convenient for use, PET is becoming popular. Studies have compared CLI and PET for cancer treatment monitoring and revealed that they are strongly relevant in terms of drug efficacy. To utilize CLI as a high-throughput method for preclinical treatment monitoring and drug screening, more investigations are required. In the groundbreaking study by Xu et al. [42], to compare the efficacy of both methods in therapeutic monitoring, two mouse tumor models (large cell lung cancer cell line H460 and prostate cancer cell line PC3) were given bevacizumab versus vehicle treatments. Two common radiotracers, 3′-deoxy-3′-^{18}F-fluorothymidine (^{18}F-FLT) and ^{18}F-FDG, were used to assess bevacizumab therapy efficacy [42].

7 Future Prospects of Light-Emitting Materials in Point-of-Care (POC) Diagnostics

Progressive mindsets of researchers are unknotting the knots of POC diagnostics and shading lights on novel POC healthcare solutions with successful utilizations of light-emitting materials. Researchers are exploiting the roles of material science and engineering to address the gaps in terms of sensitivity, stability, and device scalability.

7.1 Eco-friendly and Hybrid Materials for POC

Next-generation perovskites are lead-free and environmentally friendly. They reduce toxicity but retain excellent photoluminescence efficiency. These materials are particularly used in ultrasensitive detection, where the diagnostic platforms are relatively smaller. Organic–inorganic hybrid materials provide improved stability and functionality. They have already been used in optoelectronic devices like lasers, solar cells, and LEDs. With their versatile designs and properties, they contribute to high-performance diagnostic technology. Ikram et al. [43] address that, in numerical modeling, the $CsSnI_3$-based perovskite solar cell has the best power conversion efficiency of any lead-free perovskite-based device, at 28.97% [43].

7.2 Quantum Dots in Diagnostics in POC

QDs are tiny semiconductors. QDs and similar nanoparticles possess a high surface area-to-volume ratio (due to their small size) and functional groups that can be associated with a variety of diagnostic (e.g., optical, radioisotopic, or magnetic) and therapeutic (e.g., anticancer) agents.

They exhibit higher optical and electrical properties. They are promisingly used to diagnose cancer in early stages and treat the disease. However, Guo et al. [44] revealed their concerns mentioning that, toxicity is a major associated problem. That's why researchers are leaning towards non-toxic QDs such as carbon (CQDs), graphene (GQDs), black phosphorus (BPQDs), and perovskite (PQDs). Functionalized QDs are modified with proteins, lipids, and other components. Customization of characteristics according to specific diagnostic requirements improves their clinical applicability [44].

7.3 Self-healing and Stretchable Materials in POC

In resource-constrained environments, self-healing materials crucially contribute to POC devices by increasing their lifespan. Self-healing, stretchy, electroluminescent devices are being made from carbon nanotube/polyurethane composites. Similar to natural systems, these materials are able to repair photodegradation or mechanical damage autonomously. These developments lower the failure rates of those POC devices and promise a long-term future for POC diagnostics. The self-healing and stretchable electroluminescent device mentioned by Shi et al. [45] maintains a consistent luminance after 10 cycles of cutting and healing, as well as 350 cycles of stretching and releasing [45].

7.4 AI Integration in POC Diagnostics

AI has the capability to evaluate complex signal patterns. They have explicabilities in biochemical sensing. They increase diagnostic accuracy. According to Khan et al. [46], predictive healthcare and tailored therapy are possible with AI, as they can synthesize material, diagnose at the molecular level, and study imaging. Integrating AI in wearable devices allows for real-time monitoring. Pathogen-based infections, bacterial diagnostics, and therapy make use of modified nanobiosensors (NBs) that have been augmented with electrochemistry, acoustics, electromagnetism, and photothermal resonance [46].

As data analysis gets improved, and remote clinical decision-making can be performed, it becomes helpful for people who reside in rural areas and belong to disadvantaged populations.

7.5 Wearable POC Devices in POC

Real-time monitoring of crucial biomarkers, including glucose, lactate, and hydration levels, can be performed with wearable POC devices. Wearables can be skin-, textile-, and biofluidics-based. They can be widely applicable, ranging from monitoring physiological health to neuropsychological problems. Optical and electrochemical sensors and flexible microfluidic technologies improved noninvasive biomarker detection processes. These innovative ideas promote individualized treatments. By identifying disease in early stage, socioeconomic burdens can be reduced. Prakashan et al. [47] found that wearable sensors are becoming increasingly popular due to their capacity to provide regular and continuous monitoring of physiological data through dynamic, non-invasive assessments of biomarkers in biofluids such as tears, perspiration, interstitial fluid, and saliva [47].

7.6 3D Printing in Diagnostics in POC

3D printing technologies are getting incorporated into POC devices. 3D printing reduces the costs of production. They accurately incorporate light-emitting materials into customized diagnostic equipment used in POC. With the use of this technology, healthcare organizations are structuring frameworks for personalized medicines that adhere to quality and do not violate regulatory norms. Bastawrous et al. [48] show that by adding 3D scanning of surface topologies, they can conformally print devices onto curved surfaces like contact lenses [48].

7.7 Sustainability and Eco-friendly Solutions in POC

With advanced light-emitting materials, POC diagnostics become sustainable, eco-friendly, and green solutions. Water-based luminous nanoparticles synthesis are innovative hydrothermal synthesis methods. They can be used safely as an alternative to conventional chemical processes. Rhodamine B-doped fluorescent paints are mitigating the aggregation-caused quenching (ACQ). Li et al. [49] conclude that when the emulsion starts to polymerize, Rhodamine B forms bonds to the latex particles. It ensures that a stable fluorescence is obtained and boosts their diagnostic applications [49].

Medical waste and contamination are global issues. Alternatively, biodegradable and recyclable materials can be used in POC devices to resolve the issues. Disposable diagnostic technologies are important to maintaining global health. However, they make the waste management complicated. Biodegradable polymers promote environmentally friendly disposal techniques. Landfill dependency can be reduced by using biodegradable polymers. As these materials get disintegrated in controlled circumstances, they become viable for reducing environmental effects. Ongaro et al. [50] reported that advanced nanotechnology and polymer science show the path to developing biodegradable materials that are more durable and functionally stable [50].

7.8 Expanded Diagnostic Applications in POC

Light-emitting materials have expanded their diagnostic capabilities by addressing health disparities in low-income communities. POC devices should be affordable and efficient for combating neglected tropical diseases (NTDs). Manyazewal et al. [51] reviewed that countries in Africa experiencing sociopolitical instability also face a significant burden of NTDs, with the continent placing second globally in NTD burden (33%, 578 million people) and first in internal displacement (50%, 31.6 million people) by 2023 [51].

As the vulnerable populations have limited diagnostic access, they are still being affected disproportionately. Especially in places like Africa, healthcare efforts are impeded by persistent sociopolitical instability. Early and exact identification at the point of care is critically important for reducing the physical, economic, and societal consequences.

Heidt et al. [52] strongly recommended that nanotechnology, telemedicine, drones, wearable sensors, and augmented reality can improve healthcare systems in those circumstances. Mobile-operated health apps and improved POC diagnostics provide care more promptly. With the improvement of stability, we can hope that these technologies will be advanced and be able to promote long-term health development by minimizing global inequities [52].

However, light-emitting POC diagnostics are positively contributing to both high- and low-income communities. In developed countries, they are streamlining the procedures, saving costs, and increasing diagnosis efficiency. In low-income areas where laboratories may be hours away, light-emitting POC instruments are frequently the only realistic choice for providing fast diagnosis, particularly for infectious diseases.

7.9 Emerging Technologies for Pathogen Detection in POC

Light-emitting materials can identify novel biological targets and developing infections. Therefore they can fight against novel viruses and antibiotic-resistant bacterial strains. Traditional bacterial detection methods are dependent upon central laboratories and specialized technicians. It delays the diagnosis by several hours or even days. Advanced biosensors, microfluidic chips, and integrated diagnostic systems enable monitoring of infection loads in food, water, and environmental samples in real time. Nnachi et al. [53] further added that multiplexed and sensitive sensors should be the parts of future studies that will help in the simultaneous detection of multiple infections [53]. By integrating analytical technology, food safety, environmental monitoring, and public health will be improved, ultimately addressing biological hazards.

8 Conclusion

Revolution in POC diagnostics is being achieved by light-emitting materials' fast, accurate, and budget-friendly medical testing. Light-emitting materials exhibit unique optical features. Tunable emission spectra and excellent photoluminescence efficiency suitably fit them in a variety of diagnostic approaches. Incorporating these materials into portable devices potentially alters healthcare services, which is crucial in low-resource countries and rural areas. Water-based QDs and organic–inorganic hybrids are breakthroughs that are eco-friendly and biodegradable. They confirm the global demand for sustainable healthcare solutions. Diagnoses are being done more accurately by integrating AI technologies into light-emitting materials. This is crucial for providing tailored and predictive healthcare services. Stability, scalability, biocompatibility, and cost-effectiveness are some of the persisting issues. Future studies should focus on designing ergonomic devices, integrating strategies, and investigating the possibilities of synergistic relationship buildings between sensing technologies for establishing comprehensive diagnostic platforms.

Declaration: Conflict of Interest The author declares no competing interests.

References

1. Lubin, I.M., Astles, J.R., Bunn, J.D., Cornish, N.E., Lazaro, G., Marshall, A.A., et al.: The clinical laboratory is an integral component to health care delivery: an expanded representation of the total testing process. Am. J. Clin. Pathol. **160**, 124–129 (2023). https://doi.org/10.1093/ajcp/aqad038
2. Luppa, P.B., Müller, C., Schlichtiger, A., Schlebusch, H.: Point-of-care testing (POCT): current techniques and future perspectives. TrAC, Trends Anal. Chem. **30**, 887–898 (2011). https://doi.org/10.1016/j.trac.2011.01.019
3. Chan, J.T.N., Nguyen, V., Tran, T.N., Nguyen, N.V., Do, N.T.T., van Doorn, H.R., et al.: Point-of-care testing in private pharmacy and drug retail settings: a narrative review. BMC Infect. Dis. **23**, 551 (2023). https://doi.org/10.1186/s12879-023-08480-w
4. Engel, N., Ganesh, G., Patil, M., Yellappa, V., Pant Pai, N., Vadnais, C., et al.: Barriers to point-of-care testing in India: results from qualitative research across different settings, users and major diseases. PLoS ONE **10**, e0135112 (2015). https://doi.org/10.1371/journal.pone.0135112
5. Drancourt, M., Michel-Lepage, A., Boyer, S., Raoult, D.: The point-of-care laboratory in clinical microbiology. Clin. Microbiol. Rev. **29**, 429–447 (2016). https://doi.org/10.1128/CMR.00090-15
6. Holtgrewe, L.M.L., Jain, S., Dekova, R., Broger, T., Isaacs, C., Theron, G., et al.: Innovative COVID-19 point-of-care diagnostics suitable for tuberculosis diagnosis: a scoping review. J. Clin. Med. **13**, 5894 (2024). https://doi.org/10.3390/jcm13195894
7. Shang, M., Guo, J., Guo, J.: Point-of-care testing of infectious diseases: recent advances. Sensors & Diagnostics **2**, 1123–1144 (2023). https://doi.org/10.1039/D3SD00092C
8. Point-of-Care Diagnostics Market Size to Reach USD 72.26 Billion by 2027 Growing at 11.92% CAGR (2022)
9. Hu, H., Salim, T., Chen, B., Lam, Y.M.: Molecularly engineered organic-inorganic hybrid perovskite with multiple quantum well structure for multicolored light-emitting diodes. Sci. Rep. **6**, 33546 (2016). https://doi.org/10.1038/srep33546
10. Tao, Y., Chan, H.F., Shi, B., Li, M., Leong, K.W.: Light: a magical tool for controlled drug delivery. Adv. Funct. Mater. **30** (2020). https://doi.org/10.1002/adfm.202005029
11. Zhang, Z.: Light-emitting materials for wearable electronics. Nat. Rev. Mater. **7**, 839–840 (2022). https://doi.org/10.1038/s41578-022-00502-4
12. Zhu, C., Chen, Z., Gao, S., Goh, B.L., Samsudin, I.B., Lwe, K.W., et al.: Recent advances in non-toxic quantum dots and their biomedical applications. Prog. Nat. Sci.: Mater. Int. **29**, 628–640 (2019). https://doi.org/10.1016/j.pnsc.2019.11.007.
13. Bajwa, J., Munir, U., Nori, A., Williams, B.: Artificial intelligence in healthcare: transforming the practice of medicine. Futur. Healthc. J. **8**, e188–e194 (2021). https://doi.org/10.7861/fhj.2021-0095

14. Nayak, S., Blumenfeld, N.R., Laksanasopin, T., Sia, S.K.: Point-of-care diagnostics: recent developments in a connected age. Anal. Chem. **89**, 102–123 (2017). https://doi.org/10.1021/acs.analchem.6b04630
15. Katchman, B.A., Smith, J.T., Obahiagbon, U., Kesiraju, S., Lee, Y.-K., O'Brien, B., et al.: Application of flat panel OLED display technology for the point-of-care detection of circulating cancer biomarkers. Sci. Rep. **6**, 29057 (2016). https://doi.org/10.1038/srep29057
16. Recent trends in emerging infectious diseases. Int. J. Health Sci. (Qassim) **3**, V–VIII (2009)
17. Jethva, P., Momin, M., Khan, T., Omri, A.: Lanthanide-doped upconversion luminescent nanoparticles—evolving role in bioimaging, biosensing, and drug delivery. Materials **15**, 2374 (2022). https://doi.org/10.3390/ma15072374
18. Wu, J., Wu, J., Wei, W., Zhang, Y., Chen, Q.: Upconversion nanoparticles based sensing: from design to point-of-care testing. Small **20** (2024). https://doi.org/10.1002/smll.202311729
19. Dong, Y., Tang, X., Zhang, Z., Song, J., Niu, T., Shan, D., et al.: Perovskite nanocrystal fluorescence-linked immunosorbent assay methodology for sensitive point-of-care biological test. Matter **3**, 273–286 (2020). https://doi.org/10.1016/j.matt.2020.05.004
20. Al-Hawat, M., Cherifi, K., Tricou, L., Lamontagne, S., Tran, M., Ngu, A.C.Y., et al.: Fluorescent pH-sensing bandage for point-of-care wound diagnostics. Aggregate **5** (2024). https://doi.org/10.1002/agt2.472
21. Zhu, H., Fan, J., Du, J., Peng, X.: Fluorescent probes for sensing and imaging within specific cellular organelles. Acc. Chem. Res. **49**, 2115–2126 (2016). https://doi.org/10.1021/acs.accounts.6b00292
22. Chen, J., Ho, W.K.H., Yin, B., Zhang, Q., Li, C., Yan, J., et al.: Magnetic-responsive upconversion luminescence resonance energy transfer (LRET) biosensor for ultrasensitive detection of SARS-CoV-2 spike protein. Biosens. Bioelectron. **248**, 115969 (2024). https://doi.org/10.1016/j.bios.2023.115969
23. Weihs, F., Anderson, A., Trowell, S., Caron, K.: Resonance energy transfer-based biosensors for point-of-need diagnosis—progress and perspectives. Sensors **21**, 660 (2021). https://doi.org/10.3390/s21020660
24. Liu, F., Zou, J., Luo, X., Liu, Y., Huang, C., He, X., et al.: A point-of-care chemiluminescence immunoassay for pepsinogen I enables large-scale community health screening. Anal. Bioanal. Chem. **413**, 4493–4500 (2021). https://doi.org/10.1007/s00216-021-03412-6
25. Ying, X., Zhou, L., Fu, W., Wang, Y., Su, B.: Electrochemiluminescence devices for point-of-care testing. Sens. Diagn. **2**, 480–491 (2023). https://doi.org/10.1039/D2SD00232A
26. Wei, C., Xu, B., Zhang, M., Su, Z., Gu, J., Guo, W., et al.: Highly ordered inkjet-printed quantum-dot thin films enable efficient and stable QLEDs with EQE exceeding 23%. EScience **4**, 100227 (2024). https://doi.org/10.1016/j.esci.2023.100227
27. Zhang, F., Yi, D., Sun, H., Zhang, H.: Cadmium-based quantum dots: preparation, surface modification, and applications. J. Nanosci. Nanotechnol. **14**, 1409–1424 (2014). https://doi.org/10.1166/jnn.2014.8751
28. Storti, F., Bonfadini, S., Criante, L.: Battery-free fully integrated microfluidic light source for portable lab-on-a-chip applications. Sci. Rep. **10**, 12910 (2020). https://doi.org/10.1038/s41598-020-69581-z
29. Ravi, K., Manoharan, T.J.M., Wang, K.-C., Pockaj, B., Nikkhah, M.: Engineered 3D ex vivo models to recapitulate the complex stromal and immune interactions within the tumor microenvironment. Biomaterials **305**, 122428 (2024). https://doi.org/10.1016/j.biomaterials.2023.122428
30. Trautmann, A., Roth, G.-L., Nujiqi, B., Walther, T., Hellmann, R.: Towards a versatile point-of-care system combining femtosecond laser generated microfluidic channels and direct laser written microneedle arrays. Microsyst. Nanoeng. **5**, 6 (2019). https://doi.org/10.1038/s41378-019-0046-5
31. Mousavi, S.M., Kalashgrani, M.Y., Gholami, A., Omidifar, N., Binazadeh, M., Chiang, W.-H.: Recent advances in quantum dot-based lateral flow immunoassays for the rapid, point-of-care diagnosis of COVID-19. Biosensors (Basel) **13**, 786 (2023). https://doi.org/10.3390/bios13080786

32. Liu, H.-Y., Wang, Z.-G., Liu, S.-L., Pang, D.-W.: Single-virus tracking with quantum dots in live cells. Nat. Protoc. **18**, 458–489 (2023). https://doi.org/10.1038/s41596-022-00775-7
33. Ge, L., Yu, J., Ge, S., Yan, M.: Lab-on-paper-based devices using chemiluminescence and electrogenerated chemiluminescence detection. Anal. Bioanal. Chem. **406**, 5613–6530 (2014). https://doi.org/10.1007/s00216-014-7756-1
34. Babin, B.M., Fernandez-Cuervo, G., Sheng, J., Green, O., Ordonez, A.A., Turner, M.L., et al.: Chemiluminescent protease probe for rapid, sensitive, and inexpensive detection of live *Mycobacterium tuberculosis*. ACS Cent. Sci. **7**, 803–814 (2021). https://doi.org/10.1021/acscentsci.0c01345
35. Chen, X., Wang, X., Fang, Y., Zhang, L., Zhao, M., Liu, Y.: Long-lasting chemiluminescence-based POCT for portable and visual pathogenic detection and in situ inactivation. Anal. Chem. **94**, 8382–8391 (2022). https://doi.org/10.1021/acs.analchem.2c00877
36. Li, K., Hong, E., Wang, B., Wang, Z., Zhang, L., Hu, R., et al.: Advances in the application of upconversion nanoparticles for detecting and treating cancers. Photodiagnosis Photodyn. Ther. **25**, 177–192 (2019). https://doi.org/10.1016/j.pdpdt.2018.12.007
37. Srichan, C., Srichan, W., Danvirutai, P., Ritsongmuang, C., Sharma, A., Anutrakulchai, S.: Non-invasively accuracy enhanced blood glucose sensor using shallow dense neural networks with NIR monitoring and medical features. Sci. Rep. **12**, 1769 (2022). https://doi.org/10.1038/s41598-022-05570-8
38. Sang, M., Cho, M., Lim, S., Min, I.S., Han, Y., Lee, C., et al.: Fluorescent-based biodegradable microneedle sensor array for tether-free continuous glucose monitoring with smartphone application. Sci. Adv. **9** (2023). https://doi.org/10.1126/sciadv.adh1765
39. Singh, V., Nerimetla, R., Yang, M., Krishnan, S.: Magnetite-quantum dot immunoarray for plasmon-coupled-fluorescence imaging of blood insulin and glycated hemoglobin. ACS Sens. **2**, 909–915 (2017). https://doi.org/10.1021/acssensors.7b00124
40. Ripoll, C., Orte, A., Paniza, L., Ruedas-Rama, M.J.: A quantum dot-based FLIM glucose nanosensor. Sensors **19**, 4992 (2019). https://doi.org/10.3390/s19224992
41. Son, J.H., Cho, B., Hong, S., Lee, S.H., Hoxha, O., Haack, A.J., et al.: Ultrafast photonic PCR. Light Sci. Appl. **4**, e280–e280 (2015). https://doi.org/10.1038/lsa.2015.53
42. Xu, Y., Chang, E., Liu, H., Jiang, H., Gambhir, S.S., Cheng, Z.: Proof-of-concept study of monitoring cancer drug therapy with cerenkov luminescence imaging. J. Nucl. Med. **53**, 312–317 (2012). https://doi.org/10.2967/jnumed.111.094623
43. Ikram, M., Malik, R., Raees, R., Imran, M., Wang, F., Ali, S., et al.: Recent advancements and future insight of lead-free non-toxic perovskite solar cells for sustainable and clean energy production: a review. Sustainable Energy Technol. Assess. **53**, 102433 (2022). https://doi.org/10.1016/j.seta.2022.102433
44. Guo, W., Song, X., Liu, J., Liu, W., Chu, X., Lei, Z.: Quantum dots as a potential multi-functional material for the enhancement of clinical diagnosis strategies and cancer treatments. Nanomaterials **14**, 1088 (2024). https://doi.org/10.3390/nano14131088
45. Shi, X., Zhou, X., Zhang, Y., Xu, X., Zhang, Z., Liu, P., et al.: A self-healing and stretchable light-emitting device. J. Mater. Chem. C Mater. **6**, 12774–12780 (2018). https://doi.org/10.1039/C8TC02828A
46. Khan, H., Jan, Z., Ullah, I., Alwabli, A., Alharbi, F., Habib, S., et al.: A deep dive into AI integration and advanced nanobiosensor technologies for enhanced bacterial infection monitoring. Nanotechnol. Rev. **13** (2024). https://doi.org/10.1515/ntrev-2024-0056
47. Prakashan, D., Ramya, P.R., Gandhi, S.: A systematic review on the advanced techniques of wearable point-of-care devices and their futuristic applications. Diagnostics **13**, 916 (2023). https://doi.org/10.3390/diagnostics13050916
48. Bastawrous, S., Wu, L., Liacouras, P.C., Levin, D.B., Ahmed, M.T., Strzelecki, B., et al.: Establishing 3D printing at the point of care: basic principles and tools for success. Radiographics **42**, 451–468 (2022). https://doi.org/10.1148/rg.210113
49. Li, W., Wang, J., Xie, Y., Tebyetekerwa, M., Qiu, Z., Tang, J., et al.: Water-based fluorescent paint: presenting a novel approach to study and solve the aggregation caused quench (ACQ) effect in traditional fluorescent materials. Prog. Org. Coat. **120**, 1–9 (2018). https://doi.org/10.1016/j.porgcoat.2018.03.003

50. Ongaro, A.E., Ndlovu, Z., Sollier, E., Otieno, C., Ondoa, P., Street, A., et al.: Engineering a sustainable future for point-of-care diagnostics and single-use microfluidic devices. Lab Chip **22**, 3122–3137 (2022). https://doi.org/10.1039/D2LC00380E
51. Manyazewal, T., Davey, G., Hanlon, C., Newport, M.J., Hopkins, M., Wilburn, J., et al.: Innovative technologies to address neglected tropical diseases in African settings with persistent sociopolitical instability. Nat. Commun. **15**, 10274 (2024). https://doi.org/10.1038/s41467-024-54496-4
52. Heidt, B., Siqueira, W., Eersels, K., Diliën, H., van Grinsven, B., Fujiwara, R., et al.: Point of care diagnostics in resource-limited settings: a review of the present and future of PoC in Its most needed environment. Biosensors (Basel) **10**, 133 (2020). https://doi.org/10.3390/bios10100133
53. Nnachi, R.C., Sui, N., Ke, B., Luo, Z., Bhalla, N., He, D., et al.: Biosensors for rapid detection of bacterial pathogens in water, food and environment. Environ. Int. **166**, 107357 (2022). https://doi.org/10.1016/j.envint.2022.107357

Light-Emitting Materials for Wearable Bioelectronics

Aisha Okmi

Abstract Light-emitting materials in wearable biosensors have transformed health monitoring technology in many aspects. Since the discovery of light-emitting diodes (organic and inorganic), they have been utilized in various medical applications, enabling more accurate and long-term monitoring of essential vital signs. As material fabrication progressed, more promising light-emitting materials were integrated into wearable biosensors, developing significant possibilities for targeting potential diseases. Photoplethysmography (PPG) is a technique employed widely in wearable bioelectronics, operating light with different wavelengths (such as green, red, and infrared) to measure physiological parameters, such as heartbeat and blood pressure, for bio and medical applications. The health benefits of light-emitting medical-based technologies extended to the early prediction of crucial diseases relying on accurate long-term records leading to precise diagnosis of those diseases. The capability to continually track essential signs and diagnose diseases in their early stages leads to a more comprehensive recording of each patient's health profile, opening up possibilities for personalized medicine. This chapter discusses how light-emitting materials in wearable bioelectronics convey precise real-time health monitoring and continuous health tracking, improving patients' treatment and leading to customizing medicine, where long-term monitoring data tailors therapies.

Keywords Bioelectronics · Diodes · Photoplethysmography · Heartbeat · Cardiovascular

A. Okmi (✉)
Department of Physical Sciences, Physics Division, College of Science, Jazan University, Jazan, Kingdom of Saudi Arabia
e-mail: aokmi@jazanu.edu.sa

© The Author(s), under exclusive license to Springer Nature Switzerland AG 2025

N. O. Etafo (ed.), *Tailored Light Emitters For Biomedical Applications*, Engineering Materials, https://doi.org/10.1007/978-3-031-88731-4_7

1 Introduction: The Concepts and Their Applications in Healthcare

The use of light-emitting materials in bio-optoelectronics emerged at the beginning of 1980. Since then, scientists have achieved countless experiments to enhance the performance of those materials, making them suitable for different types of applications, including healthcare [1]. Wearable bioelectronics based on light-emitting elements are known for emitting light when exposed to changes in the surrounding environment. Those materials instantly respond to physical changes in the human body once in contact with the skin and offer noninvasive techniques to track health issues. For example, the mechanism of the pulse oximeter, a small device that can be used regularly to measure blood pressure, depends on the principles of photoplethysmography (PPG) [2], which uses the absorbed light from light-emitting material such as light-emitting diodes (LED) to measure the changes of the blood volume in the blood vessels [3, 4] The simplicity of the fabrication from different types of noncomplicated and inexpensive precursors makes it facilitated to improve their performance in several kinds of medical applications. Most produced light-emitting substances are transparent, flexible, and highly effective for microdevice applications, enabling the innovative development of comfortable vitals signal monitors. All these advantages make them excellent candidates for health monitoring, such as blood pressure detection and glucose increase besides detecting fatal diseases in their early stages. The options of materials that emit light at specific wavelengths for wearable health monitoring devices include various categories of organic and inorganic materials; however, four distinct types of those materials were reported in the last 15 years to be widely integrated into the medical devices, as listed in Table. 1. Organic light-emitting diodes (OLED) [1, 5] were massively studied and reported to be one of the most promising light-emitting materials integrated into wearable devices for health purposes and have created a revolutionary approach in this field. Although inorganic light-emitting diode LEDs, developed over 40 years ago and reached a mature stage in most technological aspects, OLEDs excelled as flexible, transparent, and energy-efficient in fabricating health monitor devices [3, 6]. Murawski and Gather reported several unique benefits of OLEDs include minimal heat emission, instant response, fast refresh, excellent visuality, and durability [1]. These unique aspects make the OLEDs one of the most promising materials for integration into health monitor devices. Quantum dots (QDs) are one of the cutting-edge light-emitting materials in the field of health signals tracking [7, 8]. The use of QDs in bio-sensing applications is a new emergent as it is stated in a recent study by Abdel-Hakim et al., which discusses the use of carbon quantum dots as cancer marker detector in biosensing platform [9]. The list of light-emitting materials includes a wide variety, such as Micro LEDs, Perovskite LEDs (PeLEDs), Organic–Inorganic Hybrid Materials, Silicon Photonics, Bio-LEDs, and Electroluminescent Polymers (ELPs) [4, 10, 11]. While these materials remain an affluent spot of exploration for noninvasive medical and bio-applications, each possesses distinctive aspects that make them an excellent match for integration into health sensors.

Table. 1. A list of the most usable light-emitting materials in the field of the wearable-bio-sensors

Type of light-emitting material	Techniques in medical wearable devices	Wavelength-emitting (nm)	Usage (health signs detected)	Examples of wearable devices	Reference
Organic Light-Emitting Diodes (OLEDs)	Flexible displays, PPG sensors	448, 527, 620–633, and725 nm	Heart rate and oxygen levels	Flexible OLED wristbands, smart patches	[1, 5]
Inorganic Light-Emitting Diodes (LEDs)	PPG, SpO2 sensors, heart rate monitoring	500–600 nm green 600–680 nm red 800–950 nm IR	Heart rate, blood oxygen levels, respiration rate	Smartwatches and PPG ring	[12]
Quantum Dot Light-Emitting Diodes (QD-LEDs)	PPG sensors	Tunable wavelengths several different, RGB, UV to NIR	Heart rate and blood oxygen levels	Fingertips and ear clips	[8, 13]
Perovskite Light-Emitting Diodes (PeLEDs)	Emerging optoelectronic devices	Tunable from visible to NIR	Heart rate, stress levels, blood oxygen	Emerging smart patches	[11, 14]

This chapter focuses on using light-emitting materials in wearable bioelectronics and how this technology transforms traditional health monitoring, leading to greater precision in real-time data collection, improving patient outcomes, and enhancing accessibility to continuous health tracking. The most incredible result researchers in this field may hope for is reaching an utterly personalized medicine when patients can tailor their treatment based on long-term monitoring results. However, several challenges remain to be addressed, including ensuring user comfort, optimizing power efficiency, maintaining devices regularly, and protecting patient privacy. Figure 1 highlights the progress made in the field of biosensors based on the most studied light-emitting materials, and the related challenges.

2 Monitoring the Vital Signs Using Light-Emitting Wearable Devices

Wearable technology incorporates light-emitting components, such as green, red, or infrared LEDs, to emit light that is absorbed by the skin for medical applications [15]. Light interacts with blood in the microvascular system during transmission, resulting in absorption by blood constituents such as hemoglobin or reflection. These interactions depend on the light's wavelength and the tissue's optical properties,

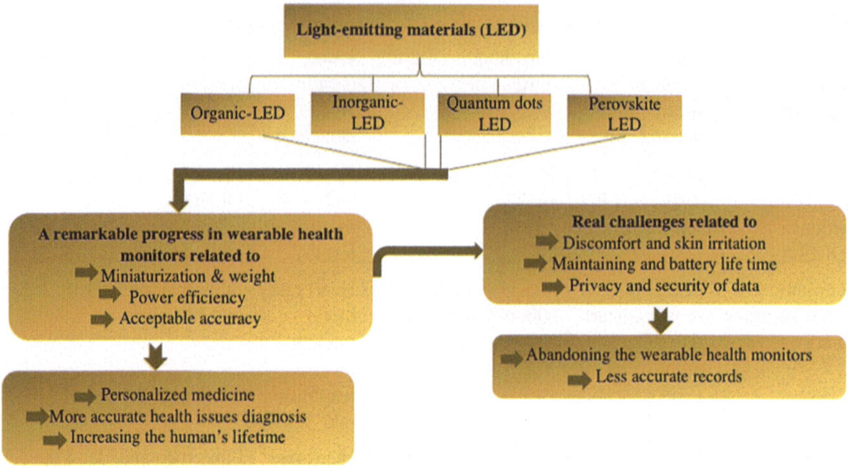

Fig. 1 A schematic description of the wearable bio-electronics based on light-emitting materials highlighting the advantages and the challenges

providing essential insights into physiological factors such as blood oxygenation and circulation [15]. Most of the techniques for vital signs monitoring includes a photodetector captures reflected or transmitted light, and alterations in light intensity are analyzed to measure various physiological factors such as heart rate, oxygen saturation (SpO_2), or respiratory rate. Although the materials for health monitoring purposes follow the same principles, differences related to the type of light-emitting components, such as wavelength and how light interacts with the human body parts, would create a different mechanism. Before describing how these techniques work within health monitoring devices, it is worth to review their origins in the medical realm and operating principles.

As it is known, the heart rate record is the most important vital sign because it provides essential insight into the overall health system. Decades ago, manual heartbeat records, including palpation and stethoscope, were the first health tests for illness detection [16]. While methods like electrocardiography (ECG or EKG) [17], sphygmomanometers, and conventional Holter monitors remain vital tools for health evaluation, they are often time-consuming, require specialized interpretation, and are not user-friendly for immediate or routine use [15]. Although these techniques leverage the benefits of light-emitting materials for monitoring health indicators, only a few are well-suited for integration into wearable devices due to challenges such as bulky equipment, complex wiring, and difficulties in component replacement. This highlights that not all light-emitting-based devices are easily adaptable for miniaturization and wearable applications.

The fascinating discovery of light absorption by human tissues was critical in most new health monitor wearable devices. Initially, the integrated light into PPG devices can be classified into two types based on its interaction with the human body

[2, 18]. Tamura et al. reviewed that LEDs in PPG can emit either infrared, transmitting into the human tissues, or green, reflecting from the human skin. In both cases, the resultant beam can be read out by a photodetector, precisely evaluating the blood circulation, oxygen saturation, or blood pressure [12]. Although the integration of PPG techniques into wearable devices was successfully achieved at the beginning of the current century, the emergence and use of these PPG in healthcare centers appeared nearly 50 years ago [19]. The discovery of light-emitting materials drastically improved PPG techniques in several ways, from massive size to carry-on devices to wearable devices, the most desirable development. Light-emitting materials have contributed to the massive advancement in the bio-electronic wearable monitors in many aspects, such as miniaturization, wavelength control, energy efficiency, fixability, and the accuracy of the results.

2.1 Vital Sign Monitoring: Measure Physiological Parameters Such as Heart Rate, Blood Pressure, and Oxygen Saturation.

Heartbeat:

Heartbeat record provides an instant identifier for the patient's health, making it one of the most significant vital signs. The need for more precise and long-term records increases as the patient ages. Consequently, the demand for wearable bioelectronic devices for these urgent cases has become a demand. As it had been demonstrated before, PPG is an optical technique that operates light to measure the changes in blood volume in the microvascular bed, providing information related to heart pulse records, blood pressure, and oxygen rate [20]. Depending on specific principles, all three vital signs—heartbeat, blood pressure, and oxygen rate—can be monitored regularly with PPG wearable devices; however, a few changes regarding the configuration and supporting technology can be made based on the target health indicators.

Heartbeat-observing devices use a wearable lightweight wristband that looks like a watch, Fig. 2. The PPG technology behind these devices includes the following essential parts: First, the wavelength source comprises a wide range of choices, as shown in Table 1. As Maeda et al. reported, the standard wristbands monitors enable the green LED (525 nm wavelength) to be a light source since it does not penetrate deep into the skin [21]. The reflected beam can be measured with a simple photodetector, the second fundamental part of the heartbeat monitor in wristband device. The detected resultant signal is challenging to read or analyze immediately, which makes it a requirement to process the signal properly. At this step, the signal analyzer contains a series of noise filters and amplifiers that deliver an instant, precise read [20, 21]. Now, the question is, how does the PPG function light to measure the heartbeat? The answer to this question is simple, although it passes through several technical processes. The LED in the wristband shines a light with a specific

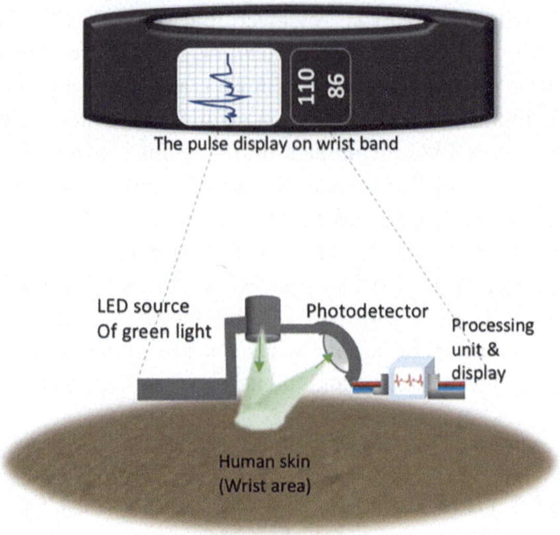

Fig. 2 Simple illustration of the PPG mechanism in wearable device based on green LED

wavelength to the skin in the wrist area, where it partially penetrates the skin and is absorbed by the blood, as Fig. 2, indicated. The light absorption by the blood alters as the blood volume changes due to the heartbeats, creating a train of signals (fluctuations) that can be detected and recorded by the photodetectors [22]. The simplicity of the principles led to health monitors becoming accessible devices for individuals across various lifestyles. They serve as critical tools for tracking heart health and monitoring athletic performance, significantly contributing to the increase in the average human lifespan.

Blood pressure:

Due to modern lifestyles, blood pressure is a significant health indicator that is challenging to control. As a result, wearable health sensors to track changes in blood pressure are critically important. Zhou et al. reviewed that PPG technique which relies on fluctuations in reflected light caused by its interaction with the skin, which result from changes in blood volume within the cardiovascular bed during each heartbeat [23]. According to the same article, this method can be integrated with advanced techniques, such as pulse transit time (PTT) and pulse wave analysis (PWA), to develop wearable devices capable of effectively monitoring blood pressure. The role, again, is similar to what was mentioned in the last section. The LED in the PPG device generates the light that interacts with the blood fluctuations in every single heartbeat; however, in the blood pressure device setup, there is an extra requirement to measure the time interval between the ventricular contraction points (R-wave peek, measured by ECG) and the arrival of the pulse wave (detected by the photodetector in the PPG device) [18, 23]. The pulse wave analyzer is an alternative technique that can be combined with light-emitting materials through PPG devices to measure blood pressure. One of the main differences between PPT and PWA is that PWA measures wave features such as peak timing, slope, and width without measuring the R-points, which means there is no need for the ECG sensor. On the other hand, PPT and PWA are significant strategies that can operate separately when combined with light-emitting materials in wearable devices, offering accurate, exact blood pressure records. The two technologies broadly use LED green wavelength, red, and infrared light sources [24, 25].

Oxygen saturation:

Oxygen saturation (SpO_2) is a physiological indicator of how much oxygen binds to blood hemoglobin. SpO_2 is a vital sign of the same importance as the biological signs discussed in the previous subsections [26]. Detecting early heart failure and acute respiratory diseases such as COVID-19 and lung dysfunction, and tracking fitness are all monitored and managed by measuring oxygen levels in the blood [27]. In this regard, wearable devices based on light-emitting materials afford excellent manners to track the related physiological parameters, saving human life. Fu et al. describe a noninvasive technique known as pulse oximetry uses red and infrared LED as a light source in the SpO_2 monitoring devices, and can be combined with the PPG devices. Pulse oximetry wearable device include three primary elements: LED dual-wavelength (red and infrared), photodetector, and signal processing unit. Each of those components has a particular role in SpO_2 tracking and recording [28]. As light from red and infrared LEDs passes through human tissue, blood is either oxygenated or deoxygenated. Hemoglobin absorbs these wavelengths differently; in other words, oxygenated hemoglobin absorbs infrared light and reflects red light, while deoxygenated hemoglobin absorbs red light and reflects infrared light. The sequence absorption and the reflection of different wavelengths produces fluctuations in light intensity, producing a waveform signal corresponding to pulsatile blood flow. The photodetector captures the intensity of each waveform, and the oxygen levels can be identified using an internal algorithm converter [26, 28].

As can be shown, the three essential vital signs—heart rate, blood pressure, and oxygen saturation—are identifiable and trackable using the same technology (PPG), with only minor adjustments to the configuration and supplemental techniques. The Apple Watch is one of the most compromising examples of a health monitor wristband [29]. Apple watch is designed to function with light-emitting materials LED with multiple wavelengths to interact with human blood and measure the essential vital signs simultaneously.

2.2 *Disease Detection: Early Detection of Health Conditions Using Wearable Sensors*

Wearable devices based on light-emitting materials have been widely used to detect particular diseases in their early stages. Techniques including PPG and pulse oximetry can detect cardiovascular diseases in their early appearance and assist in diagnosing them accurately to void critical consequences [30–32]. However, the details regarding the detection of the diseases are more complicated than those of the vital signs recording. In other words, in the case of functioning light-emitting materials in wearable devices to monitor bio-indicators, the job is simple, relying on the instant records that give a fast glimpse of the body's health situation. On the other hand, detecting disease often does not depend on simple data collection and analysis or instant records; instead, it requires deep analysis and prolonged regular data collection, which usually demands extra parts in the wearable devices that do not exist in the essential signs monitors. In the following subsections, the focus will be on some of the techniques that function light-emitting materials in the field of disease detection and how they differ from vital monitoring based on similar methods.

Cardiovascular Diseases

Cardiovascular disease is a type of heart dysfunction and blood vessel disease that is known to be the leading cause of death worldwide. Signs of heart failure, hypertension, arrhythmias, and arterial stiffness are aspects of cardiovascular disease [33]. These issues can be assessed through heart health monitoring, often employing PPG techniques [24]. However, subtle variations in the application of PPG are crucial for the early detection of cardiovascular abnormalities and associated health indicators [24]. Feukeu states that the irregular heartbeat pattern, such as sudden spikes in a heartbeat unaccompanied by physical effort, arrhythmias, and reduced heart rate variation, can be seen in the severe health condition of the PPG signals. While detecting those three symptoms, either green LED (530 nm) or infrared LED (940 nm) functions as a light source for PPG in bio-wearable devices, and each produces distinguishable marks on the PPG readings [34, 35]. Cardiovascular diseases often can be reflected clearly in the signal analysis of the time variations in the connective heartbeats, known as heart rate variability (HRV). In abnormal cases, reduced HRV indicates stress fatigue, which means that the heart is effectively unresponsive to the varying physiological demands. Compared to reduced HRV, arrhythmias show more bio-marks related to the heart's electrical signals that would be displayed on PPG as erratic and unpredictable intervals and waveform patterns. On the other hand, an irregular heartbeat is identified on PPG as either an extra heartbeat or a missing heartbeat, which is associated with anomalies in timing intervals between peaks [7, 36]. It can be concluded that PPG, based on LEDs as a light source, utilizes an effective and non-invasive method to detect cardiovascular abnormalities, including irregular heartbeats, arrhythmias, and changes in heart rate variability, enabling significant potential for continuous health monitoring and early disease detection.

Diabetes

Combining near-infrared spectroscopy (NIR) with wearable devices is a promising technique for measuring glucose in blood. NIR has a wavelength between 700 and 2500 nm and can penetrate skin tissue to interact with blood ingredients [37, 38]. Glucose in the blood absorbs light at a specific wavelength, showing a spectrum with distinct peaks at determined wavelengths, such as 940, 1025, and 1560–1590 nm. The analysis of those peaks provides an excellent early detection of diabetic cases

[22, 39]. Gutiérrez et al. revealed that combining luminescent metal–organic frameworks (MOFs) into biosensors affords another noninvasive method to detect high glucose levels. Although this method works by detecting acetone, one of the diabetes biomarkers offering an indirect method for the early detection of diabetes, it is a promising research area for creating small and straightforward wearable devices [40].

Hypertension (High Blood Pressure)

Wearable devices using light-emitting materials like infrared and green LEDs are widely used to predict hypertension (high blood pressure) [21]. Wearables typically emit either infrared LEDs (850–940 nm) or green LEDs (530 nm) to the skin, where they interact with blood vessels. Hypertension detection requires PPG to be combined with PWA and PPT to analyze blood flow patterns and arterial stiffness [20, 21]. The critical factor in the detection of high blood pressure is examining the resultant shape of the PPG form, which is created by heartbeat fluctuations. The question that arises now is how wearable devices based on light-emitting materials detect hypertension, which differs from those used to measure it. Answering this question relies on understanding the principles in both cases. Detection of hypertension focuses on changes of health patterns in vascular health patterns. For example, once PTT or PWV values display regular increases, it may suggest potential hypertension, provoking patients to seek a proper diagnosis [23, 41]. The methods used to measure hypertension using PPG devices are more likely to measure changes in blood pressure related to heartbeats. Consequently, it does not measure hypertension directly; instead, it measures the trends in the blood that correlate with hypertension risk.

In addition to hypertension, diabetes, and cardiovascular illness, light-emitting materials in wearable devices can assist in detecting additional health issues at home, particularly those that make physiological changes detectable by optical sensors as illustrated below.

Detecting other symptoms and diseases with wearable light-emitting devices

Mirjalali et al. reviewed that optical fiber technologies, mentioned in the article as Fiber Bragg Grating (FBG), can be incorporated into wearable devices for the early detection of COVID-19 [42]. Likewise, sleep disorders, including sleep apnea, are detectable by monitoring SpO_2 changes and abnormal heart rate variability HRV during sleep. PPG-based wearables are also known to detect chronic stress and mental health conditions like stress and depression by tracking HRV [31, 42, 43]. Chronic stress usually correlates with reduced HRV values, which estimate the body's low ability to adapt to stress, providing signs of overall mental health and stability. Tracking rare low HRV may also indicate a reduction in the human body's liquid percentage, resulting in insights into the risk of dehydration and heat stress [44]. It is worth mentioning that low hemoglobin levels or consistently decreased SpO_2 readings that are unaccompanied with respiratory infections may indicate anemia. In this regard, pulse oximetry equipped with either red 660 nm or infrared 940 nm LED can provide an initial indication to anemia, reducing the need for immediate blood tests [45]. Consequently, wearing a bio-monitor device combining multiple light-emitting materials (green, red, and infrared LEDs) and pulse oximetry is growing as an essential demand for comprehensive, real-time health monitoring. This integration improves accessibility to critical health data and enables the early detection and prevention of various medical conditions, highlighting its potential to revolutionize personal healthcare management.

2.3 Personalized Medicine: Tailor Treatments Based on Real-Time Data from Wearable Devices

As highlighted in the sections above, wearable devices using light-emitting materials drive a significant shift from standardized medicine—where treatments are based on symptoms similarities—to personalized treatment approaches that rely on the unique differences identified through real-time, long-term biomarker monitoring [46]. Bizzarri and Pensotti stated that targeting treatments based on specific, consistent health records and an individual's genetic background is referred to personalized medicine [47]. The concept of customized medicine began taking shape in the early twentieth century and has evolved significantly over the last 20 years, especially with advancements in genomics and the emergence of wearable devices that enable continuous health monitoring. The evaluation of this concept is correlated with the discovery of DNA [47], biosensors, wearable devices, and light-emitting materials, which will allow continuous real-time health monitoring. Particular methods and best practices are crucial and can be summarized as the following [48]. First, preserving accuracy over time, calibrate devices against clinical-grade equipment, especially for measures like blood pressure or SpO_2. Second, Personalized baseline metrics for each user, including normal ranges for heart rate, SpO_2, and HRV. This can be conducted by obtaining data over an extended period and in different circumstances (rest, activity, and sleep) to construct an entire health profile. Third, Establish personalized thresholds for metrics based on baselines, with automated alerts for significant deviations such as low SpO_2 or irregular heart rate. This is achievable by notifying patients and healthcare providers for immediate action when indicators indicate potential issues. Fourth, the treatment plans can be modified to adapt to the patient's progress or alterations in health status by placing regular check-ups with healthcare providers to improve treatment methods based on the patient's changing requirements. Finally, Provide simple instructions or training sessions to ensure individuals understand their wearable data and can respond accurately to cautions or recommendations by regularly training patients on interpreting device information, including HRV, SpO_2, and heart rate variations, and the consequences for their health [36, 46, 49–51].

The following subsection focuses on the following topics: types of wearable biosensors and their capabilities, data collection, analysis, and interpretation techniques, applications in disease management and early detection, and progress toward personalized medicine.

Types of wearable biosensors and their capabilities

Pulse oximetry (red and infrared LEDs) is essential in personalized medicine and its sequential processes. Continuous SpO_2 monitoring via pulse oximetry enables customized therapy of respiratory disorders, especially for individuals with Chronic Obstructive Pulmonary Disease (COPD), asthma, or COVID-19 [31, 43]. Real-time data allows medical professionals to notice rapid falls in oxygen levels, indicating respiratory distress and allowing for fast action. This monitoring sustains tailored treatment by entitling doctors to change drugs, oxygen therapy, or other treatments based on each patient's baseline oxygen requirements and daily movements, resulting in individualized care plans that address fluctuations in respiratory function [52]. Pulse oximetry can detect sleep apnea through frequent reductions in SpO_2 phases, indicating interrupted breathing [31]. By examining these differences, personalized medicine can lead to a precise determination of the frequency and severity of apnea episodes specific to each patient, enabling customized CPAP machine settings. Adjusting treatment intensity to individual demands improves success in decreasing apnea episodes. Pulse oximetry can help manage anemia by recognizing ongoing low SpO_2 levels, indicating effective oxygen transport throughout the body without frequent blood tests. Identifying SpO_2 patterns associated with low hemoglobin allows doctors to adapt therapies, such as iron supplements or dietary alterations, to each patient's needs. Treatment can be modified as oxygen levels improve. Pulse oximetry enables tailored workout or rehabilitation programs by providing real-time SpO_2 feedback during physical activity. Setting individualized criteria guarantees that individuals recuperating from respiratory illnesses or managing chronic diseases can engage in safe activities. Pulse oximetry enables direct evaluation of SpO_2 levels, permitting physicians to customize treatment plans for each patient, which can be one of the pioneer methods for promoting the view of personalizing medicine [53, 54]

Photoplethysmography (PPG) detects blood volume changes with each heartbeat using green or infrared LEDs, effectively monitoring heart rate and heart rate variability. This approach is beneficial for tracking cardiovascular health since it allows healthcare providers to monitor HRV, heart rate, and pulse wave velocity (PWV) to detect arrhythmias, hypertension, and other cardiovascular problems [46]. For example, changes in HRV can point out abnormal heart rhythms like atrial fibrillation, which are crucial for determining a patient's cardiovascular stability and risk factors. PPG also has a vital role in controlling chronic stress and mental health issues. The correlation between law records of HRV and chronic anxiety or autonomic dysfunction, permitting clinicians to observe and handle disorders such as tension and depression, can establish precise health profiles [30, 55]. By understanding the scanned HRV patterns, clinicians can comprehend a patient's stress levels and autonomic balance, permitting them to change lifestyle advice, therapies, or drugs to improve mental well-being. Furthermore, PPG can assist in identifying early indications of diabetes-related cardiovascular health issues. By evaluating pulse wave patterns, PPG can detect changes in artery stiffness frequently linked with diabetes and its impact on vascular function. Overall, PPG-based wearable devices provide comprehensive health data that supports customized therapy by allowing for real-time monitoring and focused interventions for cardiovascular disease, mental health disorders, and diabetes-related vascular health [56]. By integrating PPG into wearable devices, healthcare can shift towards proactive, patient-centric care, enhancing outcomes across various health domains.

Continuous glucose monitors (CGM) equipped with near-infrared spectroscopy (NIR) have revolutionized diabetes care and metabolic health by providing continuous, real-time insights into blood glucose levels.

These devices use near-infrared wavelengths, typically around 940 and 1045 nm, to measure glucose levels in interstitial fluid, as glucose molecules absorb light at specific wavelengths in the NIR range. CGMs can accurately estimate glucose concentrations by analyzing the light absorption patterns without requiring frequent finger pricks or blood samples [37, 39, 57]. This technique effectively transforms glucose management, allowing individuals to scan blood glucose tendencies and immediately adjust insulin doses and physical activity. By providing instant feedback, CGMs support a highly personalized approach to diabetes care, aiding people to maintain stable glucose levels and avoid dangerous highs (hyperglycemia) or lows (hypoglycemia) [37]. Individuals can pay more attention to understand better how their lifestyle options, such as meals, training, and stress, impact their glucose levels, allowing them to create proactive adjustments to their habits and treatments by tracking real-time glucose information.

Additionally, to managing established diabetes, CGMs also play a critical role in monitoring and intervening in prediabetes and metabolic syndrome [58]. Following glucose oscillations, CGMs can detect early signs of insulin resistance and blood sugar instability that often precede type 2 diabetes. This early detection enables patients and doctors to cooperate to apply preventative strategies like lifestyle changes, dietary adjustments, and focused physical exercise to stop or slow down the development of full-fledged diabetes [59]. CGMs with NIR technology thus support not only treatment for those with diabetes but also preventive health measures for those at risk, fostering a proactive approach to managing metabolic health.

Personalized medicine is inextricably linked to advances in light-emitting materials and biosensor technology, as these instruments give the real-time, continuous data required to tailor treatment to each individual's specific needs.

Light-emitting biosensors, such as those used in PPG and near-infrared spectroscopy (NIR), allow for noninvasive, precise monitoring of critical biomarkers such as heart rate, blood oxygen levels, glucose, and other physiological indications. These sensors continuously gather crucial insights, providing more than isolated pictures of health; they indicate patterns, fluctuations, and rapid responses to lifestyle choices and therapies [46]. This data enables patients to manage their health problems proactively, including real-time glucose monitoring for diabetes, measuring SpO_2 and heart rate variability for respiratory and cardiovascular health, and assessing vascular function to prevent consequences of metabolic syndrome. By leveraging these biosensors' unique light absorption properties, healthcare providers may give completely individualized treatment, altering therapies based on dynamic, real-time data rather than conventional averages. In summary, light-emitting biosensors enable the advancement of personalized medicine by providing the foundational technology that transforms tailored healthcare from a concept to a realistic, daily reality for patients worldwide.

3 Design Considerations and Challenges

The future of biosensor wearable devices for health monitoring holds exciting advancements alongside significant challenges to overcome. Enhancing accuracy and increasing the buttery lifetime are also fields for expanding improvement. Despite the considerable progress researchers have made in developing wearable biomonitors based on light-emitting materials to enable long-term vital sign monitoring and advance personalized medicine with its many advantages, several critical challenges still need to be addressed thoughtfully. The following subsections focus on the main challenging aspects of light-emitting wearable devices, including examples and statistics [20, 57].

3.1 Physical Challenges Including Comfort and Wearability

Direct contact with the skin can cause discomfort, such as excessive sweating and irritation. Despite the efforts to synthesize wearable devices from easily vandalized and anti-allergic materials, wearing them for hours always causes discomfort. A poll conducted by Gartner scanned millions of consumers in the USA. It showed that around one-third of American consumers who owned a wearable technology ceased using it within six months, primarily due to pain leading to the discontinuation of the records [60]. According to the article published in 2019, users abandoned their wearable devices for several reasons: lack of GPS, uncomfortable size and weight, poor buttery, lack of waterproofing, and failure to integrate into their daily routine. A study by Stuart et al. released in 2024 indicated that a remarkable number of wearable technology users experience skin discomfort and irritation, resulting in decreased usage or abandonment of the device. Although light-emitting wearable devices are designed to be light, flexible, and comfortable to wear long, they still can impact daily life activities like swimming and particular cardio activities [61]. A review published in the Journal of Medical Internet Research has pointed out that participants perceived wearables as intrusive in daily activities, influencing their motivation to persist in usage [62]. Age is crucial when feeling discomfort or pain when wearing health monitor devices. As indicated by [63], the usage significantly declines with age, with individuals aged 50–64 and older being 43% less likely to use these devices than those aged 18–34, indicating that discomfort and ergonomic issues were key factors in this decline. These studies and data collection, which were conducted between 2019 and 2024, unequivocally show that physical difficulties like discomfort and ergonomic problems are significant barriers to using health monitors for persistent and reliable record-keeping.

3.2 Technical Challenges Including Power Efficiency and Battery Life and Regular Maintenance

Arya at el. reviewed that sustained operation is key in increasing biosensors' wearability and enabling continuous monitoring without frequent recharging. Sensors, including LEDs utilized in PPG or pulse oximetry, necessitate a constant power source, pushing the need for efficient power economy of wearable devices [64]. The efforts to design the type of batteries that can last for long periods are remarkable; however, it is still vital to balance several aspects, including the device's operational power requirements, with small, light batteries because larger batteries might make the device heavier and less comfortable. Self-powered wearables that use motion or body heat to generate electricity have advanced, but these technologies still require maturity for consistent, long-term energy efficiency [65, 66].

Implementing strategies like integrating low-power LEDs and refining wavelength choices to tackle power efficiency issues can reduce energy consumption while preserving signal accuracy. Furthermore, advancements in rechargeable batteries and energy-harvesting technologies, including body heat and motion-based charging, are expected to enhance gadget longevity and decrease the frequency of recharging [67, 68]. However, the substantial power requirements of light-emitting biosensors may lead to diminished battery longevity, requiring frequent recharging or battery replacements—an especially notable annoyance for implantable or long-term wearable devices.

Implantable biodegradable biosensors need help balancing how much energy they use with how small their devices are [69, 70]. To keep working, they need small, efficient power sources. Likewise, routine maintenance, including battery replacement or recharging, might be intrusive and impracticable for these devices. In specialized applications, such as tear-based ocular wearable biosensors, technological constraints hinder the development process, including miniaturization, power consumption, and long-term stability [64–66]. Addressing these challenges necessitates innovative, energy-efficient designs to reduce maintenance requirements and enhance user adherence, enabling wearable and implanted biosensors to realize their full promise for sustained health monitoring. Advancing energy-efficient designs can fully realize the potential of wearable and implantable biosensors, thereby transforming health monitoring into a smooth and dependable component of daily life.

3.3 Accuracy and Reliability

As wearable biosensors play an increasingly central role in health monitoring and personalized medicine, achieving high accuracy and reliability of those devices is a real challenge. The need for precise data collection and interpretation is paramount because inaccuracies can lead to misdiagnosis, ineffective treatments, or a loss of user trust. Several factors contribute to this challenge, including environmental interference, and the devices' technical limitations.

Environmental Factors and Noise: Salehizadeh indicated that wearable biosensors' operation principles work in dynamic environments where external circumstances interfere with signal accuracy. For example, ambient light can disrupt PPG readings, while motion artifacts caused by physical activity can introduce noise into the data [32, 71]. These inevitably produced interferences can alter the accuracy of measurements such as heart rate, blood oxygen saturation (SpO_2), or glucose levels. Accordingly, advanced signal processing algorithms and hardware designs are crucial to filter out noise and isolate meaningful data from irrelevant signals [72]. As a result, strategies such as multi-wavelength sensing and adaptive filtering are under consideration to improve reliability, but maintaining consistent accuracy across diverse environments remains difficult.

Technical Limitations and Miniaturization: Regarding technical obstacles, biosensors possess several technical limitations related to their size and sensitivity, as well as the challenges to accuracy and reliability that accompany depreciation [69, 73]. While essential for user comfort and wearability, miniaturization often compromises sensor sensitivity and resolution [74, 75]. The strangulation needed to detect small changes in biomarkers escalates with device miniaturization, hence diminishing measurement precision. Advancements in materials science and associated technologies, including nanomaterials and flexible substrates, are extensively investigated to improve the sensitivity of tiny sensors while maintaining their usefulness.

Calibration and Long-Term Stability: Over long durations of use, constant calibration is required to ensure the accuracy of wearable biosensors [76]. However, frequent recalibration might limit user compliance and present obstacles, such as the need for human intervention, which may raise other concerns, such as data privacy risks. To solve this, creating durable materials and self-calibrating technologies is critical to assure accuracy while reducing the need for frequent manual adjustments [77].

Battery Life and Signal Quality: The operation of wearable biosensors, specifically light-emitting-based materials like LEDs, requires significant energy, which can adversely affect accuracy [78]. As battery levels deplete, signal strength and quality tend to degrade, resulting in less reliable readings [79]. To mitigate this, energy-efficient designs that incorporate low-power LEDs and advanced power management systems are essential for maintaining consistent performance and reliability.

3.4 Data Privacy and Security

Bouderhem highlighted that health data collected by wearable devices are sensitive since they reflect an individual's physiological and biological state, encompassing essential information that impacts all activities. For this matter, handling those data must conducted with much care about privacy [80]. General regulations and land policies like the Health Insurance Portability and Accountability Act (HIPAA) and General Data Protection Regulation (GDPR), which set standards for handling and storing personal health information, have to be followed strictly [81, 82]. Consequently, data sharing of those records must be preceded by obtaining a user's consent. Although the data collected by light-emitting wearable devices can still be available for specific types of health studies and surveys, implementing anonymization techniques for collected data can protect user identity, mainly when devices are used in broader research studies or healthcare analytics [83, 84]. With the rise of IoT-connected devices, security challenges also extend to preventing unauthorized access, requiring regular firmware updates and strong authentication processes.

References

1. Murawski, C., Gather, M.C.: Emerging biomedical applications of organic light-emitting diodes. Adv. Opt. Mater. **9** (2021). https://doi.org/10.1002/adom.202100269
2. Kyriacou, P.A., Allen, J. (eds.): Photoplethysmography: Technology, Signal Analysis and Applications (2021)
3. Cha, G.D., Kim, D.-H., Kim, D.C.: Wearable and implantable light-emitting diodes and their biomedical applications. Korean J. Chem. Eng. **41**, 1–24 (2024). https://doi.org/10.1007/s11814-023-00006-z
4. Bae, S.-H., Kim, D., Chang, S.-Y., Hur, J., Kim, H., Lee, J.-W., et al.: Hybrid integrated photomedical devices for wearable vital sign tracking. ACS Sens. **5**, 1582–1588 (2020). https://doi.org/10.1021/acssensors.9b02529
5. Jeon, Y., Choi, H., Lim, M., Choi, S., Kim, H., Kwon, J.H., et al.: A wearable photobiomodulation patch using a flexible red-wavelength OLED and its in vitro differential cell proliferation effects. Adv. Mater. Technol. **3** (2018). https://doi.org/10.1002/admt.201700391
6. Li, Y.: Organic Optoelectronic Materials, vol. 91 (2015)
7. Chen, S., Qi, J., Fan, S., Qiao, Z., Yeo, J.C., Lim, C.T.: Flexible wearable sensors for cardiovascular health monitoring. Adv. Healthc. Mater. **10** (2021). https://doi.org/10.1002/adhm.202100116
8. Kim, J., Shim, H.J., Yang, J., Choi, M.K., Kim, D.C., Kim, J., et al.: Ultrathin quantum dot display integrated with wearable electronics. Adv. Mater. **29** (2017). https://doi.org/10.1002/adma.201700217
9. Abdel-Hakim, A., Belal, F., Hammad, M.A., Kishikawa, N., El-Maghrabey, M.: Adoption of self-exothermic reaction for synthesis of multifunctional carbon quantum dots: applications to vincristine sensing and cell imaging. Talanta **282**, 126971 (2025). https://doi.org/10.1016/j.talanta.2024.126971
10. Hee Lee, J., Lee, S., Kim, D., Jae, L.K.: Implantable Micro-Light-Emitting Diode (μLED)-based optogenetic interfaces toward human applications. Adv. Drug Deliv. Rev. **187**, 114399 (2022). https://doi.org/10.1016/j.addr.2022.114399

11. Pathania, A., RA, RB, WF, TP, and TA: Biomedical Applications of Perovskites: The Era of Bio-piezoelectric Systems. Bentham Science Publishers (2024). https://doi.org/10.2174/978 98152563831240101
12. Tamura, T., Maeda, Y., Sekine, M., Yoshida, M.: Wearable photoplethysmographic sensors—past and present. Electronics (Basel) **3**, 282–302 (2014). https://doi.org/10.3390/electronics3 020282
13. Shabbir, H., Csapó, E., Wojnicki, M.: Carbon quantum dots: the role of surface functional groups and proposed mechanisms for metal ion sensing. Inorganics (Basel) **11**, 262 (2023). https://doi.org/10.3390/inorganics11060262
14. Chun, F., Wang, F.: Recent advances in perovskite-based flexible electroluminescent devices. ACS Nano (2024). https://doi.org/10.1021/acsnano.4c06587
15. Mao, P., Li, H., Yu, Z.: A review of skin-wearable sensors for non-invasive health monitoring applications. Sensors **23**, 3673 (2023). https://doi.org/10.3390/s23073673
16. Neuman, M.R.: Vital signs: heart rate. IEEE Pulse **1**, 51–55 (2010). https://doi.org/10.1109/ MPUL.2010.939179
17. Tasli, H.E., Gudi, A., den Uyl, M.: Remote PPG based vital sign measurement using adaptive facial regions. In: 2014 IEEE International Conference on Image Processing (ICIP), pp. 1410–1414. IEEE (2014). https://doi.org/10.1109/ICIP.2014.7025282.
18. Alian, A.A., Shelley, K.H.: Photoplethysmography. Best Pract. Res. Clin. Anaesthesiol. **28**, 395–406 (2014). https://doi.org/10.1016/j.bpa.2014.08.006
19. Barnes, R.W., Garrett, W.V., Slaymaker, E.E., Reinertson, J.E.: Doppler ultrasound and supraorbital photoplethysmography for noninvasive screening of carotid occlusive disease. Am. J. Surg. **134**, 183–186 (1977). https://doi.org/10.1016/0002-9610(77)90339-7
20. Kim, K.B., Baek, H.J.: Photoplethysmography in wearable devices: a comprehensive review of technological advances, current challenges, and future directions. Electronics (Basel) **12**, 2923 (2023). https://doi.org/10.3390/electronics12132923
21. Maeda, Y., Sekine, M., Tamura, T.: The advantages of wearable green reflected photoplethysmography. J. Med. Syst. **35**, 829–834 (2011). https://doi.org/10.1007/s10916-010-9506-z
22. Jain, P., Maddila, R., Joshi, A.M.: A precise non-invasive blood glucose measurement system using NIR spectroscopy and Huber's regression model. Opt. Quantum Electron. **51**, 51 (2019). https://doi.org/10.1007/s11082-019-1766-3
23. Zhou, Z.-B., Cui, T.-R., Li, D., Jian, J.-M., Li, Z., Ji, S.-R., et al.: Wearable continuous blood pressure monitoring devices based on pulse wave transit time and pulse arrival time: a review. Materials **16**, 2133 (2023). https://doi.org/10.3390/ma16062133
24. Almarshad, M.A., Islam, M.S., Al-Ahmadi, S., Bahammam, A.S.: Diagnostic features and potential applications of PPG signal in healthcare: a systematic review. Healthcare (Switzerland) **10** (2022). https://doi.org/10.3390/healthcare10030547
25. Elgendi, M., Fletcher, R., Liang, Y., Howard, N., Lovell, N.H., Abbott, D., et al.: The use of photoplethysmography for assessing hypertension. NPJ Digit. Med. **2**, 60 (2019). https://doi.org/10.1038/s41746-019-0136-7
26. Ma, G., Zhu, W., Zhong, J., Tong, T., Zhang, J., Wang, L.: Wearable ear blood oxygen saturation and pulse measurement system based on PPG. In: IEEE SmartWorld, ubiquitous intelligence & computing, advanced & trusted computing, scalable computing & communications, cloud & big data computing, internet of people and smart city innovation (SmartWorld/SCALCOM/UIC/ATC/CBDCom/IOP/SCI), pp. 111–116. IEEE (2018). https://doi.org/10.1109/SmartW orld.2018.00054
27. Zhang, Z., Khatami, R.: Can we trust the oxygen saturation measured by consumer smartwatches? Lancet Respir. Med. **10**, e47–e48 (2022). https://doi.org/10.1016/S2213-2600(22)001 03-5
28. Fu, Y., Liu, J.: System design for wearable blood oxygen saturation and pulse measurement device. Procedia Manuf. **3**, 1187–1194 (2015). https://doi.org/10.1016/j.promfg.2015.07.197
29. Monitor your heart rate with apple watch. Apple Support (2024)

30. Namvari, M., Lipoth, J., Knight, S., Jamali, A.A., Hedayati, M., Spiteri, R.J., et al.: Photoplethysmography enabled wearable devices and stress detection: a scoping review. J. Pers. Med. **12**, 1792 (2022). https://doi.org/10.3390/jpm12111792
31. Deviaene, M., Lazaro, J., Huysmans, D., Testelmans, D., Buyse, B., Van Huffel, S., et al.: Sleep apnea detection using pulse photoplethysmography (2018). https://doi.org/10.22489/CinC.2018.134
32. Salehizadeh, S.: Motion and noise artifact detection and vital signal reconstruction in ECG/PPG based wearable devices (2015)
33. Chue, C.D., Townend, J.N., Steeds, R.P., Ferro, C.J.: Republished paper: arterial stiffness in chronic kidney disease: causes and consequences. Postgrad. Med. J. **86**, 560–566 (2010). https://doi.org/10.1136/pgmj.2009.184879rep
34. Feukeu, E.A., Winberg, S.: Photoplethysmography: light emitter diode wavelength derivation from the absorption spectra of haemoglobin. In: 2019 International Multidisciplinary Information Technology and Engineering Conference (IMITEC), pp. 1–6. IEEE (2019). https://doi.org/10.1109/IMITEC45504.2019.9015874
35. Cusini, I., Rinaldi, R., Castiglioni, P., Faini, A., Villa, F.: Multi-wavelength SPAD photoplethysmography for cardio-respiratory monitoring. Front. Phys. **11** (2023). https://doi.org/10.3389/fphy.2023.952103
36. Hughes, A., Shandhi, M.M.H., Master, H., Dunn, J., Brittain, E.: Wearable devices in cardiovascular medicine. Circ. Res. **132**, 652–670 (2023). https://doi.org/10.1161/CIRCRESAHA.122.322389
37. Hina, A., Saadeh, W.: Noninvasive blood glucose monitoring systems using near-infrared technology—a review. Sensors **22**, 4855 (2022). https://doi.org/10.3390/s22134855
38. Di Filippo, D., Sunstrum, F., Khan, J., Welsh, A.: Non-invasive glucose sensing technologies and products: a comprehensive review for researchers and clinicians. Sensors **23**, 9130 (2023). https://doi.org/10.3390/s23229130
39. Naresh, M., Peddakrishna, S., Thirupathi, M.: Non-invasive Glucose Measurement with 940 nm Sensor Using Short Wave NIR Technique, pp. 95–103 (2023). https://doi.org/10.1007/978-3-031-36246-0_10
40. Gutiérrez, M., Möslein, A.F., Tan, J.-C.: Facile and fast transformation of nonluminescent to highly luminescent metal-organic frameworks: acetone sensing for diabetes diagnosis and lead capture from polluted water. ACS Appl. Mater. Interfaces **13**, 7801–7811 (2021). https://doi.org/10.1021/acsami.0c22307
41. Gesche, H., Grosskurth, D., Küchler, G., Patzak, A.: Continuous blood pressure measurement by using the pulse transit time: comparison to a cuff-based method. Eur. J. Appl. Physiol. **112**, 309–315 (2012). https://doi.org/10.1007/s00421-011-1983-3
42. Mirjalali, S., Peng, S., Fang, Z., Wang, C., Wu, S.: Wearable sensors for remote health monitoring: potential applications for early diagnosis of Covid-19. Adv. Mater. Technol. **7** (2022). https://doi.org/10.1002/admt.202100545
43. Michard, F., Shelley, K., L'Her, E.: COVID-19: pulse oximeters in the spotlight. J. Clin. Monit. Comput. **35**, 11–14 (2021). https://doi.org/10.1007/s10877-020-00550-7
44. Porto, A.A., Benjamim, C.J.R., da Silva Sobrinho, A.C., Gomes, R.L., Gonzaga, L.A., da Silva, R.G., et al.: Influence of fluid ingestion on heart rate, cardiac autonomic modulation and blood pressure in response to physical exercise: a systematic review with meta-analysis and meta-regression. Nutrients **15**, 4534 (2023). https://doi.org/10.3390/nu15214534
45. McLintic, A., Wong, A.: Oximetry. Physics and Measurement for Anesthesia, pp. 57–64. Springer Nature Switzerland, Cham (2024). https://doi.org/10.1007/978-3-031-65060-4_8
46. Chau, D., Osborne, T.F., Gass, A.P., Kaye, L.W., Singer, C., Nerenberg, L.: Critical Topics in an Aging Society • Homeless Older Populations: A Practical Guide for the Interdisciplinary Care Team and Elder Abuse (n.d.)
47. Bizzarri, M., Pensotti, A., Cucina, A., Monti, N., Fedeli, V.: Personalized Treatments: Where Patient's History and Biological Background Meet, pp. 63–86 (2022). https://doi.org/10.1007/978-3-030-74804-3_4.

48. Cinti, C., Trivella, M.G., Joulie, M., Ayoub, H., Frenzel, M.: The roadmap toward personalized medicine: challenges and opportunities. J. Pers. Med. **14**, 546 (2024). https://doi.org/10.3390/jpm14060546
49. Masoumian Hosseini, M., Masoumian Hosseini, S.T., Qayumi, K., Hosseinzadeh, S., Sajadi Tabar, S.S.: Smartwatches in healthcare medicine: assistance and monitoring; a scoping review. BMC Med. Inform. Decis. Mak. **23** (2023). https://doi.org/10.1186/s12911-023-02350-w
50. Shajari, S., Kuruvinashetti, K., Komeili, A., Sundararaj, U.: The emergence of AI-based wearable sensors for digital health technology: a review. Sensors **23**, 9498 (2023). https://doi.org/10.3390/s23239498
51. Olyanasab, A., Annabestani, M.: Leveraging machine learning for personalized wearable biomedical devices: a review. J. Pers. Med. **14**, 203 (2024). https://doi.org/10.3390/jpm14020203
52. Angus, D.C.: Your mileage may vary. JAMA **331**, 1179 (2024). https://doi.org/10.1001/jama.2024.0972
53. Shah, S.A., Velardo, C., Gibson, O.J., Rutter, H., Farmer, A., Tarassenko, L.: Personalized alerts for patients with COPD using pulse oximetry and symptom scores. In: 2014 36th Annual International Conference of the IEEE Engineering in Medicine and Biology Society, pp. 3164–3167. IEEE (2014). https://doi.org/10.1109/EMBC.2014.6944294
54. Buekers, J., Theunis, J., De Boever, P., Vaes, A.W., Koopman, M., Janssen, E.V., et al.: Wearable finger pulse oximetry for continuous oxygen saturation measurements during daily home routines of patients with Chronic Obstructive Pulmonary Disease (COPD) over one week: observational study. JMIR Mhealth Uhealth **7**, e12866 (2019). https://doi.org/10.2196/12866
55. Dzedzickis, A., Kaklauskas, A., Bucinskas, V.: Human emotion recognition: review of sensors and methods. Sensors **20**, 592 (2020). https://doi.org/10.3390/s20030592
56. Medina, A., Lopez, N., Galdos, J., Supo, E., Rendulich, J., Sulla, E.: Continuous blood pressure estimation in wearable devices using photoplethysmography: a review. Int. J. Emerg. Technol. Adv. Eng. **12**, 104–113 (2022). https://doi.org/10.46338/ijetae1022_12
57. Jain, P., Joshi, A.M., Mohanty, S.P., Cenkeramaddi, L.R.: Non-invasive glucose measurement technologies: recent advancements and future challenges. IEEE Access **12**, 61907–61936 (2024). https://doi.org/10.1109/ACCESS.2024.3389819
58. Ahmed, I., Jiang, N., Shao, X., Elsherif, M., Alam, F., Salih, A., et al.: Recent advances in optical sensors for continuous glucose monitoring. Sens. Diagn. **1**, 1098–1125 (2022). https://doi.org/10.1039/D1SD00030F
59. Ghosh, N., Verma, S.: Technological advancements in glucose monitoring and artificial pancreas systems for shaping diabetes care. Curr. Med. Res. Opin., 1–13 (2024). https://doi.org/10.1080/03007995.2024.2422005
60. Fadhil, A.: Perceived User Behavior in Abandoning Wearable Health & Wellness Trackers (2019)
61. Stuart, S., de Kok, M., O'Searcoid, B., Morrisroe, H., Serban, I.B., Jagers, F., et al.: Critical design considerations for longer-term wear and comfort of on-body medical devices. Bioengineering **11** (2024). https://doi.org/10.3390/bioengineering11111058
62. Moore, K., O'Shea, E., Kenny, L., Barton, J., Tedesco, S., Sica, M., et al.: Older adults' experiences with using wearable devices: qualitative systematic review and meta-synthesis. JMIR Mhealth Uhealth **9**, e23832 (2021). https://doi.org/10.2196/23832
63. Nagappan, A., Krasniansky, A., Knowles, M.: Patterns of ownership and usage of wearable devices in the united states, 2020–2022: survey study. J. Med. Internet Res. **26**, e56504 (2024). https://doi.org/10.2196/56504
64. Arya, S., Sharma, A., Singh, A., Ahmed, A., Dubey, A., Padha, B., et al.: Review—energy and power requirements for wearable sensors. ECS Sens. Plus **3** (2024). https://doi.org/10.1149/2754-2726/ad54d2
65. Reid, R.C., Mahbub, I.: Wearable self-powered biosensors. Curr. Opin. Electrochem. **19**, 55–62 (2020). https://doi.org/10.1016/j.coelec.2019.10.002
66. Song, Y., Mukasa, D., Zhang, H., Gao, W.: Self-powered wearable biosensors. Acc. Mater. Res. **2**, 184–197 (2021). https://doi.org/10.1021/accountsmr.1c00002

67. Yin, L., Kim, K.N., Trifonov, A., Podhajny, T., Wang, J.: Designing wearable microgrids: towards autonomous sustainable on-body energy management. Energy Environ. Sci. **15**, 82–101 (2022). https://doi.org/10.1039/D1EE03113A
68. Magno, M., Polonelli, T., Benini, L., Popovici, E.: A low cost, highly scalable wireless sensor network solution to achieve smart LED light control for green buildings. IEEE Sens. J. **15**, 2963–2973 (2015). https://doi.org/10.1109/JSEN.2014.2383996
69. Alam, F., Ashfaq Ahmed, M., Jalal, A., Siddiquee, I., Adury, R., Hossain, G., et al.: Recent progress and challenges of implantable biodegradable biosensors. Micromachines (Basel) **15**, 475 (2024). https://doi.org/10.3390/mi15040475
70. Hosseini, E.S., Dervin, S., Ganguly, P., Dahiya, R.: Biodegradable materials for sustainable health monitoring devices. ACS Appl. Bio Mater. **4**, 163–194 (2021). https://doi.org/10.1021/acsabm.0c01139
71. Crescentini, M., Bennati, M., Carminati, M., Tartagni, M.: Noise limits of CMOS current interfaces for biosensors: a review. IEEE Trans. Biomed. Circuits Syst. **8**, 278–292 (2014). https://doi.org/10.1109/TBCAS.2013.2262998
72. Sharma, A., Badea, M., Tiwari, S., Marty, J.L.: Wearable biosensors: an alternative and practical approach in healthcare and disease monitoring. Molecules **26**, 748 (2021). https://doi.org/10.3390/molecules26030748
73. Mohamed, M.A.: Wearable Miniaturized Electrochemical Sensors: Benefits and Challenges, pp. 147–185 (n.d.). https://doi.org/10.1039/9781788013895-00147
74. Soleymani, L., Li, F.: Mechanistic challenges and advantages of biosensor miniaturization into the nanoscale. ACS Sens. **2**, 458–467 (2017). https://doi.org/10.1021/acssensors.7b00069
75. dos Santos, C.C., Lucena, G.N., Pinto, G.C., Júnior, M.J., Marques, R.F.C.: Advances and current challenges in non-invasive wearable sensors and wearable biosensors—a mini-review. Med. Devices Sens. **4** (2021). https://doi.org/10.1002/mds3.10130.
76. Nasiri, S., Khosravani, M.R.: Progress and challenges in fabrication of wearable sensors for health monitoring. Sens. Actuators A Phys. **312**, 112105 (2020). https://doi.org/10.1016/j.sna.2020.112105
77. Lorestani, F., Zhang, X., Abdullah, A.M., Xin, X., Liu, Y., Rahman, M.M., et al.: A highly sensitive and long-term stable wearable patch for continuous analysis of biomarkers in sweat. Adv. Funct. Mater. **33** (2023). https://doi.org/10.1002/adfm.202306117
78. Magno, M., Boyle, D.: Wearable energy harvesting: from body to battery. In: 2017 12th International Conference on Design & Technology of Integrated Systems in Nanoscale Era (DTIS), pp. 1–6, IEEE (2017). https://doi.org/10.1109/DTIS.2017.7930169
79. Chong, Y.-W., Ismail, W., Ko, K., Lee, C.-Y.: Energy harvesting for wearable devices: a review. IEEE Sens. J. **19**, 9047–9062 (2019). https://doi.org/10.1109/JSEN.2019.2925638
80. Bouderhem, R.: Privacy and Regulatory Issues in Wearable Health Technology. ECSA 2023, p. 87. MDPI, Basel Switzerland (2023). https://doi.org/10.3390/ecsa-10-16206
81. Isibor, E.: Regulation of Healthcare Data Security: Legal Obligations in A Digital Age (2024). https://doi.org/10.2139/ssrn.4957244
82. Shah, W.F.: Preserving privacy and security: a comparative study of health data regulations—GDPR vs. HIPAA. Int. J. Res. Appl. Sci. Eng. Technol. **11**, 2189–2199 (2023). https://doi.org/10.22214/ijraset.2023.55551.
83. Mehdi, S.H., Rezazadeh, J., Ampani, R., Varghese, B.: Privacy and Security Issues of IoT Wearables in Smart Healthcare, pp. 423–433 (2023). https://doi.org/10.1007/978-3-031-29078-7_37
84. Awotunde, J.B., Jimoh, R.G., Folorunso, S.O., Adeniyi, E.A., Abiodun, K.M., Banjo, O.O.: Privacy and Security Concerns in IoT-Based Healthcare Systems, pp. 105–134 (2021). https://doi.org/10.1007/978-3-030-75220-0_6

Applications in Therapeutics

Photoluminescence-Based Phototherapy

Renad Almughathawi, Meri Algarni, Nessrin Awadhallah Kattan, and Mazen R. Alrahili

Abstract Photoluminescence-based phototherapy is an innovative and minimally invasive approach to treat various medical conditions such as cancer and bacterial infections. The technology allows for precise targeting of affected tissues by exploiting the controlled absorption and emission properties of luminescent materials such as quantum dots and upconversion nanoparticles. Recent advances in luminescent materials have improved therapeutic outcomes through mechanisms such as Förster resonance energy transfer (FRET) and reactive oxygen species (ROS) generation, enabling applications in antibacterial therapy, immune system activation, and cancer treatment. However, challenges remain regarding materials biocompatibility, tissue penetration, and clinical scalability. This report provides a comprehensive overview of the mechanisms, applications, and future directions of luminescence therapy, focusing on its transformative potential in modern medicine.

Keywords Photoluminescent · Cancer treatment · Phototherapy · And light emitters

1 Introduction

Photoluminescent phototherapy offers a cutting-edge way to treat many health issues, from infections to cancer [1–5]. This treatment uses special light-emitting materials like quantum dots and up-conversion nanoparticles to create specific effects in targeted body parts [6–9]. These effects include making reactive oxygen species (ROS) heating small areas or getting the immune system to work. This approach has benefits over usual treatments like chemotherapy and antibiotics such as being less invasive more targeted, and causing fewer side effects throughout the body [9]. At its

R. Almughathawi · N. A. Kattan · M. R. Alrahili (✉)
Physics Department, School of Science, Taibah University, Medina, Saudi Arabia
e-mail: mrahili@taibahu.edu.sa

M. Algarni
Faculty of Science, Department of Physics, Al-Baha University, Alaqiq, Saudi Arabia

© The Author(s), under exclusive license to Springer Nature Switzerland AG 2025
N. O. Etafo (ed.), *Tailored Light Emitters For Biomedical Applications*, Engineering Materials, https://doi.org/10.1007/978-3-031-88731-4_8

core, photoluminescence works by controlling how light is absorbed and given off at certain wavelengths, which allows it to be used on both surface and deep tissues [10]. Scientists can design luminescent materials for different healing purposes, including killing bacteria fighting cancer, and boosting the immune system. While this method shows promise, it still faces hurdles. These include how deep the light can reach in the body making sure the materials are safe for the body and figuring out how to use it on a larger scale in hospitals and clinics.

This chapter reviews various aspects of luminescence-based phototherapy. The article begins by discussing the mechanism of phototherapy with light emitters, including the fundamentals of luminescence, energy transfer processes such as Förster resonance energy transfer (FRET), and the activation of therapeutic agents. The chapter then reviews applications of antibacterial phototherapy, highlighting the mechanism of action, types of photosensitizers, and clinical efficacy against multidrug-resistant pathogens. Next, the focus is on photoimmunotherapy, which combines phototherapy with immune activation to target tumors through synergistic interactions with immune cells. The discussion continues with cancer phototherapy, where nanoparticle-based targeting and photosensitizer localization enable selective killing of tumor cells with minimal damage to healthy tissue. Finally, the chapter addresses future directions and challenges, emphasizing the need for biocompatible materials, overcoming tissue penetration limitations, and exploring multimodal therapies that combine phototherapy with other treatment modalities as schematically illustrated in Fig. 1. This chapter aims to highlight its potential for translation in modern medicine and its promising future as the basis of innovative treatment strategies by providing a comprehensive overview of the mechanisms, applications, and challenges of photoluminescence therapy.

2 Mechanism of Phototherapy with Light Emitters

Photoluminescence (PL) in phototherapy relies on materials that absorb photons and emit light to activate therapeutic agents. The main materials used are quantum dots, switchable nanoparticles, and rare-earth-doped nanocrystals, which can be engineered to emit light at specific wavelengths suitable for medical applications. The main mechanism involves energy transfer, typically via Förster resonance energy transfer (FRET). FRET is an extremely sensitive physical phenomenon in which energy is non-radiatively transferred from an excited fluorescent donor molecule to a nearby acceptor molecule by dipole–dipole coupling. This energy transfer occurs over a short range, typically 1–10 nm, making FRET a powerful tool for studying molecular interactions and distances at the nanoscale. Through this controlled energy release, PL materials allow precise targeting of affected areas, minimizing damage to surrounding healthy tissue. Recent advances have shown that nanoparticles with tunable emissivity can target deeper tissues, improving the versatility of phototherapy. The efficiency of FRET depends on several factors, including the spectral overlap between donor emission and acceptor absorption, the distance

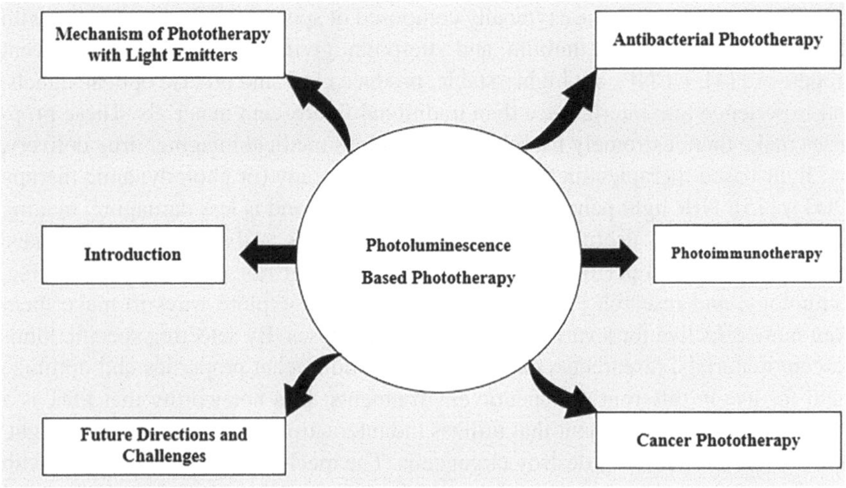

Fig. 1 An overview of photoluminescence-based phototherapy, highlighting its applications and advancements, including mechanisms with light emitters, antibacterial phototherapy, photoimmunotherapy, cancer phototherapy, and future directions and challenges

between donor and acceptor, and the relative orientation of their dipoles. Widely used in biochemistry and molecular biology, FRET allows the study of dynamic processes such as protein–protein interactions, conformational changes, and intracellular signaling. Modern techniques combining FRET with fluorescence microscopy or spectroscopy have further expanded its applications in live-cell imaging and high-throughput analysis. Its precision and versatility have made FRET an indispensable method for improving our understanding.

2.1 Photoluminescence Fundamentals

Photoluminescence is the process by which certain materials absorb photons and re-emit them, usually at different wavelengths depending on their composition and structure. This phenomenon is central to many biomedical applications, especially phototherapy, due to its ability to produce controlled light emission in response to an external light source [11, 12]. Commonly used materials in light-emitting applications include quantum dots, upconversion nanoparticles, and rare-earth doped nanoparticles, each with unique properties that allow their emission to be precisely tuned for specific medical purposes. For example, quantum dots are semiconductor nanocrystals that emit bright and stable light in a wide color spectrum, making them ideal for precision imaging and therapy. Upconversion nanoparticles (UCNPs) are small materials that can convert low-energy near-infrared (NIR) light into high-energy visible or ultraviolet (UV) light through a process called photon upconversion

[13]. These nanoparticles are typically composed of special matrices combined with elements such as erbium, thulium, and ytterbium, giving them unique luminescent properties [14]. UCNPs are highly stable, produce clear and precise optical signals, and experience less interference than traditional fluorescent materials. These properties make them extremely useful in areas such as medical imaging, drug delivery, and light-based therapies such as photodynamic therapy (or photodynamic therapy (PDT)) [15]. NIR light penetrates deeper into tissues and is less damaging, making UCNPs particularly useful for biological applications. Advances in design have improved safety and performance, allowing for a wider range of uses in medicine, technology, and research [16]. Scientists continue to explore ways to make them even more effective for a variety of innovative purposes. By selecting specific luminescent materials, researchers can control the luminescent properties and optimize them for use in different therapeutic environments. It is noteworthy that PDT is a minimally invasive treatment that utilizes the interaction of a photosensitizer, light, and oxygen to selectively destroy target cells. The mechanism of action begins with the administration of a photosensitizer, which preferentially accumulates in diseased tissues such as tumors and infection sites. When irradiated with light of a specific wavelength, the photosensitizer enters an excited state, enabling it to transfer energy to surrounding molecular oxygen.

This process generates reactive oxygen species (ROS), such as singlet oxygen and free radicals, which can cause oxidative damage to cellular components such as membranes, proteins, and DNA, as shown in Fig. 2. The resulting cell death occurs through mechanisms like apoptosis, necrosis, or autophagy, depending on the intensity of ROS generation and the cellular context. PDT also triggers secondary effects, such as immune system activation and vascular damage, further contributing to its therapeutic efficacy. The selective nature of PDT, combined with its ability to preserve surrounding healthy tissue, makes it a versatile option for treating various cancers, skin disorders, and microbial infections.

2.2 Energy Transfer Mechanisms

Energy transfer mechanisms play an important role in enhancing or modulating luminescence, allowing precise control of light energy in a therapeutic context. Förster resonance energy transfer (FRET) is a key process in which energy is transferred from an excited donor molecule to a nearby acceptor molecule (typically 1–10 nm away) without photon emission, thus allowing controlled energy release at target sites [17]. FRET is widely used in phototherapy and imaging applications due to its high short-range efficiency, allowing local treatment with minimal collateral damage. In addition to FRET, other mechanisms such as Dexter energy transfer, which involve electron exchange and require closer proximity between the donor and acceptor, are also used in special cases to enhance or inhibit luminescence as needed. In recent studies, these mechanisms have been incorporated into nanoparticle systems to increase energy transfer efficiency in cancer phototherapy, antibacterial treatment,

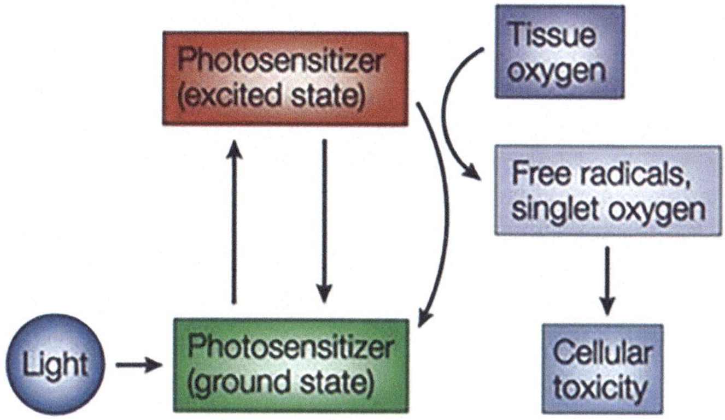

Fig. 2 Photodynamic therapy (PDT) relies on three key components: light, a photosensitizer, and oxygen. When the photosensitizer absorbs light of specific wavelengths, it transitions from its ground state to an excited state. As it relaxes back to the ground state, it releases energy that interacts with oxygen, producing reactive oxygen species (ROS) such as singlet oxygen and free radicals. These ROS are highly reactive and induce cellular toxicity, leading to targeted cell damage. Copyright 2003 Nature Publishing Group [8]

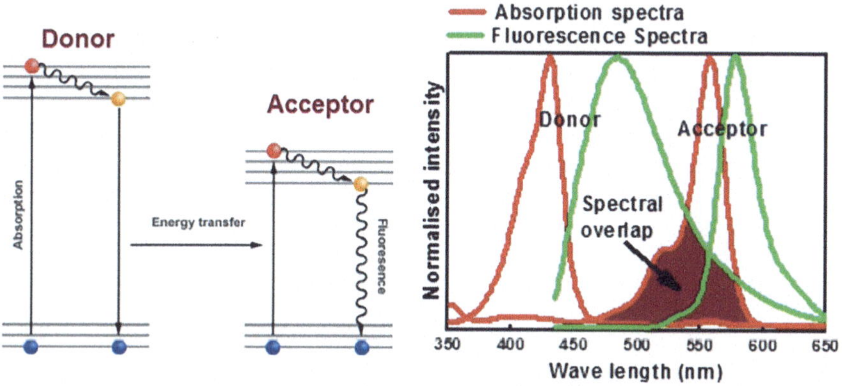

Fig. 3 (left) Illustration of the FRET process and (right) Absorption and fluorescence spectra of an ideal donor–acceptor pair. Copyright from Cornell University reprinted archive [18]

and imaging, providing better control of emission rate and wavelength for specific therapeutic applications as illustrated in Fig. 3.

2.3 Photoactivation of Therapeutic Agents

Photoactivation of therapeutic agents is a process by which light activates or enhances the therapeutic effect of a drug or photosensitizer, allowing controlled treatment at targeted sites of the body. When activated by light, photosensitizers generate reactive oxygen species (ROS) that damage nearby cells, a mechanism used in photodynamic therapy for antibacterial and anticancer treatments. Additionally, drug delivery systems can be designed to precisely release therapeutic agents when exposed to specific wavelengths of light, thereby reducing systemic toxicity and side effects. Nanoparticles play an important role in this process because they can be designed to encapsulate drugs and release them when activated by light, thereby increasing the stability and concentration of the drug at the target site. This controlled activation and release mechanism has shown great promise in clinical applications, allowing clinicians to achieve high therapeutic efficacy while minimizing the impact on healthy tissues.

2.4 *Antibacterial Phototherapy*

Antibacterial phototherapy uses light-activated photosensitizers to generate reactive oxygen species (ROS) that disrupt bacterial cell structures, effectively eliminating pathogens, including antibiotic-resistant strains. Photosensitizers such as porphyrins and chlorins are commonly used because of their high ROS production when exposed to light, but recent developments in the field of luminescent nanoparticles have further improved their effectiveness by increasing ROS production and allowing for precise bacterial targeting. Studies have demonstrated that these nanoparticles not only reduce bacterial load but also minimize damage to surrounding tissues due to their selective activation. Antibacterial phototherapy is particularly useful in treating skin infections, wounds, and even infections caused by drug-resistant bacteria, providing an alternative to traditional antibiotic treatments [19].

2.4.1 Mechanism of Action

The antibacterial mechanism of phototherapy mainly involves photosensitizers generating reactive oxygen species (ROS). When exposed to specific wavelengths of light, photosensitizers generate singlet oxygen and other ROS, which interact with bacterial cells by oxidizing important cellular structures including cell walls, membranes, and intracellular proteins. This oxidative damage disrupts cell integrity and metabolic functions, ultimately leading to bacterial cell death. Importantly, ROS-based killing is not limited to bacteria, making it effective against a wide range of pathogens, including antibiotic-resistant strains such as MRSA and Pseudomonas aeruginosa. Unlike traditional antibiotics, this approach does not induce resistance, as ROS generation directly destroys bacterial structures rather than targeting specific proteins that bacteria are capable of mutating through mutations.

2.4.2 Types of Photosensitizers

The efficacy of antibacterial phototherapy depends largely on the choice of photosensitizer, among which porphyrin, chlorine, and phthalocyanine are commonly used because they generate high levels of ROS when activated by light. Porphyrin, a natural pigment, is highly effective in generating ROS that disrupt bacterial cells. Chlorine, a porphyrin derivative, is particularly effective because of its strong absorption in the red spectrum, allowing deeper tissue penetration [20]. Recent advances have combined these photosensitizers with luminescent nanoparticles, such as gold and silver nanoparticles, which stabilize the photosensitizers and enhance ROS generation by amplifying the local electromagnetic field, thereby improving the efficacy of the antibacterial effect. This nanoparticle-assisted phototherapy approach also allows for the controlled release of ROS, improving bacterial target selectivity while minimizing damage to host cells.

2.4.3 Applications and Effectiveness

Antibacterial phototherapy is used in a variety of clinical and healthcare settings for the treatment of topical infections, wound disinfection, and surface disinfection [21]. For example, in wound care, phototherapy is effective in reducing bacterial counts in infected wounds and accelerating healing by preventing reinfection, a benefit that is particularly important for chronic wounds in diabetic patients. Another application is in dental care, where phototherapy helps control biofilm-associated infections that are often resistant to conventional antibiotics. In healthcare settings, phototherapy is also being investigated as a surface disinfection tool, where light-activated photosensitizers applied to surfaces can kill bacteria, reducing the risk of hospital-acquired infections. Studies consistently report high efficacy in reducing bacterial counts in these applications, demonstrating the versatility and effectiveness of phototherapy as an antibacterial.

2.5 Photoimmunotherapy

Photoimmunotherapy enhances the eradication of cancer cells by combining immunological stimulation with phototherapy [22, 23]. In this approach, light-sensitive agents are used to target cancer cells. When exposed to light, these agents produce reactive oxygen species (ROS), which damage cancer cells and trigger an immunological response. Thus, ROS production triggers the release of tumor antigens, which recruit immune cells to the site and boost the body's immunological response to cancer cells. Recent research indicates that nanoparticles can enhance the selectivity of this response, resulting in more efficient targeted treatments. Clinical trials have shown that photoimmunotherapy is effective in treating cancers such as melanoma, emphasizing its potential as a minimally invasive, immune-activating cancer therapy.

2.5.1 Mechanism of Photoimmunotherapy

The mechanism of photoimmunotherapy involves selectively targeting photosensitisers to cancer cells. When light activates, these photosensitizers generate reactive oxygen species (ROS) that damage cancer cells and release tumor antigens. The immune system then recognizes these tumor antigens, initiating an immune response that targets the remaining cancer cells. One of the crucial aspects of this mechanism is the accurate activation of the photosensitizers using near-infrared (NIR) light, which penetrates deep into tissues, allowing effective treatment of tumors situated below the skin's surface [24]. One crucial aspect of this mechanism is the accurate activation of the photosensitizers using near-infrared (NIR) light. This light penetrates deep into tissues, effectively treating tumors below the skin's surface. The targeted ROS production induces localized cell death (necrosis or apoptosis) while also releasing tumor-associated antigens, thereby transforming the tumor into a vaccine that aids the immune system in recognizing and eliminating similar cells throughout the body. This accuracy and ability to activate the immune system are advantageous for treating difficult-to-reach or resistant cancers.

2.5.2 Synergy with Immune Cells

The immune response initiated in photoimmunotherapy is considerably enhanced by the production of ROS and the subsequent recruitment of immune cells to the tumor site [25]. When ROS destroy cancer cells, they release tumor-specific antigens and create a pro-inflammatory environment that attracts immune cells, for example, dendritic cells, macrophages, and T-cells, to the damage site. Furthermore, Dendritic cells grasp tumor antigens and deliver them to T-cells, boosting the immune system's ability to identify and destroy cancer cells. The synergy between immune activation and ROS production transforms the tumor into a hub of robust immune activity, efficiently using the body's natural defenses that would attack cancerous cells beyond the treated area. This procedure, known as the "abscopal effect," is especially promising for treating metastatic cancer. It allows the immune system to locate and destroy distant tumor cells that the initial light therapy may not directly target.

2.5.3 Clinical Applications

Clinical applications of photoimmunotherapy have demonstrated notable advancements, especially in treating skin cancers and tumors that are challenging to address through conventional therapies. In clinical trials, photoimmunotherapy has shown promising results for head and neck cancers, as well as glioblastoma, a highly aggressive brain cancer with limited treatment options. These trials have highlighted photoimmunotherapy's precision and reduced side effects, with NIR light used to activate photosensitizers that specifically bind to cancer cells, sparing surrounding healthy tissue. For instance, the Food and Drug Administration (FDA) has granted fast-track designation to certain photoimmunotherapy agents for advanced head and neck cancer, a testament to the technology's potential for translation into widespread clinical practice [26]. Furthermore, ongoing research aims to apply photoimmunotherapy in combination with immune checkpoint inhibitors, enhancing the body's immune response even further and opening new pathways for tackling metastatic and recurrent cancers.

2.6 Cancer Phototherapy

Cancer phototherapy, particularly photodynamic therapy (PDT), uses photosensitizers that concentrate on tumor cells and produce cytotoxic ROS upon light exposure, destroying the cells. This approach has significant advantages over standard therapies, such as high specificity for cancer cells and minimal systemic toxicity, making it suitable for superficial and some internal cancers. Nanoparticles have revolutionized cancer phototherapy by providing controlled delivery of photosensitizers, allowing treatment to penetrate deeper tumors using near-infrared (NIR) light. PDT's applications are being expanded through research, and recent clinical trials have shown that it is effective in treating cancer resistant to chemotherapy and radiation [27].

2.6.1 Mechanism of Cancer Phototherapy

HI Pass reported that the mechanism of cancer phototherapy includes the selective accumulation of photosensitizers in cancer cells, which remain inactive until exposed to light of a specific wavelength [28]. Once activated, these photosensitizers generate ROS, which damage cellular components, such as cell membranes, proteins, and DNA, ultimately leading to cell death. This cytotoxic effect is often limited to the area exposed to light, allowing for precise tumor targeting with minimal impact on surrounding healthy tissue. The efficacy of this mechanism relies on the efficient localization of photosensitizers within the tumor; several techniques, for instance conjugating photosensitizers with tumor-targeting molecules, have been developed to enhance this selectivity. This therapy method has successfully treated superficial tumors and early-stage cancers when light can easily penetrate the affected cells.

2.6.2 Targeted Treatment

Nanoparticle-based light emitters have changed the landscape of cancer phototherapy by allowing highly targeted treatment with reduced systemic toxicity [12]. Consequently, nanoparticles can be engineered to deliver photosensitizers selectively to tumor sites by passive targeting through the enhanced permeability and retention (EPR) effect. In contrast, nanoparticles accumulate more readily in tumors due to their leaky vasculature or by active targeting, using surface ligands that bind specifically to receptors on cancer cells. Furthermore, nanoparticles can increase the stability and solubility of photosensitizers to improve selectivity, reducing the requirement for high drug doses and minimizing side effects. For instance, gold nanorods and up-conversion nanoparticles are particularly effective because they enable phototherapy in deeper tissues using near-infrared (NIR) light, penetrating tissues more effectively than visible light. These advances highlight nanoparticles' potential to improve the precision and safety of cancer phototherapy, particularly for tumors located beyond superficial layers.

2.6.3 Current Applications and Effectiveness

Photodynamic therapy (PDT) has demonstrated considerable promise in treating superficial cancers, including basal cell carcinoma, non-melanoma skin cancers, and certain head-and-neck cancers, with established effectiveness in obtaining high local tumor control and patient tolerance. Therefore, PDT has an advantage over conventional therapies, including chemotherapy and radiation, since it is more targeted and has fewer side effects. In contrast to chemotherapy, which may damage healthy cells throughout the body, PDT targets cells exposed to light, making it suited for localized treatments. In addition, PDT has been proven to stimulate immunological responses against treated cancers, which may reduce recurrence rates. Research into NIR-emitting photosensitizers and new delivery systems that improve light penetration and beneficial effectiveness expands PDT's applicability for deeper-seated cancers. As clinical trials are ongoing, PDT is increasingly viewed as a feasible complement or alternative to conventional treatment, particularly for patients with treatment-resistant or recurring tumors [29].

3 Cancer Detection and the Role of Luminescent MOFs in Biosensing and Bioimaging

Recently, cancer detection has been recognized as an essential challenge in public health worldwide, as both the incidence and mortality rates of cancer continue to rise annually. Early diagnosis is essential for improving treatment outcomes and survival rates. Several diagnostic technologies and tumor imaging approaches have been developed, including computed tomography (CT) scans, magnetic resonance imaging (MRI), enzyme-linked immunosorbent assays (ELISA), and tissue biopsy. Despite widespread adoption, these technologies face high costs, lengthy measurement times, complex sample preparation, and skilled operators' requirements. To address these obstacles, advancements in bioanalysis and bioimaging are creating new chances to improve cancer diagnosis efficiency. Biomarkers, for example, deoxyribonucleic acid (DNA), microribonucleic acid (miRNA), proteins, metabolites, and exosomes, provide crucial cytogenetic and dynamic information about tumor cells [30]. Nevertheless, their insignificant concentrations in cells, blood, and serum during the early stages of cancer make detection difficult, necessitating the creation of highly sensitive and selective biosensors based on innovative functional materials. Furthermore, bioimaging has significant potential for biomolecular detection applications, drug tracking, disease diagnostics, early cancer detection, and image-guided therapy.

Metal–organic frameworks (MOFs), crystalline porous nanomaterials of metal ions and organic ligands, have enormous potential in this area. MOFs are distinguished by their several morphologies, involving one-dimensional, two-dimensional, and three-dimensional structures. They outperform typical porous nanomaterials due to their vast surface area, configurable pore size, and rich active sites. MOFs have arisen as a rapidly growing research topic, with applications including catalysis, sensors, drug delivery, gas storage, gas separation, bioimaging, and water treatment.

Because of their outstanding optical properties, Luminescent MOFs (LMOFs), a subgroup of MOFs, hold significant promise for biosensing and bioimaging applications. Despite their considerable development potential, detailed assessments of LMOFs have been limited. LMOFs have distinct benefits, such as (i) Structure-dependent performance and modularity enable precise creation and adjustment of luminous features like fluorescence color; (ii) reversible structural alterations in response to external stimuli, which include temperature, pressure, or adsorption while retaining crystallinity; and (iii) post-synthetic modifications, for example, ligand exchange or host–guest reactions, that improve functionality. Subsequently, LMOFs have been used in several sensing and imaging applications, such as electrochemiluminescence (ECL), chemiluminescence (CL), and fluorescence/photoluminescence (FL/PL). Their luminosity can be classified into two types: self-luminescent MOFs, which have inherent luminescence due to metal centers and organic ligands, and composite luminescent materials, which have guest molecules added to improve luminescence.

3.1 The Role of Photothermal Conversion Efficiency for Cancer Applications

Photothermal conversion efficiency (PCE) determines the ability of photothermal agents to transform the absorbed electromagnetic radiation, particularly near-infrared

(NIR) light, into a heat mechanism central to the efficacy of photothermal therapy (PTT) in cancer treatment. From a conceptual viewpoint, PCE's technique involves the absorption of light energy by photothermal agents, including gold nanoparticles, carbon-based nanomaterials, or semiconductors, which have unique optical characteristics suited to NIR wavelengths. These agents undergo electronic transitions when excited by NIR light, resulting in non-radiative relaxation processes. In the case of plasmonic materials such as gold nanoparticles, the absorbed light energy excites electrons from their ground state to a higher energy state, resulting in electron–hole pairs or localized surface plasmon resonance (LSPR). As a result, these excited electrons relax to the ground state, releasing energy in the form of heat through phonon–phonon interactions or vibrational energy dissipation.

PCE can be quantitatively evaluated as the ratio of thermal energy produced to the total energy input, which depends on factors including the agent's absorption cross-section, the quantum yield of non-radiative decay, and the efficiency of energy transmission to the surrounding medium. Moreover, this method is further influenced by the photothermal agent's material properties, including its shape, size, and surface modifications, which dictate its absorption efficiency and thermal conductivity. High PCE benefits cancer treatment by generating enough heat to create localized hyperthermia within tumor tissues, resulting in protein denaturation, membrane disruption, and cell death. Additionally, high PCE agents reduce the requirement for NIR light dose and exposure duration, decreasing the potential risk of overheating healthy tissues while improving the safety and precision of PTT. As the research progresses, understanding and refining the PCE process is critical for developing next-generation photothermal treatments with enhanced biocompatibility, tumor selectivity, and clinical application.

In recent years, the experimental technique to determine PCE has been increased dramatically to examine the ability of a given nanomaterial to convert the absorbed light into heat in the NIR light (808 nm). Therefore, we would like to briefly discuss this technique. The heating of the solution can lead to a change in the thermal energy of a colloidal nanomaterials suspension (such as gold nanoparticles and carbon nanotubes) within a glass cuvette. This change is described by the rate of the input heat from laser power (Q_{in}), and the rate of the heat dissipation (Q_{out}), which satisfies the energy balance equation as reported by Alrahili et al. [31–34]

$$\sum_i m_i C_i \frac{dT}{dt} = Q_{in} - Q_{out}, \tag{1}$$

where m_i and C_i are the mass and specific heat capacity of the component of the system, T is the temperature of the solution, and t is time. The input heat that is absorbed by the nanomaterials is given as

$$Q_{in} = hA(T - T_{amb}), \tag{2}$$

where I_0 is the incident laser power, I_{tr} is the transmitted laser power, and η is the photothermal conversion efficiency.

The output heat that is dissipated to the environment can be written as

$$Q_{out} = hS(T(t) - T_0), \tag{3}$$

where h is the heat transfer coefficient, S is the surface area of the cuvette, $T(t)$ is the temperature at time t, and T_0 is the ambient temperature.

Using Eqs. (2) and (3) and accounting for the fact that the mass and specific heat capacity of GNMs are much smaller than that of water, the Eq. (1) can be simplified as

$$\frac{d\Delta T}{dt} = \frac{(I_0 - I_{tr})}{m_W C_w}\eta - B\Delta T, \tag{4}$$

where m_W and C_W are the mass and specific heat capacity of the aqueous solution (such as water), respectively. Here we define $\Delta T = T(t) - T_0$ as the change in temperature, and $B = \frac{hS}{m_W C_w}$ as the constant rate associated with the heat loss, which can be determined by tracing the temperature decay profile to the ambient temperature after the laser is turned off. In this regime $(I_0 - I_{tr}) = 0$ and from Eq. (4) one can be found

$$T(t) = T_0 + (T_{\max} - T_0)\exp(-Bt), \tag{5}$$

where we applied the initial condition that is when the laser is turned off at $t = 0$ we have the maximum temperature $T_{\max}$ (see Table 1).

For thermal equilibrium, the temperature is constant. Hence Eq. (4) gives us the expression for the photothermal conversion efficiency

$$\eta = \frac{(T_{\max} - T_0)}{(I_0 - I_{tr})} m_W C_W B. \tag{6}$$

Table 1 Comparison of photothermal efficiency of different nanomaterials

Nanomaterial types	Operating wavelength (nm)	PCE (%)	References
Gold nanoparticle	808	20–88	[38]
Carbon dots	808	30–86	[39]
Single-walled carbon nanotubes	808	84	[37]
Polymer nanoparticles	808	71	[40]
Multi-walled carbon Nanotubes	808	50	[41]
Metal sulphides	808	45	[42]
Iron oxide	808	20	[43]
Organic molecules	808	9	[44]

4 Future Directions and Challenges

The future of photoluminescence-based phototherapy has enormous potential, but obstacles remain in material development, tissue penetration, and clinical translation. Developing biocompatible, tunable photoluminescent materials is a prominent priority since it allows for better control over light output and tissue penetration, particularly with near-infrared (NIR) emitters. Tissue absorption and scattering of light are still critical limits, particularly for deep-seated cancers, but improvements in NIR materials and fibre-optic delivery systems provide intriguing alternatives. Furthermore, regulatory and clinical limitations such as large-scale production, long-term safety, and cost are essential to the broadest therapeutic possibilities—spread use. Combining phototherapy with other modalities, such as immunotherapy, is an ongoing development that could result in synergistic effects that improve treatment efficacy and expand therapeutic possibilities.

4.1 Material Development Based on Nanomaterials

One of the most pressing needs in photoluminescent phototherapy is the development of new, biocompatible based on nanomaterials that can emit light efficiently within the therapeutic wavelength range and penetrate deeper into tissues. Current materials, such as quantum dots and metal nanoparticles, are promising but often require improvements in safety, stability, and emission tunability [35]. For instance, quantum dots offer excellent light emission properties but may contain toxic elements like cadmium, necessitating further research into safer alternatives. The development of organic and inorganic nanoparticles and other biocompatible materials with tunable emission properties can enable more precise control over light activation, potentially allowing for better treatment outcomes with fewer side effects. Furthermore, efforts are underway to create nanoparticles that respond to multiple stimuli (such as pH or enzyme levels), enhancing their ability to selectively activate in specific tissue environments and expanding the possibilities for targeted phototherapy applications [36]. Materials development for cancer detection and treatment has witnessed remarkable advancements, leveraging interdisciplinary approaches to improve diagnostic precision and therapeutic efficacy. Nanomaterials with the help of nanotechnologies have emerged as a cornerstone in this field due to their tunable physicochemical properties and unique interactions with biological systems. Gold nanoparticles, for instance, have been extensively utilized and used for early cancer detection through enhanced imaging techniques such as surface-enhanced Raman scattering (SERS) and photoacoustic imaging, allowing for the identification of malignancies at the molecular level [37]. Similarly, polymeric nanocarriers and liposomes are engineered for targeted drug delivery, ensuring the precise release of chemotherapeutic agents to tumor sites while minimizing systemic toxicity. Beyond nanoparticles, hybrid materials integrating biomolecules and synthetic scaffolds have facilitated the development of biosensors for real-time monitoring of tumor biomarkers, enabling dynamic assessments of disease progression. In cancer immunotherapy, biomaterials such as dendritic cell scaffolds and hydrogel matrices have been tailored to modulate immune responses, enhancing the efficacy of checkpoint inhibitors and adoptive T-cell therapies. Furthermore, advancements in smart materials, including stimuli-responsive hydrogels and shape-memory alloys, provide innovative platforms for the localized and controlled delivery of therapeutics, especially in precision oncology applications. These developments underscore the transformative potential of materials science in revolutionizing cancer detection and treatment, bridging gaps between traditional modalities and cutting-edge biomedical innovations.

Nanomaterials used in cancer applications can be broadly classified into inorganic and organic categories based on their composition and origin. Inorganic nanomaterials include gold nanoparticles, magnetic nanoparticles such as iron oxide, carbon-based nanomaterials like carbon nanotubes and graphene oxide, quantum dots, silica-based nanoparticles, and ceramic nanoparticles (e.g., zirconia and alumina) as seen in the schematic illustration of the Fig. 4. These materials are characterized by their stability, tunable physicochemical properties, and unique interactions with electromagnetic fields, making them suitable for imaging, photothermal therapy, and drug delivery. On the other hand, organic nanomaterials encompass lipid-based nanoparticles, polymeric nanoparticles, dendrimers, and protein-based nanoparticles. These materials are primarily derived from biological or organic sources, offering enhanced biocompatibility and versatility for applications such as controlled drug delivery, gene therapy, and immunotherapy. The classification of nanomaterials into these categories underscores their diverse roles in improving cancer diagnosis and treatment through tailored functionalities.

4.2 *Tissue Penetration Limitations*

Tissue penetration is a crucial obstacle in photoluminescent phototherapy because biological tissues absorb and scatter light, limiting treatment depth and efficacy. While effective for surface uses, visible light cannot penetrate deeply enough to treat internal organs or large tumors. To address this, researchers have focused on near-infrared (NIR) emitting materials that function within a "therapeutic window" (650–900 nm) where tissue absorption is minimal, which could enable light to reach deeper structures. NIR-emitting up-conversion nanoparticles and other biocompatible materials are being developed to leverage this window, allowing for effective phototherapy at greater depths. Another promising approach involves using optical fibres to deliver light directly to the target site within the body, further extending the reach of phototherapy to previously inaccessible areas.

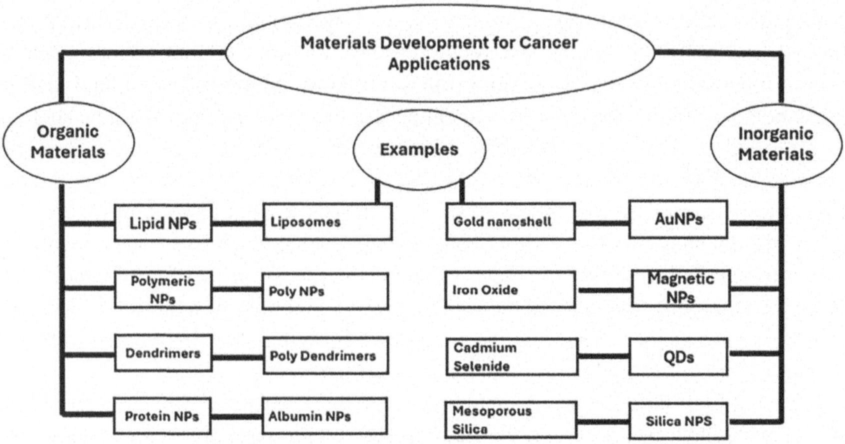

Fig. 4 An infographic illustrating the development of materials for cancer applications, categorizing organic and inorganic materials. Subcategories include innovative approaches like lipid nanoparticles, polymeric nanoparticles, dendrimers, and protein-based nanoparticles for organic materials, alongside gold nanoshells, iron oxide, cadmium selenide, and mesoporous silica for inorganic materials, emphasizing their potential in advancing cancer therapies

4.3 Clinical Translation

The translation of photoluminescent phototherapy into clinical practice faces significant regulatory and manufacturing challenges. Ensuring the long-term safety of photoluminescent materials, especially nanoparticles, is a major regulatory concern, as they may accumulate in tissues or elicit unforeseen biological responses. Regulatory agencies require extensive testing and data on toxicity, biodegradability, and elimination pathways, which can slow the path to approval. Additionally, scaling up the production of complex nanoparticles with precise optical properties presents both technical and cost-related challenges, potentially limiting widespread adoption. Developing cost-effective synthesis methods and scalable production processes will be essential for making these therapies more accessible. Finally, establishing robust clinical data on efficacy across diverse patient populations is necessary to ensure both regulatory approval and integration into standard care protocols.

4.4 Multi-modal Therapies

Combining phototherapy with other treatments, such as chemotherapy, immunotherapy, or gene therapy, is promising for enhancing therapeutic outcomes. Multi-modal therapies leverage the unique strengths of each treatment, such as the localized cytotoxic effects of phototherapy with the systemic tumor suppression of chemotherapy or the immune-stimulating properties of immunotherapy. For instance, photodynamic therapy (PDT) has been shown to work synergistically with immune checkpoint inhibitors, enhancing the immune response and increasing the body's ability to recognize and destroy cancer cells that have spread beyond the primary tumor site. Such approaches are particularly valuable for tackling metastatic or treatment-resistant cancers, as they can provide comprehensive coverage and prevent recurrence. Additionally, researchers are exploring photothermal and photodynamic combinations, which use light both to heat and produce ROS in targeted regions, enhancing cancer cell destruction and reducing the need for high drug doses. These integrative approaches have shown promising results in preclinical studies and are now being investigated in clinical trials.

References

1. Ahmad, F., Varghese, R., Panda, S., Ramamoorthy, S., Areeshi, M.Y., Fagoonee, S., Haque, S.: Smart nanoformulations for brain cancer theranostics: challenges and promises. Cancers **14**(21), 5389 (2022)
2. Tam, L.K., Chu, J.C., He, L., Yang, C., Han, K.C., Cheung, P.C., Ng, D.K., Lo, P.C.: Enzyme-responsive double-locked photodynamic molecular beacon for targeted photodynamic anticancer therapy. J. Am. Chem. Soc. **145**(13), 7361–7375 (2023)
3. Wang, C., Tao, H., Guo, Y.: Emerging materials for photodynamic therapy. Theranostics **9**(2), 223–245 (2019)
4. Sekar, R., Basavegowda, N., Thathapudi, J.J., Sekhar, M.R., Joshi, P., Somu, P., Baek, K.H.: Recent progress of gold-based nanostructures towards future emblem of photo-triggered cancer theranostics: a special focus on combinatorial phototherapies. Pharmaceutics **15**(2), 433 (2023)
5. Sun, J., Xing, F., Braun, J., Traub, F., Rommens, P.M., Xiang, Z., Ritz, U.: Progress of phototherapy applications in the treatment of bone cancer. Int. J. Mol. Sci. **22**(21), 11354 (2021)
6. Wang, Y., Staudinger, J.N., Mindt, T.L., Gasser, G.: Theranostics with photodynamic therapy for personalized medicine: to see and to treat. Theranostics **13**(15), 5501 (2023)
7. Mitsunaga, M., Ogawa, M., Kosaka, N., Rosenblum, L.T., Choyke, P.L., Kobayashi, H.: Cancer cell–selective in vivo near infrared photoimmunotherapy targeting specific membrane molecules. Nat. Med. **17**(12), 1685–1691 (2011)
8. Dolmans, D.E., Fukumura, D., Jain, R.K.: Photodynamic therapy for cancer. Nat. Rev. Cancer **3**(5), 380–387 (2003)
9. Hu, T., Wang, Z., Shen, W., Liang, R., Yan, D., Wei, M.: Recent advances in innovative strategies for enhanced cancer photodynamic therapy. Theranostics **11**(7), 3278 (2021)
10. Lucky, S.S., Soo, K.C., Zhang, Y.: Nanoparticles in photodynamic therapy. Chem. Rev. **115**(4), 1990–2042 (2015)
11. Mohammad-Hadi, L., Mohammad-Hadi, M.: Applications of Minimally Invasive Nanomedicine-Based Therapies in 3D in vitro Cancer Platforms. Morgan & Claypool Publishers (2020)
12. Shoaib, A., Javed, S., Tabish, M., Khan, M.E., Zaki, M., Alqahtani, S.S., Sultan, M.H., Ahsan, W., Afzal, M.: Applications of nanomedicine-integrated phototherapeutic agents in cancer theranostics: a comprehensive review of the current state of research. Nanotechnol. Rev. **13**(1), 20240023 (2024)
13. Xie, J., Zheng, Y., Ying, J.Y.: Protein-directed synthesis of highly fluorescent gold nanoclusters. J. Am. Chem. Soc. **131**(3), 888–889 (2009)
14. Haase, M., Schäfer, H.: Upconverting nanoparticles. Angew. Chem. Int. Ed. **50**(26), 5808–5829 (2011)

15. Alivisatos, A.P.: Perspectives on the physical chemistry of semiconductor nanocrystals. J. Phys. Chem. **100**(31), 13226–13239 (1996)
16. Wang, F., Liu, X.: Recent advances in the chemistry of lanthanide-doped upconversion nanocrystals. Chem. Soc. Rev. **38**(4), 976–989 (2009)
17. Förster, T.: Zwischenmolekulare energiewanderung und fluoreszenz. Ann. Phys. **437**(1–2), 55–75 (1948)
18. Hussain, S.A.: An introduction to fluorescence resonance energy transfer (FRET) (2009). arXiv: 0908.1815
19. Zhao, B., Wang, H., Dong, W., Cheng, S., Li, H., Tan, J., Zhou, J., He, W., Li, L., Zhang, J., Luo, G.: A multifunctional platform with single-NIR-laser-triggered photothermal and NO release for synergistic therapy against multidrug-resistant Gram-negative bacteria and their biofilms. J. Nanobiotechnol. **18**, 1–25 (2020)
20. Zhao, X., Liu, J., Fan, J., Chao, H., Peng, X.: Recent progress in photosensitizers for overcoming the challenges of photodynamic therapy: from molecular design to application. Chem. Soc. Rev. **50**(6), 4185–4219 (2021)
21. Dai, T., Huang, Y.Y., Hamblin, M.R.: Photodynamic therapy for localized infections—state of the art. Photodiagn. Photodyn. Ther. **6**(3–4), 170–188 (2009)
22. Dai, Y., Xu, C., Sun, X., Chen, X.: Nanoparticle design strategies for enhanced anticancer therapy by exploiting the tumour microenvironment. Chem. Soc. Rev. **46**(12), 3830–3852 (2017)
23. Hamblin, M.R., Hasan, T.: Photodynamic therapy: a new antimicrobial approach to infectious disease? Photochem. Photobiol. Sci. **3**(5), 436–450 (2004)
24. Kharkwal, G.B., Sharma, S.K., Huang, Y.Y., Dai, T., Hamblin, M.R.: Photodynamic therapy for infections: clinical applications. Lasers Surg. Med. **43**(7), 755–767 (2011)
25. Kobayashi, H., Choyke, P.L.: Near-infrared photoimmunotherapy of cancer. Acc. Chem. Res. **52**(8), 2332–2339 (2019)
26. Nagaya, T., Friedman, J., Maruoka, Y., Ogata, F., Okuyama, S., Clavijo, P.E., Choyke, P.L., Allen, C., Kobayashi, H.: Host immunity following near-infrared photoimmunotherapy is enhanced with PD-1 checkpoint blockade to eradicate established antigenic tumors. Cancer Immunol. Res. **7**(3), 401–413 (2019)
27. Alsaab, H.O., Alghamdi, M.S., Alotaibi, A.S., Alzhrani, R., Alwuthaynani, F., Althobaiti, Y.S., Almalki, A.H., Sau, S., Iyer, A.K.: Progress in clinical trials of photodynamic therapy for solid tumors and the role of nanomedicine. Cancers **12**(10), 2793 (2020)
28. Pass, H.I.: Photodynamic therapy in oncology: mechanisms and clinical use. JNCI: J. Natl. Cancer Inst. **85**(6), 443–456 (1993)
29. Aebisher, D., Czech, S., Dynarowicz, K., Misiołek, M., Komosińska-Vassev, K., Kawczyk-Krupka, A., Bartusik-Aebisher, D.: Photodynamic therapy: past, current, and future. Int. J. Mol. Sci. **25**(20), 11325 (2024)
30. Liu, C.M., Hsieh, C.L., Shen, C.N., Lin, C.C., Shigemura, K., Sung, S.Y.: Exosomes from the tumor microenvironment as reciprocal regulators that enhance prostate cancer progression. Int. J. Urol. **23**(9), 734–744 (2016)
31. Alrahili, M., Peroor, R., Savchuk, V., McNear, K., Pinchuk, A.: Morphology dependence in photothermal heating of gold nanomaterials with near-infrared laser. J. Phys. Chem. C **124**(8), 4755–4763 (2020)
32. Alrahili, M.R.: Insights into gold nanoparticle optical behavior: size-dependent absorption and extinction peaks. J. Nanoelectron. Optoelectron. **19**(8), 783–790 (2024)
33. Alrahili, M.: Single silver nanoparticles: local refractive index response to localized surface plasmon resonance and molar attenuation coefficient. Colloid J. **86**(1), 138–152 (2024)
34. Alrahili, M.: Light to heat conversion efficiency of single-walled carbon nanotubes. J. Taibah Univ. Sci. **16**(1), 923–932 (2022)
35. Zhou, Z., Sun, Y., Shen, J., Wei, J., Yu, C., Kong, B., Liu, W., Yang, H., Yang, S., Wang, W.: Iron/iron oxide core/shell nanoparticles for magnetic targeting MRI and near-infrared photothermal therapy. Biomaterials **35**(26), 7470–7478 (2014)

36. Yoon, H.J., Lee, H.S., Lim, J.Y., Park, J.H.: Liposomal indocyanine green for enhanced photothermal therapy. ACS Appl. Mater. Interfaces **9**(7), 5683–5691 (2017)
37. Yang, Z., Gao, M., Wu, W., Yang, X., Sun, X.W., Zhang, J., Wang, H.C., Liu, R.S., Han, C.Y., Yang, H., Li, W.: Recent advances in quantum dot-based light-emitting devices: challenges and possible solutions. Mater. Today **1**(24), 69–93 (2019)
38. Clapp, A.R., Medintz, I.L., Mattoussi, H.: Förster resonance energy transfer investigations using quantum-dot fluorophores. ChemPhysChem **7**(1), 47–57 (2006)
39. Dexter, D.L.: A theory of sensitized luminescence in solids. J. Chem. Phys. **21**(5), 836–850 (1953)
40. Chen, H., Shao, L., Ming, T., Sun, Z., Zhao, C., Yang, B., Wang, J.: Understanding the photothermal conversion efficiency of gold nanocrystals. Small. **6**(20), 2272–2280 (2010)
41. Lan, M., Zhao, S., Zhang, Z., Yan, L., Guo, L., Niu, G., Zhang, J., Zhao, J., Zhang, H., Wang, P., Zhu, G.: Two-photon-excited near-infrared emissive carbon dots as multifunctional agents for fluorescence imaging and photothermal therapy. Nano Res. **10**, 3113–3123 (2017)
42. Lyu, Y., Zeng, J., Jiang, Y., Zhen, X., Wang, T., Qiu, S., Lou, X., Gao, M., Pu, K.: Enhancing both biodegradability and efficacy of semiconducting polymer nanoparticles for photoacoustic imaging and photothermal therapy. ACS Nano **12**(2), 1801–1810 (2018)
43. Maestro, L.M., Haro-González, P., Del Rosal, B., Ramiro, J., Caamano, A.J., Carrasco, E., Juarranz, A., Sanz-Rodríguez, F., Solé, J.G., Jaque, D.: Heating efficiency of multi-walled carbon nanotubes in the first and second biological windows. Nanoscale **5**(17), 7882–7889 (2013)
44. Chen, Y., Cheng, L., Dong, Z., Chao, Y., Lei, H., Zhao, H., Wang, J., Liu, Z.: Degradable vanadium disulfide nanostructures with unique optical and magnetic functions for cancer theranostics. Angew. Chem. **129**(42), 13171–13176 (2017)

Tailored Organic Light-Emitting Diodes (OLEDs) for Next-Generation Biomedicine

Maida Mobeen, Akim Oladokoun, Maryam Hussain, Ishrat Fatima, Jamila Naz, Muhammad Anas, Waseem Ahmed Khattak, Muhammad Majeed, Aftab Umar, Rikza Saleem, Laiba, and Fredrick Kayusi

Abstract The interaction between light and matter is driving some of the most groundbreaking advancements in modern biomedicine. By tapping into the unique properties of light, researchers have developed sophisticated tools for diagnostics, therapy, and real-time biological monitoring. Looking ahead, the future of OLEDs in healthcare is incredibly promising. Ongoing research into biocompatible materials and innovative manufacturing techniques will only expand their capabilities

---

M. Mobeen · M. Majeed (✉)
Department of Botany, University of Gujrat, Punjab 50700, Pakistan
e-mail: m.majeed@uog.edu.pk; majeedmohal@gmail.com

A. Oladokoun
Laboratory of Botany and Ecology Vegetable (LBEV), University of Lome (UL), Lomé, Togo

M. Hussain
Department of Biotechnology and Genetic Engineering, University of Mansehra, Dhodial, Pakistan

I. Fatima
Department of Biological Sciences, University of Veterinary and Animal Sciences Lahore, Punjab, Pakistan

J. Naz
Department of Forestry and Range Management, Bahauddin Zakariya Uinversity, Multan, Punjab, Pakistan

M. Anas · W. A. Khattak
Faculty of Biological Sciences, Department of Plant Sciences, Quaid-I-Azam University, Islamabad, Pakistan

M. Anas
Department of Soil Science and Plant Nutrition, University of Selcuk, Konya, Turkey

A. Umar
Department of Botany, University of Agriculture, Faisalabad, Punjab, Pakistan

R. Saleem
Department of Radiology and Imaging Technology, Government College University, Faisalabad, Punjab, Pakistan

© The Author(s), under exclusive license to Springer Nature Switzerland AG 2025
N. O. Etafo (ed.), *Tailored Light Emitters For Biomedical Applications*, Engineering Materials, https://doi.org/10.1007/978-3-031-88731-4_9

further. As these technologies advance, OLEDs are poised to revolutionize wearable diagnostics, implantable therapies, and cutting-edge biosensors, bringing us closer to practical, real-world medical solutions. The integration of light-emitting technologies into biomedicine has fundamentally transformed the way diagnostics and treatments are performed, offering an unprecedented combination of precision, non-invasiveness, and efficiency. Technologies such as lasers, light-emitting diodes (LEDs), and advanced quantum dot devices leverage specific wavelengths of light to interact with biological tissues in highly controlled ways. Tailored organic light-emitting diodes (OLEDs) represent a significant advancement in the field of biomedicine, offering innovative solutions for diagnostics and therapeutic applications. This chapter explores the design and engineering of OLEDs with specific properties to enhance their functionality in biological environments. By optimizing the materials and structures used in these devices, researchers aim to improve their efficiency, stability, and biocompatibility. The integration of tailored OLEDs into biomedical systems holds promise for real-time imaging, targeted drug delivery.

Keywords Organic · Technology · LED · Medicals · Technologies advance

1 Custom Organic Light-Emitting Diodes (OLEDs) for Advanced Biomedicine Applications

Organic light-emitting diodes (OLEDs) are making waves in the biomedical field, offering a glimpse into the future of healthcare technologies. Thanks to their unique features (mechanical flexibility, biocompatibility, and tunable wavelengths), OLEDs are becoming a go-to choice for innovative medical applications. Unlike conventional light sources, OLEDs use organic semiconductors, allowing them to be lightweight, thin, and energy-efficient [1]. This flexibility makes them easy to customize for specific medical needs, paving the way for exciting advancements in areas like wearable devices, implantable sensors, and opt genetics. OLEDs' flexibility is particularly useful in wearable systems designed for continuous health monitoring or therapeutic treatments. One standout application is in phototherapy, where wavelength-tunable near-infrared (NIR) OLEDs have shown tremendous potential. By emitting light in the NIR spectrum, these devices can stimulate cellular processes like wound healing and tissue regeneration. Research has shown that NIR OLEDs not only enhance cell growth but are also robust enough to withstand repeated bending and stretching,

Laiba
Department of Orthotics and Prosthetics, Government College University, Faisalabad, Punjab, Pakistan

F. Kayusi
Department of Environmental Studies, Geography and Planning, Maasai Mara University, Narok, Kenya

making them ideal for wearable biomedical devices. Moreover, their low operational temperatures ensure they're safe for extended use [2].

In implantable devices, OLEDs shine just as brightly—literally and figuratively. Opto-genetics, a technique that uses light to control nerve cell activity, relies on precise light delivery, and OLEDs are perfect for this. They can emit light at specific wavelengths with pinpoint accuracy, helping researchers and clinicians develop advanced treatments for neurological conditions. Additionally, the use of biocompatible materials in OLEDs ensures they can be implanted safely without triggering harmful reactions in the body. For example, studies have shown that OLEDs integrated into neural interfaces could transform how we approach neurological therapy [3].

Another area where OLEDs excel is in overcoming challenges related to durability and efficiency. Innovations in electrode design, such as swapping brittle indium tin oxide for flexible silver-based alternatives, have significantly boosted their mechanical strength and electrical performance [4]. These improvements allow OLEDs to remain bright and efficient, even when bent or flexed repeatedly. Furthermore, the introduction of thermally activated delayed fluorescence (TADF) emitters has made OLEDs more energy-efficient, a critical factor for battery-powered medical devices. What's even more exciting is the versatility of OLEDs in medical applications. Tiny, micro-scale OLEDs have been developed for minimally invasive devices, delivering high brightness while consuming very little power [5]. These devices can be fine-tuned to emit specific wavelengths, making them ideal for tasks like targeted cancer therapies or fluorescence-based biosensors [6]. Their customizable optical properties also make them invaluable in precision medicine, where treatments are tailored to individual patients [7].

Looking ahead, the future of OLEDs in healthcare is incredibly promising. Ongoing research into biocompatible materials and innovative manufacturing techniques will only expand their capabilities further. As these technologies advance, OLEDs are poised to revolutionize wearable diagnostics, implantable therapies, and cutting-edge biosensors, bringing us closer to practical, real-world medical solutions. With their adaptability and wide-ranging applications, OLEDs are set to become a cornerstone of next-generation biomedical innovation [8].

1.1 Revolutionizing Light-Matter Interaction in Biomedicine

The interaction between light and matter is driving some of the most groundbreaking advancements in modern biomedicine. By tapping into the unique properties of light, researchers have developed sophisticated tools for diagnostics, therapy, and real-time biological monitoring. These tools are precise, non-invasive, and incredibly effective, reshaping how we understand and treat various health conditions [8]. Recent progress in photonics has given scientists unprecedented control over how light interacts with biological tissues, unlocking a new wave of diagnostic and therapeutic possibilities (Fig. 1).

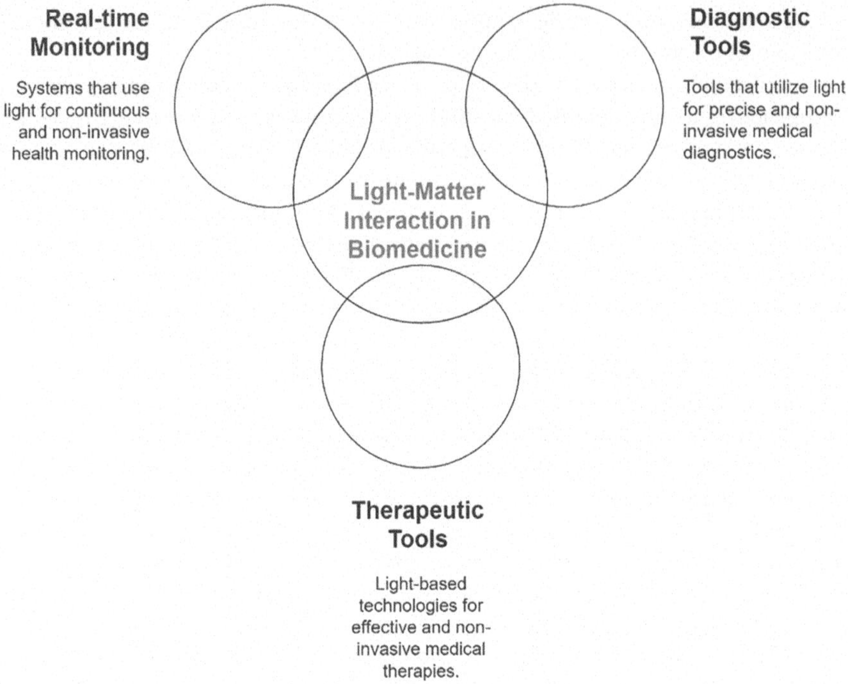

Fig. 1 Revolutionizing biomedicine with light-based technologies

1.2 Light: The Key to Revolutionary Imaging

One of the most profound ways light-matter interaction is transforming biomedicine is through imaging. Techniques like fluorescence microscopy, super-resolution microscopy, and stimulated Raman scattering have redefined how we study cells and tissues [9]. These methods exploit light's ability to excite molecules, enabling scientists to visualize biochemical processes at a molecular scale. Take super-resolution microscopy, for example. By surpassing the traditional diffraction limit of light, it allows researchers to observe cellular structures and dynamics with astonishing nanometer-level precision. This capability has been crucial for understanding disease mechanisms at their roots, providing insights that are essential for developing targeted therapies. Beyond cellular imaging, innovative technologies like photoacoustic imaging and optical coherence tomography (OCT) have opened new avenues for non-invasive diagnostics [10]. Photoacoustic imaging combines the strengths of optical and ultrasound imaging, creating high-resolution images of tissues deep within the body. This technique has proven invaluable for detecting conditions like cancer and cardiovascular diseases at their earliest stages, when treatment is most effective [11].

1.3 Light-Powered Therapies

The therapeutic potential of light is equally transformative. Photodynamic therapy (PDT) is a standout example. By using light to activate photosensitizing agents, PDT generates reactive oxygen species that selectively destroy diseased tissues, such as cancer cells. The integration of near infrared (NIR) light has further enhanced PDT by enabling deeper tissue penetration, making it effective for treating tumors in challenging locations [12]. Nanotechnology has taken this a step further with the development of NIR-responsive nanostructures like up conversion nanoparticles. These tiny structures amplify the effects of light, enabling greater precision and depth in photodynamic treatments. Such advancements are particularly promising for addressing cancers and other conditions in hard-to-reach areas of the body, where traditional therapies often fall short [13].

1.4 Precision Medicine with Nanotechnology

Nanotechnology has also introduced light-activatable nano-platforms that can modulate cellular behaviors with remarkable accuracy. These platforms are designed to control processes such as immune responses, signal cascades, and stem cell differentiation by delivering light stimulation in a highly targeted and time-specific manner [14]. This approach is revolutionizing precision medicine by enabling interventions that are finely tuned to an individual's unique biological makeup [6]. For example, these light-responsive nano-platforms can minimize off-target effects, ensuring that treatments focus exclusively on the intended cells or tissues [15]. The result is safer, more effective therapies that have the potential to transform patient outcomes (Fig. 2).

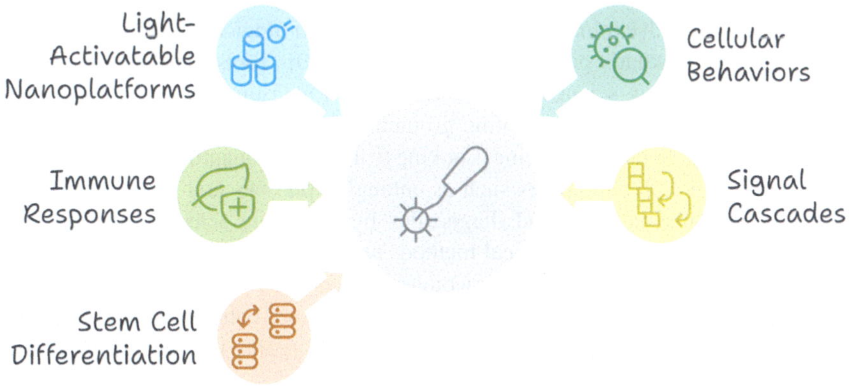

Fig. 2 Nanotechnology precision medicines

1.5 The Opto-genetics Breakthrough

Opto-genetics is another field that highlights the power of light-matter interaction. By genetically engineering cells to express light-sensitive proteins, researchers can manipulate cellular activities (neuron firing) with extraordinary precision [16]. Recent advancements, like up conversion nanoparticles that convert NIR light into visible light, have overcome the challenge of limited light penetration in opto-genetics. These innovations make it possible to activate light-sensitive proteins deep within tissues, expanding the reach of opto-genetics in neuroscience and beyond. Imagine treating neurological disorders, restoring vision, or even repairing brain circuits with pinpoint accuracy all thanks to light's unique properties [17].

1.6 Light-Activated Drug Delivery

The precise control offered by light has also been applied to drug delivery systems. Light-activated platforms use photosensitive materials that release therapeutic agents only when exposed to specific wavelengths of light [18]. This approach ensures that drugs are delivered directly to their target, minimizing side effects and maximizing treatment efficacy. For instance, gold Nano rods and plasmatic nanoparticles can absorb specific wavelengths of light to trigger the release of encapsulated drugs [6]. This targeted approach has already shown promise in cancer therapy, offering a way to treat tumors with fewer side effects compared to traditional chemotherapy [19].

1.7 The Frontier of Bio-photonics and Quantum Photonics

Bio-photonics, which explores light's interaction with biological systems, is pushing the boundaries of what's possible in biomedicine [20]. Tools like biosensors and optical tweezers allow scientists to manipulate and measure biological molecules with extraordinary precision, enabling groundbreaking research in areas like drug discovery and regenerative medicine. Looking to the future, quantum photonics holds immense potential. Technologies such as entangled photons and quantum sensors could revolutionize imaging and diagnostics by achieving sensitivity and precision levels far beyond what classical methods can offer [21]. Quantum sensors, for example, could detect subtle changes in biological systems, enabling the early detection of diseases at a molecular level. Similarly, quantum-enhanced imaging could provide clearer, more detailed views of tissues and organs, improving diagnostic accuracy and patient care (Fig. 3).

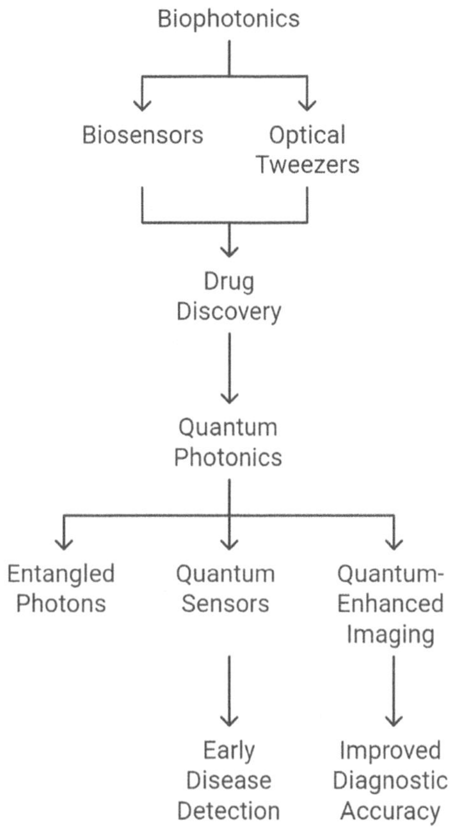

Fig. 3 Advancements in bio-photonics and quantum photonics

1.8 Shaping the Future of Medicine

The possibilities for light-matter interaction in biomedicine are endless. From wearable light-based diagnostic devices to implantable therapeutic systems, the integration of light into healthcare is creating new opportunities to improve human health. These advancements not only make treatments more effective but also empower patients with tools for earlier detection and personalized care [22].

2 Illuminating the Path to Diagnosis and Treatment

The integration of light-emitting technologies into biomedicine has fundamentally transformed the way diagnostics and treatments are performed, offering an unprecedented combination of precision, non-invasiveness, and efficiency. Technologies such as lasers, light-emitting diodes (LEDs), and advanced quantum dot devices leverage specific wavelengths of light to interact with biological tissues in highly controlled ways. These interactions enable critical applications, including imaging, photodynamic therapy (PDT), and photo-bio modulation (PBM), and continue to inspire new innovations in healthcare. By exploiting the unique properties of light, researchers and clinicians are developing tools that improve patient outcomes, enhance the accuracy of diagnoses, and minimize invasive procedures [23].

In diagnostic imaging, light emitters play a pivotal role in enabling deep tissue visualization and high-resolution imaging. Near-infrared (NIR) light emitters, for example, have demonstrated an exceptional ability to penetrate biological tissues by reducing light scattering and absorption, resulting in clearer images and better contrast. These capabilities are further enhanced by lanthanide-based nanoparticles (UCNPs), which convert NIR light into visible emissions, improving resolution while minimizing tissue auto-fluorescence. Similarly, semiconductor broadband light emitters are widely used in optical coherence tomography (OCT) systems, a high-resolution imaging technology capable of detecting early-stage diseases such as cancers and retinal disorders [24]. These advanced light-emitting devices provide clinicians with a more accurate understanding of tissue structures, enabling earlier and more effective intervention.

In therapeutic applications, light-emitting technologies have revolutionized treatments by offering targeted and minimally invasive solutions. PDT, for example, relies on light to activate photosensitizing agents that produce reactive oxygen species, selectively destroying diseased tissues such as tumors. Quantum dot light-emitting devices (QLEDs) have emerged as particularly promising for PDT due to their tunable wavelength specificity, which can be optimized for precise cancer treatments. Meanwhile, PBM uses low-level light to stimulate cellular activity, promoting wound healing, reducing inflammation, and enhancing recovery. Flexible organic LEDs (OLEDs) and NIR OLEDs have further advanced wearable phototherapy devices, offering highly adaptable and patient-friendly solutions that deliver specific wavelengths of light to enhance therapeutic outcomes while minimizing side effects.

Biocompatibility has become a cornerstone of integrating light-emitting devices into medical applications, especially for long-term use. Recent advancements in biodegradable and biocompatible materials have led to the development of implantable light emitters, constructed from polymers and nanomaterials that interact safely with biological tissues. These devices are now being used in applications ranging from opto-genetics to minimally invasive diagnostics. Biodegradable light-emitting systems have been particularly successful in opto-genetics, where light is used to control cellular activities such as neuronal firing with extraordinary precision. The ability to integrate these systems seamlessly into the body has opened new avenues for treating neurological disorders and advancing our understanding of brain function [25].

One of the greatest strengths of light-emitting technologies is their adaptability to diverse medical scenarios. Tunable light sources, such as LEDs, provide precise control over both wavelength and intensity, allowing clinicians to customize their use for various applications. For instance, tunable LEDs have been employed in dermatology and endoscopy to enhance tissue differentiation, optimize color rendering, and improve diagnostic accuracy. Such versatility makes light-emitting devices invaluable tools in modern medicine, empowering healthcare professionals to address a wide range of challenges with tailored solutions. Despite these advancements, the widespread adoption of light emitters in biomedicine faces certain challenges. Standardizing key parameters such as wavelength, power, and exposure time remains critical to ensuring consistent results across both research and clinical settings. Inconsistent documentation of these parameters in scientific studies has been identified as a barrier to reproducibility, underscoring the need for rigorous protocols and best practices. Addressing these challenges will be essential to unlocking the full potential of light-emitting technologies in healthcare [26].

Looking ahead, the future of light emitters in medicine is being shaped by the convergence of material science, nanotechnology and bioengineering. Emerging technologies such as flexible and bio integrated light-emitting devices promise to redefine therapeutic and diagnostic paradigms. These devices, often incorporating advanced materials like perovskites and metal nanoclusters, are pushing the boundaries of efficiency, tenability, and mechanical flexibility [27]. Wearable and implantable light emitters are already showing immense promise in delivering patient-specific care, while innovations in light-emitting materials continue to expand the scope of applications in diagnostics and treatment. By harnessing these cutting-edge developments, researchers and clinicians are poised to transform the landscape of modern medicine, offering groundbreaking solutions to some of the most pressing healthcare challenges.

2.1 Bio-imaging

Bioimaging has transformed biomedical research and clinical diagnostics, offering non-invasive, real-time visualization of biological processes with exceptional precision. The evolution of tailored light emitters, including quantum dots, lanthanide-based nanoparticles, and near-infrared (NIR) fluorescent probes, has greatly expanded the capabilities of bioimaging. These innovations have enhanced imaging resolution, increased penetration depth, and minimized issues such as phototoxicity and autofluorescence, positioning bioimaging as an essential tool in modern medicine. Among these advancements, the use of NIR light, particularly in the NIR-II window (1000–1700 nm), has addressed significant limitations of conventional imaging methods by reducing light scattering and absorption. This allows for deeper tissue visualization and improved contrast, making NIR technologies indispensable in applications ranging from diagnostics to therapeutic interventions [28].

One of the most groundbreaking innovations in bioimaging is the development of lanthanide-based up conversion nanoparticles (UCNPs), which convert low-energy NIR photons into higher-energy emissions. These nanoparticles exhibit high sensitivity, stability, and low cytotoxicity, making them ideal for imaging applications such as cancer diagnostics and opto-genetics. Similarly, persistent luminescence nanoparticles (PLNPs), which emit light long after external excitation, have revolutionized long-term imaging by eliminating the need for continuous illumination. This not only reduces background auto-fluorescence but also enables precise tracking of biological processes over extended periods. PLNPs emitting in the NIR range have shown great promise in tumor imaging and theranostics, acting as both diagnostic tools and therapeutic agents. Advances in surface engineering and energy transfer optimization have further expanded their potential, enabling highly functionalized Nano probes for targeted applications [29].

Carbon dots (CDs) have also emerged as a versatile and biocompatible tool in bioimaging. Their excellent water solubility and tunable photoluminescence properties make them particularly suitable for deep tissue imaging in the NIR-II region, where they enable high-resolution imaging with minimal photo-toxicity. Recent breakthroughs in CDs have led to rapid renal clearance, high quantum yields, and the ability to integrate with photo-thermal cancer therapy. Similarly, quantum dots (QDs) remain a cornerstone of bio-imaging, known for their size-tunable emission, photostability, and narrow spectral bands. These properties allow for multiplexed imaging, where multiple targets are visualized simultaneously. Despite concerns about the toxicity of cadmium-based QDs, alternative materials such as graphene quantum dots (GQDs) have been developed, offering comparable optical performance with improved biocompatibility and safety [30].

Rare-earth-doped nanomaterials emitting in the NIR-II region have further broadened the scope of bio-imaging by facilitating imaging beyond visible wavelengths. These materials excel in reducing photon scattering and absorption, enabling high-resolution imaging of deep tissues. Advances in their design have led to multimodal imaging techniques that combine NIR fluorescence with magnetic resonance imaging (MRI) or computed tomography (CT), enhancing diagnostic accuracy and providing a more comprehensive understanding of biological systems. Fluorescent nanostructures, including up conversion and down conversion materials, have also improved the resolution and sensitivity of bio-imaging. By converting NIR light into visible or ultraviolet emissions, these materials achieve precise imaging with minimal tissue damage. Current research focuses on optimizing energy transfer processes within these materials to produce brighter emissions and higher contrast, further pushing the boundaries of imaging technology [31].

Despite these remarkable advances, several challenges remain in translating these technologies into widespread clinical use. Key issues such as biocompatibility, stability, and scalability must be addressed to ensure the safe and effective application of imaging agents in humans. Surface modifications, such as the addition of bio functional polymers or targeting ligands, have been employed to enhance the specificity and stability of these agents. These modifications not only improve the interaction between nanoparticles and biological targets but also minimize nonspecific binding and potential toxicity, paving the way for safer and more reliable bio-imaging solutions [32].

As bioimaging technologies continue to evolve, their applications in disease diagnosis, monitoring, and treatment are rapidly expanding. From real-time visualization of cellular processes to image-guided cancer therapy, tailored light emitters are unlocking new possibilities in precision medicine. The integration of bioimaging with advanced therapeutic modalities such as photothermal and photodynamic treatments underscores its multifunctional potential in healthcare. Future research will likely focus on developing more efficient, scalable, and biocompatible imaging agents while exploring new wavelengths and multimodal approaches. These efforts promise to enhance the utility of bioimaging technologies and redefine their role in the diagnosis and treatment of complex medical conditions [33].

3 Treatment of Phototherapeutic

A modern fast developing method in biomedical uses, phototherapeutic therapy is distinguished by its high precision, low invasiveness, and capacity to target tissues that are diseased while preserving tissues that are healthy. Both of its main modalities—photodynamic treatment (PDT) and photo-thermal treatment (PTT)—use light-responsive substances that, when activated by particular wavelengths of light, produce warmth or reactive oxygen species (ROS). Due to developments in the fields of materials and nanotechnology, such treatments—which are mostly utilized in oncology—are becoming more widely applied in other medical specialties. To cause cell death, PDT uses photosensitizers, which release reactive oxygen species (ROS) in response to light. Research has demonstrated that this approach has a lot of potential for treating cancer because of its accuracy and low risk of affecting nearby tissues. Recent advancements in photosensitizer chemicals, including aza-boron-dipyrromethene colors, have shown increased ROS formation and higher photo-thermal efficiency during conversion, for example, which results in more successful tumor removal without regrowth. Enzyme-activatable photosensitizers have also surfaced, improving targeted therapy by decreasing adverse reactions and improving tumor selectivity [34].

PTT, on the contrary hand, kills cancer cells specifically by converting sunlight into heat using photothermal reagents. Because of their special catalytic and plasmatic qualities, nanomaterials like gold-semiconductor composites have been developed to maximize this process, allowing for high-efficiency generation of heat and superior biocompatibility. Furthermore, because they provide greater penetration into tissues and less harm to cells that are healthy, NIR, or near-infrared and light-responsive nanoparticles are emerging as a key component of PTT. Enhancing the therapeutic chemicals' biocompatibility and focusing capabilities is a significant difficulty in phototherapy. To improve the immune response and ensure accurate transmission of phototherapeutic drugs, biomimetic nanomaterials were produced, drawing inspiration from cell membranes. These substances decrease immunological clearance, prolong flow duration in vivo, and enhance therapeutic results. The capacity of hydrogels containing photosensitizers to localize therapy at the tumor site, reducing systemic harm and improving therapeutic effectiveness, has also drawn interest [35].

The goal of new approaches to improve phototherapeutic results is also to get beyond the tumor microenvironment's drawbacks, namely hypoxia. The Nano platforms with the ability to alter this environment by means of activation processes or targeted distribution have enormous opportunities for PIT and PDT optimization. ROS-sensitive drugs and heat activatable nanoparticles, for example, have been developed to enhance responses to therapy in hypoxic environments, increasing effectiveness while lowering systemic negative impacts [36]. Phototherapy's adaptability is further demonstrated by its use in conjunction with other treatments including chemotherapy, immunotherapy, and radiation. By combining these strategies, phototherapy lowers the risk of metastasis and recurrence by stimulating immune system reactions in addition to directly eliminating tumor cells. The opportunity for synergy emphasizes the need it is to keep developing phototherapeutic techniques to solve current clinical issues and broaden their use. A potential area of biomedical uses is phototherapeutic therapy, which uses light-activated substances to deliver simple, targeted, and efficient treatments. Future developments in the field of materials, nanotechnology, and personalized medicine will likely overcome existing constraints and improve the effectiveness and safety of this significant therapeutic approach.

3.1 Opto-genetics

The use of light to precisely regulate the activity of cells has transformed the fields of neurology and biomedical research due to opto-genetics. This novel method enables spatiotemporal accuracy in biological system modulation by combining genetic engineering and optical activation. By the introduction of photosensitive proteins, including halorhodopsins, channelrhodopsins, and other light-activated ion channels, into certain cells, scientists can precisely alter or promote biological functions. Understanding the intricacies of brain networks, diagnosing neurological conditions, and creating cutting-edge treatment approaches are all made possible by technological advances. Optogenetics' capacity to attain cellular specificity is one of its primary characteristics. By genetic targeting, which is researchers may influence certain neuronal communities by selectively expressing light-sensitive proteins in certain kinds of cells or brain areas. This is accomplished by using transgenic models of animals or vectors of viruses, which assure the precise transmission of genetic components. Once produced, such proteins react to certain wavelengths of light that may be transmitted using wireless optoelectronic surgical procedures, microscale light-emission diodes (led) and optical fibers [37].

Optogenetics has several uses outside of fundamental neuroscience. Modern advances indicate the importance it is for solving a variety of biological problems. Chronic discomfort, Parkinson's illness, and epilepsy were all treated with optogenetic methods. Scientists may regain typical activity rates without the need of pharmaceutical therapies by carefully addressing dysfunctional brain circuitry. Additionally, optogenetic approaches have been investigated for tissues that are not neurons. By specifically activating optogenetics, cardiomyocytes, for instance, has been employed to control heart rhythms and may provide remedies for arrhythmias along with different cardiac conditions. Combining nanotechnology and electronic devices to get over conventional constraints constitutes one of the most exciting advancements in optogenetics. The use of connected optical fibers in traditional optogenetic studies limited animal mobility and presented difficulties for ongoing studies [38]. Disconnected operation is now possible with flexible, multifunctional optoelectronic equipment, which are emerging advances. With the use of wireless power transmission, these gadgets may simultaneously monitor cerebral activity and provide light to remote brain areas. For instance, subdermal implantation was created that combine led with magnetic wire antennas to provide strong visual command in animals that are free to move around. The creation of nanomaterials that transmit light is a further advance in optogenetics. With the use of non-invasive techniques like near-infrared (NIR) illumination, which can enter tissues more deeply than light that is visible, such substances allow the wireless stimulation of highly photosensitive proteins. The utilization of light-transducing nanoparticles for high-quality optogenetic regulation was covered by studies, that also highlighted the potential of these materials in therapeutic settings, such as regenerative healthcare and cancer treatment. These nanoparticles allow minimally invasive tissue-level optogenetics by transforming near-infrared light into localized visible light. Although its immense promise, optogenetics has a number of issues that need to be resolved before it can be used more widely in therapeutic settings. The requirement for genetic alteration to insert receptive to proteins into the desired cells is one significant drawback. Vectors that transmit viruses have shown promise, however there are still issues with immune reactions and inaccurate consequences. Additionally, there are technical difficulties in delivering light to precise areas, especially in interior organs or tissue. These problems are being addressed with the aid of developments in biocompatible illumination, microlens lists, and optical fiber technologies [39].

Researchers have opened the door for more accurate and adaptable light delivery methods by demonstrating the effective application of organic LEDs (OLEDs) for excellent quality optogenetics. Additionally, new opportunities for personalized treatment have been made possible by the combination of optogenetics and bioelectronics. For example, bioelectronic inserts that combine wearable technology with optogenetic technologies have the ability to detect and treat illnesses in instantaneously [40]. These devices enable automated and traceless treatments by using light as a specific trigger to regulate treatments. These applications hold great promise for the treatment of long-term illnesses like diabetes or cardiovascular disease, where it is essential to dynamically regulate physiological variables. A revolutionary method for comprehending and managing intricate biological systems is optogenetics [41]. This technique offers unmatched regulation of biological functions by using photosensitive proteins and cutting-edge optical technology, opening the door to discoveries in cancer, cardiology, neurology, and other fields. Addressing present issues and realizing the full promise of optogenetics in medical applications will need continual advances in genetic engineering, materials science, and device manufacture. Optogenetics has the potential to be a key component of next-generation healthcare research and treatment because of its exceptional capacity to integrate accuracy, specificity, and adaptability [42].

4 Future Engineering: Challenges and Possibilities

Light emitter engineering for biological applications offers a unique combination of potential and problems. These technologies, which include nanomaterial and organic light-emitting diodes (OLEDs) consisting of as lanthanide-based up-conversion nanoparticles (UCNPs), have the potential to completely transform imaging, treatment, and diagnostics. But to fully use such technologies' enormous scope for clinical application, it is necessary to overcome technological, material, and legal barriers. Optimizing light emitters' effectiveness in biological contexts is a major task [43]. Conventional emitters, like inorganic LEDs, frequently find it difficult to strike a compromise between biocompatibility and high efficiency. Innovations that reduce toxicity and improve incorporation with soft tissues, such as UCNPs and elastic organic LEDs, demonstrate promise. For instance, when near-infrared (NIR) activation occurs, UCNPs release bright or ultraviolet light, a characteristic that permits photodynamic treatment and deep cell imaging with less photo damage to neighboring tissues. But there is still a critical problem with precisely tailoring these substances to provide better stability, adjustable wavelengths, and superior signal-to-noise levels [44].

There are several advantages to integrating biocompatible and biodegradable light-emitting substances, but there are also certain challenges. Biodegradable producers, like biodegradable small particles and resorbable Polymers include have made it possible for short-term implants to disintegrate innocuously once their purpose is fulfilled. These substances have demonstrated potential for use in anything from medication delivery to injury healing. Still, thorough testing of materials is necessary to guarantee its durability in biological contexts while preserving functionality, like constant light emission. Miniaturizing light emitters for used or implanted devices presents another difficulty. In optogenetics, whereby specific light transmission may either stimulate or repress brain activity, technologies like microscale LEDs (μLEDs) have proven useful. However, creating flexible, long-lasting, and wirelessly driven μLEDs adds complexity to the manufacturing process [45]. Device efficiency has been greatly enhanced by developments in thin-film transistors and biocompatible packaging techniques, enabling less intrusive implantation and longer usefulness. For example, siloxane-encapsulated elastic LEDs have outstanding thermal and mechanical durability, which makes them perfect for ongoing biomedical applications. Regulatory issues can have a significant impact on the biological light emitter research pipeline [46].

When devices are authorized for use in clinical settings, regulatory agencies like the FDA need thorough safety assessments that include photostability, biocompatibility, and cytotoxicity assessment. Although these strict regulations are necessary to guarantee security for patients, they may impede innovation. For instance, to address particular issues, like for a long-time tissue contact and the environmental effects of device deterioration, novel regulatory structures are required for developing technologies such as ubiquitous OLEDs and near-infrared emitters. Considering these difficulties, there are a ton of potential. Because near-infrared (NIR) emitters can reach deep into tissues that are living, they hold great promise for light therapy and diagnosis [47]. Developments in wavelength-tunable and wearable techniques have made it possible to use them for healing wounds and growth of hair stimulation, highlighting the broad range of therapeutic advantages of this kind of technology. Additionally, there is potential for powering implanted biomedical technology by integrating devices that emit light with nanotechnology, like reflectors, to improve light utilization effectiveness. Another level of innovation is introduced by new developments such as light-driven micro-nanomotors. Such tiny devices can give exact, targeted treatments while navigating biological surroundings. With the remarkable temporal and spatial accuracy that comes from using light as a signal for control, nanomotors can carry out complex operations like tailored administration of medicine or Nano surgery. But because of issues with transportation efficiency and biological compatibility, their move from indoor proof-of-concept research to in actual use continues to be a major obstacle [48].

For customized light emitters to reach their full capabilities, interdisciplinary cooperation will be crucial in addition to technological advancements. Designing devices which satisfy practical clinical demands requires close collaboration between researchers, bioengineers, materials scientists, and doctors. For example, precise medicine's use of devices that emit light depends on the smooth fusion of diagnosis and treatment, necessitating developments in computing algorithms and equipment. Personalized and adaptable technologies that react constantly to biological inputs are the direction the field is heading towards in the future. By modifying their light intensity in response to immediate input from tissues or detectors, smart gadgets may improve therapeutic results while reducing adverse effects. Additionally, using AI and machine learning in data analysis and design of devices might speed up manufacturing processes and enhance results for patients [49]. To sum up, designing light emitters for applications in medicine is a quickly developing field with enormous obstacles and revolutionary possibilities. A new age of healthcare equipment is being paved by researchers tackling regulatory challenges and improving material qualities. The upcoming decade of biomedical research promises safer, effective, and extremely customized medical treatments by addressing these obstacles and using the potential of cutting-edge light-emitting gadgets [50].

4.1 Therapeutics Applications

Customized light emitters, like quantum dot light-emitting devices (QLEDs), near-infrared light-emission diodes (NIR OLEDs) and LEDs, are revolutionizing the pharmaceutical industry by providing new methods of treating illnesses with never-before-seen accuracy and effectiveness. Such methods are becoming more and more popular because they offer great regional and temporal precision, controlled parameters like wavelength, extent, and duration, and tailored light administration with less invasiveness. Uses in photodynamic treatment (PDT), photo-bio-modulation, photo-thermal therapy (PTT), healing wounds, and other fields are made possible by these characteristics. Photodynamic treatment (PDT), which uses photo-responsive devices to activate photosensitizers at certain wavelengths, is a significant therapeutic use of customized light emitters. The use of PDT in malignancies has shown great promise since light-induced activity produces reactive oxygen species (ROS), which kill malignant cells despite leaving healthy tissue intact. Comparing nanoparticle-based technologies that react to near-infrared (NIR) light to conventional Ultraviolet or visible-light frameworks, the former have shown better deep-tissue absorption and less photo toxicity [51]. Such advances are fundamental to the agnostic for cancer because they limit side effects while simultaneously improving treatment effectiveness [52].

QLEDs are versatile, wavelength-specific systems for photo bio modulation and photodynamic therapy, among other photo medical uses. With its deep-red spectrum output, excellent emission effectiveness, and versatility in focusing on particular photosensitizer absorption spikes QLEDs can improve wound healing and cancer therapy results. Recent research, for instance, has shown a wide range of therapeutic possibilities by successfully killing Staphylococcus aureus that is resistant to meth and encouraging the growth of new tissue [53]. Phototherapy is also being revolutionized by organic LEDs (NIR OLEDs) and near-infrared light-emission diodes (NIR LEDs). They are perfect for treating illnesses that are found in thick tissues because of their capacity to penetrate deep tissue. By encouraging cell growth and enhancing recovery results, like in human follicles for hair epidermal papilla tissues, by precisely calibrated exposure to light, recent developments in wearing and wavelength-tunable NIR OLEDs have made it possible for further uses in therapy. They are much more useful in portable medical devices because of their adaptability and lower temperatures during operation [54].

LEDs, or diodes that emit light, are used in a variety of medical procedures. Their wavelengths range from UV to infrared light in tumor models, blue-colored LEDs have shown anti-metastatic and anti-proliferative properties, offering a non-invasive way to manage tumor growth. Utilizing photo-bio-modulation processes to promote repair of tissues and regulate responses to inflammation, red and infrared light-emitting devices are extensively utilized in pain treatment and healing of wounds. Another advancement in customized light delivery, especially in photodynamic treatment, is the use of elastic light-emitting textiles. Active keratosis as well as experimental models of cancer can be effectively treated using such structures, which incorporate optical fibers into fabrics to distribute light uniformly. These developments demonstrate the way light-based therapies may be used in a variety of clinical settings. Another important area of research is the use of customized cylindrical diffusion devices for interstitial transmission of light. By limiting light intensities to specified tissue volumes, such devices reduce collateral harm and increase the efficacy of cancer treatment regimens [55].

Customizing light-emitted profiles opens up new opportunities for minimally or non-invasive treatments and fits in nicely with personalized medicine's objectives. Last but not least, sophisticated light-responsive drug delivery structures (DDSs) use the spatiotemporal management that light provides to precisely release medications for treatment [56]. Particularly intriguing for deep-tissue uses include nanostructured DDSs triggered by NIR rays, which provide dual-mode treatments including photodynamic and photothermal techniques, regulated release of drugs, and bioimaging. New therapeutic approaches that integrate diagnostics and treatments into one device are being made possible by such systems. Medicinal techniques are being revolutionized by customized light emitters, which provide extremely effective, accurate, and less intrusive therapies. These forms of technology have enormous promise to solve difficult medical issues in a variety of domains, from photothermal and photodynamic treatments to photo-bio modulation and sophisticated systems for delivering drugs. It is anticipated that when they are progressively incorporated into implantable, versatile, and wearable technology, their clinical influence will increase and revolutionize medicine in the coming years [57].

5 Conclusion

In conclusion, tailored organic light-emitting diodes (OLEDs) represent a transformative advancement in biomedicine, offering unprecedented opportunities for innovative diagnostic and therapeutic applications. Their unique properties, such as flexibility, lightweight design, and tunable emission spectra, pave the way for enhanced imaging techniques and targeted treatments that can significantly improve patient outcomes. As research continues to evolve, the integration of OLED technology into biomedical devices promises not only to advance our understanding of biological processes but also to revolutionize the delivery of healthcare. Customizing light emitted profiles opens up new opportunities for minimally or non-invasive treatments and fits in nicely with personalized medicine's objectives. Last but not least, sophisticated light-responsive drug delivery structures (DDSs) use the spatiotemporal management that light provides to precisely release medications for treatment. Particularly intriguing for deep-tissue uses include nanostructured DDSs triggered by NIR rays. The potential for OLEDs to facilitate real-time monitoring and personalized medicine underscores their importance in the future of medical technology, making them a vital component in the quest for more effective and efficient healthcare solutions. This convergence of technology and medicine is likely to lead to breakthroughs that enhance diagnostic accuracy, streamline treatment protocols, and ultimately provide patients with more tailored healthcare experiences. As research continues to advance, the integration of OLED technology into wearable devices and smart medical equipment will likely transform patient engagement and empower individuals to take charge of their health like never before.

References

1. Righini, G.C., Krzak, J., Lukowiak, A., Macrelli, G., Varas, S., Ferrari, M.: From flexible electronics to flexible photonics: a brief overview. Opt. Mater. **115**, 111011 (2021)
2. Osman, W.N.A.W., Rosli, M.H., Mazli, W.N.A., Samsuri, S.: Comparative review of biodiesel production and purification. Carbon Capture Sci. Technol. **13**, 100264 (2024)
3. Cho, Y., Park, S., Lee, J., Yu, K.J.: Emerging materials and technologies with applications in flexible neural implants: a comprehensive review of current issues with neural devices. Adv. Mater. **33**, 2005786 (2021)
4. El Guerraf, A., Ziani, I., Ben Jadi, S., El Bachiri, A., Bazzaoui, M., Bazzaoui, E.A., et al.: Smart conducting polymer innovations for sustainable and safe food packaging technologies. Compr. Rev. Food Sci. Food Saf. **23**, e70045 (2024)
5. Murawski, C., Gather, M.C.: Emerging biomedical applications of organic light-emitting diodes. Adv. Opt. Mater. **9**, 2100269 (2021)
6. Mourtzis, D., Angelopoulos, J.: Development of an extended reality-based collaborative platform for engineering education: operator 5.0. Electronics (Basel) **12**, 3663 (2023)
7. Sharma, A., Majdinasab, M., Khan, R., Li, Z., Hayat, A., Marty, J.L.: Nanomaterials in fluorescence-based biosensors: defining key roles. Nano-Struct. Nano-Objects **27**, 100774 (2021)
8. Yang, X., Mu, G., Weng, K., Tang, X.: Advances in high-efficiency blue OLED materials. In: Photonics, vol. 11, p. 864 (2024)
9. Insero, G., Fusi, F., Romano, G.: The safe use of lasers in biomedicine: principles of laser-matter interaction. J. Public Health Res. **12**, 22799036231187076 (2023)
10. Zheludev, N.I., Yuan, G.: Optical superoscillation technologies beyond the diffraction limit. Nat. Rev. Phys. **4**, 16–32 (2022)
11. Choi, W., Park, B., Choi, S., Oh, D., Kim, J., Kim, C.: Recent advances in contrast-enhanced photoacoustic imaging: overcoming the physical and practical challenges. Chem. Rev. **123**, 7379–7419 (2023)
12. Li, D., Liu, P., Tan, Y., Zhang, Z., Kang, M., Wang, D., et al.: Type I photosensitizers based on aggregation-induced emission: a rising star in photodynamic therapy. Biosensors **12**, 722 (2022)
13. Kohar, D., Ray, D.K., Nepal, R., Phogat, J.: Revolutionizing therapeutics: the power of nanotechnology in precision medicine. J. Pharma Insights Res. **1**, 24–29 (2023)
14. Bag, A., Maheshwari, R.: Advances in polymer-centric nanomedicines for theranostic cancer treatment. J. Drug Deliv. Sci. Technol. **100**, 106105 (2024)
15. Kang, W., Liu, Y., Wang, W.: Light-responsive nanomedicine for cancer immunotherapy. Acta Pharmaceutica Sinica B **13**, 2346–2368 (2023)
16. Bouzin, M., Zeynali, A., Marini, M., Sironi, L., Scodellaro, R., D'Alfonso, L., et al.: Multiphoton laser fabrication of hybrid photo-activable biomaterials. Sensors **21**, 5891 (2021)
17. Camcıoglu, E., Mohammadrezaloo, D.G., Dinc, B.: Optogenetics and its transformative role in tissue engineering and regenerative medicine. Nano Select **5**, e202400013 (2024)
18. Abdelmohsen, H.A.M., Copeland, N.A., Hardy, J.G.: Light-responsive biomaterials for ocular drug delivery. Drug Deliv. Transl. Res. **13**, 2159–2182 (2023)
19. Reddy, K.T.K., Reddy, A.S.: Recent breakthroughs in drug delivery systems for targeted cancer therapy: an overview. Cell. Mol. Biomed. Rep. **5**, 13–27 (2025)
20. Karlo, J., Prasad, R., Singh, S.P.: Biophotonics in food technology: quo vadis? J. Agric. Food Res. **11**, 100482 (2023)
21. Simone, G.: Trends of biosensing: plasmonics through miniaturization and quantum sensing. Crit. Rev. Anal. Chem. **54**, 2183–2208 (2024)
22. Villazon, J.I., Jang, H., Shi, L.: Nonlinear optical imaging modalities in biomedicine. GEN Biotechnol. **3**, 290–298 (2024)
23. Ran, C., Pu, K.: Molecularly generated light and its biomedical applications. Angew. Chem. Int. Ed. **63**, e202314468 (2024)

24. Yang, Y., Jiang, Q., Zhang, F.: Nanocrystals for deep-tissue in vivo luminescence imaging in the near-infrared region. Chem. Rev. **124**, 554–628 (2023)
25. Lee, G., Choi, H.E., Hong, S.H., Choi, M., Han, D.-W., Lee, J., et al.: Upconversion nanomaterials and delivery systems for smart photonic medicines and healthcare devices. Adv. Drug Deliv. Rev. **188**, 114419 (2022)
26. Molani, A., Pennati, F., Ravazzani, S., Scarpellini, A., Storti, F.M., Vegetali, G., et al.: Advances in portable optical microscopy using cloud technologies and artificial intelligence for medical applications. Sensors **24**, 6682 (2024)
27. Yang, X., McGlynn, E., Das, R., Paşca, S.P., Cui, B., Heidari, H.: Nanotechnology enables novel modalities for neuromodulation. Adv. Mater. **33**, 2103208 (2021)
28. Lahoti, H.S., Jogdand, S.D.: Bioimaging: evolution, significance, and deficit. Cureus **14** (2022)
29. Shi, S., Chen, J., Wang, X., Xiao, M., Chandrasekaran, A.R., Li, L., et al.: Biointerface engineering with nucleic acid materials for biosensing applications. Adv. Func. Mater. **32**, 2201069 (2022)
30. Wang, B., Cai, H., Waterhouse, G.I.N., Qu, X., Yang, B., Lu, S.: Carbon dots in bioimaging, biosensing and therapeutics: a comprehensive review. Small Sci. **2**, 2200012 (2022)
31. Khonina, S.N., Kazanskiy, N.L., Skidanov, R.V., Butt, M.A.: Advancements and applications of diffractive optical elements in contemporary optics: a comprehensive overview. Adv. Mater. Technol., 2401028 (2024)
32. Shukla, M., Verma, N.V., Mohanta, Z., Tripathi, S., Pandya, A.: A review on tunable multifunctional Prussian blue nanoparticles; their promising biological applications & future directions. Coord. Chem. Rev. **496**, 215414 (2023)
33. Liu, Z.: Visualized Medicine: Emerging Techniques and Developing Frontiers (2023)
34. Cai, Y., Lv, Z., Chen, X., Jin, K., Mou, X.: Recent advances in biomaterials based near-infrared mild photothermal therapy for biomedical application: a review. Int. J. Biol. Macromol., 134746 (2024)
35. Shi, S., Zhong, H., Zhang, Y., Mei, Q.: Targeted delivery of nano-radiosensitizers for tumor radiotherapy. Coord. Chem. Rev. **518**, 216101 (2024)
36. Jiang, W., Liang, M., Lei, Q., Li, G., Wu, S.: The current status of photodynamic therapy in cancer treatment. Cancers **15**, 585 (2023)
37. Liu, K., Yao, Y., Xue, S., Zhang, M., Li, D., Xu, T., et al.: Recent advances of tumor microenvironment-responsive nanomedicines-energized combined phototherapy of cancers. Pharmaceutics **15**, 2480 (2023)
38. Zhang, H., Fang, H., Liu, D., Zhang, Y., Adu-Amankwaah, J., Yuan, J., et al.: Applications and challenges of rhodopsin-based optogenetics in biomedicine. Front. Neurosci. **16**, 966772 (2022)
39. Emiliani, V., Entcheva, E., Hedrich, R., Hegemann, P., Konrad, K.R., Lüscher, C., et al.: Optogenetics for light control of biological systems. Nat. Rev. Methods Prim. **2**, 55 (2022)
40. Chang, S., Koo, J.H., Yoo, J., Kim, M.S., Choi, M.K., Kim, D.-H., et al.: Flexible and stretchable light-emitting diodes and photodetectors for human-centric optoelectronics. Chem. Rev. **124**, 768–859 (2024)
41. Yadav, S., Mittal, P., Negi, S.: Recent advancements over a decade for organic light-emitting diodes: from structural diversity, role of layers, colour emission, material classification, performance improvement, fabrication to applications. Bull. Mater. Sci. **45**, 109 (2022)
42. Park, S., Takakuwa, M., Fukuda, K., Lee, S., Yokota, T., Someya, T.: Toward ultraflexible organic electronic devices. MRS Bull. **48**, 999–1012 (2023)
43. Li, Y., Guo, C., Yuan, J., Yang, X., Wu, M., Wu, L., et al.: Recent advances and prospects of persistent luminescent materials in public health applications. Chem. Eng. J., 150424 (2024)
44. Cha, G.D., Kim, D.-H., Kim, D.C.: Wearable and implantable light-emitting diodes and their biomedical applications. Korean J. Chem. Eng. **41**, 1–24 (2024)
45. Islam, A., Shah, S.H.U., Haider, Z., Imran, M., Amin, A., Haider, S.K., et al.: Biological interfacial materials for organic light-emitting diodes. Micromachines **14**, 1171 (2023)
46. Kong, D., Zhang, K., Tian, J., Yin, L., Sheng, X.: Biocompatible and biodegradable light-emitting materials and devices. Adv. Mater. Technol. **7**, 2100006 (2022)

47. Khan, M.I., Hossain, M.I., Hossain, M.K., Rubel, M.H.K., Hossain, K.M., Mahfuz, A., et al.: Recent progress in nanostructured smart drug delivery systems for cancer therapy: a review. ACS Appl. Bio Mater. **5**, 971–1012 (2022)
48. Parvin, N., Kumar, V., Joo, S.W., Mandal, T.K.: Emerging trends in nanomedicine: carbon-based nanomaterials for healthcare. Nanomaterials **14**, 1085 (2024)
49. Pelucchi, E., Fagas, G., Aharonovich, I., Englund, D., Figueroa, E., Gong, Q., et al.: The potential and global outlook of integrated photonics for quantum technologies. Nat. Rev. Phys. **4**, 194–208 (2022)
50. Fidan, I., Huseynov, O., Ali, M.A., Alkunte, S., Rajeshirke, M., Gupta, A., et al.: Recent inventions in additive manufacturing: holistic review. Inventions **8**, 103 (2023)
51. Arshad, F., Waheed, M., Harun, N., Fatima, K., Khan, B.A., Fatima, K., et al.: Indigenous farmer's perception about fodder and foraging species of semi-arid lowlands of Pakistan: a case study of district Kasur, Pakistan. Taiwania **67**, 510–523 (2022)
52. Wang, Y., Wen, Y., Zhuang, X., Liu, S., Zhang, L., Xie, W.: Flexible organic optoelectronic devices: design, fabrication, and applications. APL Photonics **9** (2024)
53. Jayan, K.D., Babu, K.: Luminescent perovskite quantum dots: progress in fabrication, modelling and machine learning approaches for advanced photonic and quantum computing applications. J. Lumin., 120906 (2024)
54. Sadia, H., Malik, K., Naqvi, S.A.M., Hassan, A., Abbas, S.: Botany, ethnomedicine, phytochemistry and pharmacology of musk cucumber (sicana odorifera)-a review. Ethnobot. Res. Appl. **27**, 1–38 (2024)
55. Thakur, M., Modi, V.K.: Biocolorants in food: sources, extraction, applications and future prospects. Crit. Rev. Food Sci. Nutr. **64**, 4674–4713 (2024)
56. Puccetti, M., Pariano, M., Schoubben, A., Giovagnoli, S., Ricci, M.: Biologics, theranostics, and personalized medicine in drug delivery systems. Pharmacol. Res., 107086 (2024)
57. Yang, D., Lee, Y., Kang, H., Vu, Q.H., Kang, G., Lee, S.E., et al.: Green manufacturing of electrically-tunable smart light-weight planar optics: a review. Int. J. Precis. Eng. Manuf.-Green Technol., 1–23 (2024)

Engineering Hydrogel-Based Composites for Photoluminescent Biomaterials

Moses Kumi and Onome Ejeromedoghene

Abstract The engineering of hydrogel-based composites for photoluminescent biomaterials presents a promising frontier in material science, offering significant advancements in bioimaging, drug delivery, and tissue engineering. Hydrogels, known for their high-water content and biocompatibility, open new possibilities for dynamic interactions with biological systems when combined with photoluminescent properties. This chapter explores the strategic selection of materials and fabrication methods for developing photoluminescent hydrogel composites, emphasizing the trade-offs between stability, biocompatibility, and photoluminescent efficiency. A particular focus is given to photoluminescent eutectogels, a class of composite materials that combine distinct phases to enhance luminescent properties, offering novel avenues for biomedical applications. These biomaterials have been shown to exhibit remarkable potential in imaging, sensing, and therapeutic interventions, where their interactions with biological systems are critically evaluated, revealing mechanisms that govern cellular uptake, biocompatibility, and in vivo performance. Finally, the chapter outlines the future directions of this field, including the development of multifunctional hydrogels capable of integrating therapeutic and diagnostic functions in a single system, paving the way for next-generation biomedical technologies. Through a comprehensive review of material selection, fabrication strategies, and biomedical applications, this chapter provides a thorough understanding of the evolving landscape of photoluminescent hydrogel composites and their transformative impact on biomedicine.

Keywords Hydrogel composites · Biomaterials · Photoluminescence · Eutectogels

M. Kumi
Frontiers Science Center for Flexible Electronics (FSCFE), Xi'an Institute of Flexible Electronics (IFE), Xi'an Institute of Biomedical Materials and Engineering (IBME), Northwestern Polytechnical University (NPU), Xi'an, Shaanxi, P. R. China

O. Ejeromedoghene (✉)
State and Local Joint Engineering Laboratory for Novel Functional Polymeric Materials, College of Chemistry, Chemical Engineering and Materials Science, Soochow University, Suzhou, Jiangsu Province, P. R. China
e-mail: oejeromedoghene@suda.edu.cn

© The Author(s), under exclusive license to Springer Nature Switzerland AG 2025
N. O. Etafo (ed.), *Tailored Light Emitters For Biomedical Applications*, Engineering Materials, https://doi.org/10.1007/978-3-031-88731-4_10

1 Introduction

The integration of photoluminescent materials into hydrogel matrices has emerged as a transformative approach in the development of advanced biomaterials. Hydrogels are well known for their high-water content and biocompatibility, and they have long been recognized for their versatile applications in the biomedical field, ranging from drug delivery systems to tissue engineering [1]. The incorporation of photoluminescent properties into these hydrogels further enhances their utility, enabling them to interact with biological systems in a variety of ways. Photoluminescence, the emission of light from a material upon excitation, serves as a valuable tool for real-time imaging, biosensing, and therapeutic monitoring [2]. By leveraging this property, hydrogel composites can be engineered to respond dynamically to physiological environments, facilitating a range of diagnostic and therapeutic applications.

Hydrogels are inherently suited for biomedical applications due to their structural similarity to biological tissues, which enables effective integration with living systems [3]. Their unique ability to maintain high water content, mimicking the extracellular matrix, makes them an ideal candidate for the delivery of drugs, growth factors, and other therapeutic agents [4]. However, one of the challenges faced by traditional hydrogels in biomedical applications is their limited ability to provide real-time feedback or enable non-invasive monitoring of their interactions within biological environments. The addition of photoluminescent components to hydrogel systems addresses this limitation, enabling the tracking of materials in vivo and enhancing the functionality of the biomaterials [5].

The engineering of photoluminescent hydrogel composites involves the careful selection of materials that not only impart photoluminescence but also maintain the inherent properties of the hydrogel, such as biocompatibility, biodegradability, and tunable mechanical strength. These composites often combine organic molecules, inorganic nanoparticles, or hybrid materials, each contributing unique advantages and posing distinct challenges [6]. The choice of photoluminescent agents plays a critical role in determining the spectral properties, stability, and overall effectiveness of the composite material [7]. Furthermore, the fabrication methods used to integrate photoluminescent materials into the hydrogel matrix must balance the need for high photoluminescent efficiency with the retention of the hydrogel's desirable biological properties.

A key subset of photoluminescent hydrogel composites is the class of materials known as eutectogels. These eutectic systems are composed of two or more phases that interact synergistically to enhance the overall properties of the material, particularly in terms of photoluminescent performance [8]. Eutectogels present a promising approach to the fabrication of photoluminescent hydrogels by offering increased luminescent intensity, improved stability, and more effective interaction with biological systems. These composites have shown particular promise in applications such as bioimaging and photodynamic therapy, where precise control over the light emission and absorption properties of the material is required.

Biomedical applications of photoluminescent hydrogel composites are diverse, ranging from non-invasive imaging techniques to targeted drug delivery and wound healing [9]. The ability to monitor the distribution and behavior of these materials in real-time provides a significant advantage over traditional methods, allowing for more accurate diagnostics and personalized treatments. Additionally, the potential for combining photoluminescence with therapeutic functions, such as in photodynamic therapy or drug release, represents an exciting area of research [10]. The interaction of photoluminescent hydrogels with biological systems is complex, involving mechanisms such as cellular uptake, fluorescence resonance energy transfer (FRET), and phototoxicity, all of which influence the efficacy of the material in vivo [11].

In this chapter, we will explore the fundamental principles behind the engineering of photoluminescent hydrogel composites, detailing the material selection and fabrication strategies that underpin their design. Herein, the unique properties of photoluminescent eutectogels and their potential in a range of biomedical applications, particularly in imaging, sensing, and therapy were examined. Finally, the plausible mechanisms by which these hydrogels interact with biological systems and consider future directions for their development, with an emphasis on enhancing their multifunctionality and clinical applicability are discussed. Through this exploration, we aim to provide a comprehensive understanding of the advances in photoluminescent hydrogel technology and its transformative impact on biomedical research and applications.

2 Material Selection and Fabrication Strategies of Photoluminescent Hydrogel Composites

The development of photoluminescent hydrogel composites requires a careful selection of materials that not only impart the desired luminescent properties but also maintain the inherent biological and mechanical properties of hydrogels. The biocompatibility, biodegradability, and high-water content of hydrogels make them an ideal candidate for a wide range of biomedical applications such as drug delivery, tissue engineering, and bioimaging [12]. The incorporation of photoluminescent materials enhances these hydrogels, allowing them to be used for real-time tracking, imaging, and therapeutic monitoring within biological systems [13]. In general, three primary types of materials are employed in photoluminescent hydrogel composites: organic photoluminescent materials, inorganic nanoparticles, and hybrid systems that combine both organic and inorganic components [14–16].

Organic photoluminescent materials, such as organic dyes, conjugated polymers, and small molecules, are widely used for their tunable photoluminescent properties, flexibility, and cost-effectiveness [17]. Common examples include fluorescent dyes such as fluorescein, rhodamine, and cyanine, as well as conjugated polymers like polyfluorene and polyphenylenevinylene (Fig. 1). These materials offer a broad range of emission wavelengths and can be easily customized to suit specific applications

[18]. However, the primary limitation of organic materials lies in their relatively low photostability and susceptibility to photobleaching under prolonged exposure to light, which may compromise their performance in long-term applications [19]. Furthermore, the biocompatibility of these materials can be a concern depending on their chemical structure, as some may exhibit cytotoxicity.

Inorganic materials, particularly nanoparticles like quantum dots (QDs), lanthanide-doped nanoparticles, and silica-based particles, are increasingly integrated into hydrogel composites for their superior photoluminescent efficiency, narrow emission spectra, and enhanced stability compared to organic materials [20]. Quantum dots, for instance, are semiconducting nanocrystals that can be tuned to emit light at specific wavelengths by adjusting their size, making them highly suitable for multi-modal imaging and diagnostic applications [21]. Despite their advantages, inorganic nanoparticles present challenges, including potential toxicity—especially with cadmium-based quantum dots—and the complexity involved in surface functionalization to improve biocompatibility. These nanoparticles often require careful engineering to ensure that their surface coating does not degrade in physiological environments and that they do not elicit an immune response.

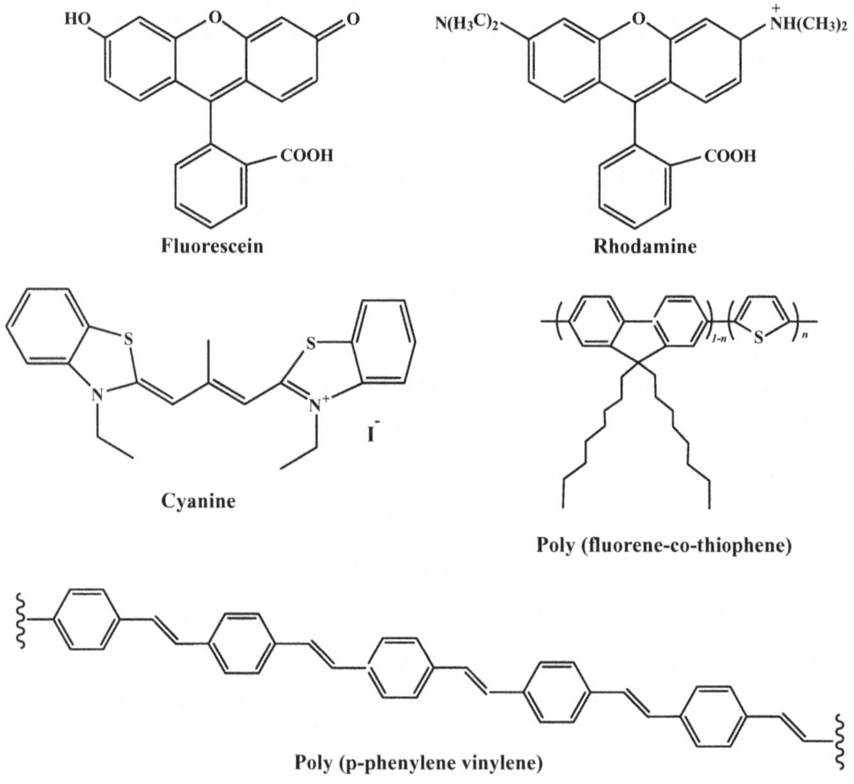

Fig. 1 Common examples of organic photoluminescent materials

Hybrid photoluminescent materials, which combine both organic and inorganic components, aim to leverage the advantages of each class of material. For example, organic dyes can be functionalized onto the surface of quantum dots to enhance their biocompatibility while preserving their high photoluminescent efficiency [22]. Similarly, hybrid materials can include photoluminescent dyes embedded within a silica nanoparticle or a polymeric matrix, offering better dispersion and stability in aqueous environments [20]. These hybrid systems generally provide a balance between the high efficiency of inorganic materials and the ease of handling and tunability of organic materials. However, the synthesis of hybrid materials can be complex, and maintaining the stability and performance of both organic and inorganic components can be challenging, especially over extended periods of use.

In addition to material selection, the fabrication methods used to incorporate these photoluminescent materials into hydrogel matrices play a crucial role in determining the properties of the final composite. Several fabrication strategies are employed, each with specific advantages and limitations (Fig. 2). The sol–gel method, for example, is frequently used to integrate inorganic nanoparticles such as quantum dots into the hydrogel matrix [23]. This technique involves the transition of a sol (a colloidal suspension of nanoparticles) into a gel (a three-dimensional network structure), allowing for high control over the material composition and morphology [24]. However, this method is primarily limited to inorganic materials and may face issues related to nanoparticle agglomeration, which can reduce the uniformity and performance of the composite.

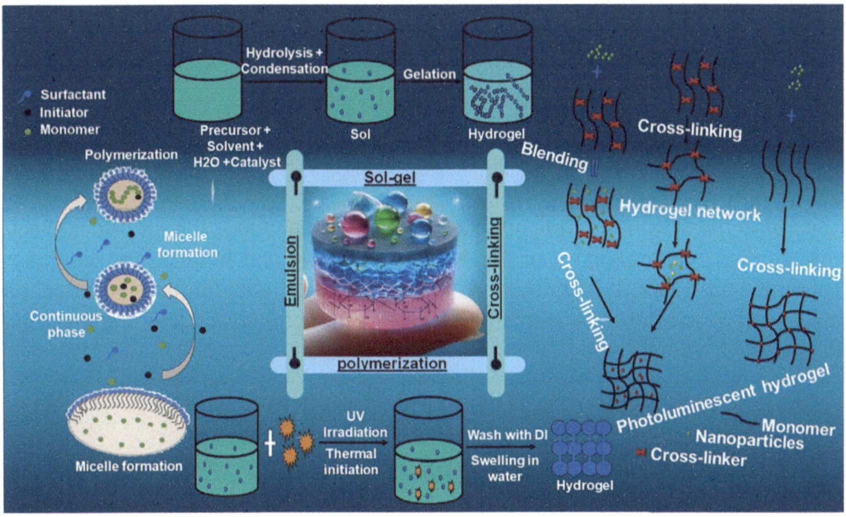

Fig. 2 Fabrication strategies for photoluminescent hydrogel composites

Polymerization techniques, such as free radical polymerization, UV-initiated polymerization, or ring-opening polymerization, offer another common route for fabricating photoluminescent hydrogel composites [25]. These methods enable the incorporation of organic dyes, conjugated polymers, or hybrid composites into a polymeric matrix. Polymerization allows for customization of the hydrogel's mechanical properties, crosslinking density, and overall stability, making it suitable for a wide range of applications [26]. However, some polymerization methods require harsh conditions, such as ultraviolet light or high temperatures, which can degrade the photoluminescent materials, especially those that are organic or sensitive to heat [27]. Therefore, careful optimization of these conditions is necessary to preserve the luminescent properties.

Chemical crosslinking is another widely used method to fabricate photoluminescent hydrogel composites [23]. In this process, crosslinking agents such as glutaraldehyde or genipin are used to form covalent bonds between polymer chains, creating a stable three-dimensional network structure [28]. Crosslinking can enhance the mechanical strength of the hydrogel and improve its stability in biological environments, making it ideal for drug delivery or tissue engineering applications [29, 30]. However, crosslinking agents may pose potential toxicity concerns, and achieving uniform crosslinking throughout the hydrogel can be challenging. Furthermore, the crosslinking process can sometimes alter the photoluminescent properties of the embedded materials, especially in the case of organic dyes or hybrid systems.

Finally, emulsion polymerization offers another strategy for fabricating photoluminescent hydrogel composites. This technique involves the emulsification of monomers in water, followed by polymerization in the presence of surfactants, which results in the formation of hydrogel composites [31]. Emulsion polymerization allows for the efficient incorporation of both hydrophilic and hydrophobic photoluminescent materials, making it highly versatile [32]. However, the need for surfactants and stabilizers can affect the biocompatibility of the final composite, and the stability of the emulsion system must be carefully controlled to avoid aggregation or phase separation of the materials.

To aid in the selection of materials and fabrication methods for specific applications, a comparative analysis of the various materials and fabrication techniques is provided in Table 1, highlighting their advantages and limitations based on factors such as stability, biocompatibility, ease of fabrication, and photoluminescent efficiency.

3 Photoluminescent Eutectogels

Deep eutectic solvents (DES) are a class of ionic solvents formed by the eutectic mixture of two or more components that, when combined, exhibit a significantly lower melting point than the individual constituents. Typically, DES is composed of a hydrogen bond donor (e.g., urea or glycerol) and a hydrogen bond acceptor (e.g., a quaternary ammonium salt) [43]. This unique interaction results in a liquid state

Table 1 Comparison of Photoluminescent Materials and Fabrication Methods for Hydrogel Composites

Material	Advantages	Limitations	Fabrication method	Advantages	Limitations	References
Organic materials (e.g., dyes, polymers)	High tunability of emission spectra, wide variety of materials, cost-effective	Low photostability, photobleaching, biocompatibility concerns	Sol–gel	High control over nanoparticle size, excellent dispersion of materials	Limited to inorganic materials, issues with nanoparticle agglomeration	[33–36]
			Polymerization	Flexibility in designing custom matrices, scalable, tunable properties	Harsh conditions (UV/heat) may degrade photoluminescent materials	
Inorganic nanoparticles (e.g., quantum dots, nanocrystals)	High photoluminescent efficiency, long-term stability, narrow emission spectra	Potential toxicity (e.g., Cd-based QDs), surface functionalization challenges	Chemical crosslinking	Enhanced mechanical strength, stable structure	Potential toxicity of crosslinking agents, uneven crosslinking	[37–39]
			Emulsion polymerization	Good dispersion of hydrophobic and hydrophilic materials, efficient	Need for surfactants, which may affect biocompatibility	
Hybrid materials (organic + inorganic)	Combines the advantages of both materials (e.g., high efficiency and biocompatibility)	Complex synthesis, challenges in maintaining stability of both components	Polymerization	Allows for incorporation of both organic and inorganic components	Potential incompatibility between organic and inorganic components	[40–42]
			Sol–gel	Superior control over morphology, stable nanocomposite formation	Complex synthesis procedures, risk of nanoparticle agglomeration	

at ambient temperatures and imparts DES with exceptional properties such as low volatility, high thermal stability, and biodegradability. DES is highly versatile and can dissolve a wide range of substances, including polymers, salts, and biomolecules [44]. This versatility, combined with their tunable physicochemical properties, has made DES a key component in various scientific fields, including green chemistry, electrochemistry, and biomedical engineering. In the context of material science, DES has emerged as a vital precursor for the development of eutectogels.

Eutectogels are hydrogels imbued with DES as the primary solvent phase [45]. The incorporation of DES into the gel matrix introduces unique dual-phase interactions, which significantly enhance the material's mechanical strength, ionic conductivity, and functional versatility. These features make eutectogels particularly suited for applications demanding robust and adaptive materials, such as flexible sensors, bioelectronics, and photoluminescent systems (Fig. 3). Eutectogels represent an emerging class of materials that have garnered significant attention for their unique and versatile properties, particularly when incorporated into photoluminescent hydrogel composites [46]. These gels are distinguished by their dual-phase structure, in which two distinct phases co-exist in a homogeneous gel network. The term "eutectogel" draws from the concept of eutectic systems, typically seen in materials science, where two phases exhibit enhanced properties due to their interaction, resulting in a highly stable and functional composite material [47]. The key feature of eutectogels is the interaction between these phases, which may be composed of organic or inorganic components, to create synergistic effects that enhance their photoluminescent capabilities, mechanical properties, and overall performance.

One of the defining characteristics of eutectogels is the presence of two or more materials that form a co-continuous network within the gel, allowing for improved dispersion and compatibility between phases [48]. In the context of photoluminescent composites, this dual-phase interaction is pivotal for optimizing the photoluminescence properties of the material. The photoluminescent efficiency of eutectogels often exceeds that of conventional hydrogel composites due to the synergistic interactions between the organic and inorganic phases [49]. These interactions enable

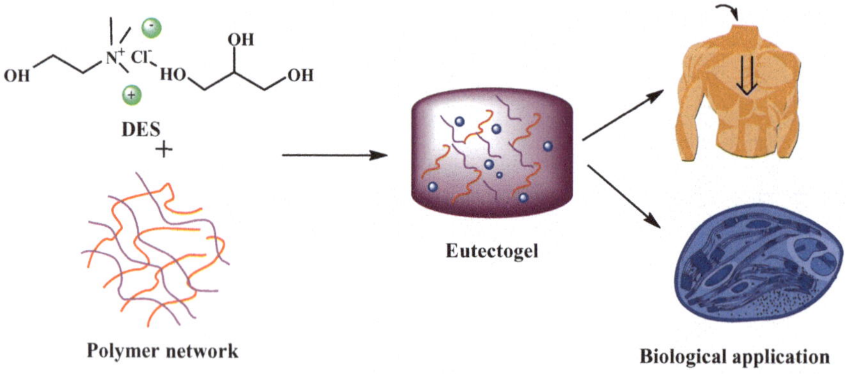

Fig. 3 Functional Eutectogel network for biological application

the creation of photoluminescent systems that possess enhanced stability, longer emission lifetimes, and improved resistance to photobleaching—critical factors for biomedical applications that require long-term stability. For instance, An et al. [50]. employed a dual catalytic redox system involving $FeCl_3$ and Vitamin C (VC) to create a highly viscous, ultra-stretched deep eutectic solvent (DES)/poly(acrylic acid) (PAA) eutectogel for detecting finger movements, thereby demonstrating the eutectogel's potential for use in flexible wearable devices. Wang et al. [51]. created a self-adaptive, multi-responsive thermochromic hydrogel (PHC-Gel) designed for dual-modal digital and visual sensing. Jiang et al. [52]. Developed a piezo-electrochromic tactile-sensation display (PETSD) that combines piezoelectric modulus with an electrochromic system to enable real-time human–computer interaction.

The organic phase of a eutectogel typically consists of a photoluminescent polymer or dye, while the inorganic phase may be composed of nanoparticles such as quantum dots or lanthanide-doped materials. These two phases are carefully selected to complement each other in terms of photophysical properties [53]. For example, the organic phase may provide a tunable emission spectrum or offer high energy absorption, while the inorganic phase can enhance quantum yield and stability. The interaction between these phases can lead to energy transfer processes, such as Förster resonance energy transfer (FRET), which further amplifies the photoluminescent signal [54]. Zhang et al. [55]. developed a reversible fluorescent eutectogel by integrating anthracene groups as photoswitchable fluorescent units, enabling applications in conformal encryption and anti-counterfeiting. Chen et al. [56]. introduced an anthracene-based organohydrogel capable of recording fluorescence patterns and reconfiguring stereostructures, designed for dual encryption purposes.

In addition to the enhanced photoluminescence properties, eutectogels offer several other unique benefits. The dual-phase structure imparts increased mechanical strength, flexibility, and environmental stability to the hydrogel composite. These characteristics make eutectogels especially attractive for applications such as bioimaging, sensor technologies, and drug delivery, where both the mechanical properties and photoluminescent behavior of the material are of paramount importance [57].

Moreover, the design of eutectogels allows for tunable properties such as viscosity, transparency, and responsiveness to external stimuli, such as temperature, pH, or ionic strength [58–60]. This versatility enables the fine-tuning of the material's characteristics to meet the specific needs of diverse biomedical applications. Vo et al. [61]. created a highly stretchable and tough eutectogel using polyvinylpyrrolidone (PVP) dissolved in a deep eutectic solvent (reline). The material, with 40 wt% PVP, offers excellent stretchability (1410% strain), toughness (544.8 kJ/m^3), and ionic conductivity (0.015 S/m), along with self-healing properties. Li et al. [62]. developed a one-pot method to create high-performance eutectogels by copolymerizing acrylic acid (AA) and DMAEMA in a deep eutectic solvent (DES). The resulting PAA-co-PDMAEMA eutectogels exhibited tunable mechanical properties, high transparency, favorable conductivity, and excellent anti-freezing and adhesion properties. These materials show potential for use in flexible sensors, with excellent strain durability and high temperature sensitivity, making them suitable for wearable electronics.

The photoluminescent properties of eutectogels are further enhanced by the spatial arrangement of the organic and inorganic components within the hydrogel matrix [63]. By optimizing the size, shape, and distribution of the particles, it is possible to maximize the interaction between the two phases, leading to better energy transfer efficiency and stronger photoluminescence [64]. The hybrid system also helps to mitigate the limitations typically associated with each phase when used in isolation. For example, the photostability of organic materials, which may suffer from rapid photobleaching, can be significantly improved by the addition of inorganic nanoparticles, which have a much higher resistance to photobleaching.

The unique structure of eutectogels also plays a role in improving their biocompatibility [65]. The interaction between organic and inorganic phases can result in a more favorable surface morphology, reducing the risk of toxicity when the material is introduced into biological systems. Moreover, the gel-like consistency of eutectogels enhances their ability to mimic biological tissues, offering a more natural environment for cell growth and interaction [66]. As a result, eutectogels are increasingly used in tissue engineering and regenerative medicine, where their combination of mechanical strength, biocompatibility, and photoluminescent properties is highly beneficial.

In summary, photoluminescent eutectogels represent a promising class of materials for advanced biomedical applications due to their dual-phase systems and enhanced photoluminescent properties. By leveraging the unique interactions between the organic and inorganic components, eutectogels offer improved stability, photoluminescent efficiency, and biocompatibility. Their ability to be fine-tuned for specific applications further enhances their potential, making them ideal candidates for a range of cutting-edge technologies, from bioimaging to smart drug delivery systems.

4 Biomedical Applications and Plausible Mechanisms of Interaction with Biosystems

Photoluminescent hydrogels, particularly those enhanced with photoluminescent eutectogels, have garnered significant attention for their potential in a range of biomedical applications. The combination of the hydrophilic nature of hydrogels and the luminescent properties provided by organic and inorganic materials creates an ideal platform for various biomedical technologies, including drug delivery systems, wound healing, tissue engineering, and biosensors (Fig. 4). These applications take advantage of both the inherent biocompatibility of hydrogels and the unique, enhanced properties of photoluminescence, offering exciting new possibilities for diagnostics, therapy, and tissue regeneration [67].

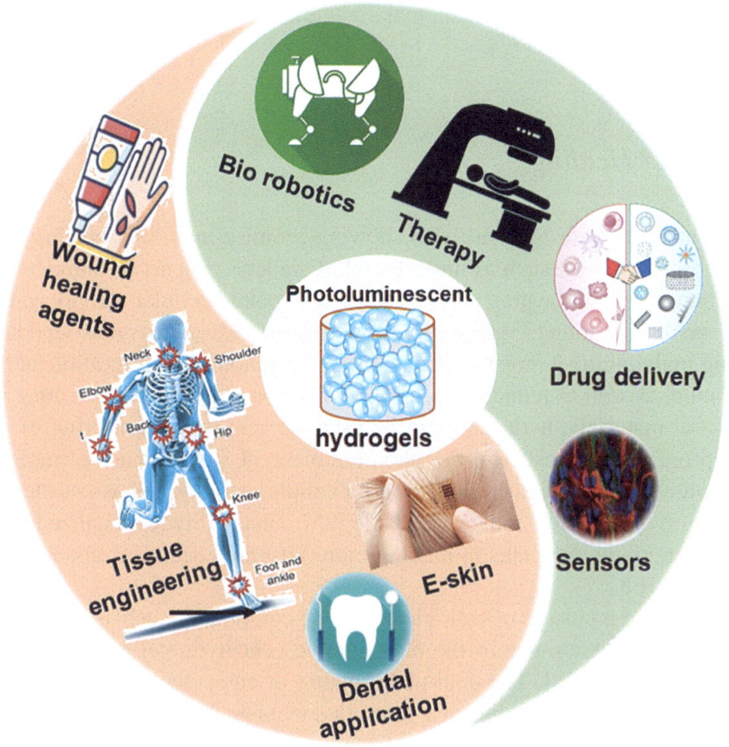

Fig. 4 Biomedical applications of photoluminescent hydrogels

4.1 *Drug Delivery Systems*

One of the most promising applications of photoluminescent hydrogel composites is in controlled drug delivery systems. The high-water content and tunable network structure of hydrogels make them ideal carriers for hydrophilic drugs, while their biocompatibility ensures minimal adverse effects on the body [68]. Photoluminescence, in this case, serves a dual function: it enables real-time tracking of drug release and distribution, and it can be used for site-specific targeting in response to external stimuli.

In the case of stimuli-responsive drug delivery, photoluminescent eutectogels can be engineered to release therapeutic agents in response to changes in the local environment, such as variations in pH, temperature, or ionic strength [69]. For example, when the hydrogel matrix is embedded with photosensitive materials, exposure to light can induce changes in the structure of the hydrogel, leading to controlled drug release [70]. The photoluminescence allows clinicians to monitor the spatial and temporal distribution of the drug, improving the precision and effectiveness of the treatment [71]. Additionally, the incorporation of inorganic nanoparticles, like quantum dots, enhances the stability of the system, making it less susceptible to degradation during the drug delivery process [72].

4.2 Wound Healing

Photoluminescent hydrogels are also showing promise in wound healing applications. Chronic wounds, such as those found in diabetic patients or individuals with burns, often have poor healing outcomes due to impaired cellular activity and inefficient tissue regeneration [73]. Hydrogels offer several advantages in wound healing, including maintaining a moist environment that promotes cell migration and tissue regeneration, as well as reducing the risk of infection [74]. By incorporating photoluminescent materials, hydrogels can be used for real-time monitoring of wound healing progress. For instance, the photoluminescent signals can be employed to track the rate of tissue regeneration, monitor cellular activity, and assess the level of inflammation or infection at the wound site [75]. This ability to visualize healing in real-time can guide clinicians in making more informed decisions about treatment adjustments [76].

Moreover, the inclusion of biologically active compounds such as growth factors or antimicrobial agents within the photoluminescent hydrogel can accelerate the healing process [77, 78]. The dual-phase nature of eutectogels also allows for the co-delivery of these compounds in a controlled manner, enhancing their therapeutic effects.

4.3 Tissue Engineering

In tissue engineering, photoluminescent hydrogels can be used as scaffolds for cell growth and tissue regeneration. The biocompatibility and structural similarity of hydrogels to the extracellular matrix (ECM) make them ideal candidates for supporting cellular growth and promoting tissue formation. Photoluminescent materials embedded within these hydrogels allow for non-invasive imaging and tracking of cells or tissues over time [79]. The ability to monitor cell behavior, such as migration, differentiation, or proliferation, in real-time is crucial for optimizing the design of tissue-engineered constructs. For example, quantum dots and conjugated polymers can be used to tag specific cell types within the hydrogel scaffold, enabling real-time tracking of cellular activities during the tissue regeneration process [80–85].

Furthermore, photoluminescent hydrogels can be engineered to mimic the native tissue environment more closely, enhancing the survival and function of implanted cells. The interaction between the hydrogel matrix and the encapsulated cells is critical, and the photoluminescent properties can help assess cell-hydrogel interactions and evaluate the mechanical properties of the tissue-engineered constructs [86]. In addition, photothermal therapy (using light to induce localized heating) can be integrated into the hydrogel system, providing a method for promoting cell differentiation or enhancing vascularization in tissue engineering applications [87].

4.4 Biosensors

Photoluminescent hydrogels have found exciting applications in biosensors due to their ability to exhibit changes in photoluminescence in response to biological or chemical stimuli. For example, hydrogels can be designed to detect changes in pH, ionic concentration, or specific biomolecules such as glucose, proteins, or DNA [88]. The photoluminescent signal provides a direct readout of these changes, offering a non-invasive and real-time detection method that can be particularly useful for diagnostics and disease monitoring [89, 90].

Photoluminescent biosensors can be applied in a variety of medical fields, including glucose monitoring in diabetic patients, pathogen detection, and cancer diagnostics. The high sensitivity and specificity of photoluminescent signals make these sensors highly reliable for detecting low concentrations of target analytes [91]. In addition, the biocompatibility and flexibility of hydrogels allow these sensors to be implanted in vivo or used in wearable devices for continuous health monitoring [92, 93].

4.5 Dental Application

Photoluminescent hydrogels are rapidly gaining attention in the field of dentistry due to their versatility and ability to integrate both therapeutic and diagnostic functions. One promising application is in the development of restorative dental fillings and coatings. Photoluminescent hydrogels can be designed to mimic the mechanical and physical properties of natural tooth structures, making them ideal for use in dental restorations such as fillings, crowns, and coatings [94]. The photoluminescence properties of these hydrogels enable real-time monitoring of the restoration's integrity, allowing dentists to detect any degradation or wear early, which can help prevent further damage and improve the longevity of the restoration. Another key application lies in tracking tissue regeneration following dental procedures such as periodontal surgery, gum grafts, or implant placements. Photoluminescent materials embedded in hydrogels allow for non-invasive monitoring of the healing process, providing valuable insights into cell migration, tissue growth, and inflammation levels [95]. This ability to monitor healing in real-time aids clinicians in making more informed treatment decisions, optimizing recovery, and improving patient outcomes. Photoluminescent hydrogels are also being explored as advanced dental biomaterials with embedded sensors capable of detecting changes in the oral environment [96]. For example, these sensors can measure pH levels, bacterial activity, or inflammation, which are critical markers for diagnosing dental diseases like caries (tooth decay) or gingivitis (gum disease) [97]. The ability to detect such changes early through photoluminescent signals could lead to more proactive and personalized dental care, enabling patients to address oral health issues before they require invasive treatments [97]. In the realm of early disease detection, photoluminescent hydrogels offer the potential for identifying subtle changes in dental tissues that might otherwise go unnoticed [98]. For instance, a photoluminescent hydrogel applied to an area of the mouth with suspected decay could provide immediate feedback on the presence of demineralization or bacterial activity, helping to diagnose dental issues at an early stage and enabling quicker, less invasive interventions [99]. Additionally, these hydrogels can be used as coatings for dental implants, where the photoluminescent signals can monitor the integration process between the implant and surrounding tissue [100]. This real-time tracking ensures that any complications, such as inflammation or infection, are detected early, improving the success rates of dental implants. Photoluminescent hydrogels could also be incorporated into oral care products like toothpaste, mouthwash, or dental strips [101]. In these applications, the hydrogels could provide real-time feedback on the effectiveness of the oral care regimen by detecting bacterial levels or other oral health parameters, offering users valuable insights into their hygiene practices [102, 103]. Furthermore, these hydrogels hold promise for enhancing photodynamic therapy (PDT) in the treatment of oral cancers. By delivering photosensitizing agents to tumor sites within the oral cavity, photoluminescent hydrogels can improve the targeting and efficacy of PDT, enabling clinicians to monitor the distribution and accumulation of the agent through luminescent signals, ensuring precise treatment and minimizing damage to healthy tissues [104]. Finally, photoluminescent hydrogels could revolutionize oral drug delivery systems. These hydrogels can be tailored to release drugs locally within the oral cavity in response to specific stimuli like pH or light, offering controlled and targeted delivery of medications such as antimicrobial agents or anti-inflammatory drugs. The photoluminescent properties enable clinicians to track the drug's release and distribution, ensuring the treatment is effective and reaches the intended site of action.

4.6 Bio Robotics

Bio robotics, a field that combines biology, robotics, and biomedical engineering, has been significantly enhanced by the integration of photoluminescent hydrogels. These advanced materials are particularly suited for applications in biorobotics due to their flexibility, biocompatibility, and unique ability to interact with biological systems [105]. One of the most promising areas of application is in the development of soft robotics, which are robots made from highly flexible materials that can mimic the movements and behaviors of biological organisms [106]. Photoluminescent hydrogels can be used to create soft actuators and sensors that can respond to biological stimuli, such as changes in pH, temperature, or ionic concentration. These actuators can simulate the dynamic and adaptable movements seen in living organisms, offering a significant advantage over traditional rigid robotic systems in applications that require fine motor control and adaptability, such as prosthetics, surgical tools, or therapeutic devices [107].

Photoluminescent hydrogels also enable non-invasive monitoring of biorobotic systems in real-time. By embedding photoluminescent materials into the hydrogel, researchers can track the movement and behavior of biorobotic devices, providing valuable feedback during testing and deployment [108]. This capability is particularly beneficial in prosthetics and exoskeletons, where it is important to monitor both the function of the device and the interaction with the wearer's body [109]. In these systems, the photoluminescence can offer insights into the device's response to external stimuli, such as pressure or force, allowing for adjustments to be made for improved comfort, functionality, and safety.

Moreover, biorobotic systems in the medical field, such as surgical robots or autonomous diagnostic tools, can greatly benefit from the incorporation of photoluminescent hydrogels. These hydrogels can be used in bio robotic implants, where their ability to respond to light or other environmental changes allows for more precise control and adaptation during surgeries or other medical procedures. For instance, bio-robots equipped with photoluminescent hydrogels could be used for minimally invasive surgeries, where real-time imaging of the robot's position within the body is crucial. The photoluminescence allows clinicians to track the surgical tools or implants visually, ensuring accuracy and reducing the risk of complications [110–112].

In the realm of biorobotics, photoluminescent hydrogels can also contribute to the development of bio-hybrid systems—robots that are partially made from living cells or tissues [113]. These bio-hybrid robots can use photoluminescent hydrogels as scaffolds to support and guide the growth of living cells, enabling the creation of systems that have both biological and mechanical components [114]. The photoluminescence of these hydrogels can help researchers monitor the development of these bio-hybrid robots, tracking the integration of living tissues with synthetic materials, and providing valuable data for the improvement of tissue-engineered devices [115].

The use of photoluminescent hydrogels in biorobotics also has significant potential in the field of rehabilitation. For example, soft biorobotic gloves or wearable exoskeletons designed to assist individuals with mobility impairments can be equipped with photoluminescent hydrogels that help monitor the performance of the system and its interaction with the user's body [116]. These systems could adapt to the user's movements in real-time, providing feedback that ensures proper functionality and comfort. Photoluminescence could also enable the continuous monitoring of the user's physical therapy progress, ensuring that the robotic system delivers the appropriate level of support as recovery progresses [117–119].

Additionally, bio-robots equipped with photoluminescent hydrogels could be used for environmental monitoring in medical or industrial applications. These robots could autonomously detect changes in biological or chemical parameters, providing real-time data that can be used for early diagnosis, environmental hazard detection, or even monitoring patients' health parameters in real-time [120]. Photoluminescent hydrogels would enable these robots to operate autonomously while continuously monitoring the biological signals around them, offering non-invasive and high-precision data collection [121].

4.7 Therapy

Photoluminescent hydrogels hold considerable promise in the field of therapy, particularly in the development of innovative treatment strategies that combine therapeutic delivery with real-time monitoring. Their unique properties make them ideal candidates for use in various therapeutic applications, including photodynamic therapy (PDT), wound healing, cancer treatment, and tissue regeneration.

In photodynamic therapy, photoluminescent hydrogels are utilized to deliver photosensitizing agents to targeted areas within the body, where they can be activated by light to produce reactive oxygen species that damage cancerous or infected cells. These hydrogels enhance the precision of PDT by providing localized treatment, minimizing the impact on surrounding healthy tissues [122]. The ability to track the distribution and accumulation of the photosensitizer via photoluminescence signals significantly improves treatment outcomes. Clinicians can monitor the effectiveness of the therapy in real-time, adjusting parameters like light dosage and duration to optimize therapeutic efficacy [123]. This real-time feedback system also reduces the risk of complications such as skin damage or overexposure to light, allowing for more controlled and personalized cancer treatments [124].

Moreover, the flexibility of photoluminescent hydrogels enables them to be used in combination with other therapeutic modalities, such as gene therapy or immunotherapy [125]. For instance, photoluminescent hydrogels can be used as carriers for gene delivery systems, where the photoluminescence enables the tracking of gene transfer efficiency and expression levels in real time [126]. In immunotherapy, these hydrogels can deliver immunomodulatory agents to specific sites in the body, enhancing the immune response against tumors or infections [127]. By monitoring the hydrogel's behavior and the distribution of the therapeutic agent through photoluminescence, clinicians can optimize the treatment regimen to maximize.

5 Mechanisms of Interaction with Biological Systems

The successful application of photoluminescent hydrogels in biomedical fields hinges on their ability to interact effectively with biological systems. Understanding the mechanisms of interaction is critical for ensuring their safety, efficacy, and biocompatibility. These mechanisms generally encompass cell uptake, biocompatibility, and immune response, each of which plays a key role in the material's performance in vivo (Fig. 5).

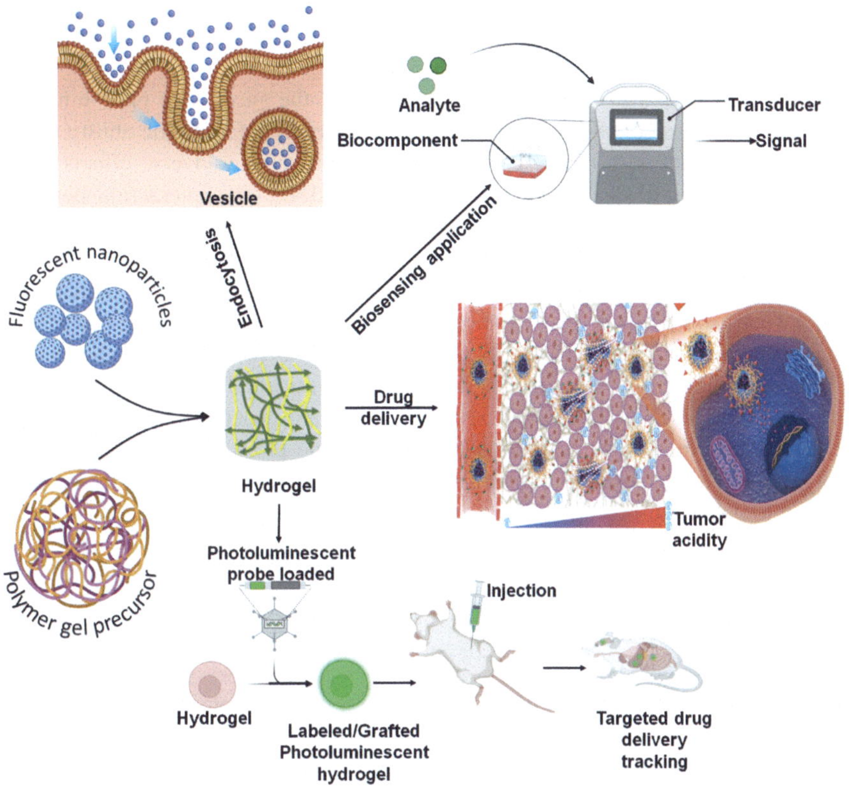

Fig. 5 Interaction of photoluminescent hydrogels with biological systems

5.1 *Cell Uptake and Bioavailability*

Cellular uptake is one of the fundamental mechanisms by which hydrogels interact with biological systems [128]. The incorporation of photoluminescent materials such as quantum dots or organic dyes within hydrogel matrices can enhance the uptake of these materials by cells. This uptake can be mediated through various endocytic pathways, including clathrin-mediated endocytosis, pinocytosis, or phagocytosis. The physicochemical properties of the hydrogel matrix, such as its surface charge, porosity, and molecular weight, directly influence the efficiency of cellular uptake [129].

In photoluminescent hydrogels, the photoluminescent signal also allows for the non-invasive tracking of the internalization process. This is particularly valuable for drug delivery or gene therapy applications, where it is important to monitor the location and quantity of the delivered material within target cells or tissues.

5.2 Biocompatibility and Toxicity

Biocompatibility is a critical factor in determining the success of photoluminescent hydrogels in medical applications. Biocompatibility refers to the ability of the material to interact with biological systems without causing adverse effects, such as inflammation, cell death, or immune rejection [130]. The interaction between photoluminescent hydrogels and cells can be influenced by the composition of the hydrogel, as well as the characteristics of the photoluminescent materials used [131]. Inorganic materials like quantum dots may raise concerns about toxicity, particularly with certain heavy metals like cadmium, which can leach from the nanoparticles [132]. However, surface modification strategies, such as coating the quantum dots with biocompatible polymers or peptides, can help mitigate these risks.

In contrast, organic photoluminescent materials are generally considered more biocompatible, though their stability can be an issue [133]. The development of hybrid materials that combine both organic and inorganic components is an emerging strategy to balance biocompatibility and photoluminescent efficiency [134].

5.3 Immune Response

Another important consideration is the immune response to photoluminescent hydrogels. While hydrogels are typically designed to be non-immunogenic, the presence of foreign materials such as inorganic nanoparticles or synthetic polymers may trigger an immune reaction [135]. The encapsulation of these materials within the hydrogel matrix can reduce their direct interaction with the immune system, minimizing inflammatory responses [136, 137]. Moreover, functionalization of the hydrogel surface with targeting ligands or peptides can promote selective interactions with specific cell types, helping to further reduce unwanted immune activation [138, 139].

In conclusion, photoluminescent hydrogels exhibit significant potential across a wide array of biomedical applications due to their dual functionality, combining therapeutic delivery with imaging capabilities. The mechanisms of interaction with biological systems—ranging from cellular uptake and biocompatibility to immune responses—are critical to their success in these applications. Ongoing research into the optimization of these interactions and the development of new photoluminescent materials will further enhance the utility of these composites in advancing personalized medicine and therapeutic monitoring.

6 Conclusion and Future Directions

In recent years, photoluminescent hydrogels, particularly those incorporating eutectogels, have emerged as a highly promising class of biomaterials with a broad range of biomedical applications. The ability to harness both the unique mechanical properties of hydrogels and the photoluminescent capabilities of organic and inorganic materials has positioned these composites at the forefront of research in areas such as drug delivery systems, wound healing, tissue engineering, and biosensing. Photoluminescent eutectogels, with their dual-phase structure and enhanced photoluminescent efficiency, offer substantial advantages in terms of stability, tunability, and biocompatibility, making them ideal candidates for addressing the challenges faced by conventional biomaterials in these fields.

Key findings from this review underscore the versatility of photoluminescent hydrogels in advancing personalized medicine. Their ability to be engineered for specific applications, from real-time tracking of drug release to monitoring tissue regeneration, positions these materials as powerful tools in clinical settings. Furthermore, the photoluminescent properties of these hydrogels provide new avenues for non-invasive diagnostics, allowing for the monitoring of disease progression and therapy effectiveness through advanced imaging techniques. By combining therapeutic delivery with diagnostic imaging, these materials open the door to the development of theranostics, an integrated approach to treatment and monitoring that has the potential to revolutionize healthcare, particularly in cancer and chronic disease management.

Looking ahead, several exciting directions for future research and development in photoluminescent hydrogels are emerging. As the field progresses, further optimization of material properties—such as improving photostability, minimizing toxicity, and enhancing the specificity of targeting—will be crucial for the broader clinical adoption of these systems. Additionally, there is a growing interest in personalized medicine, where photoluminescent hydrogels can be tailored to meet the unique needs of individual patients. For example, the development of responsive hydrogels that adapt to the patient's changing biological conditions, such as inflammation levels or tissue regeneration needs, could significantly improve therapeutic outcomes.

The integration of nanotechnology with photoluminescent hydrogels also holds immense promise. The use of advanced nanoparticles, including quantum dots, nanocapsules, and nanoscale sensors, could enable more efficient drug encapsulation, targeted delivery, and real-time monitoring of therapeutic efficacy. This nanohybrid approach may further enhance the material's photoluminescent properties, while simultaneously improving the functional integration of photoluminescence with the biological environment. Furthermore, as the understanding of the immune response to these materials deepens, strategies to improve their biocompatibility—such as functionalizing hydrogel surfaces with bioactive molecules or biomimetic peptides—will continue to play a crucial role in their clinical translation.

Another key area for development lies in the scalability and commercialization of photoluminescent hydrogels. While the research is highly promising, challenges related to the large-scale synthesis, cost-effectiveness, and reproducibility of these materials remain. Advances in 3D printing technologies and biomanufacturing processes could provide new ways to fabricate customized hydrogel composites, making them more accessible for clinical use.

Finally, multimodal imaging is a rapidly evolving field where photoluminescent hydrogels could make significant contributions. By combining photoluminescence with other imaging modalities such as MRI, CT, or ultrasound, it may be possible to create hybrid diagnostic systems that offer enhanced resolution and depth of information. These advances could be particularly beneficial in oncology, where precise tumor identification, drug tracking, and monitoring of therapeutic response are critical for improving patient outcomes.

In summary, photoluminescent hydrogels, particularly eutectogels, represent a highly innovative and versatile class of materials with vast potential in the biomedical field. Their ability to combine therapeutic and diagnostic capabilities offers a unique opportunity to revolutionize personalized medicine and theranostic approaches. Continued advancements in material design, optimization, and clinical application are expected to drive further breakthroughs, ultimately leading to more effective, targeted, and non-invasive treatment options for patients. With ongoing research and development, photoluminescent hydrogels are poised to play a transformative role in the future of healthcare, offering new solutions for disease diagnosis, treatment, and monitoring.

References

1. Guimarães, C.F., Ahmed, R., Marques, A.P., Reis, R.L., Demirci, U.: Engineering hydrogel-based biomedical photonics: design, fabrication, and applications. Adv. Mater. **33**, 2006582 (2021)
2. Zhang, K.Y., Yu, Q., Wei, H., Liu, S., Zhao, Q., Huang, W.: Long-lived emissive probes for time-resolved photoluminescence bioimaging and biosensing. Chem. Rev. **118**, 1770–1839 (2018)
3. Kumi, M., Ejeromedoghene, O., Dana, W., Zhang, Z.: Unlocking the biological response of smart Stimuli-Responsive hydrogels and their application in biological systems. Eur. Polym. J. **209**, 112906 (2024). https://doi.org/10.1016/j.eurpolymj.2024.112906
4. Subbiah, R., Guldberg, R.E.: Materials science and design principles of growth factor delivery systems in tissue engineering and regenerative medicine. Adv. Healthc. Mater. **8**, 1801000 (2019)
5. Cheng, Q., Hao, A., Xing, P.: Stimulus-responsive luminescent hydrogels: design and applications. Adv. Colloid Interface Sci. **286**, 102301 (2020). https://doi.org/10.1016/j.cis.2020.102301
6. Liu, W., Lustig, W.P., Li, J.: Luminescent inorganic-organic hybrid semiconductor materials for energy-saving lighting applications. EnergyChem **1**, 100008 (2019)
7. Algar, W.R., Massey, M., Rees, K., Higgins, R., Krause, K.D., Darwish, G.H., et al.: Photoluminescent nanoparticles for chemical and biological analysis and imaging. Chem. Rev. **121**, 9243–9358 (2021)

8. Tomé, L.C., Mecerreyes, D.: Emerging ionic soft materials based on deep eutectic solvents. J. Phys. Chem. B **124**, 8465–8478 (2020). https://doi.org/10.1021/acs.jpcb.0c04769
9. Chen, Z., Chen, T., Guo, B., Yang, F.: Advances in photo-responsive hydrogel integrated with biomedical materials for antitumor applications. Eur. Polym. J. 113431 (2024)
10. Chen, J., Fan, T., Xie, Z., Zeng, Q., Xue, P., Zheng, T., et al.: Advances in nanomaterials for photodynamic therapy applications: status and challenges. Biomaterials **237**, 119827 (2020)
11. Yan, Z., Kavanagh, T., da Silva Harrabi, R., Lust, S.T., Tang, C., Beavil, R.L., et al.: FRET sensor-modified synthetic hydrogels for real-time monitoring of cell-derived matrix metalloproteinase activity using fluorescence lifetime imaging. Adv. Funct. Mater. **34** (2024). https://doi.org/10.1002/adfm.202309711
12. Li, X., Su, X.: Multifunctional smart hydrogels: potential in tissue engineering and cancer therapy. J. Mater. Chem. B **6**, 4714–4730 (2018)
13. Yang, Y., Zhang, Y., Xie, S., Tang, Y., Zeng, Z., Tang, B.Z.: Hydrogel-derived luminescent scaffolds for biomedical applications. Mater. Chem. Front. **5**, 3524–3548 (2021)
14. Omidian, H., Wilson, R.L.: Enhancing hydrogels with quantum dots. J. Compos. Sci. **8**, 203 (2024). https://doi.org/10.3390/jcs8060203
15. Li, B., Yu, J., Niu, Q., Li, Z., Zhang, Y., Yang, D., et al.: Organic–inorganic hybrid luminescent hydrogel glued by a cationic polymeric binder. Macromol. Rapid Commun. **42** (2021). https://doi.org/10.1002/marc.202100562
16. Wang, X., Wei, W., Guo, Z., Liu, X., Liu, J., Bing, T., et al.: Organic–inorganic composite hydrogels: compositions, properties, and applications in regenerative medicine. Biomater. Sci. **12**, 1079–1114 (2024). https://doi.org/10.1039/D3BM01766D
17. Wang, J., Yang, Y., Li, K., Zhang, L., Li, Z.: Purely organic fluorescence afterglow: visible-light-excitation, inherent mechanism, tunable color, and practical applications with very low cost. Angew. Chemie Int. Ed. **62** (2023). https://doi.org/10.1002/anie.202304020
18. Ahumada, G., Borkowska, M.: Fluorescent polymers conspectus. Polymers (Basel) **14**, 1118 (2022)
19. Demchenko, A.P.: Photobleaching of organic fluorophores: quantitative characterization, mechanisms, protection. Methods Appl. Fluoresc. **8**, 22001 (2020)
20. Fernandes, N.B., Nayak, Y., Garg, S., Nayak, U.Y.: Multifunctional engineered mesoporous silica/inorganic material hybrid nanoparticles: theranostic perspectives. Coord. Chem. Rev. **478**, 214977 (2023)
21. Castro, R.C., Ribeiro, D.S.M., Santos, J.L.M.: Visual detection using quantum dots sensing platforms. Coord. Chem. Rev. **429**, 213637 (2021)
22. Pandey, S., Bodas, D.: High-quality quantum dots for multiplexed bioimaging: a critical review. Adv. Colloid Interface Sci. **278**, 102137 (2020)
23. Zhou, W., Hu, Z., Wei, J., Dai, H., Chen, Y., Liu, S., et al.: Quantum dots-hydrogel composites for biomedical applications. Chinese Chem. Lett. **33**, 1245–1253 (2022)
24. Lu, B., Cheng, H., Qu, L.: Inorganic hydrogel based on low-dimensional nanomaterials. ACS Nano **18**, 2730–2749 (2024)
25. Dalei, G., Das, S.: Polyacrylic acid-based drug delivery systems: a comprehensive review on the state-of-art. J. Drug Deliv. Sci. Technol. **78**, 103988 (2022)
26. Gao, Y., Peng, K., Mitragotri, S.: Covalently crosslinked hydrogels via step-growth reactions: crosslinking chemistries, polymers, and clinical impact. Adv. Mater. **33**, 2006362 (2021)
27. Liu, B., Zhao, H., Wang, Y.: Advanced flame-retardant methods for polymeric materials. Adv. Mater. **34**, 2107905 (2022)
28. Yu, Y., Xu, S., Li, S., Pan, H.: Genipin-cross-linked hydrogels based on biomaterials for drug delivery: a review. Biomater. Sci. **9**, 1583–1597 (2021)
29. Xue, X., Hu, Y., Wang, S., Chen, X., Jiang, Y., Su, J.: Fabrication of physical and chemical crosslinked hydrogels for bone tissue engineering. Bioact. Mater. **12** (2022). https://doi.org/10.1016/j.bioactmat.2021.10.029
30. Xue, X., Hu, Y., Deng, Y., Su, J.: Recent advances in design of functional biocompatible hydrogels for bone tissue engineering. Adv. Funct. Mater. **31** (2021). https://doi.org/10.1002/adfm.202009432

31. El Sayed, M.M.: Production of polymer hydrogel composites and their applications. J. Polym. Environ. **31**, 2855–2879 (2023). https://doi.org/10.1007/s10924-023-02796-z
32. Gharieh, A., Khoee, S., Mahdavian, A.R.: Emulsion and miniemulsion techniques in preparation of polymer nanoparticles with versatile characteristics. Adv. Colloid Interface Sci. **269**, 152–186 (2019)
33. Kurek, E., Rosendale, M., Verlhac, J.-B., Marais, S., Daniel, J., Blanchard-Desce, M.: "Fruity" Dye-based Fluorescent Nanoparticles (dFONs): A Fully Organic Counterpart of Alloy and Core-Shell Metallic Nanoparticles. Tuning Topology to Maximize Nano-interfacial Promoted Fluorescence Enhancement (2024). https://doi.org/10.26434/chemrxiv-2024-42f7k
34. Lesas, J., Bienvenu, T.C.M., Kurek, E., Verlhac, J., Grivet, Z., Têtu, M., et al.: Dye-based fluorescent organic nanoparticles, new promising tools for optogenetics. Adv. Healthc. Mater. (2024). https://doi.org/10.1002/adhm.202402132
35. Yang, L.-X., Liu, Y.-C., Cho, C.-H., Chen, Y.-R., Yang, C.-S., Lu, Y.-L., et al.: A universal strategy for the fabrication of single-photon and multiphoton NIR nanoparticles by loading organic dyes into water-soluble polymer nanosponges. J. Nanobiotechnol. **20**, 311 (2022). https://doi.org/10.1186/s12951-022-01515-5
36. Mysliwiec, J., Durko-Maciag, M., Popczyk, A., Szukalska, A., Szukalski, A., Bretonniere, Y., et al.: Toward white lasers: organic widely real-time tunable emitters. In: Camposeo, A., Farsari, M., Persano, L., Busse, L.E., Rarity, J.G., Alsing, P.M., et al. (eds.) Emerging Imaging and Sensing Technologies for Security and Defence VII, p. 37. SPIE (2022). https://doi.org/10.1117/12.2637678
37. Sonam, S., Patel, P., Pandey, D., Sharma, A., Jain, K.: Quantum dots: functionalization and theranostic applications. In: Multifunctional and Targeted Theranostic Nanomedicines, pp. 215–240. Springer Nature Singapore, Singapore (2023). https://doi.org/10.1007/978-981-99-0538-6_10
38. Li, M., Tang, Q., Wan, H., Zhu, G., Yin, D., Lei, L., et al.: Functional inorganic nanoparticles in cancer: biomarker detection, imaging, and therapy. APL Mater. **12** (2024). https://doi.org/10.1063/5.0231279
39. Komsthöft, T., Bovone, G., Bernhard, S., Tibbitt, M.W.: Polymer functionalization of inorganic nanoparticles for biomedical applications. Curr. Opin. Chem. Eng. **37**, 100849 (2022). https://doi.org/10.1016/j.coche.2022.100849
40. Petrelli, V., Dell'Anna, M.M., Mastrorilli, P., Viola, V., Catauro, M., D'Angelo, A.: Synthesis by sol-gel route of organic-inorganic hybrid material: chemical characterization and in vitro release study. Appl. Sci. **13**, 8410 (2023). https://doi.org/10.3390/app13148410
41. Sousa, R.P.C.L., Figueira, R.B., Callone, E., Dirè, S., Costa, S.P.G., Raposo, M.M.M.: Amino-alcohol organic-inorganic hybrid sol-gel materials based on an epoxy bicyclic silane: synthesis and characterization. Nanomaterials **13**, 2429 (2023). https://doi.org/10.3390/nano13172429
42. Ikake, H., Hara, S., Shimizu, S.: Skillful control of dispersion and 3D network structures: advances in functional organic-inorganic nano-hybrid materials prepared using the sol-gel method. Polymers (Basel) **14**, 3247 (2022). https://doi.org/10.3390/polym14163247
43. Hou, Y.C., Yao, C.F., Wu, W.Z.: Deep eutectic solvents: green solvents for separation applications. Acta. Phys.-Chim. Sin. **34**, 873–885 (2018)
44. Kist, J.A., Zhao, H., Mitchell-Koch, K.R., Baker, G.A.: The study and application of biomolecules in deep eutectic solvents. J. Mater. Chem. B **9**, 536–566 (2021)
45. Zhang, H., Xue, K., Shao, C., Hao, S., Yang, J.: Recent progress in bioinspired design strategies for freeze resistant hydrogel platforms toward flexible electronics. Chem. Mater. (2023)
46. Peñas-Núñez, S.J., Mecerreyes, D., Criado-Gonzalez, M.: Recent advances and developments in injectable conductive polymer gels for bioelectronics. ACS Appl. Bio Mater. (2024)
47. Nicolau, A., Mutch, A.L., Thickett, S.C.: Applications of functional polymeric eutectogels. Macromol. Rapid Commun. **45**, 2400405 (2024)
48. Fang, L.: Deep eutectic solvents based ionic conductive gel fibers (2023)
49. Wu, H., Pang, Z., Ji, L., Pang, X., Li, Y., Yu, X.: Strong adhesive, high conductive and environmentally stable eutectogel based on "Water in deep eutectic Solvent": ultrasensitive flexible temperature and strain sensors. Chem. Eng. J. **497**, 154883 (2024)

50. Wang, J., Ma, Z., Wang, Y., Shao, J., Yan, L.: Ultra-stretchable, self-healing, conductive, and transparent PAA/DES ionic gel. Macromol. Rapid Commun. **42** (2021). https://doi.org/10.1002/marc.202000445
51. Xie, L., Wang, X., Zou, X., Bai, Z., Liang, S., Wei, C., et al.: Engineering self-adaptive multi-response thermochromic hydrogel for energy-saving smart windows and wearable temperature-sensing. Small **19**, 2304321 (2023)
52. Bi, S., Jin, W., Han, X., Cao, X., He, Z., Asare-Yeboah, K., et al.: Ultra-fast-responsivity with sharp contrast integrated flexible piezo electrochromic based tactile sensing display. Nano Energy **102**, 107629 (2022)
53. Qi, P., Jia, L., Yi, M., Zhao, E., Liu, Y., Song, A., et al.: Chemiluminescent gels of G-quadruplexes in deep eutectic solvents. Colloids Surf. Phys. Chem. Eng. Asp. **655**, 130319 (2022)
54. Dos Santos, M.C., Algar, W.R., Medintz, I.L., Hildebrandt, N.: Quantum dots for Förster resonance energy transfer (FRET). TrAC Trends Anal. Chem. **125**, 115819 (2020)
55. Li, C., Liu, J., Qiu, X., Yang, X., Huang, X., Zhang, X.: Photoswitchable and reversible fluorescent eutectogels for conformal information encryption. Angew. Chemie **135**, e202313971 (2023)
56. Shang, H., Le, X., Sun, Y., Shan, F., Wu, S., Zheng, Y., et al.: Integrating photorewritable fluorescent information in shape-memory organohydrogel toward dual encryption. Adv. Opt. Mater. **10**, 1–8 (2022). https://doi.org/10.1002/adom.202200608
57. Yu, D., Jiang, D., Xue, Z., Mu, T.: Deep eutectic solvents as green solvents for material preparation. Green Chem. (2024)
58. Sun, S., Yu, L., Teng, J., Gu, Y., Pang, Y., Xu, X., et al.: Eutectic gels: presentation and prospect. Appl. Mater. Today **39**, 102342 (2024)
59. Mercadal, P.A., González, A., Beloqui, A., Tomé, L.C., Mecerreyes, D., Calderón, M., et al.: Eutectogels: the multifaceted soft ionic materials of tomorrow. JACS Au **4**, 3744–3758 (2024)
60. Ejeromedoghene, O., Orege, J.I., Oderinde, O., Okoye, C.O., Alowakennu, M., Nnyia, M.O., et al.: Deep eutectic solvent-assisted stimuli-responsive smart hydrogels–a review. Eur. Polym. J. **181**, 111711 (2022)
61. Vo, T.H., Lam, P.K., Sheng, Y.-J., Tsao, H.-K.: A functional eutectogel based on ultra-high–molecular weight polymers: physical entanglements in deep eutectic solvent. J. Colloid Interface Sci. **683**, 610–619 (2025). https://doi.org/10.1016/j.jcis.2024.12.126
62. Li, S., Wu, Y., Zhang, X., Chen, D., Ma, Y., Yang, W.: Eutectogel-based strain and temperature sensor with widely tunable mechanical properties regulated by copolymerization-induced phase separation and electrostatic interaction. Mater. Today Nano **25**, 100440 (2024). https://doi.org/10.1016/j.mtnano.2023.100440
63. Cheng, Q., Hao, A., Xing, P.: Eutectogels as matrices to manipulate supramolecular chirality and circularly polarized luminescence. ACS Nano **16**, 6825–6834 (2022)
64. Ma, Y., Yang, Y., Li, T., Hussain, S., Zhu, M.: Deep eutectic solvents as an emerging green platform for the synthesis of functional materials. Green Chem. **26**, 3627–3669 (2024)
65. Vakili, S., Mohamadnia, Z., Ahmadi, E.: Self-healing, electrically conductive, antibacterial, and adhesive eutectogel containing polymerizable deep eutectic solvent for human motion sensing and wound healing. Biomacromol **25**, 7704–7722 (2024)
66. Parsana, N., Seoud, O.E., Al-Ghamdi, A., Kasoju, N., Malek, N.: Deep eutectic solvent and poly (vinyl alcohol) based self-healable, injectable and adhesive "Eutectogel": an emerging drug delivery vehicle. ChemistrySelect **9** (2024). https://doi.org/10.1002/slct.202304157
67. Lee, H.P., Gaharwar, A.K.: Light-responsive inorganic biomaterials for biomedical applications. Adv. Sci. **7** (2020). https://doi.org/10.1002/advs.202000863
68. Khan, F., Atif, M., Haseen, M., Kamal, S., Khan, M.S., Shahid, S., et al.: Synthesis, classification and properties of hydrogels: their applications in drug delivery and agriculture. J. Mater. Chem. B **10**, 170–203 (2022)
69. Harun-Ur-Rashid, M., Jahan, I., Islam, M.J., Kumer, A., Huda, M.N., Imran, A.B., et al.: Global advances and smart innovations in supramolecular polymers. J. Mol. Struct. **1304**, 137665 (2024)

70. Dong, X., Wang, C., Song, H., Shao, J., Lan, G., Zhang, J., et al.: Advancement in soft hydrogel grippers: comprehensive insights into materials, fabrication strategies, grasping mechanism, and applications. Biomimetics **9**, 585 (2024)
71. Liu, J., Lécuyer, T., Seguin, J., Mignet, N., Scherman, D., Viana, B., et al.: Imaging and therapeutic applications of persistent luminescence nanomaterials. Adv. Drug Deliv. Rev. **138**, 193–210 (2019)
72. Wagner, A.M., Knipe, J.M., Orive, G., Peppas, N.A.: Quantum dots in biomedical applications. Acta Biomater. **94**, 44–63 (2019)
73. Kumi, M., Chen, T., Zhang, Z., Wang, A., Li, G., Hou, Z., et al.: Integration of hydrogels and 3D bioprinting technologies for chronic wound healing management. ACS Biomater. Sci. Eng. (2024). https://doi.org/10.1021/acsbiomaterials.4c00957
74. Liang, Y., He, J., Guo, B.: Functional hydrogels as wound dressing to enhance wound healing. ACS Nano **15**, 12687–12722 (2021). https://doi.org/10.1021/acsnano.1c04206
75. Li, S., Mohamedi, A.H., Senkowsky, J., Nair, A., Tang, L.: Imaging in chronic wound diagnostics. Adv. Wound Care **9**, 245–263 (2020)
76. Mota, F.A.R., Pereira, S.A.P., Araujo, A.R.T.S., Passos, M.L.C., Saraiva, M.L.M.F.S.: Biomarkers in the diagnosis of wounds infection: an analytical perspective. TrAC Trends Anal. Chem. **143**, 116405 (2021)
77. Zhang, X., Qin, M., Xu, M., Miao, F., Merzougui, C., Zhang, X., et al.: The fabrication of antibacterial hydrogels for wound healing. Eur. Polym. J. **146**, 110268 (2021)
78. Xi, Y., Ge, J., Wang, M., Chen, M., Niu, W., Cheng, W., et al.: Bioactive anti-inflammatory, antibacterial, antioxidative silicon-based nanofibrous dressing enables cutaneous tumor photothermo-chemo therapy and infection-induced wound healing. ACS Nano **14**, 2904–2916 (2020)
79. Wang, L., Li, B., Xu, F., Li, Y., Xu, Z., Wei, D., et al.: Visual in vivo degradation of injectable hydrogel by real-time and non-invasive tracking using carbon nanodots as fluorescent indicator. Biomaterials **145**, 192–206 (2017)
80. Ding, N., Zhou, F., Li, G., Shen, H., Bai, L., Su, J.: Quantum dots for bone tissue engineering. Mater. Today Bio, 101167 (2024)
81. Gil, C.J., Li, L., Hwang, B., Cadena, M., Theus, A.S., Finamore, T.A., et al.: Tissue engineered drug delivery vehicles: methods to monitor and regulate the release behavior. J. Control. Release **349**, 143–155 (2022)
82. Yi, D.K., Nanda, S.S., Kim, K., Selvan, S.T.: Recent progress in nanotechnology for stem cell differentiation, labeling, tracking and therapy. J. Mater. Chem. B **5**, 9429–9451 (2017)
83. Yukawa, H., Baba, Y.: In vivo fluorescence imaging and the diagnosis of stem cells using quantum dots for regenerative medicine. Anal. Chem. **89**, 2671–2681 (2017)
84. Zhang, J., Jin, J., Wan, J., Jiang, S., Wu, Y., Wang, W., et al.: Quantum dots-based hydrogels for sensing applications. Chem. Eng. J. **408**, 127351 (2021)
85. Biswas, A., Shukla, A., Maiti, P.: Biomaterials for interfacing cell imaging and drug delivery: an overview. Langmuir **35**, 12285–12305 (2019)
86. Gao, F., Jiao, C., Yu, B., Cong, H., Shen, Y.: Preparation and biomedical application of injectable hydrogels. Mater. Chem. Front. **5**, 4912–4936 (2021)
87. Zhang, X., Tan, B., Wu, Y., Zhang, M., Liao, J.: A review on hydrogels with photothermal effect in wound healing and bone tissue engineering. Polymers (Basel) **13**, 2100 (2021)
88. Jung, I.Y., Kim, J.S., Choi, B.R., Lee, K., Lee, H.: Hydrogel based biosensors for in vitro diagnostics of biochemicals, proteins, and genes. Adv. Healthc. Mater. **6**, 1601475 (2017)
89. Hang, Y., Boryczka, J., Wu, N.: Visible-light and near-infrared fluorescence and surface-enhanced Raman scattering point-of-care sensing and bio-imaging: a review. Chem. Soc. Rev. **51**, 329–375 (2022)
90. Omidian, H., Chowdhury, S.D., Akhzarmehr, A.: Hydrogels in biosensing and medical diagnostics. J. Bioact. Compat. Polym. 08839115241253260 (2024)
91. Castro, R.C., Saraiva, M.L.M.F.S., Santos, J.L.M., Ribeiro, D.S.M.: Multiplexed detection using quantum dots as photoluminescent sensing elements or optical labels. Coord. Chem. Rev. **448**, 214181 (2021)

92. Chern, M., Kays, J.C., Bhuckory, S., Dennis, A.M.: Sensing with photoluminescent semiconductor quantum dots. Methods Appl. Fluoresc. **7**, 12005 (2019)
93. Cui, C., Fu, Q., Meng, L., Hao, S., Dai, R., Yang, J.: Recent progress in natural biopolymers conductive hydrogels for flexible wearable sensors and energy devices: materials, structures, and performance. ACS Appl. Bio Mater. **4**, 85–121 (2021). https://doi.org/10.1021/acsabm.0c00807
94. Kawatra, T., Gupta, D., Gupta, T.K., Verma, R.: Role of nanomaterials in implant dentistry. In: Emerging Sustainable Nanomaterials for Biomedical Applications, pp. 385–408. Springer (2024)
95. Sharma, C., Verma, M., Abidi, S.M.S., Shukla, A.K., Acharya, A.: Functional fluorescent nanomaterials for the detection, diagnosis and control of bacterial infection and biofilm formation: Insight towards mechanistic aspects and advanced applications. Colloids Surf. B Biointerfaces **232**, 113583 (2023)
96. Hooshiar, M.H., Moghaddam, M.A., Kiarashi, M., Al-Hijazi, A.Y., Hussein, A.F., Alrikabi, H.A., et al.: Recent advances in nanomaterial-based biosensor for periodontitis detection. J. Biol. Eng. **18**, 28 (2024)
97. Li, Y., Tang, H., Liu, Y., Qiao, Y., Xia, H., Zhou, J.: Oral wearable sensors: health management based on the oral cavity. Biosens. Bioelectron X **10**, 100135 (2022)
98. Paqué, P.N., Herz, C., Wiedemeier, D.B., Mitsakakis, K., Attin, T., Bao, K., et al.: Salivary biomarkers for dental caries detection and personalized monitoring. J. Pers. Med. **11**, 235 (2021)
99. Dewan, M., Shrivastava, D., Goyal, L., Zwiri, A., Hussein, A.F., Alam, M.K., et al.: Recent advancements and applications of nanosensors in oral health: revolutionizing diagnosis and treatment. Eur. J. Dent. (2024)
100. Lach, S., Jurczak, P., Karska, N., Kubiś, A., Szymańska, A., Rodziewicz-Motowidło, S.: Spectroscopic methods used in implant material studies. Molecules **25**, 579 (2020)
101. Aminu, N., Chan, S.-Y., Toh, S.-M.: Roles of nanotechnological approaches in periodontal disease therapy. J. Appl. Pharm. Sci. **7**, 234–242 (2017)
102. Shashikiran, N.D., Hadakar, S., Gaonkar, N., Taur, S., Gugawad, S., Maurya, A., et al.: Ozone and Nanotechnology in Dentistry. Cambridge Scholars Publishing (2022)
103. Yadav, P., Yadav, L., Laddha, H., Agarwal, M., Gupta, R.: Upsurgence of smartphone as an economical, portable, and consumer-friendly analytical device/interface platform for digital sensing of hazardous environmental ions. Trends Environ. Anal. Chem. **36**, e00177 (2022)
104. Sun, B., Rahmat, J.N.B., Zhang, Y.: Advanced techniques for performing photodynamic therapy in deep-seated tissues. Biomaterials **291**, 121875 (2022)
105. Cianchetti, M., Laschi, C., Menciassi, A., Dario, P.: Biomedical applications of soft robotics. Nat. Rev. Mater. **3**, 143–153 (2018). https://doi.org/10.1038/s41578-018-0022-y
106. Phillips, J.W., Prominski, A., Tian, B.: Recent advances in materials and applications for bioelectronic and biorobotic systems. View **3**, 20200157 (2022)
107. Jayakumar, A., Jose, V.K., Lee, J.: Hydrogels for medical and environmental applications. Small Methods **4**, 1900735 (2020). https://doi.org/10.1002/smtd.201900735
108. Banerjee, H., Suhail, M., Ren, H.: Hydrogel actuators and sensors for biomedical soft robots: brief overview with impending challenges. Biomimetics **3**, 15 (2018)
109. Zarei, M., Lee, G., Lee, S.G., Cho, K.: Advances in biodegradable electronic skin: material progress and recent applications in sensing, robotics, and human–machine interfaces. Adv. Mater. **35**, 2203193 (2023)
110. Fekete, Z., Ebrahimi, N., Bi, C., Cappelleri, D.J., Ciuti, G., Conn, A.T.: Magnetic actuation methods in bio/soft robotics. Adv. Funct. Mater. (2021)
111. Dahiya, R.S., Valle, M., Dahiya, R.S., Valle, M.: Tactile sensing technologies. Robot. Tactile Sens. Technol. Syst., 79–136 (2013)
112. Ebrahimi, N., Bi, C., Cappelleri, D.J., Ciuti, G., Conn, A.T., Faivre, D., et al.: Magnetic actuation methods in bio/soft robotics. Adv. Funct. Mater. **31**, 2005137 (2021)
113. Guo, Z., Richardson, J.J., Kong, B., Liang, K.: Nanobiohybrids: materials approaches for bioaugmentation. Sci. Adv. **6**, eaaz0330 (2020)

114. Zheng, L., Hart, N., Zeng, Y.: Micro-/nanoscale robotics for chemical and biological sensing. Lab Chip (2023)
115. Agrawal, R., Deshmukh, R., Garg, A., Mali, S.N., Prajapati, B.G., Singh, K.: Nanobots: a revolutionary technology in the development of pharmaceuticals. Bionanoscience **15**, 159 (2025)
116. Sun, Z., Zhu, M., Lee, C.: Progress in the triboelectric human–machine interfaces (HMIs)-moving from smart gloves to AI/haptic enabled HMI in the 5G/IoT era. Nanoenergy Adv. **1** (2021)
117. Meena, J.S., Choi, S.B., Jung, S.-B., Kim, J.-W.: Electronic textiles: new age of wearable technology for healthcare and fitness solutions. Mater. Today Bio **19**, 100565 (2023)
118. Servati, P., Tashakori, A., Zhang, W., Wang, Y., Jiang, Z., Servati, A., et al.: Artificial intelligence-powered, interactive, stretchable, immersive displays and wearables. IEEE Open J. Immersive Disp. (2024)
119. Arik, B.: Smart bio-textiles for medicine and healthcare applications. In: Smart Textiles from Natural Resources, pp. 495–537. Elsevier (2024)
120. Nguyen, P., Courchesne, N.-M.D., Duraj-Thatte, A., Praveschotinunt, P., Joshi, N.: Engineered living materials: engineered living materials: prospects and challenges for using biological systems to direct the assembly of smart materials. Adv. Mater. (2018)
121. Xie, M., Hisano, K., Zhu, M., Toyoshi, T., Pan, M., Okada, S., et al.: Flexible multifunctional sensors for wearable and robotic applications. Adv. Mater. Technol. **4**, 1800626 (2019)
122. Khurana, B., Gierlich, P., Meindl, A., Gomes-da-Silva, L.C., Senge, M.O.: Hydrogels: soft matters in photomedicine. Photochem. Photobiol. Sci. **18**, 2613–2656 (2019)
123. Wang, J., Dong, J.: Optical waveguides and integrated optical devices for medical diagnosis, health monitoring and light therapies. Sensors **20**, 3981 (2020)
124. Misra, R., Acharya, S.: Smart nanotheranostic hydrogels for on-demand cancer management. Drug Discov. Today **26**, 344–359 (2021). https://doi.org/10.1016/j.drudis.2020.11.010
125. Yousefiasl, S., Ghovvati, M., Mirshafiei, M., Hakimi, F., Azadi, A., Moezzi, S.M.I., et al.: Nanostructure-reinforced multifunctional hydrogels for synergistic cancer therapy. Coord. Chem. Rev. **522**, 216207 (2025)
126. Zahed, Z., Hadi, R., Imanzadeh, G., Ahmadian, Z., Shafiei, S., Zadeh, A.Z., et al.: Recent advances in fluorescence nanoparticles "quantum dots" as gene delivery system: a review. Int. J. Biol. Macromol. **254**, 127802 (2024)
127. Niu, H., Li, X., Li, H., Fan, Z., Ma, J., Guan, J.: Thermosensitive, fast gelling, photoluminescent, highly flexible, and degradable hydrogels for stem cell delivery. Acta Biomater. **83**, 96–108 (2019)
128. Vernerey, F.J., Lalitha Sridhar, S., Muralidharan, A., Bryant, S.J.: Mechanics of 3D cell–hydrogel interactions: experiments, models, and mechanisms. Chem. Rev. **121**, 11085–11148 (2021)
129. Baumann, B., Wittig, R., Lindén, M.: Mesoporous silica nanoparticles in injectable hydrogels: factors influencing cellular uptake and viability. Nanoscale **9**, 12379–12390 (2017)
130. Jurak, M., Wiącek, A.E., Ładniak, A., Przykaza, K., Szafran, K.: What affects the biocompatibility of polymers? Adv. Colloid Interface Sci. **294**, 102451 (2021). https://doi.org/10.1016/j.cis.2021.102451
131. Zhao, Y., Shi, C., Yang, X., Shen, B., Sun, Y., Chen, Y., et al.: pH-and temperature-sensitive hydrogel nanoparticles with dual photoluminescence for bioprobes. ACS Nano **10**, 5856–5863 (2016)
132. Gidwani, B., Sahu, V., Shukla, S.S., Pandey, R., Joshi, V., Jain, V.K., et al.: Quantum dots: prospectives, toxicity, advances and applications. J. Drug Deliv. Sci. Technol. **61**, 102308 (2021)
133. Du, Y., Xue, Y., Ma, P.X., Chen, X., Lei, B.: Biodegradable, elastomeric, and intrinsically photoluminescent poly (silicon-citrates) with high photostability and biocompatibility for tissue regeneration and bioimaging. Adv. Healthc. Mater. **5**, 382–392 (2016)
134. Kong, D., Zhang, K., Tian, J., Yin, L., Sheng, X.: Biocompatible and biodegradable light-emitting materials and devices. Adv. Mater. Technol. **7**, 2100006 (2022)

135. Shofolawe-Bakare, O.T., Stokes, L.D., Hossain, M., Smith, A.E., Werfel, T.A.: Immunostimulatory biomaterials to boost tumor immunogenicity. Biomater. Sci. **8**, 5516–5537 (2020)
136. Nakkala, J.R., Li, Z., Ahmad, W., Wang, K., Gao, C.: Immunomodulatory biomaterials and their application in therapies for chronic inflammation-related diseases. Acta Biomater. **123**, 1–30 (2021)
137. Kharaziha, M., Baidya, A., Annabi, N.: Rational design of immunomodulatory hydrogels for chronic wound healing. Adv. Mater. **33**, 2100176 (2021)
138. Peng, Y., Liang, S., Meng, Q., Liu, D., Ma, K., Zhou, M., et al.: Engineered bio-based hydrogels for cancer immunotherapy. Adv. Mater. 2313188 (2024)
139. Zhang, Z., He, C., Chen, X.: Designing hydrogels for immunomodulation in cancer therapy and regenerative medicine. Adv. Mater. **36**, 2308894 (2024)

Machine Learning for Custom-Designed Light Emitters in Biomedicine

Samson Olusegun Afolabi, Ekaterina V. Skorb, and Sergey Shityakov

Abstract Machine learning (ML) has emerged as a pivotal tool in the design of light-emitting materials, significantly accelerating the discovery process by enabling precise predictions of material properties. Through the analysis of extensive datasets, ML facilitates material discovery and optimization, particularly in predicting emission characteristics and designing innovative compounds. When integrated with physics-based modeling approaches such as Density Functional Theory (DFT) and molecular dynamics (MD) simulations, ML further enhances the prediction and refinement of properties like emission wavelength, efficiency, and stability. Additionally, inverse design leverages computational methods alongside ML to develop novel material structures, fine-tune properties, and optimize performance. These advancements have notably improved applications in energy-efficient organic light-emitting diodes (OLEDs), LEDs, fiber-optic communication, and biophotonics. Integration with artificial intelligence, nanotechnology, and bioinformatics expands their applications, including surgical precision and deep-tissue imaging, advancing the capabilities of biomedical technologies. Despite persistent challenges related to data quality, model interpretability, and computational costs, progress in ML algorithms and interdisciplinary collaboration continues to drive advancements in the biomedical field.

Keywords Machine learning · Biomedicine · Light emitters · Inverse design · Machine learning applications

---

S. O. Afolabi (✉) · E. V. Skorb · S. Shityakov
Infochemistry Scientific Center, ITMO University, Saint Petersburg, Russia
e-mail: olusegunafolabi2@itmo.ru

© The Author(s), under exclusive license to Springer Nature Switzerland AG 2025

N. O. Etafo (ed.), *Tailored Light Emitters For Biomedical Applications*, Engineering Materials, https://doi.org/10.1007/978-3-031-88731-4_11

1 Predicting Materials for Desired Light Emission

ML is transforming the discovery and optimization of materials for light emission in biomedical applications. These applications, including fluorescence imaging, biosensors, and phototherapy, require materials with customized optical properties, biocompatibility, and stability [1, 2]. By utilizing extensive datasets from material science, ML offers a robust approach to understanding and predicting the properties of light-emitting materials [3, 4], greatly expediting the design and development process.

One of the key contributions of ML is its ability to accelerate the search for suitable materials. Traditional experimental approaches to discovering light-emitting compounds are often labor-intensive and time-consuming, relying on trial-and-error methods [5]. In contrast, ML algorithms can analyze existing datasets to identify patterns and correlations between molecular structures and their emission properties.

This enables the prediction of emission wavelengths, intensities [6], and other critical optical features, providing researchers with a focused set of candidates for experimental validation. Besides, ML can propose novel compounds or modify existing materials, optimizing their photobiophysical properties for targeted biomedical applications [7, 8]. According to Hashizume et al. [9], ML poses ability to handle complex, multivariate optimization problems makes it invaluable for designing light-emitting materials that meet multiple requirements, such as emission spectrum, brightness, biocompatibility, and solubility [10]. Wu et al. [11] reported that ML can reveal novel light emission mechanisms, including advanced fluorescence or phosphorescence properties tailored to specific biomedical needs by analyzing relationships between molecular structures and photophysical processes.

Nevertheless, implementing ML to predict materials for desired light emission involves several critical steps. As shown in Fig. 1, the first step in using ML to predict materials for desired light emission involves gathering a dataset. This dataset typically includes materials with known light emission properties, which can come from various sources such as experimental databases, computational simulations like DFT, or published research [12, 13]. The collected data often consists of key information, including material structure, chemical composition, synthesis conditions, and optoelectronic properties such as bandgap energy or quantum efficiency [6, 14]. Assembling high-quality data is critical because the accuracy of ML models largely depends on the robustness of the data being fed into the algorithm [15]. Therefore, ensuring the data is clean and standardized through normalization and filtering processes is an essential part of the preparation phase.

Once the data is prepared, the next step is feature engineering, where important material descriptors that influence light emission are selected. These descriptors might include chemical properties such as atomic number, electronegativity, molecular orbitals, or electronic structure properties like the bandgap [16, 17]. Additionally, physical characteristics such as particle size and surface area may also play a role in determining a material's light emission behavior. Dimensionality reduction techniques, such as principal component analysis, are often employed to condense the

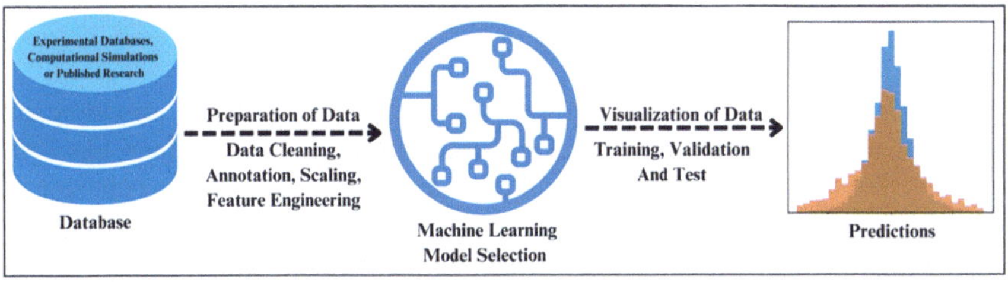

Fig. 1 Image illustrating the machine learning process. On the left, a database icon labeled "Experimental Databases, Computational Simulations or Published Research" represents data sources. An arrow points to "Preparation of Data," including data cleaning, annotation, scaling, and feature engineering. The next step is "Machine Learning Model Selection," depicted by a neural network icon. Another arrow leads to "Visualization of Data," covering training, validation, and testing. The final step is "Predictions," shown as a histogram with blue and orange bars

number of features, enabling the model to focus on the most influential factors. Reiser et al. [18] stated that materials are frequently represented in a structured format, such as graph-based representations, where atoms and bonds are modeled as nodes and edges, allowing the algorithm to process complex material structures effectively.

The choice of the ML model depends on the type of prediction task at hand. In many cases, supervised learning models are used because they work well when there is labeled data available data that includes both the input features and their corresponding emission properties [19]. Regression models like Linear Regression, Random Forests, or Support Vector Regression (SVR) are particularly useful when the goal is to predict the intensity of light emission [20]. On the other hand, classification models are suitable for tasks where materials need to be categorized, such as distinguishing between materials that emit light and those that do not, or classifying them based on their emission color. In cases where large and complex datasets exist, deep learning techniques like Convolutional Neural Networks (CNNs) can be employed to capture intricate nonlinear relationships between the input material descriptors and their emission properties [21].

Once the model is selected, the data is typically split into training, validation, and test sets. Stoean et al. [22] revealed that this division allows the ML algorithm to learn from one portion of the data (training) while using the validation set to fine-tune its hyperparameters, such as the depth of decision trees or the number of neurons in a neural network. Hyperparameter tuning is essential for optimizing the model's performance and ensuring it generalizes well to unseen data. After training, the model's performance is evaluated using metrics appropriate for the task [23]. For regression models, common evaluation metrics include Mean Squared Error (MSE) or R-squared values, while classification tasks rely on metrics such as accuracy, precision, and recall. Cross-validation techniques are often employed to further assess the model's robustness and to reduce the likelihood of overfitting [24]. Once the model demonstrates strong predictive capabilities, it can be used for design.

1.1 Physics-Based Modeling

Physics-based modeling is a cornerstone of modern materials science, providing the means to predict and optimize material properties for specific applications, like light emission. Wu and colleagues [25] highlighted that the light-emission behavior of materials is determined by the interplay of electronic, structural, and optical properties. They emphasized that an understanding of these interactions is essential for the advancement of technologies such as LEDs, organic semiconductors, and luminescent phosphors. By employing sophisticated computational techniques rooted in the principles of quantum mechanics and materials science, researchers can simulate and design materials with tailored properties, paving the way for more efficient and effective optoelectronic devices.

Central to the prediction of light-emission properties is the use of quantum mechanical methods. These approaches provide a fundamental understanding of how electrons interact within a material's atomic framework. Among these methods, DFT has emerged as a powerful tool. According to Kurth et al. [26], DFT predicts key electronic properties, such as band structure and charge density, by solving the Schrödinger equation for a system of electrons, which are directly linked to optical behavior. For applications involving light emission, the Time-Dependent DFT (TD-DFT) extension is particularly valuable. TD-DFT enables the study of excited electronic states, which are crucial for modeling the absorption and emission of light [27]. This capability makes it indispensable for designing materials with specific emission wavelengths or colors.

While DFT and TD-DFT are versatile and computationally efficient, certain systems require more precise methods to account for complex electron correlations and excitations. Post-Hartree–Fock techniques, such as Configuration Interaction (CI) and Coupled-Cluster (CC) methods, provide higher accuracy by explicitly considering electron–electron interactions [28]. These methods are particularly useful for studying the detailed photophysical mechanisms of small molecules and quantum dots, where accurate modeling of excited states is essential [29]. However, Behara [30] reported that their computational cost limits their applicability to smaller systems, prompting the development of hybrid methods that combine quantum mechanical accuracy with computational efficiency.

In addition to quantum mechanical approaches, MD simulations play a critical role in modeling light-emitting materials [31]. Unlike static quantum mechanical methods, MD simulations account for the dynamic behavior of atoms and molecules over time, providing insights into how thermal fluctuations, external stresses and molecular interactions influence a material's properties [32]. This is especially relevant for organic materials, where molecular flexibility and conformational changes can significantly impact electronic and optical behavior. Coupling MD simulations with quantum mechanics, as in QM/MM (Quantum Mechanics/Molecular Mechanics) hybrid models, enables the simultaneous exploration of large-scale dynamics and localized electronic effects [28]. This combined approach is particularly effective for studying complex systems like OLEDs, where the interplay of molecular motion and electronic transitions governs light-emission efficiency.

As reported by Segall et al. [33], a complementary approach to detailed simulations involves using first-principles calculations, which predict material properties based solely on fundamental physical laws. Ab initio molecular dynamics (AIMD) exemplifies this methodology by simulating atomic interactions in real time based on quantum mechanical principles. AIMD is particularly effective for studying how structural distortions, phase transitions, and thermal effects influence optical properties [34]. This approach has been instrumental in understanding phenomena like photoluminescence quenching and thermal degradation in light-emitting materials, providing valuable insights for improving material stability and efficiency.

Nieves et al. [35] reviewed that high-throughput computational techniques have further revolutionized the discovery and optimization of light-emitting materials. By automating the calculation of material properties across large datasets, these methods enable the rapid screening of potential candidates with desirable optical characteristics. For example, databases generated from first-principles calculations can be mined to identify materials with specific band gaps, emission wavelengths, or quantum yields. This approach significantly accelerates the development of new materials for applications ranging from displays to solid-state lighting.

Understanding the dynamics of excitons, or bound electron–hole pairs, is another critical aspect of modeling light emission. Excitons are the primary carriers of energy in many light-emitting materials, and their behavior directly influences emission efficiency and color purity [36]. Theoretical frameworks such as Marcus theory and Förster Resonance Energy Transfer (FRET) provide valuable tools for modeling exciton dynamics. Markus theory describes charge transfer processes, which are essential for understanding the recombination of electrons and holes that lead to light emission [37]. FRET, on the other hand, focuses on the migration of excitons between molecules or nanostructures, which is crucial for designing materials with efficient energy transfer and minimal non-radiative losses.

Computational spectroscopy serves as a bridge between theoretical predictions and experimental validation. By simulating absorption and emission spectra, computational spectroscopy provides a direct comparison to experimental data, enabling the refinement of models and the validation of underlying assumptions [38]. Techniques such as TD-DFT and many-body perturbation theory, including the GW (G describes electron propagation, while W represents screened electron interactions) approximation, are widely employed for this purpose. As noted by Orlando et al. [39], these methods not only predict the wavelengths and intensities of emitted light but also offer valuable insights into the electronic transitions and energy levels underlying the emission process.

This information is crucial for designing materials with targeted optical properties and for understanding the mechanisms of phenomena like phosphorescence and delayed fluorescence.

The integration of ML into physics-based modeling represents a transformative development in the field. By training algorithms on extensive datasets of material properties, ML models can predict optical characteristics with remarkable speed and accuracy [40]. For example, neural networks and regression models can be used to estimate band gaps, emission spectra, and quantum yields based on a material's structural features. This data-driven approach not only accelerates the discovery of novel materials but also enables the exploration of vast design spaces that would be computationally prohibitive using traditional methods alone. Furthermore, ML can identify patterns and correlations that may not be immediately apparent, providing new insights into the factors that govern light-emission behavior. Generally, physics-based modeling provides a powerful framework for understanding and predicting the properties of light-emitting materials by combining quantum mechanical methods, MD, computational spectroscopy, and ML techniques [41].

1.2 Inverse Design

Inverse design has emerged as a transformative approach in materials science, offering a powerful framework for tailoring materials to achieve specific properties rather than discovering materials through traditional trial-and-error methods [42]. This methodology is particularly significant in the development of light-emitting materials, where precise control over optical properties such as emission wavelength, intensity, and efficiency is critical for applications ranging from energy-efficient lighting and high-definition displays to advanced sensors and bioimaging technologies.

Figure 2 shows the schematic procedure of inverse design. The process of inverse design begins with the identification of desired light-emission properties [43]. These include parameters such as emission wavelength, which determines the color of light and is typically expressed in nanometers [44], emission intensity, which dictates brightness [45], and efficiency metrics such as photoluminescent quantum yield (PLQY) or electroluminescent efficiency [46]. Stability under operation conditions, including thermal, chemical, and photostability, also constitutes a critical requirement, as it impacts the longevity and reliability of devices incorporating these materials.

Another vital computational approach involves quantum chemistry simulations, which provide a deeper understanding of the electronic and optical properties of materials at the molecular level. By integrating these quantum and molecular insights, researchers can make informed decisions about material design and optimization [43]. Zuccarini et al. [47] noted that machine learning has transformed the field of material prediction and design [47]. Supervised learning models, trained on extensive datasets of materials and their properties, enable the prediction of material behavior under specific conditions [19]. Beyond prediction, generative models such as generative adversarial networks (GANs) and variational autoencoders (VAEs) take this a step further by creating entirely new material structures that align with the predefined property targets. These generative approaches are particularly effective in exploring

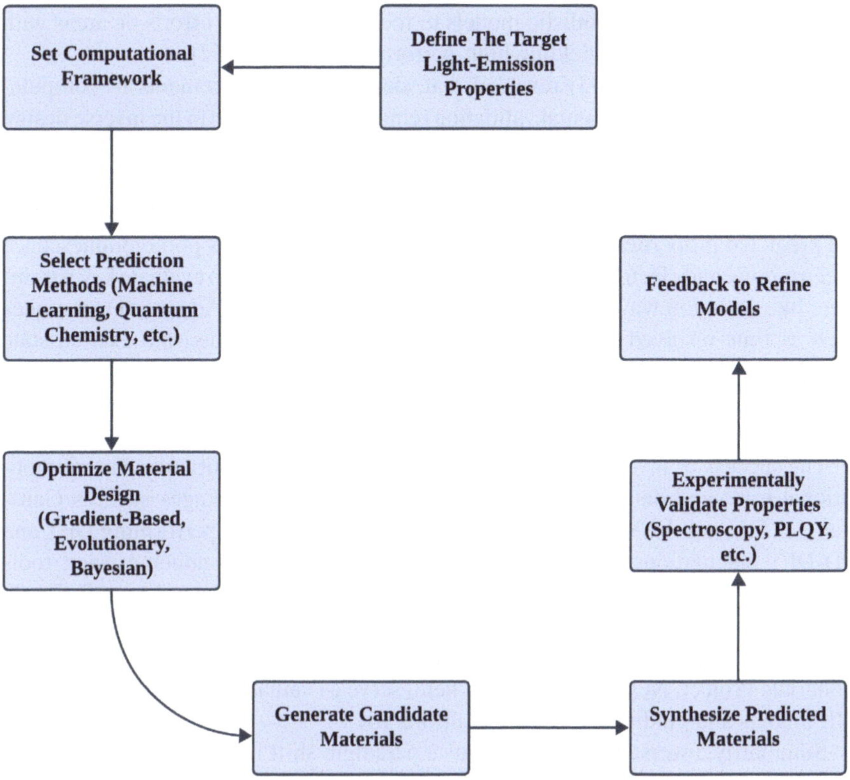

Fig. 2 Flowchart illustrating the process of inverse design of materials with specific light-emission properties. It begins with setting a computational framework and defining target properties. Prediction methods like machine learning and quantum chemistry are selected, followed by optimizing material design using gradient-based, evolutionary, or Bayesian approaches. Candidate materials are generated and synthesized. Properties are experimentally validated through methods such as spectroscopy and PLQY. Feedback is used to refine models, completing the cycle

vast chemical spaces, offering innovative solutions that may not have been conceived through conventional methods [48].

Thirunavukkarasu et al. [49] concluded that optimization techniques are crucial for refining material designs to achieve desired emission properties. Gradient-based optimization methods are particularly effective in continuous property spaces, allowing researchers to iteratively adjust molecular descriptors to improve predicted performance [50]. Evolutionary algorithms, inspired by the principles of natural selection, are better suited for exploring discrete material spaces. By applying operations such as mutation and crossover to an initial population of materials, these algorithms evolve toward candidates with optimal properties over successive generations [51]. Bayesian optimization, which balances exploration and exploitation, provides another powerful tool for efficiently navigating the material search space.

This approach uses probabilistic models to focus experimental efforts on areas with the highest likelihood of yielding high-performing materials [52].

Sun and colleagues [53] revealed that, despite the advancements in computational techniques, experimental validation remains a critical step in the inverse design process. Predicted materials must be synthesized and tested to confirm their properties and ensure their practical applicability. Synthesis techniques, ranging from chemical vapor deposition to molecular self-assembly, must be carefully optimized to preserve the predicted properties [54]. Characterization methods such as photoluminescence spectroscopy and electroluminescence measurements are used to evaluate key parameters like emission wavelength, intensity, and efficiency [55]. Advanced techniques such as time-resolved spectroscopy provide additional insights into excited-state dynamics and quantum yields [56]. Importantly, the results of these experiments feed back into the computational models, enabling iterative refinement and improving the accuracy of future predictions [57].

The success of inverse design relies heavily on the availability of robust computational tools and datasets. Quantum chemistry software packages such as Gaussian, ORCA, and VASP provide the necessary capabilities for performing DFT and TD-DFT calculations [58], while MD simulations can be conducted using tools like AMBER and GROMACS [59]. ML libraries such as TensorFlow, PyTorch, and Scikit-learn offer powerful frameworks for developing predictive models and optimization algorithms [60]. Publicly accessible material databases, including the Materials Project, NOMAD, and PubChem, serve as valuable resources for training ML models and guiding experimental efforts [61].

Summarily, inverse design represents a paradigm shift in the discovery and optimization of light-emitting materials. By starting with desired optical properties and leveraging advanced computational methods, optimization techniques, and experimental validation, researchers can accelerate the development of innovative materials with tailored characteristics.

1.3 Applications of Machine Learning-Designed Light Emitters

The application of ML in designing light emitters has revolutionized various scientific, industrial, and commercial domains. Light emitters, which include LEDs, lasers, and OLEDs, play crucial roles in everyday technologies like displays, lighting, communication, and medical devices. By integrating ML into their design process, researchers and engineers have unlocked unprecedented potential in terms of efficiency, customization, and functionality. As depicted in Fig. 3, we explore the multifaceted applications of machine-learning-designed light emitters, focusing on areas such as telecommunications, healthcare, energy efficiency, quantum computing, and advanced manufacturing.

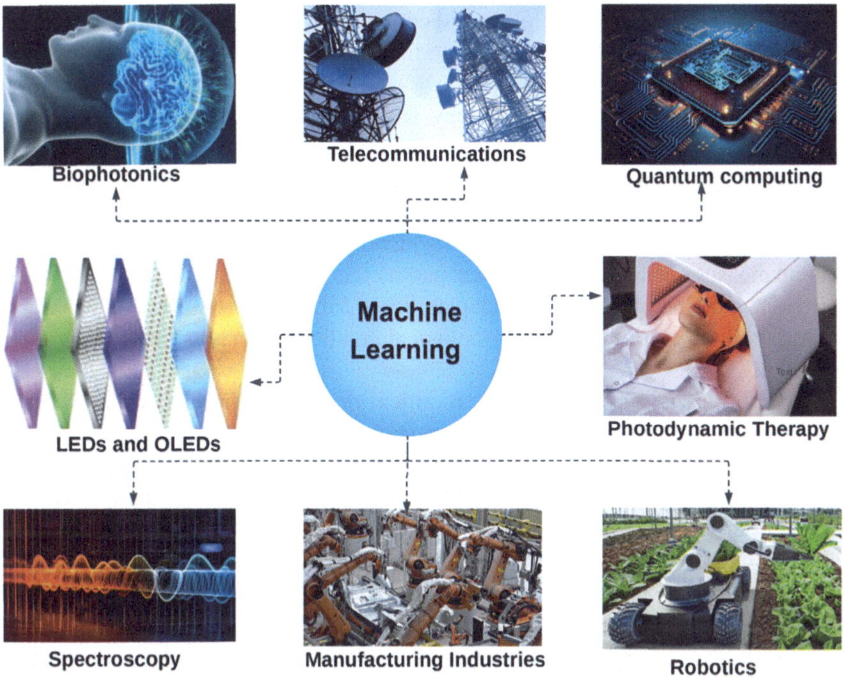

Fig. 3 Diagram illustrating the applications of machine learning, represented by a central blue circle. Arrows connect it to various fields: Biophotonics (image of a brain scan), Telecommunications (telecom towers), Quantum Computing (circuit board), Photodynamic Therapy (person under a light device), LEDs and OLEDs (colorful light patterns), Spectroscopy (light waves), Manufacturing Industries (robotic arms), and Robotics (robot in agriculture)

Nevin et al. [61] reported that machine learning has greatly enhanced the design of light emitters, particularly for fiber-optic communication systems in the field of telecommunications. These systems depend on highly efficient lasers and light sources to transmit data across vast distances at remarkable speeds. ML algorithms enable the optimization of light emitters for key factors such as wavelength stability, spectral purity, and energy efficiency [62, 63]. By leveraging ML, researchers can model and simulate the intricate dynamics of light-matter interactions in semiconductor materials [64, 65]. This ensures the development of lasers with precise emission frequencies, reducing signal distortion and improving data transmission rates [66]. Additionally, ML-powered predictive maintenance enhances the reliability of light emitters in fiber-optic networks, minimizing downtime and lowering operational costs [67].

In the fields of healthcare and biophotonics, the significance of light emitters has expanded considerably with the integration of ML techniques [68]. Light-based medical technologies, including imaging systems, diagnostic tools, and therapeutic instruments, rely on emitters specifically optimized for distinct applications. Within biophotonics, ML-driven emitter designs have enhanced fluorescence microscopy, enabling superior imaging resolution and contrast [69]. By precisely calibrating the wavelength and intensity of emitted light, researchers can now visualize biological structures with remarkable detail.

Furthermore, in photodynamic therapy, which employs light to activate drugs for cancer treatment, ML facilitates the development of emitters that maximize therapeutic outcomes while minimizing unintended harm to healthy tissues [70]. Similarly, Iqbal et al. [71] stated that wearable health-monitoring devices have benefited from ML-optimized emitters, which are frequently integrated with sensors to provide accurate measurements of physiological parameters such as heart rate, blood oxygen saturation, and glucose levels. The adaptability of ML ensures the efficient operation of these emitters across diverse physiological conditions, thereby broadening their clinical utility.

Energy efficiency has emerged as a critical priority in the modern world, and ML-designed light emitters present innovative solutions in this area. Traditional approaches to designing LEDs and OLEDs often rely on labor-intensive trial-and-error methods. In contrast, ML algorithms enable the rapid analysis of material properties, thermal dynamics, and device architectures, resulting in emitters that are both more energy-efficient and durable [72]. ML has been pivotal in the development of next-generation LEDs characterized by enhanced luminous efficacy and reduced power consumption. By optimizing material compositions, such as phosphors and quantum dots, ML-designed emitters achieve superior color rendering and optimized light distribution. These advancements play a crucial role in promoting energy conservation across residential, commercial, and industrial lighting applications.

The progression of display technologies from cathode-ray tubes to OLED and microLED displays has been significantly enhanced by ML-designed light emitters [73]. These advanced emitters offer high brightness, exceptional color accuracy, and extended lifespans, which are essential for devices such as smartphones, televisions, and augmented reality (AR) systems. ML accelerates the discovery of novel materials for emitters, including organic semiconductors and perovskites, by predicting their optical and electronic properties [74]. This predictive capability allows manufacturers to design displays with wider color gamuts, higher refresh rates, and lower power consumption. Additionally, ML algorithms ensure uniform light emission across extensive display panels, addressing challenges such as pixel inconsistency and uneven brightness.

Preskill [75] reported that quantum computing relies on the precise manipulation of quantum states, often achieved using photons emitted by specially designed light sources. ML has emerged as a vital tool in the development of these light sources, which are integral to quantum communication and cryptography. ML-designed single-photon emitters exhibit high purity, indistinguishability, and controllability characteristics that are essential for quantum key distribution and other quantum-secured communication protocols [76]. Moreover, ML facilitates the modeling of quantum dot structures and the optimization of their emission properties, enabling the fabrication of emitters that adhere to the stringent demands of quantum systems [77]. These advancements are driving the creation of more secure communication networks and fostering progress in advanced computational capabilities [78].

Environmental monitoring systems increasingly utilize light emitters integrated into sensors to detect pollutants, gases, and other environmental parameters [79]. ML significantly enhances the performance of these emitters by optimizing their spectral properties and operational stability [80]. ML-designed emitters are widely employed in LIDAR (Light Detection and Ranging) systems for applications such as terrain mapping, vegetation health assessment, and atmospheric change tracking [81]. By tailoring emitters to specific wavelengths, these systems provide highly accurate data, supporting environmental conservation initiatives [82].

In advanced manufacturing, precision and efficiency are of utmost importance. Light-based technologies, including laser cutting, welding, and additive manufacturing, depend on high-performance light emitters to achieve optimal results [83]. ML plays a crucial role in designing these emitters by optimizing parameters such as power, coherence, and beam quality [84]. ML-designed lasers enable the selective fusion or curing of materials with exceptional precision, a capability essential for producing complex geometries and intricate designs across industries such as aerospace and medical devices. Furthermore, ML algorithms facilitate real-time monitoring and dynamic adjustment of light emitters during manufacturing processes, ensuring consistent quality, reducing waste, and enhancing overall efficiency.

Spectroscopy is a widely utilized analytical technique across disciplines such as chemistry, biology, and materials science [85]. The integration of ML has significantly advanced the design of light emitters for spectroscopic applications, improving resolution, sensitivity, and operational range. ML algorithms optimize the spectral output of light emitters, ensuring their compatibility with specific analytical requirements. For instance, in Raman spectroscopy, ML-designed lasers with narrow line widths and stable wavelengths enable precise molecular identification [86]. Similarly, in mass spectrometry, ultraviolet (UV) and visible light emitters developed using ML enhance ionization efficiency, resulting in improved analyte detection and analysis accuracy [87].

Yang et al. [88] highlighted that light emitters are essential components in the sensing systems used in autonomous vehicles and robotics. LIDAR systems, which utilize light pulses to generate 3D maps of the surrounding environment, are essential for navigation and obstacle avoidance [89]. ML enhances the design of light emitters for LIDAR systems, improving their range, resolution, and power efficiency [90]. Additionally, ML algorithms facilitate the customization of emitters for specific use cases, such as indoor navigation or outdoor mapping [91]. These advancements ensure that autonomous systems can function reliably across a range of conditions, from bright sunlight to low-light environments.

ML has revolutionized the design and application of light emitters across a wide range of industries and technologies. By harnessing the predictive and analytical capabilities of ML, researchers and engineers can create light emitters that are not only more efficient and versatile but also customized to meet specific requirements. From transforming telecommunications and healthcare to driving innovations in energy efficiency and quantum computing, ML-designed light emitters are opening new possibilities and addressing critical challenges in modern society. As

ML continues to advance, its integration with light emitter design is expected to yield even greater breakthroughs, shaping the future trajectory of technology and its applications.

1.4 ML Workflows for Light Emitter Development

The development of efficient light emitters, including LEDs, lasers, and phosphors, has become increasingly critical due to their extensive applications in energy-efficient lighting, display technologies, and communication systems [92]. This process involves a complex integration of material science, optics, and electronic engineering, with a focus on understanding and optimizing the properties of materials [93]. ML is significantly accelerating the discovery, design, and optimization of light-emitting materials and devices [91]. By utilizing ML workflows (Fig. 4), researchers can streamline both experimental and computational tasks, resulting in faster innovation cycles and reduced resource consumption.

The cornerstone of any ML workflow is the availability and quality of data. In the realm of light emitter development, data sources encompass experimental measurements, computational simulations, and publicly accessible databases [94]. These datasets provide essential information on material properties, including bandgap energies, photoluminescence efficiency, thermal stability, and structural parameters [95]. However, raw data is frequently incomplete, noisy, or inconsistent, necessitating thorough preprocessing. This process involves data-cleaning measures such as removing outliers, imputing missing values, and normalizing data to ensure uniformity across diverse sources. For instance, high-throughput screening experiments may generate thousands of material candidates with varying degrees of reliability. Standardization of such data is crucial for training robust ML models. Furthermore, feature engineering plays a pivotal role in converting raw data into informative input variables. In light emitter development, these features may encompass atomic descriptors, molecular fingerprints, or device-level parameters that play a crucial role in influencing emission characteristics, as highlighted by Burner et al. [96]. Once the data is preprocessed, the subsequent step involves selecting suitable ML algorithms [97]. The choice of algorithm whether supervised learning, unsupervised learning, or reinforcement learning depends on the specific problem to be addressed, as each approach offers distinct advantages.

Supervised learning algorithms, including regression and classification models, are frequently employed to predict specific material properties. For example, regression models can be utilized to estimate parameters such as emission wavelength or quantum yield based on material descriptors [98], while classification models are adept at categorizing materials as promising or non-promising emitters [99]. In contrast, unsupervised learning techniques, such as clustering and dimensionality reduction, are valuable for exploratory data analysis [100]. These methods

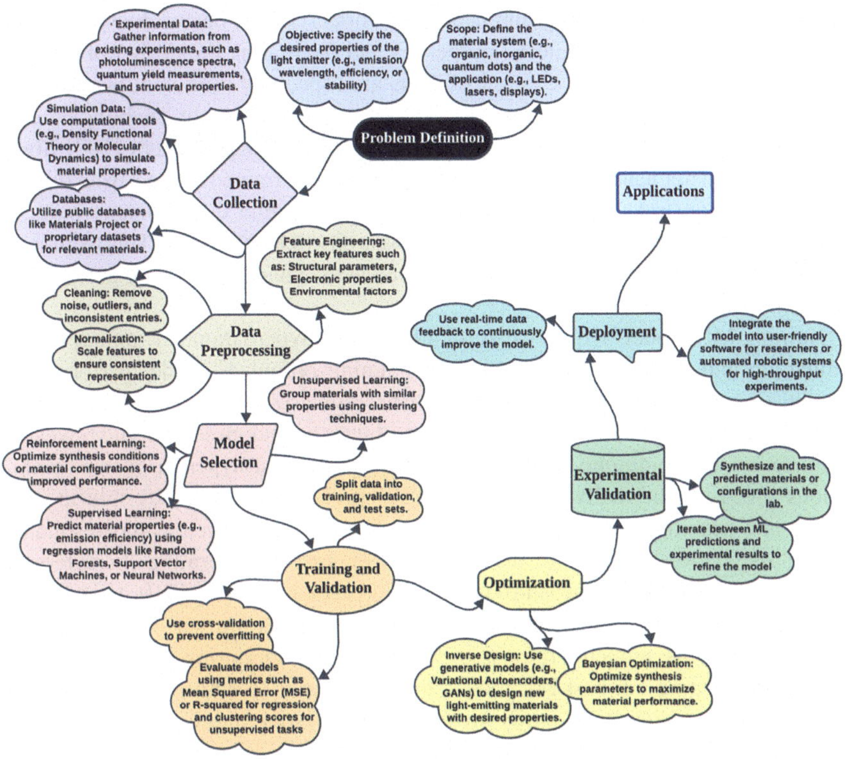

Fig. 4 Flowchart illustrating the process of developing light-emitting materials using machine learning. It begins with "Problem Definition," specifying objectives, scope, and data collection methods, including experimental, simulation, and database data. "Data Preprocessing" involves cleaning, normalization, and feature engineering. "Model Selection" includes supervised and unsupervised learning and reinforcement learning. "Training and Validation" focuses on splitting data, cross-validation, and model evaluation. "Optimization" uses inverse design and Bayesian optimization. "Experimental Validation" involves synthesizing and testing materials. "Deployment" integrates models into software for applications like LEDs and displays. Arrows indicate the iterative nature of the process, emphasizing continuous improvement and feedback

uncover latent patterns or groupings within the dataset, such as clustering materials with similar photonic properties [101]. Although less commonly applied, reinforcement learning holds promise in optimizing device architectures and fabrication processes [102]. By leveraging trial-and-error mechanisms, reinforcement learning algorithms iteratively improve performance metrics, offering a novel approach to refining complex systems [103].

The selection of an algorithm also hinges on the nature and volume of the available data. Traditional algorithms, such as linear regression and decision trees, are well-suited for smaller datasets with clearly defined relationships [104]. In contrast, advanced methods, such as deep learning, are more effective when dealing with large, complex datasets [105]. Deep neural networks, particularly convolutional neural networks (CNNs) and graph neural networks (GNNs) have achieved significant success in predicting material properties and facilitating the design of innovative light emitters [106]. For example, GNNs are especially proficient in capturing spatial and chemical relationships within crystal structures, thereby enabling precise predictions of optical properties. Additionally, Raffel and coworkers [107] highlighted that transfer learning, an approach leveraging pre-trained models from related tasks, has demonstrated significant potential in light emitter development, particularly in addressing the challenge posed by the scarcity of labeled data. This technique allows researchers to leverage existing knowledge to enhance predictive accuracy in data-limited scenarios.

Training ML models requires careful attention to hyperparameter tuning, model evaluation, and validation. Hyperparameter tuning optimizes model performance by adjusting parameters such as learning rate, regularization strength, and neural network architecture [108]. Techniques like grid search, random search, and Bayesian optimization are commonly employed to identify the best hyperparameter combinations [109]. Additionally, evaluating model performance involves splitting the dataset into training, validation, and testing subsets. Metrics such as mean squared error, classification accuracy, or the area under the receiver operating characteristic curve provide quantitative measures of a model's predictive ability [110, 111]. Cross-validation techniques further enhance reliability by assessing performance across multiple data splits, reducing the risk of overfitting or underfitting [112].

After developing a robust ML model, the focus shifts to optimization and interpretation. Optimization tasks often involve inverse design finding material compositions or device configurations that achieve desired emission properties. Generative models, including variational autoencoders (VAEs) and generative adversarial networks (GANs), are being increasingly utilized for this purpose, as noted by Karras et al. [113]. These models can generate novel material candidates with tailored properties by sampling from learned distributions. For example, a VAE trained on a dataset of phosphors could propose new compositions that maximize luminous efficiency [114]. Beyond optimization, interpreting ML models is crucial for gaining scientific insights. Techniques like feature importance analysis and SHAP (SHapley Additive exPlanations) help identify key factors influencing model predictions, offering guidance for experimental validation and further exploration [115].

Integrating ML into experimental workflows significantly enhances efficiency and innovation. Active learning, a paradigm that combines ML with experimental feedback loops, exemplifies this integration [116]. In active learning, an ML model selects the most informative experiments to perform, thereby maximizing knowledge gain while minimizing experimental costs [117]. This approach is particularly advantageous in light emitter development, where synthesis and characterization can be time-intensive and resource-intensive [118]. For instance, researchers can use active learning to prioritize testing of material compositions that are predicted to exhibit high quantum yields or thermal stability, accelerating the discovery of high-performance emitters [46].

Another critical aspect of ML workflows is the deployment of models in real-world applications. This step involves translating predictive insights into actionable recommendations for material synthesis, device fabrication, or system integration [119]. For example, an ML model might guide the fabrication of LEDs by suggesting optimal doping concentrations, layer thicknesses, or annealing temperatures [120]. Deploying such models requires user-friendly interfaces and robust computational infrastructure to support seamless interaction between researchers, engineers, and the ML system [121]. Cloud-based platforms and automated pipelines have become increasingly popular for deploying ML models, enabling real-time predictions and iterative improvements [122].

Despite its transformative potential, applying ML to light emitter development poses several challenges. According to Douglas et al. [123], a significant limitation is the quality and diversity of the available data. Experimental datasets often suffer from measurement errors, limited coverage of material space, or biases introduced during data collection. Addressing these issues requires developing standardized protocols for data generation and sharing, as well as leveraging synthetic data from computational simulations to complement experimental datasets [124]. Additionally, ensuring model interpretability remains a challenge, particularly for complex deep-learning models [125].

Ethical and environmental considerations also warrant attention. Developing energy-efficient light emitters aligns with global sustainability goals [126], but the computational resources required for training ML models can be energy-intensive [127]. Researchers are increasingly exploring ways to reduce the carbon footprint of ML workflows by optimizing algorithms, using energy-efficient hardware, and adopting green computing practices [128]. Furthermore, ethical concerns related to intellectual property and data privacy must be addressed, particularly when collaborating across industries and research institutions [129].

Schmidt et al. [32] reported that the future of machine learning in light emitter development holds immense promise, fueled by continuous advancements in algorithms, computational power, and data availability. Emerging trends include the integration of multi-modal data combining experimental, computational, and textual information to create more elaborate models [130]. Additionally, the convergence of ML with other cutting-edge technologies, such as quantum computing and high-throughput experimentation, is expected to further accelerate progress [75]. Collaborative efforts between material scientists, ML practitioners, and industry stakeholders will be instrumental in realizing the full potential of ML-driven light emitter development [131].

ML workflows provide a robust framework for accelerating the development of light emitters, addressing critical challenges in material discovery, optimization, and practical deployment. By employing data-driven methodologies, researchers can identify novel materials, enhance device performance, and streamline experimental workflows, thereby fostering innovation in energy-efficient lighting and photonics technologies.

2 Future Directions and Challenges

ML has significantly influenced the design and application of tailored light emitters in biomedicine, enabling precise control over emission properties for various diagnostic, therapeutic, and monitoring applications. Despite its successes, this field is still in its early stages, with numerous challenges and exciting directions for future development. This section explores the prospective advancements and the hurdles that ML must overcome to realize its full potential in biomedical light emitters.

2.1 Future Directions

ML has the potential to revolutionize various biomedical applications by designing advanced light emitters. In precision diagnostics and personalized medicine, ML can optimize emitters for specific medical conditions, such as tailoring fluorescence imaging emitters to enhance contrast and resolution for biomarkers [132]. As medicine increasingly focuses on personalization, ML could enable real-time adaptability of emitters to individual patient needs. Integration with advanced imaging modalities like optoacoustic imaging could further enhance the detection of early-stage cancers or microvascular abnormalities, improving diagnostic accuracy through predictive modeling and real-time data analysis.

According to Kolaříková et al. [133], ML-designed emitters have the potential to significantly enhance therapeutic applications, particularly in phototherapy methods such as photodynamic therapy and low-level light therapy. Emitters that dynamically adjust wavelength, intensity, and duration based on real-time patient feedback could reduce damage to healthy tissues and provide targeted treatments [134]. Additionally, these emitters could be incorporated into wearable or implantable devices for continuous therapeutic intervention, particularly for chronic conditions such as wound healing and degenerative diseases [135].

In the field of biosensing, ML-optimized emitters could enable highly sensitive and specific detection of biological analytes [136]. This could drive innovations in technologies like plasmonic biosensors and whispering-gallery-mode resonators, offering real-time molecular insights [137]. The combination of ML with miniaturized emitters could also facilitate the creation of portable diagnostic devices, delivering rapid and accurate results, especially in resource-limited settings or during pandemics where timely diagnostics are critical.

The convergence of ML-designed light emitters with emerging technologies such as artificial intelligence (AI), nanotechnology, and bioinformatics holds transformative potential [138]. Embedding these emitters in lab-on-a-chip devices could streamline complex assays for high-throughput screening and drug discovery. Similarly, their integration with AI-powered robotic systems could enhance visualization in autonomous surgical tools, enabling precise procedures like minimally invasive or neurosurgical interventions [139].

Expanding the spectral range of ML-designed emitters, from UV to near-infrared (NIR), could unlock new biomedical opportunities [140]. Applications may include deep-tissue imaging with NIR light for better tissue penetration or sterilization processes using UV light. Such advancements would broaden the spectrum of uses, pushing the boundaries of biomedical technology further.

2.2 Challenges

Leveraging ML for tailored light emitters in biomedicine faces several challenges. One key issue is the availability and quality of data, as the design of optimized emitters requires extensive, high-quality datasets detailing material properties, emission behaviors, and biological interactions. The absence of standardized datasets limits ML model accuracy, emphasizing the need for open-access databases and collaborative efforts across academia, industry, and healthcare institutions [141].

Computational complexity is another hurdle, as modeling intricate phenomena like light-matter interactions and biological effects demands substantial computational resources [142]. Future advancements in computational infrastructure, such as quantum or edge computing, and more efficient algorithms like federated learning, could reduce these barriers and enhance the practicality of ML in this field.

Bridging the gap between theoretical ML predictions and practical applications remains challenging due to material synthesis, fabrication constraints, and integration with biomedical systems. Addressing these issues requires interdisciplinary collaboration among engineers, material scientists, and medical professionals to ensure ML-designed emitters are feasible and deployable [143].

Regulatory and ethical considerations also play a critical role in deploying ML-designed emitters in clinical settings. The "black box" nature of some ML algorithms can hinder regulatory approval, highlighting the importance of explainable models that provide clear justifications for their predictions [144]. Moreover, ensuring equitable access and addressing environmental impacts are essential for widespread acceptance.

Finally, long-term stability and reliability are crucial for biomedical emitters, particularly for wearable or implantable devices. Emitters must maintain performance under physiological conditions such as temperature fluctuations, pH changes, and mechanical stresses. Research into robust materials, durable device architectures, accelerated aging studies, and in vivo testing will be vital for validating the longevity and dependability of ML-designed emitters.

3 Conclusions

ML is significantly transforming the development of light-emitting materials, especially in fields like biomedicine, telecommunications, and quantum computing. ML accelerates the discovery of materials by analyzing datasets to predict emission properties and suggest novel compounds. It improves material design through feature engineering, model selection, and evaluation, ultimately reducing the time and labor involved in experimental tasks. Coupled with physics-based modeling, such as quantum mechanical methods like DFT and MD simulations, ML helps optimize properties like emission wavelength, efficiency, and stability. Inverse design also plays a crucial role in customizing light-emitting materials by combining computational techniques and ML to predict material behavior, create new structures, and refine properties. Optimization strategies such as gradient-based methods, evolutionary algorithms, and Bayesian optimization further enhance the material design process. Experimental validation ensures that predicted materials meet practical standards. In various applications, ML has improved light emitters for fiber-optic communication, energy-efficient LEDs, OLEDs, quantum computing, and biophotonics. It enables precise optimization of material compositions, light stability, and energy efficiency. Although challenges remain in data quality, model interpretability, and computational costs, ongoing advancements in ML algorithms and interdisciplinary collaboration hold great promise for sustainable innovations in light-emitter technology. Addressing these challenges will be crucial to unlocking the full potential of ML-driven light emitter design.

Acknowledgements We thank project FSER-2024-0003 for the support.

References

1. Zhou, J., Huang, B., Yan, Z., et al.: Emerging role of machine learning in light-matter interaction. Light Sci. Appl. **8**, 84 (2019)
2. Gong, K., Berg, E., Cherry, S.R., Qi, J.: Machine learning in PET: from photon detection to quantitative image reconstruction. Proc IEEE Inst. Electr. Electron. Eng. **108**(1), 51–68 (2020)
3. Çadırcı, M.S., Çadırcı, M.: Machine learning models for accurately predicting properties of $CsPbCl_3$ perovskite quantum dots. arXiv preprint arXiv:2406.15515. (2024)
4. Häse, F., Roch, L.M., Friederich, P., et al.: Designing and understanding light-harvesting devices with machine learning. Nat. Commun. **11**, 4587 (2020). https://doi.org/10.1038/s41467-020-17995-8
5. Li, D., Hu, W., Wang, J., et al.: White-light emission from a single organic compound with unique self-folded conformation and multistimuli responsiveness. Chem. Sci. **9**(26), 5709–5715 (2018)
6. Bi, H., Jiang, J., Chen, J., Kuang, X., Zhang, J.: Machine learning prediction of quantum yields and wavelengths of aggregation-induced emission molecules. Materials (Basel) **17**(7), 1664 (2024)

7. Huang, G., Guo, Y., Chen, Y., Nie, Z.: Application of machine learning in material synthesis and property prediction. Materials (Basel) **16**(17), 5977 (2023)
8. Chibani, S., Coudert, F.-X.: Machine learning approaches for the prediction of materials properties. APL Mater. **8**(8), 080701 (2020)
9. Hashizume, T., Ozawa, Y., Ying, B.W.: Employing active learning in the optimization of culture medium for mammalian cells. npj Syst. Biol. Appl. **9**, 20 (2023)
10. Wu, C., Xu, Y., Fang, J., et al.: Machine learning in biomaterials, biomechanics/mechanobiology, and biofabrication: State of the art and perspective. Arch. Comput. Methods Eng. **31**, 3699–3765 (2024)
11. Prestwich, S.: Solving complex optimization problems by machine learning. AppliedMath **4**(3), 908–926 (2024)
12. Zakutayev, A., Wunder, N., Schwarting, M., et al.: An open experimental database for exploring inorganic materials. Sci Data **5**, 180053 (2018)
13. Joung, J.F., Han, M., Hwang, J., et al.: Deep learning optical spectroscopy based on experimental database: potential applications to molecular design. JACS Au. **1**(4), 427–438 (2021). https://doi.org/10.1021/jacsau.1c00035
14. Shi, X., Zhong, X., Liu, W., et al.: Prediction and exploration of emission wavelength of luminescent materials based on machine learning. SSRN Electron. J. (2024)
15. Ju, C.W., Bai, H., Li, B., Liu, R.: Machine learning enables highly accurate predictions of photophysical properties of organic fluorescent materials: emission wavelengths and quantum yields. J. Chem. Inf. Model. **61**(3), 1053–65 (2021)
16. Afolabi, S.O., Semire, B., Idowu, M.A.: Electronic and optical properties' tuning of phenoxazine-based D-A2-π-A1 organic dyes for dye-sensitized solar cells. DFT/TDDFT investigations. Heliyon (2021)
17. Semire, B., Afolabi, S.O., Latona, D.F., Oyebamiji, A.K., Adeoye, M.D., Owonikoko, A.D., Oyebamiji, O.M., Abdulsalami, I.O., Odunola, O.A.: Quantum chemical elucidation on the optoelectronic properties of N 2-(4-Aminophenyl) Pyridine-2, 5-Diamine based dyes for solar cells utilization. Chem. Afr. (2023)
18. Reiser, P., Neubert, M., Eberhard, A., et al.: Graph neural networks for materials science and chemistry. Commun Mater. **3**, 93 (2022)
19. Grill, J.B., Strub, F., Altch'e, F., et al.: Bootstrap your own latent: a new approach to self-supervised learning. Neural Inf. Process Syst. (2020)
20. Tucto, K., Aponte, W., Dulanto, J., Töfflinger, J.A., Guerra, J.A.: Combinatorial approach toward optimization of the light emission intensity of AlOxNy:Yb3+ thin films. Appl. Opt. **58**(12), 3097–3103 (2019)
21. Kattenborn, T., Leitloff, J., Schiefer, F., Hinz, S.: Review on Convolutional Neural Networks (CNN) in vegetation remote sensing. ISPRS J. Photogramm. Remote. Sens. **173**, 24–49 (2021)
22. Stoean, C., Zivkovic, M., Bozovic, A., et al.: Metaheuristic-based hyperparameter tuning for recurrent deep learning: application to the prediction of solar energy generation. Axioms. **12**, 266 (2023)
23. Schräpel, C., Kovar, L., Selzer, D., et al.: External model performance evaluation of twelve infliximab population pharmacokinetic models in patients with inflammatory bowel disease. Pharmaceutics **13** (2021)
24. Bradshaw, T., Huemann, Z., Hu, J., Rahmim, A.: A guide to cross-validation for artificial intelligence in medical imaging. Radiol Artif. Intell. **5**(4), e220232 (2023)
25. Wu, Z., Choi, H., Hudson, Z.: Achieving white-light emission using organic persistent room temperature phosphorescence. Angew. Chem. Int. Ed. Engl. (2023)
26. Kurth, S., Marques, M.A., Gross, E.K.: Electronic structure: density functional theory. (2003)
27. Ramakrishnan, R., Hartmann, M., Tapavicza, E., Von Lilienfeld, O.A.: Electronic spectra from TDDFT and machine learning in chemical space. J. Chem. Phys. **143**(8) (2015)
28. Santoro, F., Jacquemin, D.: Going beyond the vertical approximation with time-dependent density functional theory. WIREs Comput. Mol. Sci. **6**(5), 460–486 (2016). https://doi.org/10.1002/wcms.1260

29. Yang, H.L., Bai, L.F., Geng, Z.R., Chen, H., Xu, L.T., Xie, Y.C., Wang, D.J., Gu, H.W., Wang, X.M.: Carbon quantum dots: preparation, optical properties, and biomedical applications. Mater. Today Adv. **18**, 100376 (2023)
30. Behara, P.K.: Benchmarking quantum mechanical levels of theory for valence parametrization in force fields. J. Phys. Chem. B **128**(32), 7888–7902 (2024)
31. Yang, L., Horton, J.T., Payne, M.C., Penfold, T.J., Cole, D.J.: Modeling molecular emitters in organic light-emitting diodes with the quantum mechanical bespoke force field. J. Chem. Theory Comput. **17**(8), 5021–33 (2021)
32. Yazdani, M., Ghassemi, A., Shahgholi, M., Fesharaki, J.J., Galehdari, S.A.: Molecular dynamics method to investigate the interaction energy and mechanical properties of the reinforced graphene aerogel with paraffin as the phase change material in the presence of different external heat fluxes. J. Taiwan Inst. Chem. Eng. (2024)
33. Segall, M.D., Lindan, P.J., Probert, M.A., Pickard, C.J., Hasnip, P.J., Clark, S.J., Payne, M.C.: First-principles simulation: ideas, illustrations and the CASTEP code. J. Phys. Condens. Matter **14**(11), 2717 (2002)
34. Laasonen, K.: Ab initio molecular dynamics. Biomol. Simulat. 29–42 (2012)
35. Nieves, P., Arapan, S., Hadjipanayis, G., et al.: Applying high-throughput computational techniques for discovering next-generation permanent magnets. Phys Status Solidi (c) **13**, 942–950 (2016)
36. Song, S., Liu, K., Mao, X., et al.: Colorful triplet excitons in carbon nanodots for time delay lighting. Adv. Mater. **35** (2023)
37. Lawrence, J.E., Mannouch, J.R., Richardson, J.O.: Recovering Marcus theory rates and beyond without the need for decoherence corrections: the mapping approach to surface hopping. J. Phys. Chem. Lett. **15**, 707–716 (2023)
38. Yurchenko, S.: Computational Spectroscopy of Polyatomic Molecules. CRC Press (2023)
39. Orlando, R., Romaniello, P., Loos, P.: The three channels of many-body perturbation theory: GW, particle-particle, and electron-hole T-matrix self-energies. J. Chem. Phys. **159**(18) (2023)
40. Hashim, A., Hadi, A.A., Al-Aaraji, N.A.: Fabrication and augmented electrical and optical characteristics of PMMA/CoFe2O4/ZnCoFe2O4 hybrid nanocomposites for quantum optoelectronics nanosystems. Opt Quantum Electron. **55**, 1–14 (2023)
41. Lai, Z., Liu, W., Jian, X., et al.: Neural modal ordinary differential equations: Integrating physics-based modeling with neural ordinary differential equations for modeling high-dimensional monitored structures. Data-Centric Eng. **3** (2023)
42. Bastek, J.-H., Kochmann, D.: Inverse design of nonlinear mechanical metamaterials via video denoising diffusion models. Nat Mach. Intell. **5**, 1466–1475 (2023)
43. Zhang, Y., Wang, Y., Song, J., et al.: Near-infrared emitting materials via harvesting triplet excitons: Molecular design, properties, and application in organic light-emitting diodes. Adv. Opt. Mater. **6** (2018)
44. Cholsuk, C., Suwanna, S., Vogl, T.: Tailoring the emission wavelength of color centers in hexagonal boron nitride for quantum applications. Nanomaterials **12** (2022)
45. Jahanger, A., Ali, M., Balsalobre-Lorente, D., et al.: Testing the impact of renewable energy and oil price on carbon emission intensity in China's transportation sector. Environ. Sci. Pollut. Res. **30** (2023)
46. Zhao, B., Ma, H., Jia, H., et al.: Triphenylamine-derived solid-state emissive carbon dots for multicolor high-efficiency electroluminescent light-emitting diodes. Angew. Chem. Int. Ed. (2023)
47. Zuccarini, C., Ramachandran, K., Jayaseelan, D.D.: Material discovery and modeling acceleration via machine learning. APL Mater. **12**(9) (2024)
48. Ojha, U., Li, Y., Lee, Y.J.: Towards universal fake image detectors that generalize across generative models. CVPR (2023)
49. Thirunavukkarasu, M., Sawle, Y., Lala, H.: A comprehensive review on optimization of hybrid renewable energy systems using various optimization techniques. Renew. Sustain. Energy Rev. (2023)

50. Gerber, F., Furrer, R.: Optimparallel: an R package providing parallel versions of the gradient-based optimization methods of optim. arXiv preprint arXiv:1804.11058 (2018)
51. Guo, Q., Wang, R., Guo, J., et al.: Connecting large language models with evolutionary algorithms yields powerful prompt optimizers. ICLR (2023)
52. Ho, J., Jain, A., Abbeel, P.: Denoising diffusion probabilistic models. Adv. Neural. Inf. Process. Syst. **33**, 6840–51 (2020)
53. Sun, Y., Zhao, Z., Tong, H., et al.: Machine learning models for inverse design of the electrochemical oxidation process for water purification. Environ. Sci. Technol. (2023)
54. Miotello, A., Basso, L., Cazzanelli, M., Orlandi, M.: Nanodiamonds synthesis techniques. In: Proceedings of 2023 Nanodiamonds Conference. (2023)
55. Mariello, M., Kim, K., Wu, K., Lacour, S., Leterrier, Y.: Recent advances in encapsulation of flexible bioelectronic implants: materials, technologies, and characterization methods. Adv Mater. (2022)
56. Khan, J.I., Isikgor, F.H., Ugur, E., et al.: Charge carrier recombination at perovskite/hole transport layer interfaces monitored by time-resolved spectroscopy. ACS Energy Lett. (2021)
57. Huang, L., Zhang, L., Chen, X.: Updated review of advances in microRNAs and complex diseases: towards systematic evaluation of computational models. Brief Bioinform. (2022)
58. Chai, Y.-M., Zhang, H.-B., Zhang, X.-Y., Chai, L.-Q.: X-ray structures, spectroscopic, antimicrobial activity, ESP/HSA and TD/DFT calculations of Bi(III) complex containing imidazole ring. J. Mol. Struct. (2022)
59. Henin, J., Lelièvre, T., Shirts, M.R., et al.: Enhanced sampling methods for molecular dynamics simulations [Article v1.0]. Living J. Comput. Mol. Sci. (2022)
60. Tizpaz-Niari, S., Kumar, A., Tan, G., Trivedi, A.: Fairness-aware configuration of machine learning libraries. In: Proceedings of the 44th International Conference on Software Engineering (ICSE). (2022)
61. Nevin, J.W., Nallaperuma, S., Shevchenko, N.A., Li, X., Faruk, M.S., Savory, S.J.: Machine learning for optical fiber communication systems: an introduction and overview. Apl Photonics 6(12) (2021)
62. Kudyshev, Z.A., Kildishev, A.V., Shalaev, V.M., Boltasseva, A.: Machine learning–assisted global optimization of photonic devices. Nanophotonics **10**(1), 371–383 (2020)
63. Qi, T., Li, D., Fu, G., et al.: Amplification of random lasing enables a 10-kW-level high-spectral-purity Yb-Raman fiber laser. Opt. Lett. **48**(7), 1794–7 (2023)
64. Zhang, H., Liu, J., Xu, T., et al.: Recent advances on small band gap semiconductor materials ($\leq$2.1 eV) for solar water splitting. Catalysts (2023)
65. Weight, B.M., Li, X., Zhang, Y.: Theory and modeling of light-matter interactions in chemistry: current and future. Phys. Chem. Chem. Phys. (2023)
66. El-Hageen, H.M., Alatwi, A., Rashed, A.: Laser measured rate equations with various transmission coders for optimum data transmission error rates. Indones J. Electr. Eng. Comput. Sci. **20**(20), 1406–12 (2020)
67. Kliestik, T., Nica, E., Durana, P., Popescu, G.: Artificial intelligence-based predictive maintenance, time-sensitive networking, and big data-driven algorithmic decision-making in the economics of industrial internet of things. Oecon Copernicana (2023)
68. Sarbadhikary, P., George, B.P., Abrahamse, H.: Paradigm shift in future biophotonics for imaging and therapy: miniature living lasers to cellular scale optoelectronics. Theranostics **12**(17), 7335 (2022)
69. Fish, K.: Total internal reflection fluorescence (TIRF) microscopy. Curr. Protoc. (2022)
70. Teng, K.-X., Niu, L.-Y., Yang, Q.-Z.: Supramolecular photosensitizer enables oxygen-independent generation of hydroxyl radicals for photodynamic therapy. J. Am. Chem. Soc. (2023)
71. Iqbal, S.M.A., Mahgoub, I., Du, E., et al.: Development of a wearable belt with integrated sensors for measuring multiple physiological parameters related to heart failure. Sci. Rep. (2022)
72. Jin, C., Li, R., Liu, Y., Zhang, L., Zhang, J., Sun, P., et al.: Efficient and stable $Gd_3Ga_5O_{12}$:Cr^{3+} phosphors for high-performance NIR LEDs. Adv. Opt. Mater. **11** (2023)

73. Chen, Z., Li, H., Yuan, C., et al.: Color revolution: prospects and challenges of quantum-dot light-emitting diode display technologies. Small Methods **8** (2023)
74. Zhang, Y., Wang, Y., Gao, C., et al.: Recent advances in n-type and ambipolar organic semiconductors and their multi-functional applications. Chem. Soc. Rev. (2023)
75. Preskill, J.: Quantum computing in the NISQ era and beyond. Quantum (2018)
76. Cianci, S., Blundo, E., Tuzi, F., et al.: Spatially controlled single photon emitters in hBN-capped WS_2 domes. Adv. Opt. Mater. **11** (2023)
77. Oleiwi, M., Al-Nashy, B., Ajeel, S., Al-khursan, A.: InGaAsSb/GaAsSb quantum dot structures. Micro Nano Lett. (2023)
78. Xu, D.: Secure communication in wireless powered communication networks with energy accumulation. Sci. China Inf. Sci. (2021)
79. Han, T., Jang, K.Y., Dong, Y., Friend, R., Sargent, E., Lee, T.W.: A roadmap for the commercialization of perovskite light emitters. Nat. Rev. Mater. **7**, 757–777 (2022)
80. Zhou, Y., Chen, M., Zhuo, Y., Chai, Y., Xu, W., Yuan, R.: In situ electrodeposited synthesis of electrochemiluminescent Ag nanoclusters as signal probe for ultrasensitive detection of cyclin-D1 from cancer cells. Anal. Chem. **89**(12), 6787–6793 (2017)
81. Wang, J., Wang, B., Zhu, Y., Yao, T., Pan, Z., Chen, L.: Terrain mapping for autonomous trucks in surface mine. In: 2022 IEEE 25th international conference on intelligent transportation systems (ITSC) (2022)
82. Corato-Zanarella, M., Gil-Molina, A., Ji, X., Shin, M.C., Mohanty, A., Lipson, M.: Widely tunable and narrow-linewidth chip-scale lasers from near-ultraviolet to near-infrared wavelengths. Nat. Photonics **17**, 157–164 (2022)
83. Jiang, H., Jin, J., Wong, W.Y.: High-performance multi-resonance thermally activated delayed fluorescence emitters for narrowband organic light-emitting diodes. Adv. Funct. Mater. 33 (2023)
84. Ponomareva, N., Hazimeh, H., Kurakin, A., Xu, Z., Denison, C.E., McMahan, H.B., et al.: How to DP-fy ML: a practical guide to machine learning with differential privacy. J. Artif. Intell. Res. (2023)
85. Ferrari, A., Basko, D.: Raman spectroscopy as a versatile tool for studying the properties of graphene. Nat. Nanotechnol. **8**(4), 235–246 (2013)
86. Li, Z., Deng, L., Kinloch, I., Young, R.: Raman spectroscopy of carbon materials and their composites: graphene, nanotubes and fibres. Prog. Mater. Sci. (2023)
87. Khabazbashi, S., Engelhardt, J., Möckel, C., Weiss, J., Kruve, A.: Estimation of the concentrations of hydroxylated polychlorinated biphenyls in human serum using ionization efficiency prediction for electrospray. Anal. Bioanal. Chem. **414**, 7451–7460 (2022)
88. Yang, X., Ma, L., Yu, M., Chen, H., Ji, Y., Hu, A., et al.: Focus on perovskite emitters in blue light-emitting diodes. Light Sci. Appl. 12 (2023)
89. Dai, Z., Wolf, A., Ley, P.P., Glück, T., Sundermeier, M., Lachmayer, R.: Requirements for automotive LiDAR systems. Sensors (Basel) **22** (2022)
90. Chen, L., Li, Y., Huang, C., Li, B., Xing, Y., Tian, D., et al.: Milestones in autonomous driving and intelligent vehicles: survey of surveys. IEEE Trans. Intell. Veh. 8 (2023)
91. Abadi, M., Agarwal, A., Barham, P., Brevdo, E., Chen, Z., Citro, C., et al.: TensorFlow: large-scale machine learning on heterogeneous distributed systems. ArXiv. abs/1603.04467 (2016)
92. Anwar, A.R., Sajjad, M.T., Johar, M.A., Hernández-Gutiérrez, C.A., Usman, M., Łepkowski, S.P.: Recent progress in micro-LED-based display technologies. Laser Photonics Rev. **16** (2022)
93. Ariga, K.: Nanoarchitectonics: method for everything in material science. Bull. Chem. Soc. Jpn (2023)
94. Kim, H.G., Shin, H., Ha, Y., Kim, R., Kwon, S.K., Kim, Y.H., Kim, J.J.: Triplet harvesting by a fluorescent emitter using a phosphorescent sensitizer for blue organic-light-emitting diodes. ACS Appl. Mater. Interfaces **11**(1), 26–30 (2018)
95. Shtarev, D., Ryabchuk, V., Rudakova, A., Shtareva, A.V., Molokeev, M., Kirichenko, E.A., Serpone, N.: Phenomenological rule from correlations of conduction/valence band energies

and bandgap energies in semiconductor photocatalysts: calcium bismuthates versus strontium bismuthates. ChemCatChem 12 (2020)
96. Burner, J., Luo, J., White, A., Mirmiran, A., Kwon, O., Boyd, P.G., et al.: ARC–MOF: a diverse database of metal-organic frameworks with DFT-derived partial atomic charges and descriptors for machine learning. Chem. Mater. (2023)
97. Snoek, J., Larochelle, H., Adams, R.P.: Practical Bayesian optimization of machine learning algorithms. Adv. Neural Inf. Proc. Syst. 2960–2968 (2012)
98. Guzmán, J.: Regression models for categorical dependent variables using Stata. P. R. Health Sci. J. **21** (2013)
99. Simonyan, K., Vedaldi, A., Zisserman, A.: Deep inside convolutional networks: visualising image classification models and saliency maps. CoRR. abs/1312.6034 (2013)
100. Jia, W., Sun, M., Lian, J., Hou, S.: Feature dimensionality reduction: a review. Complex Intell Syst. **8**, 2663–2693 (2022)
101. Aibar, S., González-Blas, C.B., Moerman, T., Huynh-Thu, V.A., Imrichová, H., Hulselmans, G.J., et al.: SCENIC: single-cell regulatory network inference and clustering. Nat. Methods **14**, 1083–1086 (2017)
102. Han, D.-K., Mulyana, B., Stanković, V., Cheng, S.: A survey on deep reinforcement learning algorithms for robotic manipulation. Sensors (Basel) 23 (2023)
103. Wang, R., He, R., He, T., Elimelech, M., Lin, S.: Performance metrics for nanofiltration-based selective separation for resource extraction and recovery. Nat Water. **1**, 291–300 (2023)
104. Blockeel, H., Devos, L., Frénay, B., Nanfack, G., Nijssen, S.: Decision trees: from efficient prediction to responsible AI. Front. Artif. Intell. **6** (2023)
105. Isensee, F., Jaeger, P., Kohl, S.A.A., Petersen, J., Maier-Hein, K.: NnU-Net: a self-configuring method for deep learning-based biomedical image segmentation. Nat. Methods **18**, 203–211 (2020)
106. Dwivedi, V.P., Joshi, C.K., Laurent, T., Bengio, Y., Bresson, X.: Benchmarking graph neural networks. ArXiv abs/2003.00982 (2023)
107. Raffel, C., Shazeer, N.M., Roberts, A., Lee, K., Matena, M., Zhou, Y., et al.: Exploring the limits of transfer learning with a unified text-to-text transformer. J. Mach. Learn Res. 21(**140**), 1–67 (2019)
108. Ogunsanya, M., Isichei, J., Desai, S.S.: Grid search hyperparameter tuning in additive manufacturing processes. Manuf Lett. (2023)
109. Bergstra, J., Bengio, Y.: Random search for hyper-parameter optimization. J. Mach. Learn. Res. **13**, 281–305 (2012)
110. Buolamwini, J., Gebru, T.: Gender shades: intersectional accuracy disparities in commercial gender classification. FAT 77–91 (2018)
111. Çorbacıoğlu, ŞK., Aksel, G.: Receiver operating characteristic curve analysis in diagnostic accuracy studies: a guide to interpreting the area under the curve value. Turk J. Emerg. Med. **23**, 195–198 (2023)
112. Szeghalmy, S., Fazekas, A.: A comparative study of the use of stratified cross-validation and distribution-balanced stratified cross-validation in imbalanced learning. Ital. Natl. Conf. Sens. (2023)
113. Karras, T., Aittala, M., Aila, T., Laine, S.: Elucidating the design space of diffusion-based generative models. Adv. Neural Inf. Process Syst. abs/2206.00364 (2022)
114. Sun, Y., Li, Y., Zhang, W., Zhu, P., Zhu, H., Qin, W., et al.: Simultaneous synthesis, modification, and DFT calculation of three-color lead halide perovskite phosphors for improving stability and luminous efficiency of WLEDs. Adv. Opt. Mater. **10** (2021)
115. Lee, Y.-G., Oh, J., Kim, D., Kim, G.: SHAP value-based feature importance analysis for short-term load forecasting. J. Electr. Eng. Technol. **18** (2022)
116. Cacciarelli, D., Kulahci, M.: Active learning for data streams: a survey. Mach. Learn. **113**, 185–239 (2023)
117. Nöh, K., Kuhn, A., Müller, K.R.: A scalable active learning and search framework for molecular structures. J. Chem. Inf. Model. **58**(2), 201–208 (2018)

118. Hong, Y.J., Kim, J.H., Lee, J.S.: High-performance organic light-emitting diodes for display and lighting applications. Adv. Mater. **33**(1), 2001318 (2021)
119. Ji, W., Li, J., Bi, Q., Li, W., Cheng, L.: Segment anything is not always perfect: an investigation of SAM on different real-world applications. Mach. Intell. Res. (2023)
120. Wen, S., Li, D., Liu, Y., Chen, C., Wang, F., Zhou, J., et al.: Power-dependent optimal concentrations of Tm3+ and Yb3+ in upconversion nanoparticles. J. Phys. Chem. Lett. (2022)
121. Ertugrul, E., Li, P., Sheng, B.: On attaining user-friendly hand gesture interfaces to control existing GUIs. Virtual Real Intell. Hardw. **2** (2020)
122. Liu, Y., Bao, Y.: Review on automated condition assessment of pipelines with machine learning. Adv. Eng. Inform. **53** (2022)
123. Douglas, B.D., Ewell, P.J., Brauer, M.: Data quality in online human-subjects research: comparisons between MTurk, Prolific, CloudResearch, Qualtrics, and SONA. PLoS One **18** (2023)
124. Khater, M., Zhang, X., Attia, R.: Accurate computational simulations of perturbed Chen–Lee–Liu equation. Results Phys. (2023)
125. Kokhlikyan, N., Miglani, V., Martin, M., Wang, E., Alsallakh, B., Reynolds, J., et al.: Captum: a unified and generic model interpretability library for PyTorch. ArXiv (2020)
126. Fang P, Wang L, Zhan G, Yan W, Huo P, Ying A, et al. Lanthanide cerium(III) tris(pyrazolyl)borate complexes: efficient blue emitters for doublet organic light-emitting diodes. ACS Appl. Mater. Interfaces (2021)
127. Huwei, W., Shuai, C., Chien-Chiang, L.: Impact of low-carbon city construction on financing, investment, and total factor productivity of energy-intensive enterprises. Energy J. **44**, 79–102 (2023)
128. Lee, J., Yoo, H.: An overview of energy-efficient hardware accelerators for on-device deep-neural-network training. IEEE Open J. Solid-State Circuits Soc. (2021)
129. Kalyvaki, M.: Navigating the metaverse business and legal challenges: intellectual property, privacy, and jurisdiction. J Metaverse. (2023)
130. Chen, Z., Gu, Z., Cao, L., Fan, J., Madden, S., Tang, N.: Symphony: towards natural language query answering over multi-modal data lakes. Conf. Innov. Data Syst. Res. (2023)
131. Vink, K.: Sustainable life cycle design aspects: how aware are material scientists? SN Appl. Sci. (2020)
132. Wang, F., Ren, F., Ma, Z., Qu, L., Gourgues, R., Xu, C., Dai, H.: In vivo non-invasive confocal fluorescence imaging beyond 1700 nm using superconducting nanowire single-photon detectors. Nat. Nanotechnol. **17**, 653–660 (2022)
133. Kolaříková, M., Hošíková, B., Dilenko, H., Barton-Tomankova, K., Válková, L., Bajgar, R., et al.: Photodynamic therapy: Innovative approaches for antibacterial and anticancer treatments. Med. Res. Rev. **43**, 717–774 (2023)
134. Weaver, S., Paliwal, M., Phillips, M., Androski, E., Wurmser, T.: The impact of real-time patient feedback using a gamified system. Nurs. Manag. (Springhouse) (2020)
135. Capuani, S., Malgir, G., Chua, C.Y., Grattoni, A.: Advanced strategies to thwart foreign body response to implantable devices. Bioeng. Transl. Med. (2022)
136. Wang, N., Yang, J., Luo, Z., Qin, D., Wu, Y., Deng, B.: A dual-emitting immunosensor based on manganese dioxide nanoflowers and zinc sulfide quantum dots with enhanced electro-chemiluminescence performance for the ultrasensitive detection of procalcitonin. Analysis (2023)
137. Usman, F., Ghazali, K., Muda, R., Dennis, J., Ibnaouf, K.H., Aldaghri, O., et al.: Detection of kidney complications relevant concentrations of ammonia gas using plasmonic biosensors: a review. Chemosensors (2023)
138. Sacha, G.M., Varona, P.: Artificial intelligence in nanotechnology. Nanotechnology **24**(45), 452002 (2013)
139. Rhym, L.H., Manan, R., Koller, A., Stephanie, G., Anderson, D.G.: Peptide-encoding mRNA barcodes for the high-throughput in vivo screening of libraries of lipid nanoparticles for mRNA delivery. Nat. Biomed. Eng. **7** (2023)

140. Borghei, Y.S., Hosseinkhani, S.: "Semiconductor quantum dots" in biomedical opportunities. J. Lumin. (2021)
141. Ulusoy, U.: A review of particle shape effects on material properties for various engineering applications: from macro to nanoscale. Minerals (2023)
142. Ali, Y.A., Awwad, E.M., Al-Razgan, M., Maarouf, A.: Hyperparameter search for machine learning algorithms for optimizing the computational complexity. Processes (2023)
143. Schenk, T., Pesic, M., Slesazeck, S., Schroeder, U., Mikolajick, T.: Memory technology—a primer for material scientists. Rep. Prog. Phys. (2020)
144. Hassija, V., Chamola, V., Mahapatra, A., Singal, A., Goel, D., Huang, K., et al.: Interpreting black-box models: a review on explainable artificial intelligence. Cogn. Comput. **16**, 45–74 (2023)

Light-Emitting Bacteria: A Novel Platform for Biomedical Applications

Piyamson Faith Afiyos, Onyia Ifeoma Pearl, Aderemi Timothy Adeleye, and Kingsley Igenepo John

Abstract Bioluminescence is a biochemical property of living organisms which involves the generation and emission of light through chemical reactions in vivo and/or in vitro in the body of the organism. Since discovering this unique feature in a decaying fish by Robert Boyle (1668), several studies have explored this phenomenon in different organisms, the mechanism, and applications of bioluminescence. This chapter highlights the various luminous bacteria, their habitat, and their symbiotic interaction with other organisms. In principle, bioluminescence takes place in the presence of a luciferase enzyme as a catalyst for the oxidation of luciferin to emit a blue-green visible light. This property of light-emitting bacteria has been widely applied in different fields, including adenosine triphosphate (ATP) sensing, hygiene control, mapping pollution in ecosystems, preservation of artwork, gene assay, in vivo imaging, disease therapy, and sensing organic and inorganic molecules. Although advances have been made in the study of bioluminescence, the key limitations that may inform future research direction include the confines of applying bioluminescence imaging to plant metabolites, proteins and physiology. Additionally, several synthetic and natural luciferins have limitations because of their low bioavailability, stability, and cell compatibility.

Keywords Bioluminescence · Light-emitting bacteria · Luciferase · Luciferin · Quorum

---

P. F. Afiyos
Biochemistry Department, Faculty of Basic Medical Science, University of Jos, Jos, Nigeria

O. I. Pearl
Department of Pure and Applied Chemistry, College of Natural and Applied Sciences, Veritas University, Abuja, Nigeria

A. T. Adeleye
Global Centre for Environmental Remediation (GCER), College of Engineering, Science and Environment, The University of Newcastle, Callaghan, NSW, Australia

K. I. John (✉)
College of Science, Health, Engineering and Education, Murdoch University, Murdoch, Australia
e-mail: kingsleyjohn2020@gmail.com

© The Author(s), under exclusive license to Springer Nature Switzerland AG 2025

N. O. Etafo (ed.), *Tailored Light Emitters For Biomedical Applications*, Engineering Materials, https://doi.org/10.1007/978-3-031-88731-4_12

1 Introduction

Bioluminescence is the formation and release of light by living organisms, created through chemical reactions within or expelled from an organism's body. "Bio" means life, and "luminescence" means light. Bioluminescence is caused by a chemical reaction that produces light, is a form of chemiluminescence, or "chemi" from chemical, and "luminescence" or light. From the chemical reaction where light is created, toxins are a by-product of such reaction, which can cause harm to other organisms, including humans. Bioluminescence is observable in land and aquatic bacteria, which is uncommon. Light-emitting bacteria generate light and are common in seawater, aquatic animals' guts, the surface of decomposing fishes, and marine sediments [1]. These bacteria can live in terrestrial nematodes (Photorhabdus luminescens), within animals (like the Hawaiian Bobtail squid, or Aliivibrio fischeri), or freely (like Vibrio harveyi). For safety, camouflage, and attracting prey and/or mates, the host organisms use the light the bacteria produce in exchange for the bacterium's enough nutrition and comfortable dwelling. Light-emitting bacteria and other organisms have symbiotic relationships equally advantageous to both sides [2].

Table 1 lists bacteria whose genomes naturally encode the genes for bacterial luciferase and the enzymes required to generate the long-chain aldehyde substrate utilized by luciferase in light emission (luminous bacteria) [3]. For millennia, people have been able to identify light microorganisms and observe the phenomenon of bacterial luminescence. Throughout the 1700s and 1800s, light emanated from various animal items, including meat, fish, eggs, and the decomposing remains of wounds from living organisms and corpses. In 1668, Robert Boyle recorded the "uncertain shining of fishes," which was eventually ascribed to the luminous microorganisms of today. Bernard Fischer and Martin Beijerinck, two pioneering microbiologists, isolated the first light-emitting bacteria from nature in the 1880s. These bacteria have since been the subject of in-depth research from biochemistry, physiology, ecology, and, more recently, genetics. Knowing quorum sensing in bacteria, a main area of study in microbiology has greatly improved thanks to research into their light-emitting characteristics.

1.1 Symbiosis with Other Organisms

The symbiotic association between the marine gram-negative bacterium Aliivibrio fischeri and the Hawaiian bobtail squid Euprymna scolopes has been extensively documented. According to studies, the two species have a mutualistic connection in which A. Fischer's bioluminescence draws prey to the squid host, which gives *A. Fischer* a safe haven and nutrient-rich tissues [4]. According to the study by Naughton and Mandel, the bioluminescence that A. Fischer provides also helps the squid E. scolopes defend itself by acting as camouflage during its nighttime feeding activities [3]. After bacterial colonisation, a connection is formed and the squid's

Table 1 Types and environments of light-emitting bacteria [3]

Species	Habitats
Aliivibrio fisheri	Coastal area, monocentrid fish and sepiolid squids
Aliivibrio logei	Coastal aquatic region and sepiolid squids
Aliivibrio salmonicida	Atlantic salmon
Photobacterium kishitani	Marine and deep-sea fishes
Photobacterium leiognathi	Coastal water bodies, leiognathid fishes and loliginid squids
Photobacterium mandapamensis	Coastal aquatic region, apogonid and leiognathid fishes
Photobacterium phosphoreum	Marine fishes, coastal and open ocean seawater
Photorhabdus asymbiotica	Human skin lesions
Photorhabdus luminescens	Insect larvae infected with heterorhabditid nematodes

specialised organs undergo developmental modifications. Since the squid no longer needs to produce bioluminescence by daylight, it releases 90% of the bacterial population every morning [5]. The bacteria gain from this discharge because it facilitates their spread. 10,000 m^3 of saltwater can be filled with bacterial symbionts from a single bobtail squid discharge, at a concentration comparable to that of coastal waters [3]. A. fischeri is more abundant near an E. scolope population, and its abundance sharply declines as the distance from the host increases. Consequently, the symbiotic interaction between A. fischeri and E. scolopes is crucial in determining the range and abundance of E. scolopes in certain ecosystems [4].

1.2 Purpose of Bioluminescence in Light-Emitting Bacteria

Bioluminescence has been used for protection, mating, and threat awareness, according to Ruby and Morin [6]. Bioluminescence is primarily a means of dispersal for luminous bacteria, which enter fish and other marine creatures' digestive tracts and are then expelled in faecal pellets. Bioluminescence has been proposed as an efficient distribution mechanism for enteric bacteria, which are bacteria that live in the stomachs of other species, particularly those found in the ocean's depths [6]. Light-emitting bacteria can attract other creatures and encourage their consumption of these bacterial-containing faecal pellets by using their bioluminescent properties [7]. Bacteria's ability to infiltrate and populate other creatures through bioluminescence ensures their continuous existence, preservation, and dissemination.

2 Principles of Bioluminescence in Bacteria

When oxygen is present, the oxidation of an organic compound known as luciferin is catalyzed by luciferase. The chemical reaction that causes bioluminescence in light-emitting bacteria is catalyzed by the enzyme luciferase, according to Wiles et al. [8]. Different kinds of luciferin-luciferase systems exist. Using luciferase and luciferin, bioluminescence in various organisms, including bacteria, insects, and dinoflagellates, operates similarly. In particular, for bacterial bioluminescence, the biochemical mechanism entails the oxidation of an aliphatic aldehyde by a reduced flavin mononucleotide [8]. A fatty acid chain, an oxidised flavin mononucleotide, and energy in the form of blue/green visible light are the products of the oxidation reaction [9]. The bioluminescent reaction is as follows:

$$\mathrm{FMNH_2} + \mathrm{O_2} + \mathrm{R-CHOFMN} + \mathrm{H_2O} + \mathrm{R-COOH} + \mathrm{Light}(\sim 495\ \mathrm{nm}) \tag{1}$$

A thorough description of the bacterial bioluminescence mechanism is given in Fig. 1. The oxidised intermediate 1 is reduced by flavin mononucleotide (FMN) reductase to intermediate II, which then interacts with molecular oxygen, possibly via a single electron transfer (SET) pathway, as proposed for adenylated d-luciferin and oxygen [11]. An FMN-hydroperoxide species is created as a result of this reaction [12]. Intermediate IIA, which is comparatively stable without a long-chain aldehyde, was characterised using NMR spectroscopy and UV–vis absorption [13]. According to certain theories, the long-chain aldehyde produces the FMN-4a-peroxyhemiacetal species [14] by reacting with the FMN-hydroperoxide species [12], which then collapses to release the carboxylic acid [15] and the excited FMN-4a-hydroxide [16]. There is still disagreement about the excited-state species' exact genesis [5, 10]. The breakdown of the FMN-4a-peroxyhemiacetal species has been explained by a number of different mechanisms [14], such as the creation of a dioxirane intermediate or an intramolecular flavin-mediated electron transfer mechanism that starts the collapse of [14]. The intramolecular flavin-mediated electron transfer from the 5-N of the isoalloxazine ring to the distal oxygen atom of the FMN-4a-peroxyhemiacetal species is supported by additional experimental and computational research [14]. A photon of bluish-green light ($\lambda_{max} = 490$ nm) is released when the FMN-4a-hydroxide [16] relaxes to its ground state [17] (Table 2) [5]. The oxidation of the long-chain aldehyde to the equivalent carboxylic acid is another step in the cycle.

3 Quorum Sensing

Bacteria use quorum sensing, or autoinduction, to control bioluminescence [5]. Gene expression is modulated in response to variations in cell density in this phenomenon. Light-emitting bacteria continually create the autoinducer, a diffusible pheromone

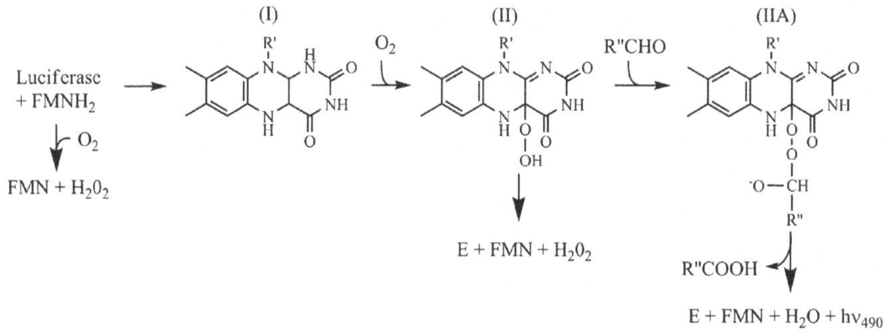

Fig. 1 Mechanism of bacterial bioluminescence [10]

Table 2 Bioluminescent system characteristics

Bacterial luciferase	Parameter
Wavelength (nm)	490
pH	~ 6.8
Temperature (°C)	2.3
Quantum yield (%)	30

that functions as an extracellular signalling molecule [5]. The expression of luciferase and other bioluminescent enzymes occurs when the concentration of autoinducer in the surrounding background achieves a maximum (>10^7 cells/mL) [5]. By measuring the amount of autoinducer in their environment, bacteria can determine their density and control their bioluminescence so that it only turns on when the cell population is large enough. The bioluminescence in the environment becomes apparent as the bacterial population grows. *A. fischeri's* interaction with its host is an illustration of quorum sensing. This mechanism is encoded and regulated by the genes luxI and luxR, respectively. LuxI is an autoinducer synthase that generates the autoinducer (AI), whereas LuxR is a transcription factor and receptor for the lux operon [5]. When LuxR attaches to AI, the two molecules work together to stimulate the copy of the lux operon and produce luciferase. This process demonstrates that *A. fischeri* only exhibits bioluminescence when the bacteria are linked to their host and have attained a high enough cell density [18]. Vibrio species also control quorum sensing by using tiny non-coding RNAs called Qrr RNAs to translate energy-intensive compounds.

4 Biomedical Applications of Light-Emitting Bacteria

4.1 ATP Sensing

In both prokaryotic and eukaryotic cells, ATP serves as the energy currency. Various ATP detection assays with varying ATP detection limits have been devised to use the firefly luciferase and d-luciferin system since Mg-ATP is a crucial co-factor in the firefly bioluminescence process. With enzymes, co-factors, buffers, and extractants meticulously balanced in each reagent mixture, suppliers provide luciferase reagent formulations customised for each system [11]. After the chemicals are mixed at 25 °C, light production peaks about 300 ms later, with a 0.25 ms lag before light emission is first noticed. According to Lundin and Eriksson, this light production is followed by a steady, continuous emission and a quick decline [12]. Either enzyme inactivity or "burst kinetics," which happens when a noteworthy quantity of the substrates (d-luciferin and ATP) is expended per minute, especially when their amount is lower than that of luciferase, is thought to be the cause of the light drop [13]. Enzyme inactivation may happen if the luciferase attaches itself to surfaces or contaminants in the d-luciferin preparation, such as l-luciferin, dehydroluciferin, or a high concentration of inhibitors like oxyluciferin. This can be avoided using a pure d-luciferin sample, like serum albumin (BSA), which is free of contaminants. Protein osmolytes, neutral detergents, and stabilising agents can also be added to keep light output constant and stop enzyme inactivation [14].

4.2 Sanitation Monitoring

Sensor technology based on bioluminescence has been used for many years to control hygiene. Specifically, grounded on the firefly bioluminescence system, the ATP-bioluminescence test is frequently applied to check the sanitation of exteriors in medical settings and meat processing industries [19, 20]. Bacterial bioluminescence is also extensively used in the food business to track the activity of Lux-tagged bacteria in situ within intricate food systems, as will be covered in greater depth later. This aids in resolving issues and enhancing storage and processing techniques [21]. Numerous studies have used ATP bioluminescence and swabbing as quick and objective ways to evaluate how clean hospital surfaces—from big objects like tables and benches to smaller ones like tweezers and other medical kits—are. In ATP-bioluminescence kits, commercially available swabs are frequently soaked with buffer. A portable luminometer equipped with an ATP-bioluminescence reagent is used to analyse the surfaces of these samples. The same manufacturer usually sells both the swabs and the portable luminometer, which complement each other. Global standardisation for this method is lacking, nevertheless. Due to discrepancies in the kits and reagents used in different investigations, there has been observed significant variability in ATP levels [22, 23]. Even with these restrictions on the comparability of data, ATP bioluminescence is still a rapid and economical way to keep an eye on hospital surface hygiene and cleanliness. It often influences housekeeping and medical staff cleaning procedures [24]. These tests have recently been applied to evaluate the cleanliness of surgical instruments, surfaces, and dentures [25, 26]. ATP bioluminescence is frequently employed in the food sector for hygiene and quality control [20]. In particular, it has been used for many years to assess the degree of contamination in fish processing plants [27].

4.3 Mapping Pollution in Ecosystems

According to a study by Widder and Falls [28], whole-cell sensors are the most popular bioluminescence sensors for tracking ecosystem toxicity. These sensors yield fast data that aid in determining toxicity levels. In order to evaluate environmental toxicity and track survival, examine creatures such as fish, crustaceans, plants, or bacteria frequently exposed to ecological tests. One benefit of light-emitting bacteria is that they can be easily identified by their light emission. Any contaminant that inhibits the breathing chain also affects illumination yield because bioluminescence and their respiratory chain are intimately related [29]. These sensors can detect organic and inorganic contaminants. Luciferin and luciferase are continuously formed when the lux gene is expressed, and the addition of the target analyte alters the baseline light intensity according to the survival capacity of the bacterial cell [3]. Bacterial bioluminescence sensors effectively detect various analytes, including uranium, zinc, and bioavailable toluene [30, 31]. Table 3 displays some bacterial bioluminescence biosensors to monitor different ecotoxicological analytes. As with other tests, meticulous pre-treatment of the sample to remove materials that can obstruct the measurement is essential for accurate findings.

Table 3 Selected bacterial bioluminescence biosensors to monitor different ecotoxicological analytes

Target	Microorganisms	Detection limits (mg L^{-1})	References
Common antibiotics	*Bacillus* WT and *E. coli* FhuAT	0.043 - 324	[32]
Mercury	*P. leiognathi*	9.87	[33]
Chlorine	*E. coli* mutants	1	[34]
$PyC_{12}Phe$ (ionic liquid)	*Vibrio fischeri*	4.17	[35]
Sucralose (sweetener)	*E. coli* mutants	1000	[36]
Terbutryn (herbicide)	*Alivibrio fischeri*	81	[37]
Arsenite	*E. coli*	39.6	[38]

4.4 Conservation of Artwork

The firefly ATP bioluminescence technique has been modified to detect ATP on surfaces to measure the number of bacteria, fungi, yeast, lichen, and algae in old artwork for historic and cultural preservation [39]. According to reports, a bioluminescence low-light technology has been used to image artwork composed of paper, stone, wood, and fibre [40, 41]. All chemicals were administered wholly to the trials, and the parameters were changed to account for the surface and geometry of the samples. The ATP bioluminescence approach and the old cultivation-based technique were recently used to evaluate microbial contamination on 17th-century murals in the nave of the old Church of the Holy Ascension (Veliki Krcimir, Serbia) [42] using commercially accessible dip slides. According to the study, ATP bioluminescence can detect "hot spots" of pollution on the artwork with speed, enabling timely assessment of areas that need more care.

4.5 Sensing Technique

Assay conditions in vitro or in vivo affect the light output in bioluminescent processes. These have been modified to sense various parameters, including pH, metal ion concentrations, glucose, reactive oxygen species, enzymes, and drug molecules. To create activity-based sensing (ABS) systems, these applications frequently use modified luciferins, such as caged luciferins, or luciferases coupled with sensing domains. The chemical activity of the bio-analytes determines the optical signal output.

Luciferin-based sensors: For particular sensing uses, luciferin-based sensors frequently employ caged luciferins, which conceal important functional groups of luciferin [43]. The analyte's presence causes light emission by uncaging the luciferin, while an external stimulus alters or exposes the functional group in this system. For example, the electron-donating -NHR or OH at the 6-position of the benzothiazole can be the masking group in luciferins. In certain instances, the masked group in d-luciferin is the carboxylic acid. These sensors are frequently made to function as turn-on probes, in which light emission is caused by the analyte uncaging the luciferin. Although they are less common, caged-coelenterazine probes have been employed to detect a variety of analytes, including thiophenols [44], β-galactosidase activities [44], and biothiols including glutathione, homocysteine, and cysteine [45]. Glycosidase inhibitors have also been used with caged-CTZ probes [46].

Luciferase-based sensors: Reactive oxygen species (ROS), metal ions, and pH can all be detected using modified firefly luciferases, which have been designed for ratiometric analysis. For example, Viviani and colleagues used mutant firefly luciferases to determine the intracellular pH in E. coli [47], and a mutant firefly luciferase was also employed for selective cadmium detection and ratiometric pH sensing [48]. A genetically encoded pH-sensitive reporter that produced light at varied wavelengths based on the pH level was recently reported [49]. It was made up of a pH-stable luciferase (Antares) and a pH-sensitive GFP. Furthermore, to detect calcium ion signaling, a genetically encoded calcium ion indicator (GECI) has been developed using Nanoluc coupled with Ca^{2+}-sensitive GCaMP6s protein. In the presence of Ca^{2+} ions, the bluish light from Nanoluc excites the GCaMP6s protein, causing it to emit yellow-green light [50].

5 Challenges on Light-Emitting Bacteria

Many bioluminescent probes have limited light output, which has made it difficult to deploy them more widely. Although systems like d-luciferin/Fluc and designed systems like Nluc/coelenterazine provide larger photon outputs, issues with stability, emission wavelength, and cell compatibility limit their use. To overcome these restrictions, research is still being done to make luciferase and luciferin combinations more effective and adaptable. The potential of bioluminescence in fields such as in vivo imaging, biosensing, and therapeutic monitoring must be expanded by improving luciferin bioavailability, stability, and emission characteristics. New luciferase-luciferin pairings with unique properties could be developed using autoluminescent systems in organisms such as fungi, providing improved solutions for applications. These advances may open up new avenues for biotechnology, environmental monitoring, and medical diagnostics advancements in areas where bioluminescent probes are currently scarce.

References

1. Nealson, K.H., Hastings, J.W.: Bacterial bioluminescence: its control and ecological significance. Microbiol. Rev. **43**(4), 496–518 (1979). https://doi.org/10.1128/mmbr.43.4.496-518.1979. ISSN 0146-0749. PMC 281490. PMID 396467
2. McFall-Ngai, M., Heath-Heckman, E.A.C., Gillette, A.A., Peyer, S.M., Harvie, E.A.: The secret languages of coevolved symbioses: insights from the Euprymna scolopes–Vibrio fischeri symbiosis. Semin. Immunol. **24**(1), 3–8 (2012). https://doi.org/10.1016/j.smim.2011.11.006. PMC 3288948. PMID 22154556
3. Naughton, L.M., Mandel, M.J.: Colonization of euprymna scolopes squid by Vibrio fischeri. J. Visual. Exp. (61):e3758 (2012). https://doi.org/10.3791/3758. ISSN 1940–087X. PMC 3399469. PMID 22414870
4. Krichevsky, A., Meyers, B., Vainstein, A., Maliga, P., Citovsky, V.: PLoS One **5**, e15461 (2010). CrossRef PubMed
5. Herring, P.J.: Review. Sex with the lights on? A review of bioluminescent sexual dimorphism in the sea. J. Mar. Biol. Assoc. U. K. **87**(4), 829–842 (2007). https://doi.org/10.1017/S0025315407056433. Bibcode:2007JMBUK.87.829H. ISSN 1469–7769. S2CID 86616254
6. Ruby, E.G., Morin, J.G.: Luminous enteric bacteria of marine fishes: a study of their distribution, densities, and dispersion. Appl. Environ. Microbiol. **38**(3), 406–411 (1979). https://doi.org/10.1128/AEM.38.3.406-411.1979. Bibcode: 1979ApEnM.38.406R. ISSN 0099–2240. PMC 243508. PMID 16345429
7. Kaskova, Z.M., Tsarkova, A.S., Yampolsky, I.V.: 1001 lights: luciferins, luciferases, their mechanisms of action and applications in chemical analysis, biology and medicine. Chem. Soc.

Rev. **45**(21):6048–6077 (2016). https://doi.org/10.1039/c6cs00296j. ISSN 1460–4744. PMID 27711774
8. Wiles, S., Ferguson, K., Stefanidou, M., Young, D.B., Robertson, B.D.: Alternative luciferase for monitoring bacterial cells under adverse conditions. Appl. Environ. Microbiol. **71**(7), 3427–3432. https://doi.org/10.1128/AEM.71.7.3427-3432.2005. Bibcode: 2005ApEnM..71.3427W. ISSN 0099–2240. PMC 1169068. PMID 16000745
9. Fisher, A.J., Thompson, T.B., Thoden, J.B., Baldwin, T.O., Rayment, I. (1996). The 1.5-Å resolution crystal structure of bacterial luciferase in low salt conditions. J. Biol. Chem. **271**(36), 21956–21968. https://doi.org/10.1074/jbc.271.36.21956. ISSN 0021–9258. PMID 8703001
10. Campbell, Z.T., Baldwin, T.O.: Two lysine residues in the bacterial luciferase mobile loop stabilize reaction intermediates. J. Biol. Chem. **284**(47), 32827–32834 (2009). https://doi.org/10.1074/jbc.M109.031716
11. DeLuca, M., McElroy, W.D.: Biochemistry. **13**, 921–925 (1974). CrossRef CAS PubMed
12. Lundin, A., Eriksson, J.: Assay Drug Dev. Technol. **6**, 531–541 (2008). CrossRef CAS
13. Lundin, A.: Methods Enzymol. **305**, 346–370 (2000). CrossRef CAS
14. Lundin, A., Styrélius, I.: Clin. Chim. Acta **87**, 199–209 (1978). CrossRef CAS
15. Lundin, A.: Adv. Biochem. Eng. Biotechnol. **145**, 31–62 (2014). CrossRef CAS
16. Amodio, E., Dino, C.: J. Infect. Public Health **7**, 92–98 (2014). CrossRef PubMed
17. Hardy, J., Francis, K.P., DeBoer, M., Chu, P., Gibbs, K., Contag, C.H.: Science **303**, 851–853 (2004). CrossRef CAS
18. Bassler, B.L.: How bacteria talk to each other: regulation of gene expression by quorum sensing. Curr. Opin. Microbiol. **2**(6), 582–587 (1999). https://doi.org/10.1016/s1369-5274(99)00025-9.ISSN1369-5274.PMID10607620
19. Dostálek, P., Brányik, T.: Czech J. Food Sci. **23**, 85–92 (2005). CrossRef
20. Hansen, C.B., Kerrouche, A., Tatari, K., Rasmussen, A., Ryan, T., Summersgill, P., Desmulliez, M.P.Y., Bridle, H., Albrechtsen, H.J.: J. Microbiol. Methods **165**, 105713 (2019). CrossRef CAS PubMed
21. Cooper, R.A., Griffith, C.J., Malik, R.E., Obee, P., Looker, N.: Am. J. Infect. Control **35**, 338–341 (2007). CrossRef PubMed
22. Lewis, T., Griffith, C., Gallo, M., Weinbren, M.: J. Hosp. Infect. **69**, 156–163 (2008). CrossRef CAS PubMed
23. Han, T., Wren, M., DuBois, K., Therkorn, J., Mainelis, G.: J. Aerosol. Sci. **90**, 114–123 (2015). CrossRef CAS PubMed
24. Rodriguez, J.A., Hooper, G.: Aorn J. **110**, 596–604 (2019). CrossRef PubMed
25. Baba, Y., Sato, Y., Owada, G., Minakuchi, S.: J. Prosthodont. Res. **62**, 353–358 (2018). CrossRef
26. Ranalli, G., Zanardini, E., Pasini, P., Roda, A.: Ann. Microbiol. **53**, 1 (2003). CrossRef CAS
27. Møretrø, T., Normann, M.A., Sæbø, H.R., Langsrud, S.: J. Appl. Microbiol. **127**, 186–195 (2019). CrossRef PubMed
28. Widder, E.A., Falls, B.: IEEE J. Sel. Top. Quantum Electron. **20**, 232–241 (2014). Search PubMed
29. Casavant, N.C., Thompson, D., Beattie, G.A., Phillips, G.J., Halverson, L.J.: Environ. Microbiol. **5**, 238–249 (2003). CrossRef CAS
30. Date, A., Pasini, P., Daunert, S.: Anal. Chem. **79**, 9391–9397 (2007). CrossRef CAS
31. Hillson, N.J., Hu, P., Andersen, G.L., Shapiro, L.: Appl. Environ. Microbiol. **73**, 7615–7621 (2007). CrossRef CAS PubMed
32. Kassim, A., Halmi, M.I.E., Gani, S.S.A., Zaidan, U.H., Othman, R., Mahmud, K., Shukor, M.Y.A.: Ecotoxicol. Environ. Saf. **196**, 1–13 (2020). CrossRef PubMed
33. Bhuvaneshwari, M., Eltzov, E., Veltman, B., Shapiro, O., Sadhasivam, G., Borisover, M.: Water Res. **164**, 1–12 (2019). CrossRef PubMed
34. Kusumahastuti, D.K.A., Sihtmäe, M., Kapitanov, I.V., Karpichev, Y., Gathergood, N., Kahru, A.: Ecotoxicol. Environ. Saf. **172**, 556–565 (2019). CrossRef CAS PubMed
35. Harpaz, D., Yeo, L.P., Cecchini, F., Koon, T.H.P., Kushmaro, A., Tok, A.I.Y., Marks, R.S., Eltzov, E.: Molecules **23**, 2454 (2018). CrossRef PubMed

36. Vermeirssen, E.L.M., Campiche, S., Dietschweiler, C., Werner, I., Burkhardt, M.: Environ. Toxicol. Chem. **37**, 2246–2256 (2018). CrossRef CAS PubMed
37. Préváral, S., Brutesco, C., Descamps, E.C.T., Escoffier, C., Pignol, D., Ginet, N., Garcia, D.: Environ. Sci. Pollut. Res. **24**, 25–32 (2017). CrossRef
38. Fukuba, T., Aoki, Y., Fukuzawa, N., Yamamoto, T., Kyo, M., Fujii, T.: Lab Chip **11**, 3508–3515 (2011). RSC
39. Ranalli, G., Pasini, P., Roda, A.: Proceedings of the 9th International Congress on Deterioration and Conservation of Stone (2000)
40. Saito, K., Chang, Y.F., Horikawa, K., Hatsugai, N., Higuchi, Y., Hashida, M., Yoshida, Y., Matsuda, T., Arai, Y., Nagai, T.: Nat. Commun. **3**, 1262 (2012). CrossRef PubMed
41. Law, J.W.F., Mutalib, N.S.A., Chan, K.G., Lee, L.H.: Front. Microbiol. **5**, 1–19 (2015). Search PubMed
42. Li, J., Chen, L., Du, L., Li, M.: Chem. Soc. Rev. **42**, 662–676 (2013). RSC
43. Lindberg, E., Mizukami, S., Ibata, K., Miyawaki, A., Kikuchi, K.: Chem. Eur. J. **19**, 14970–14976 (2013). CrossRef CAS PubMed
44. Yuan, M., Ma, X., Jiang, T., Zhang, C., Chen, H., Gao, Y., Yang, X., Du, L., Li, M.: Org. Biomol. Chem. **14**, 10267–10274 (2016). RSC
45. Nomura, N., Nishihara, R., Nakajima, T., Kim, S.B., Iwasawa, N., Hiruta, Y., Nishiyama, S., Sato, M., Citterio, D., Suzuki, K.: Anal. Chem. **91**, 9546–9553 (2019). CrossRef CAS PubMed
46. Klaubert, D.H., Meisenheimer, P., Unch, J., Zhou, W.: Eur. Pat. (2012). Search PubMed . WO2012/061477
47. Jonkers, T.J.H., Steenhuis, M., Schalkwijk, L., Luirink, J., Bald, D., Houtman, C.J., Kool, J., Lamoree, M.H., Hamers, T.: Sci. Total. Environ. **729**, 139028 (2020). CrossRef CAS PubMed
48. Kawabe, S., Uchiho, Y.: Luminescence 1–4 (2020) https://doi.org/10.1002/bio.3828. Search PubMed
49. Qian, Y., Rancic, V., Wu, J., Ballanyi, K., Campbell, R.E.: ChemBioChem **20**, 516–520 (2019). CrossRef CAS PubMed
50. Ong, T.T., Ang, Z., Verma, R., Koean, R., Tam, J.K.C., Ding, J.L.: Front. Bioeng. Biotechnol. **8**, 412 (2020). CrossRef PubMed

Multifunctional Light Emitters for Theranostics

Muyideen Olaitan Bamidele, Micheal Bola Bamikale, Motolani Adepeju Bamidele, José Sandoval Cortes, and Cristóbal Noe Aguilar

Abstract The development of multifunctional light emitters has emerged as a groundbreaking approach in the field of theranostics, providing seamless integration of diagnostics and therapeutics within a single platform. These advanced materials, including organic dyes, quantum dots, upconversion nanoparticles, and perovskites, exhibit remarkable photophysical properties such as high luminescence efficiency, photostability, and tunable emission wavelengths. By leveraging their multifunctionality, these light emitters enable precise real-time imaging, targeted drug delivery, and noninvasive therapeutic interventions, including photothermal and photodynamic therapy. Moreover, their capacity to respond to specific stimuli, such as pH, temperature, and enzyme activity, facilitates the dynamic monitoring of disease progression and treatment efficacy. Recent innovations in bioconjugation and surface engineering have enhanced biocompatibility and specificity, paving the way for applications in oncology, neurodegenerative disorders, and infectious diseases. However, challenges such as potential toxicity, scalability, and environmental impacts remain critical barriers to widespread clinical adoption. This chapter examines recent advancements, design principles, and emerging trends in multifunctional light emitters, highlighting their transformative potential in personalized medicine and sustainable theranostic strategies. By addressing the current limitations and fostering interdisciplinary collaboration, these novel light-emitting materials hold promises for redefining precision healthcare.

Keywords Diseases diagnosis · Imaging · Drug delivery · Neurological disorders · Bioluminescent imaging · Cancer

M. O. Bamidele · M. B. Bamikale · M. A. Bamidele · J. S. Cortes · C. N. Aguilar (✉)
Bioprocesses and Bioproducts Research Group, Food Research Department, School of Chemistry, Autonomous University of Coahuila, Saltillo, Mexico
e-mail: cristobal.aguilar@uadec.edu.mx

© The Author(s), under exclusive license to Springer Nature Switzerland AG 2025
N. O. Etafo (ed.), *Tailored Light Emitters For Biomedical Applications*, Engineering Materials, https://doi.org/10.1007/978-3-031-88731-4_13

1 Introduction

Multifunctional light emitters are devices used in the control, emission, and manipulation of light toward diverse applications, including advanced light-matter interaction, information encoding, and even the generation of series of wavelengths. These emitters are of utmost importance in biomedical fields for diagnosis and therapy [1]. Theragnostic on the other hand refers to a combination of therapeutic and diagnostic methods using radiopharmaceuticals in cancer imaging (Fig. 1). To this regard, two different kinds of radiopharmaceutical agents are used containing two radionuclides for the selective imaging and treatment of different cancers. It is a point to be mentioned that this technique nowadays is being applied in the diagnosis and treatment of cardiovascular, neurological and other chronic disease [2].

Multifunctional light emitters developed in the framework of theranostics are applicable in disease diagnosis and treatment [3]. They may be designed in the form of photoluminescence or electroluminescence for imaging, therapy, and biosensing. Usually fabricated from nanomaterials, these materials are capable of emitting light at specific wavelengths, thus enabling visualization of diseases while performing therapeutic functions. This enables the monitoring of a disease in real time and enhances immediate therapeutic response [4].

There are different types of multifunctional emitters, and they serve varieties of purposes. We have infrared emitters that change basically the light in the mid-infrared band for phonon-mediated, multi-purpose high-capacity encoding and display capabilities. This, if anything, adds to better-targeted drug delivery and information storage [5]. Light-emitting metasurfaces are another comprised of fully all-dielectric

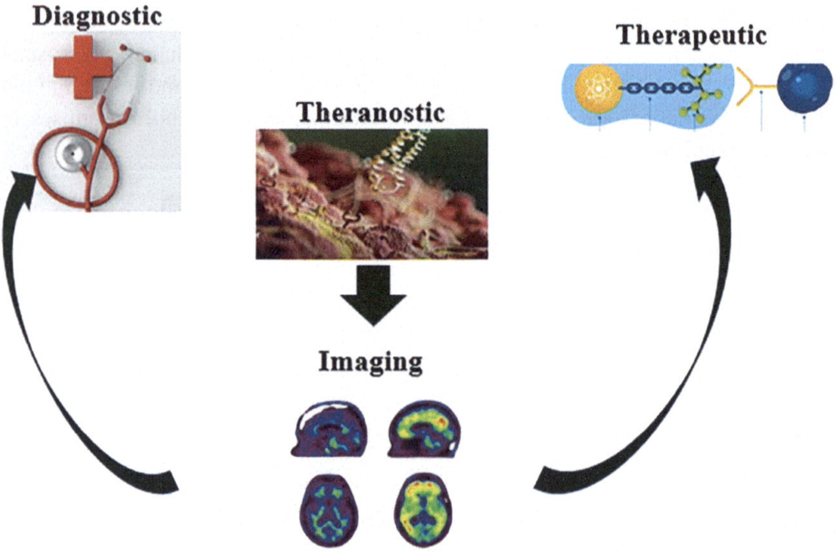

Fig. 1 Diagnostic and therapeutic approach of theranostics using imaging

materials with embedded emitters, they simultaneously address far-field radiation and spontaneous emission to improve brightness while diminishing divergence [6]. Besides there are thermally activated delayed fluorescence materials, which are designed for efficient light emission in devices like OLEDs. Their possibility of acting both as emitters and hosts for other luminescent materials allows them to reach high external quantum efficiencies while retaining stability and performance across a wide range of light colors [7]. Core–shell nanoparticles have helped to combine the luminescent property with magnetic characteristics toward biomedical applications. For example, they have been used in hyperthermia and drug delivery [8]. The last is the rare earth ion-doped perovskites which leverage the exceptional properties of rare earth ions in metal halide perovskites for applications such as near-infrared. As electrically driven emitters, they can be deployed in LEDs or applied in the field of medical imaging [9].

Most of the design strategies for these multifunctional emitters have focused on optimizing their electronic and optical characteristics because of performance improvement related to theranostics applications. Because several functionalities are included in one material, recent research aims to improve diagnostic imaging and targeted therapies, paving ways for innovative solutions for personalized medicine.

2 Theranostic Strategies with Light Emitters

Theranostic strategies involving light emitters represent an innovative hybrid of therapy and diagnostics for the targeted and real-time treatment of diseases like cancer [10], neurological disorders [11] and cardiovascular diseases [12]. These strategies involve light-emitting materials or technologies that might visualize and treat the affected area simultaneously [13]. It is clear from several research that these strategies have been applied to treat various diseases and the strategies through which these were done have been clearly seen to be different. In other words, the various ways to how these strategies work and how they are applied differ.

2.1 Quantum Dots and Nanoparticles

Nanoparticles and quantum dots are opening new channels of discovery in new imaging capabilities and are changing the mode of drug delivery systems and diagnostics. This is because of their ability to interact with the body at a microscopic level and this quite differentiate them from those that can be obtained from conventional approaches. They are evidently at the leading edge of medical research [14]. Because of the enhanced solubility, stability, and bioavailability that nanoparticles provide to medications, they aid in better drug delivery and as a result, patients who receive therapy in this form recovers faster with fewer side effects [15]. Quantum dots (QDs) are semiconductor nanoparticles with optical characteristics that make them useful for medical research and therapy. Due to their size-dependent emission, QDs may be changed or adjusted for imaging applications. These materials allow for prolonged imaging without degradation due to their greater stability when compared to conventional fluorescent dyes. For targeted detection in diagnostics, including cancer therapy, QDs can be coupled with biomolecules [16]. Since they enhance medication delivery, diagnostic methods, and real-time imaging in theranostic applications, nanoparticles and QDs both constitute a substantial breakthrough in medical technology [17].

There have been a lot of studies conducted in this area. Research on the movement of negatively charged plasmids into the inside of cells using certain inorganic nanomaterials and artificially altered cationic polymers is one example. Due to their ability to allow plasmids to pass across a variety of naturally occurring biological obstacles, the mentioned vectors are permitted for gene delivery. This has brought a lot of interest to the use of fluorescent nanocrystals in biological and biomedical imaging applications for gene transfer [18]. In another research on the application of gold nanoparticles in detecting and treating breast cancer, it was reported that the gold nanoparticle carrier thus helps to improve drug uptake into the breast tumor and the hyperthermic stimulation help to improve drug release [19].

2.2 *Bioluminescent Imaging*

Bioluminescence imaging is a sensitive tool for visualizing biological processes in vivo using light-emitting molecules secreted from living organisms. This imaging modality is one of the most efficient techniques available currently. The true value of this technique is that it can conduct non-destructive, instantaneous monitoring of the biological processes particularly gene therapy and cell-based therapies. Since gene therapies alter cells by inserting genes with light-producing proteins, these therapies are extremely important for instantaneous monitoring. This allows the imaging devices to detect the emitted light with precise data on the position, distribution, and efficiency or usefulness of the therapeutic cells [20].

This capability is of utmost importance during preclinical research, wherein sensitive monitoring of gene expression, bioluminescent signals, and tumor growth is crucial for diagnostics and therapy evaluation. As a matter of fact, through the detection of very minute changes in either gene activity or tumor progressions, bioluminescent imaging can allow one to evaluate treatment efficacies rather earlier. Applications range from disease surveillance to drug optimization; therefore, bioluminescent imaging has become a critical tool in the study of underlying complex biological processes and optimizing therapeutic outcomes [21]. A study investigated the effect of 5-fluorouracil treatment on a mouse with colorectal cancer induced by the CT26 mouse-derived CRC cancer cell line, using the combined imaging modalities of bioluminescent and micro-computed tomography. It was found that this parameter can monitor and evaluate the growth of tumors in vivo continuously. It also revealed that 5-fluorouracil injected intravenously reduced the viability of metastatic CRC cells and resulted in prolonged survival [22].

2.3 Fluorescent Proteins

Genetically modified fluorescent proteins (FPs) often gotten from marine organisms are used to monitor cellular functions and the course of disease. In addition to being employed in targeted therapies like gene therapy, FPs can be incorporated into cells to track the effectiveness of treatment. Because of this integration, researchers can see how therapies are working in real time, which gives them valuable information on how effective therapeutic interventions are, especially in clinical trials [23]. Engineered near-infrared fluorescent protein complexes, for instance, have demonstrated potential in monitoring tumour metastases and enabling medication administration in cancer diagnosis and treatments [24]. The capacity of FPs to generate light allows for the non-invasive, real-time imaging of living cells within biological tissues, which is the basis for their diagnostic potential. In cancer research, where FPs are used to visualize tumour cells and track their behaviour over time, this is especially advantageous. Instantaneous imaging, cancer research, and tracking therapy responses through detectable fluorescence changes are important diagnostic applications [25].

A novel fluorescent protein-based probe was developed to detect lead ions in human and animal serum. The probe has a linear detection range of 0.25–3500 nM and a wide dynamic response range of about 37-fold, allowing for more efficient lead poisoning screening processes [26].

2.4 Fluorescence-Guided Surgery

The surgical method known as Fluorescence-Guided Surgery improves tumour visualisation during oncology treatments by using light-emitting dyes or nanoparticles [27]. This focused strategy aids surgeons in identifying and distinguishing tumours from healthy tissue, guaranteeing successful tumour excision with the least amount of harm to surrounding structures and enhancing total therapeutic results [28]. This helps to improve surgical results by enabling improved tumour margin identification, lowering recurrence rates, and increasing patient prognosis. It also gives surgeons real-time imaging [29]. Comparing fluorescence-guided surgery to surgery without fluorescent agents, the former is safe and successful in reducing intraoperative blood loss and postoperative complication rates during surgical operations. It is crucial to note that this method can identify greater numbers of molecules, has better resolution, and is less expensive than other forms of medical imaging as such is widely applied by research [30].

2.5 *Photoactivatable Drugs*

Drugs known as photoactivatables are inert substances that become active when illuminated by light of a favourable wavelength, allowing for dose and action control. They are specifically suitable for treating cancerous cells and other chronic diseases [31].

By selectively activating at the target site, these drugs provide a therapeutic advantage by lowering systemic exposure and possible harm to other organs of the body or other cells. When they get illuminated, they change chemically, increasing their effectiveness and reducing their detrimental impacts [32, 33]. Fluorescence from photoactivatable drugs helps to identify where they are in the body, thus making it possible to see how they are acting in real time and as such improve diagnostic skills, enable physicians to track therapy efficacy and modify medicines as may be required [33].

The caged glutamate compound (JF-NP-26), which is light-activated, is one example. The compound JF-NP-26 is a modified form of raseglurant with an active drug, while its active part is "caged" by a coumarin group. mGlu5 is targeted; this receptor in the brain takes part in pain regulation. A photoprotecting coumarin group is added to the molecule of the drug that protects it until it reaches the target site, where, upon light exposure, it becomes active. The raseglurant, when inside the body, remains dormant until JF-NP-26 is exposed to light; thus, the drug will only be active at the time and place it needs to be. Mice were given the medication while LED lights were directed at the brain where action was supposed to take place. The medication helped lessen discomfort from inflammation and nerves when the light struck these locations. According to the findings, this medication may be helpful in treating various chronic illnesses where physicians require extremely exact control over the timing and location of a medication's action [34]. Another example of a photoactivatable chemical used to investigate nicotinic acetylcholine receptors is photoactivatable nicotine, helpful over a wide range of experimental setups and timescales. Photon is required for the excitation of this compound [35].

3 Drug Delivery and Responsive Release

Drug delivery has advanced significantly with the development of enhanced response-release mechanisms in precision medicine. These systems utilize stimuli-responsive mechanisms to administer therapeutic agents at optimal times and locations within the body, ensuring spatiotemporal precision, while minimizing systemic exposure [36]. This approach addresses the limitations associated with conventional medications, such as systemic toxicity, off-target effects, and poor absorption [37]. These technologies enhance treatment efficacy and patient compliance by reducing the dosing frequency and improving drug targeting [38]. These represent the convergence of engineering, materials science, and clinical expertise in the development of personalized therapeutic interventions [39].

3.1 Drug Delivery Systems

Traditional drug delivery methods, such as oral, injectable, and topical routes, have been the foundation of medical treatment, owing to their simplicity and broad applicability [40]. However, these methods often face limitations, such as rapid drug degradation, poor targeting, and uncontrolled release profiles, leading to suboptimal treatment outcomes [41]. These challenges are particularly relevant for diseases that require high precision and long-term management [42]. Conventional methods are effective for simple conditions, such as acute infections or pain relief, but they struggle with complex diseases, such as cancer therapies, neurodegenerative disorders, and chronic inflammatory diseases [43]. These limitations underscore the need for advanced delivery systems that offer improved stability, targeting capabilities, and controlled release, thereby enabling more effective and personalized treatment strategies [44].

- **Controlled Drug Delivery Systems**

Modern controlled drug delivery systems aim to sustainably and regularly release therapeutic agents, reduce the need for frequent dosing, and ensure that drug levels remain within the therapeutic window for longer periods [45]. These systems use advanced technologies, such as polymer-based implants, hydrogels, and microencapsulation, to control drug release rates [46]. Polymer-based implants allow for continuous, localized delivery, whereas hydrogels respond to physiological changes and release drugs only when required [47]. Microencapsulation involves encapsulating a drug in a protective coating and gradually releasing its active ingredients [48]. These systems offer benefits, such as enhanced patient compliance, improved therapeutic efficacy, and reduced side effects [49].

- **Responsive Release Systems**

Responsive release systems are advanced drug delivery technologies that release therapeutic agents in response to internal and external stimuli [50]. These systems are commonly used for treating localized diseases such as cancer, where the tumor microenvironment can trigger controlled drug release [51]. External stimuli, such as light, ultrasound, or magnetic fields, can dynamically control the release process, providing a noninvasive way to target treatment with high precision [52]. These systems offer advantages over traditional methods by enabling targeted and on-demand drug delivery, improving therapeutic efficacy, and minimizing systemic side effects [53]. pH-sensitive drug carriers can release their payload in the acidic environment of a tumor, thereby reducing toxicity to healthy tissues [54]. Light-responsive systems offer spatial and temporal control, allowing for drug release at specific sites and times [10]. Despite challenges such as designing predictably responsive systems, stability issues, and clinical development costs, these systems hold great promise for advancing precision medicine and improving patient outcomes across various therapeutic areas [18].

3.2 *Mechanisms of Responsive Release*

Responsive release systems use external or internal stimuli to trigger the release of therapeutic agents, thereby ensuring precise drug delivery [55]. These systems are designed to respond to specific changes in the biological environment or external interventions, allowing for controlled release that can be modulated in real-time [56]. Release mechanisms typically rely on chemical, physical, or biological changes that affect the drug carrier, causing drug release only when and where it is required [57].

3.2.1 Physiological Triggers

Responsive drug delivery systems that utilize physiological triggers have been designed to release therapeutic agents under specific conditions in the body. These systems offer a high degree of precision in drug delivery and improve therapeutic efficacy, while minimizing side effects. The release of drugs in response to physiological changes is particularly advantageous for targeting localized diseases or conditions in which the physiological environment is altered, such as cancer, inflammation, or infection [58, 59].

- **pH-Sensitive Systems**

Acidic microenvironments are characteristic of tumors, inflamed tissues, and infection sites, and provide an ideal trigger for pH-sensitive drug delivery systems [52]. These systems leverage pH variations to achieve selective and localized drug release, thus minimizing the systemic side effects [60]. Polymers such as poly (lactic-co-glycolic acid) (PLGA) and poly (ethylene glycol) (PEG) are often engineered with pH-sensitive linkers or functional groups that undergo protonation, hydrolysis, or conformational changes in response to acidic conditions [52]. This triggers the degradation of the carrier matrix or the release of encapsulated therapeutic agents. Advanced materials, including polymer-lipid hybrids, metal–organic frameworks (MOFs), and hydrogels, are also being integrated to enhance precision and drug-loading efficiency [61].

- **Enzyme-Responsive Systems**

Enzyme-responsive drug delivery systems exploit overexpression of specific enzymes under pathological conditions to achieve targeted and controlled drug release [62]. Matrix metalloproteinases (MMPs), which are commonly overexpressed in tumor microenvironments, can cleave peptide-based linkers or degrade polymeric matrices, triggering the release of therapeutic agents at the disease site [63]. Enzymes such as proteases, phospholipases, and glycosidases, which are prevalent in inflammation, infection, and cancer, have been utilized to create precision drug delivery platforms [64]. Materials, such as peptides, hydrogels, dendrimers, and nanocarriers, are often functionalized with enzyme-cleavable bonds or linkers that respond specifically to enzymatic activity [65]. These systems offer advantages, such as improved targeting, reduced systemic toxicity, and enhanced efficacy. MMP-responsive nanoparticles have been explored for the delivery of chemotherapeutics to metastatic tumors to minimize off-target effects [57].

- **Redox-Responsive Systems**

Redox-responsive systems exploit the differential redox potentials of healthy and pathological cells to achieve targeted drug delivery [66]. Cancer cells exhibit elevated intracellular glutathione (GSH) levels, which are up to 1000 times higher than extracellular concentrations [67]. This unique redox environment activates redox-sensitive bonds, such as disulfide linkages, within the drug delivery system, triggering the intracellular release of therapeutic agents [68]. Common materials used in redox-responsive systems include nanoparticles, micelles, hydrogels, and dendrimers functionalized with disulfide bonds or other redox-cleavable linkers [69]. These systems offer advantages, such as enhanced targeting, controlled release, and minimal systemic toxicity. Beyond cancer therapy, redox-responsive systems have shown promise in managing oxidative stress-related diseases such as cardiovascular disorders and neurodegenerative conditions [70].

3.2.2 External Triggers

- **Light-Responsive Systems**

Light-responsive drug delivery systems utilize photosensitive materials to achieve spatially and temporally controlled drug releases [71]. These systems operate through mechanisms such as photo-induced cleavage of linkers, photothermal effects, or photochemical reactions, enabling precise therapeutic interventions [72]. Near-infrared (NIR) light is advantageous because of its ability to penetrate deep into tissues with minimal scattering and reduced phototoxicity compared with UV light [73]. The materials commonly used in light-responsive systems include photochromic molecules, upconversion nanoparticles, and hydrogels functionalized with photosensitive groups [74]. NIR light-triggered nanoparticles have been employed in cancer therapy for the localized drug release and photothermal ablation of tumor cells. Light-responsive systems have been explored for applications in tissue engineering, wound healing, and antimicrobial treatment [75].

- **Magnetically Guided Systems**

Magnetically guided drug delivery systems utilize functionalized magnetic nanoparticles (MNPs) to achieve the precise localization and controlled release of therapeutic agents [57]. Magnetic nanoparticles, typically composed of biocompatible iron oxide, exhibit superparamagnetic properties, allowing them to be directed to specific sites using external magnetic fields [76]. Once localized, therapeutic release can be triggered by mechanisms such as heat generation via alternating magnetic fields (magnetic hyperthermia) or by environmental stimuli (e.g., pH or enzyme activity) [72]. These systems have been extensively studied for applications in cancer therapy, where magnetic hyperthermia not only induces drug release but also causes localized tumor cell death [77]. Magnetically guided systems are being developed for thrombolysis, tissue engineering, and theranostics, which integrate drug delivery with diagnostic imaging (e.g., MRI) [78].

- **Ultrasound-Responsive Systems**

Ultrasound-responsive drug delivery systems leverage the mechanical and thermal effects of ultrasound waves to achieve a controlled and targeted drug release [79]. Low-frequency ultrasound induces cavitation, that is, rapid formation and collapse of microbubbles, which disrupts carrier structures, such as liposomes, micelles, or nanoparticles [80]. High-frequency ultrasound generates localized thermal effects, enhances carrier permeability, and triggers drug release [81]. These systems are particularly advantageous for delivering drugs to deep-seated tissues or across biological barriers such as the blood–brain barrier (BBB). Ultrasound-mediated microbubble cavitation has shown promise in enhancing drug delivery to brain tumors [82]. These can be combined with imaging modalities for theranostic applications, thereby enabling simultaneous diagnosis and treatment [79].

3.3 Materials for Drug Delivery and Responsive Release

Responsive drug delivery systems utilize advanced materials capable of undergoing specific changes in response to external or internal stimuli, thereby enabling the controlled and targeted release of therapeutic agents. These materials have been engineered to possess biocompatibility, tunable responsiveness, and multifunctionality to optimize drug delivery efficacy [55]. The principal classes of materials employed in drug delivery and their characteristics are as follows:

3.3.1 Nanocarriers

- **Liposomes**: Liposomes are spherical vesicles composed of one or more phospholipid bilayers with the unique ability to encapsulate both hydrophilic drugs within their aqueous core and hydrophobic drugs within the lipid bilayer. Their biocompatibility, biodegradability, and versatility make them ideal candidates for use in modern drug delivery systems. Liposomes with conventional, stealth, and stimuli-responsive formulations are used for drug delivery, cancer therapy, vaccines, and gene therapy. They can be functionalized with targeting ligands to enhance their uptake and reduce side effects [72, 83].

- **Polymeric Nanoparticles**: Polymeric nanoparticles, composed of biodegradable polymers such as poly (lactic-co-glycolic acid) (PLGA), chitosan, polycaprolactone (PCL), and polylactic acid (PLA), offer versatile platforms for controlled and stimuli-responsive drug delivery. These nanoparticles have been engineered to enhance drug stability, improve bioavailability, and enable targeted therapeutic actions. Polymeric nanoparticles enable controlled, stimuli-responsive, and enzyme-dependent drug release mechanisms, enhancing applications in cancer therapy, gene therapy, and vaccine delivery, reducing off-target toxicity, and improving immune responses [84, 85].
- **Metal–Organic Frameworks (MOFs)**: MOFs are highly porous crystalline materials composed of metal ions or clusters coordinated to organic ligands. Their unique structural properties such as tunable porosity, high surface area, and chemical versatility make them promising candidates for advanced drug delivery and responsive release applications. MOFs offer tunable porosity, functionalization, and high surface area for precise drug loading and release. They can be designed for responsive drug release in response to various stimuli, and are used in cancer therapy, antibacterial treatments, and theranostics [86, 87].

3.3.2 Hydrogels

Hydrogels are three-dimensional hydrophilic polymer networks capable of absorbing and retaining significant amounts of water while maintaining their structure. Their biocompatibility, tunable properties, and stimuli-responsive behavior render them highly suitable for localized and sustained drug delivery. Hydrogels are biocompatible, tunable, and responsive to various stimuli, making them ideal for wound healing, cancer therapy, regenerative medicine, and eye-related drug delivery. They mimic the natural extracellular matrix, allowing for cell encapsulation and controlled drug release. They also respond to pH, temperature, enzymes, and light, rendering them suitable for various applications [88, 89].

3.3.3 Microneedles

Microneedles are micron-scale projections designed to penetrate the outermost layers of the skin, thereby facilitating pain-free and minimally invasive drug delivery [90]. These devices can either encapsulate drugs within their matrices or can be coated with therapeutic agents, offering precise control over drug release. Microneedles enable controlled and stimuli-responsive drug administration, responding to triggers, such as pH, temperature, enzymes, light, or electrical stimuli. Fabricated from biocompatible and degradable materials [91]. Microneedles have diverse applications, including vaccine delivery, diabetes management, cancer therapy, and cosmetic treatments such as anti-aging solutions [92]. Depending on their design and functionality, microneedles can be classified into solid, coated, dissolvable, and hollow types, each tailored to specific medical or cosmetic needs. Their versatility, combined with minimal patient discomfort, makes them a transformative technology in modern healthcare and beyond [93].

4 Multimodal Imaging

Multimodal imaging represents a groundbreaking approach in biomedical sciences by integrating multiple imaging techniques, such as PET-MRI, CT-ultrasound, or fluorescence imaging with MRI, to provide complementary insights into biological systems [94]. Single-modality imaging often struggles with inherent limitations such as poor spatial resolution in PET or lack of molecular specificity in CT [95]. Multimodal imaging combines the strengths of different modalities to deliver enhanced spatial resolution, molecular specificity, and comprehensive understanding of both structure and function [96]. This integration has led to significantly advanced disease diagnosis, treatment planning, and real-time monitoring, particularly in oncology, neurology, and cardiovascular research [97]. Despite its transformative potential, multimodal imaging faces challenges, such as high cost, technical complexity, and the need for sophisticated data integration, which must be addressed to fully realize its benefits in clinical and research settings [98]

4.1 The Concept and Principles of Multimodal Imaging

Multimodal imaging involves a synergistic combination of two or more imaging modalities to gain a more comprehensive understanding of biological phenomena. These modalities include structural imaging (e.g., MRI and CT), functional imaging (e.g., PET and fMRI), and molecular imaging (e.g., optical imaging and SPECT). By integrating these techniques, researchers and clinicians can visualize the anatomy, assess physiological processes, and track molecular interactions simultaneously or sequentially [98, 99].

- **MRI and PET**: MRI provides high-resolution anatomical images and can also offer functional insights through techniques like fMRI or diffusion imaging [100]. PET complements this by detecting metabolic and molecular activities using radiotracers, thereby enabling comprehensive evaluation of physiological and pathological processes [101]. Combining these modalities facilitates the precise localization of metabolic or molecular abnormalities within detailed anatomical contexts, which is particularly valuable in applications such as tumor detection, neurodegenerative disorder assessment, and cardiac viability studies [102].

- **CT and Optical Imaging**: CT provides high-resolution structural information, enabling detailed visualization of anatomical features such as bone, tissue, and organ morphology [103]. In contrast, optical imaging using techniques such as fluorescence and bioluminescence captures molecular and cellular dynamics with high sensitivity, albeit with limited tissue penetration [104]. By integrating these modalities, researchers have achieved a complementary "hybrid view" that correlates structural data from CT with functional or molecular activity from optical imaging. This synergy is particularly advantageous in preclinical research, enabling the precise tracking of tumor progression, assessment of vascular remodeling, and evaluation of drug delivery efficacy[105].

4.2 Technological Innovations Enabling Multimodal Imaging

Multimodal imaging combines two or more imaging techniques to obtain complementary information and offers a more comprehensive understanding of biological processes, disease mechanisms, and therapeutic responses [98]. Recent technological innovations have enabled the seamless integration of multiple modalities, improving resolution, sensitivity, and functional capabilities [105]. These advancements are crucial in oncology, neuroscience, and regenerative medicine [106].

4.2.1 Hardware Integration

The integration of hardware into multimodal imaging systems is critical for achieving precise synchronization between distinct imaging modalities. By unifying technologies such as PET-MRI or CT-optical imaging into a single platform, hardware advancements facilitate the simultaneous acquisition of complementary anatomical, functional, and molecular data. These innovations improve spatial alignment through advanced co-registration techniques, enhance signal detection via optimized sensor designs, and streamline the user experience with intuitive interfaces and real-time data integration [107, 108].

- **Hybrid Scanners**: Hybrid scanners such as PET/MRI and SPECT/CT integrate two distinct imaging modalities into a single platform to provide comprehensive diagnostic insights [109]. These systems enable simultaneous or sequential acquisition of datasets, combining anatomical, functional, and molecular information to enhance clinical precision. PET/MRI and SPECT/CT are imaging techniques that combine metabolic imaging capabilities with MRI and CT, offering improved spatial and temporal resolution, enhanced disease characterization, and reduced patient discomfort [110]. They also feature advanced shielding techniques, shared detector technologies, and real-time data-fusion algorithms [109].

- **Miniaturized Detectors**: Recent advancements in detector technology have led to the development of miniaturized high-performance detectors that are pivotal for the development of compact multimodal imaging systems. These detectors are crucial for applications ranging from preclinical research to point-of-care diagnostics, as they enable high-resolution imaging in inaccessible or constrained environments [111]. Advanced semiconductor detectors and nanoscale scintillators have improved sensitivity and miniaturization, making them suitable for preclinical research and point-of-care diagnostics [112]. These smaller, lighter detectors enhance the image resolution, detect low-abundance targets, and reduce system costs, making advanced imaging more accessible and affordable. They also facilitate the development of portable imaging systems, making them ideal for remote, resource-limited environments [113].

4.2.2 Software and Computational Advances

The rapid evolution of software and computational techniques has led to the development of multimodal imaging systems. These innovations have enabled more efficient data acquisition, processing, and interpretation, facilitating the integration of complex imaging modalities to enhance the diagnostic accuracy and precision [114]. Advanced software and computational advancements in imaging include real-time image reconstruction, multimodal image fusion, artificial intelligence (AI), machine learning algorithms, and data compression and transmission. These advancements have been used in personalized medicine, image-guided surgery, and quantitative imaging for disease characterization and monitoring [115].

- **Image Registration**: Image registration algorithms are crucial for integrating datasets from different imaging modalities such as CT, MRI, PET, and ultrasound [116]. By aligning these datasets, the algorithms ensure that the corresponding structures are accurately matched in both the spatial and temporal dimensions, enabling comprehensive analysis and interpretation of complex data [98]. Spatial and temporal registrations are key concepts in image registration that ensure the accuracy of aligning images based on anatomical landmarks. Applications include oncology for precise tumor targeting, neurology for a detailed understanding of brain activity, and surgical planning for precise incisions in image-guided surgery. These concepts are crucial for accurate and consistent imaging at multiple timepoints [117].
- **Data Fusion**: Data fusion is a computational technique that combines images from various imaging modalities such as CT, MRI, PET, and ultrasound. This process improved interpretability and provided a comprehensive view of the study participants. It leverages the strength of each modality by merging the anatomical, functional, and molecular data into a unified representation. Data fusion methods include pixel-, feature-, and decision-level fusion, which are employed

to achieve specific study goals. Applications include cancer diagnosis and treatment, neuroimaging, cardiovascular disease assessment, and the enhancement of precision, accuracy, and patient outcomes. This process enhances the understanding of structure and function, leading to better clinical or research outcomes [98, 118].

- **AI and Machine Learning**: Artificial intelligence and machine learning have revolutionized the interpretation of complex multimodal datasets by identifying patterns, anomalies, and correlations. These technologies use vast amounts of data from imaging modalities like MRI, CT, PET, and ultrasound to enhance diagnostic accuracy, predict outcomes, and personalize treatment plans. Techniques, such as deep learning, supervised and unsupervised learning, and reinforcement learning, are used in medical imaging, personalized medicine, and precision diagnostics. Deep learning algorithms analyze high-dimensional imaging data, extract features, and predict the disease progression. Reinforcement learning offers personalized recommendations based on the feedback [98, 115].

4.2.3 Multifunctional Contrast Agents

Multifunctional contrast agents enhance diagnostic imaging and provide therapeutic functions, enabling a combination of imaging and treatment known as theranostics. These agents integrate multiple functionalities such as improved image contrast, targeted drug delivery, and therapeutic actions into a single platform, thereby providing a comprehensive solution for disease detection and treatment [119]. They are used in various imaging techniques, such as MRI, CT, PET, and ultrasound, to enhance contrast and deliver drugs, genes, or therapeutic molecules directly to the target site. Multifunctional contrast agents include nanoparticles (NPs), polymeric micelles, and quantum dots (QDs) [120]. They are widely used in cancer imaging, cardiovascular disease, and neuroimaging. Recent innovations include multimodal imaging and AI-integrated contrast agents, which provide real-time analysis for improved diagnostics and the monitoring of therapeutic responses [121].

- **Nanoparticle-Based Agents**: Multifunctional contrast agents enhance diagnostic imaging and provide therapeutic functions, enabling a combination of imaging and treatment known as theranostics. These agents integrate multiple functionalities such as improved image contrast, targeted drug delivery, and therapeutic actions into a single platform, thereby providing a comprehensive solution for disease detection and treatment. They are used in techniques like MRI, CT, PET, and ultrasound, and have applications in cancer imaging, cardiovascular disease, and neuroimaging [122, 123].
- **Bioconjugates**: Bioconjugates, molecules functionalized with radiolabels, fluorophores, and magnetic tags, serve as powerful tools for multimodal imaging, allowing real-time tracking of complex biological processes with high specificity and sensitivity [120]. These conjugates combine the strengths of different imaging techniques, enabling the detailed visualization and monitoring of disease progression, drug delivery, and therapeutic responses [124]. Bioconjugates are

used in various applications including disease diagnosis, therapy, immunology, and neurology. They are functionalized with radiolabels for PET imaging, fluorophores for fluorescence imaging, and magnetic tags for magnetic resonance imaging (MRI). These bioconjugates offer multimodal imaging advantages, enhancing spatial and temporal resolution [125].

4.2.4 Applications of Multimodal Imaging

Multimodal imaging combines different imaging techniques to provide complementary information, resulting in enhanced diagnostic accuracy, better spatial and temporal resolutions, and more detailed insights into biological processes. This integrated approach has become increasingly important for various medical, clinical, and research applications. The following are some key areas in which multimodal imaging is applied [98, 115].

4.2.5 Oncology

Oncology is concerned with the diagnosis, treatment, and prevention of cancer and has significantly benefited from advances in multimodal imaging technologies. By combining different imaging techniques, multimodal imaging provides comprehensive and complementary data essential for early cancer detection, accurate diagnosis, precise treatment planning, and monitoring of the therapeutic response. The integration of functional, anatomical, and molecular imaging offers a detailed understanding of tumor biology and aids in better clinical decision-making [96, 110].

- **Tumor Detection and Staging**: Combining Positron Emission Tomography (PET) with Magnetic Resonance Imaging (MRI) is a powerful tool for tumor detection and staging. PET offers functional insights into tumor metabolism, such as glucose uptake or receptor expression, whereas MRI delivers high-resolution anatomical details, allowing precise localization and characterization of the tumor. This synergistic approach enhances sensitivity, enables the early detection of tumors and micrometastases, and provides valuable information for accurate staging, which is critical for personalized treatment planning [15, 123].
- **Therapy Monitoring**: Multimodal imaging, such as PET/CT or PET/MRI, plays a critical role in monitoring therapeutic efficacy by tracking both structural and functional changes in tumors. While structural imaging reveals alterations in tumor size, metabolic imaging through PET provides insights into the functional response of the tumor to therapy, including changes in glucose metabolism or receptor expression. This integrated approach allows for the early detection of treatment responses, such as reduced metabolic activity or altered blood flow, before significant changes in tumor size are observed, offering a more accurate and timely evaluation of therapeutic effectiveness [25, 113].

4.2.6 Neurology

Multimodal imaging plays a pivotal role in neurology by enhancing diagnosis and monitoring of various neurological conditions. Combining MRI with PET or functional MRI (fMRI) allows for a detailed assessment of both anatomical and functional brain activity, which is crucial for understanding neurodegenerative diseases such as Alzheimer's and Parkinson's. In stroke management, PET/MRI imaging helps in assessing tissue viability and perfusion and in guiding therapeutic decisions. Additionally, multimodal approaches are invaluable for brain tumor diagnosis and monitoring, offering insights into tumor location, metabolism, and response to treatment. This integration of multiple imaging modalities provides a more comprehensive understanding of neurological disorders, thereby improving the diagnostic accuracy and treatment planning [26, 72].

- **Brain Function Mapping**: Functional MRI (fMRI) and Positron Emission Tomography (PET) are powerful tools for mapping brain function, each offering complementary insights. fMRI detects changes in blood oxygenation and neural activity, providing real-time information on brain function, whereas PET measures glucose metabolism, highlighting regions of high metabolic activity that are critical for understanding brain functions. These modalities enable a more comprehensive view of neural activity and metabolism, which are essential for studying brain function in both health and neurological disorders. This combined approach is particularly valuable for early disease detection, monitoring disease progression, and evaluating treatment responses in conditions such as Alzheimer's disease, epilepsy, and brain tumors [35, 72].

4.2.7 Neurodegenerative Disorders

Combining Single-Photon Emission Computed Tomography (SPECT) with Magnetic Resonance Imaging (MRI) is a powerful approach to study neurodegenerative disorders. MRI provides detailed structural imaging, revealing brain atrophy and degeneration in regions such as the hippocampus in Alzheimer's disease. On the other hand, SPECT detects molecular changes, such as the deposition of amyloid plaques and tau tangles, as well as altered brain perfusion or neurotransmitter activity. This multimodal approach allows for a comprehensive understanding of both the anatomical and molecular changes associated with neurodegeneration, aiding in the early diagnosis and monitoring of diseases such as Alzheimer's, Parkinson's, and Huntington's disease [10, 82].

4.2.8 Cardiology

Multimodal imaging plays a crucial role in cardiology, enabling comprehensive assessment of both the anatomical and functional aspects of the heart. For instance, combining magnetic resonance imaging (MRI) with positron emission tomography (PET) provides valuable insights into myocardial viability, perfusion, and metabolism in conditions, such as coronary artery disease and heart failure. The integration of computed tomography (CT) with echocardiography allows for precise evaluation of heart structure and function, aiding in the diagnosis of valvular diseases, arrhythmias, and congenital heart defects. Multimodal imaging not only enhances diagnostic accuracy but also supports treatment planning, monitoring disease progression, and assessing therapeutic efficacy, ultimately improving patient outcomes in cardiovascular care [16, 82].

- **Ischemia and Infarction**: Multimodal imaging using PET/CT offers comprehensive assessment of myocardial ischemia and infarction by combining metabolic and structural information. PET provides functional insights into myocardial viability by measuring metabolic activity such as glucose utilization, whereas CT offers detailed anatomical imaging and blood flow evaluation, particularly through contrast-enhanced coronary angiography and perfusion imaging. Together, these techniques help clinicians assess the extent of ischemic damage, identify viable myocardium, and guide treatment strategies, such as revascularization in patients with coronary artery disease and post-infarction evaluation [63, 82].
- **Vascular Imaging**: CT angiography, combined with advanced optical imaging techniques such as optical coherence tomography (OCT), provides a detailed, multidimensional view of vascular architecture and plaque composition. CT angiography offers high-resolution images of the blood vessels, allowing the assessment of stenosis, aneurysms, and overall vascular integrity. Optical imaging techniques, such as OCT, provide in-depth visualization of plaque morphology and composition, including lipid-rich or fibrous plaques, which can help predict plaque stability and the risk of rupture. Together, these modalities offer a comprehensive approach for diagnosing and managing vascular diseases such as atherosclerosis, enabling more precise risk stratification and treatment planning [45, 54].

4.2.9 Immunology and Inflammation

Multimodal imaging has become a powerful tool in immunology and inflammation research, enabling detailed, real-time visualization of immune responses and inflammatory processes at both cellular and molecular levels. Techniques such as PET/CT and MRI are used to assess the extent of inflammation in diseases like rheumatoid arthritis and inflammatory bowel disease, while optical imaging can provide high-resolution images of immune cell trafficking and cytokine activity in vivo. Additionally, the integration of molecular imaging modalities, such as radiolabeled antibodies, in PET imaging allows for the precise tracking of immune cell activity, aiding in the understanding of autoimmune diseases, infections, and chronic inflammatory disorders. By combining structural, functional, and molecular data, multimodal imaging enhances early diagnosis, personalized treatment, and monitoring of therapeutic responses in inflammatory and immune-mediated diseases [117, 122]).

- **Immune Cell Tracking**: Multimodal imaging enables the tracking of specifically labeled immune cells, such as T-cells, macrophages, or dendritic cells, providing detailed insights into their migration, activation, and interaction with tissues during inflammation or immune-mediated diseases. Techniques such as PET/CT or MRI can be used to visualize immune cell dynamics in vivo, allowing real-time monitoring of immune responses during conditions such as rheumatoid arthritis, multiple sclerosis, and cancer immunotherapy. This ability to track immune cells offers valuable information for understanding disease progression, assessing the efficacy of treatments, and personalizing therapies for autoimmune and inflammatory diseases [42, 62].
- **Infection Imaging**: PET/CT imaging, combined with specialized tracers such as radiolabeled antimicrobial agents or leukocyte-specific markers, enables the visualization of infected tissues and differentiation between infection and inflammation [74, 76]. These tracers selectively target the sites of infection or inflammatory responses, allowing for the accurate localization of pathogens and assessment of tissue responses [37]. The ability to distinguish between infection and inflammation is crucial for guiding treatment decisions for conditions such as osteomyelitis, endocarditis, and sepsis. Additionally, multimodal approaches that integrate PET/CT with MRI or optical imaging can provide complementary information, thereby enhancing diagnostic accuracy and monitoring of infection-related diseases [12, 72].

4.3 *Preclinical Research*

Multimodal imaging plays a critical role in preclinical research by providing non-invasive, real-time insights into disease progression, treatment efficacy, and biological mechanisms [12]. Techniques, such as PET, MRI, and bioluminescence imaging, are used to monitor tumor growth, assess drug distribution, and track immune responses in animal models [86]. These imaging modalities allow researchers to visualize cellular and molecular processes, evaluate therapeutic strategies, and optimize drug formulations before clinical trials. By combining structural, functional, and molecular imaging, multimodal imaging enhances the translation of preclinical findings into clinical applications, improving the success rate of drug development and the understanding of disease mechanisms [18, 109].

- **Animal Models**: Multimodal imaging in small animal models enables detailed longitudinal studies on disease progression and therapeutic responses, providing both structural and functional insights [54]. Techniques such as PET/MRI and SPECT/CT allow researchers to track molecular changes, visualize tumor growth, and assess drug biodistribution over time in the same subjects. This approach reduces the number of animals required for experiments and improves data reliability by eliminating inter-animal variability [56]. Multimodal imaging is particularly valuable in preclinical models of cancer, cardiovascular diseases, and neurodegenerative disorders as it aids in understanding disease mechanisms and optimizing therapeutic strategies. These insights bridge the gap between preclinical findings and clinical applications, thereby accelerating drug development and personalized medicine [123].

- **Drug Development**: Combining imaging modalities significantly enhances drug development by providing complementary insights into pharmacokinetics, biodistribution, and target engagement of new drugs [43]. For instance, PET/CT allows precise quantification of drug distribution at the molecular level while correlating it with anatomical localization. Similarly, PET/MRI integrates functional imaging with high-resolution structural data, enabling detailed evaluation of drug delivery to specific tissues [44]. Multimodal imaging accelerates the screening of drug candidates, optimizes dosing strategies, and identifies off-target effects early in the development process. These capabilities not only reduce time and cost but also improve the success rate of translating preclinical findings into effective clinical therapies [118].

4.3.1 Advantages of Multimodal Imaging

- **Comprehensive Data Acquisition**: Multimodal imaging minimizes diagnostic uncertainties and enhances the accuracy of clinical decision-making by simultaneously capturing structural, functional, and molecular data. This innovative approach streamlined data acquisition and provided a holistic view of patient health within a single session [120].
- **Enhanced Sensitivity and Specificity**: The Integration of imaging modalities significantly enhances the diagnostic accuracy by combining complementary strengths. For instance, while MRI provides detailed anatomical visualization, pairing it with PET introduces critical metabolic insights, enabling more precise disease characterization and early detection [123].
- **Non-Invasive and Minimally Invasive Options** Multimodal imaging techniques prioritize patient comfort and safety by reducing reliance on invasive procedures. For example, combining ultrasound with MRI enables precise diagnosis without the need for biopsies under certain conditions, minimizes risks, and enhances the overall patient experience [62].
- **Dynamic Monitoring**: By enabling the continuous tracking of biological processes, multimodal imaging provides critical insights into disease progression and treatment efficacy. Real-time PET-MRI allows the precise monitoring of tumor metabolism and structural changes during therapy, facilitating timely adjustments to improve patient outcomes [76].

5 Challenges

Multifunctional light emitters represent groundbreaking innovations in theranostics and bridge the realms of diagnostics and therapy through light-driven mechanisms. Despite their transformative potential, numerous challenges have impeded their widespread clinical adoption and optimization [15, 123]. These challenges arise from their design, synthesis, functionalization, biocompatibility, and translational scalability. Addressing these issues is paramount for realizing their full potential in advanced healthcare systems.

- **Biocompatibility and Toxicity**

Nanomaterials, such as quantum dots, metal nanoparticles, and lanthanide complexes, can cause cytotoxicity because of their heavy metal content or degradation byproducts [18]. Therefore, it is crucial to ensure safe interactions with biological systems. The immune system may recognize these substances as foreign, triggering an inflammatory response. Non-biodegradable materials can persist in tissues, causing long-term adverse effects or systemic toxicity [75].

- **Photostability and Photobleaching**

Illumination exposure can lead to photobleaching or degradation of light-emitting materials, thereby affecting their functionality in diagnostic or therapeutic procedures. Uncontrolled production of reactive oxygen species (ROS) can also degrade the emitter and cause damage to healthy tissues, thereby affecting photodynamic therapy [48, 56].

- **Optical Properties and Tissue Penetration**

Biological tissues absorb and scatter light, thereby reducing the effectiveness of the light-based theranostic systems. Designing emitters for deeper tissue penetration in the near-infrared region is challenging. Intrinsic fluorescence can interfere with signal detection and reduce imaging precision. Despite these advances, achieving precise spectral emission for simultaneous imaging and therapy in complex biological environments remains a challenge [69].

- **Complexity in Material Design and Functionalization**

The multifunctionality of light-emitting materials requires sophisticated design strategies that balance imaging, therapy, and drug delivery. Surface functionalization is technically demanding to improve biocompatibility and targeting efficiency without altering the optical properties of the material. Size and shape optimization is crucial for achieving uniform and optimized dimensions at a scale, as these factors significantly influence optical properties, biodistribution, and cellular uptake [113].

- **Energy Efficiency and Photothermal Heating**

The high-intensity excitation of light in light-emitting systems can cause excessive energy consumption and overheating, potentially damaging healthy tissues.

Photothermal therapy requires a precise increase in temperature to selectively ablate diseased tissues without harming adjacent healthy structures [66].

- **Scalability and Cost**

High-quality multifunctional light emitters require complex synthetic processes and often require rare or expensive raw materials, making large-scale production economically unfeasible for many applications. Maintaining consistency in the material properties across large batches is a persistent issue. Infrastructure and equipment costs, including specialized excitation sources, imaging systems, and therapeutic apparatus, add to overall expenses [81].

- **Integration and Translational Barriers**

Multifunctional light emitters face several challenges in terms of regulatory approval, clinical validation, and ease of use. They must navigate through multiple categories, including medical devices, diagnostics, and drugs, and must undergo extensive validation in diverse patient populations to account for biological responses. The integration of these systems into routine clinical workflows requires simplified operational protocols and minimal training of healthcare professionals [107].

- **Environmental and Ethical Concerns**

The synthesis and disposal of light-emitting materials, particularly those containing rare-earth elements or toxic metals, raise environmental concerns. Ethical considerations include the use of animal models for preclinical testing and the potential inequitable access to advanced technologies in resource-limited settings [107, 119].

6 Future Direction

The advancement of multifunctional light emitters has significant transformative potential in theranostics, and offers promising unparalleled integration of diagnosis, therapy, and real-time monitoring within a single platform. Although the current achievements are noteworthy, the future of this technology will be shaped by the pursuit of enhanced precision, efficiency, and adaptability. Future research should focus on interdisciplinary innovations and emerging technologies to redefine theranostic applications [118].

- **Development of Next-Generation Materials**

Future research will focus on biodegradable and biocompatible emitters, including organic fluorophores, polymer-based nanoparticles, and hybrid organic–inorganic systems [113]. Carbon-based nanomaterials, such as graphene quantum dots, carbon nanodots, and nanotubes, are lightweight, biocompatible emitters with tunable optical properties and minimal toxicity. Research into lead-free perovskite nanocrystals addresses environmental concerns and offers high quantum yield, narrow emission spectra, and broad tunability for advanced theranostics. Smart emitters can alter their optical properties in response to specific biological cues, thereby enhancing the precision of targeted therapy and imaging [122].

- **Integration with Artificial Intelligence and Machine Learning**

AI-driven material design, enhanced imaging, and analysis have been developed using various computational algorithms. These algorithms can predict the properties of light-emitting materials, optimize their synthesis for theranostic applications, and process real-time imaging data with exceptional accuracies. Machine learning models can also predict individual patient responses and tailor light emitter use for personalized therapeutic regimens [114].

- **Multimodal and Multifunctional Platforms**

Future light emitters will be integrated with other therapeutic and diagnostic modalities, such as MRI, ultrasound, and radiotherapy, to provide synergistic effects for comprehensive treatment strategies. Simultaneous imaging and therapy platforms can minimize treatment delays and improve patient outcomes. Implantable light-emitting devices can provide continuous monitoring and on-demand therapeutic intervention, especially for chronic diseases [115, 116].

- **Advancements in Light-Tissue Interactions**

The use of near-infrared (NIR-II) emitters for deep-tissue penetration and photoacoustic integration will enable precise imaging and therapy in deep-seated tissues. This technology will overcome the limitations of purely optical techniques and improve imaging clarity and therapeutic efficacy in heterogeneous tissues by dynamically adjusting light emission to compensate for tissue scattering and absorption [18, 44].

- **Energy Efficiency and Sustainable Practices**

Future light emitters will require lower excitation energies to minimize the photothermal damage and energy consumption. Research on solar-powered emitters can lead to the development of self-sustaining devices for remote settings. Green synthesis methods focus on environment-friendly and scalable processes, reducing the ecological footprint of producing multifunctional light emitters [54].

- **Real-Time Monitoring and Feedback Systems**

Light emitters enable dynamic therapy adjustment, ensuring maximum efficacy and minimal side effects. Future systems should detect and quantify specific biomarkers in real time to provide insights into disease progression and therapeutic effectiveness [47].

- **Clinical Translation and Accessibility**

Theranostic platforms will provide advanced diagnostics and therapy to underresourced regions and democratize access to advanced healthcare technologies. Collaborative efforts among researchers, industry, and regulatory agencies will streamline the approval process for multifunctional light emitters, ensuring their safe integration into clinical practice. Advances in scalable manufacturing techniques and material optimization will reduce production costs, making theranostic technologies affordable and widely accessible [18].

- **Applications Beyond Medicine**

Light emitters can be used for environmental monitoring, agricultural diagnostics, and wearable devices, providing continuous health monitoring and early disease detection for preventive healthcare. They can detect environmental toxins, pathogens, and pollutants and can be integrated into wearable technologies to improve health outcomes [86].

7 Recommendations

To realize the transformative potential of multifunctional light emitters in theranostics, a strategic recommendation roadmap is crucial. These recommendations address the technical, clinical, regulatory, and societal aspects required to advance cutting-edge technologies. Light-emitting platforms can become a cornerstone of future precision medicine by fostering innovation, improving scalability, and enhancing accessibility [15, 123].

- **Prioritize Biocompatibility and Safety**

Research should focus on the development of biodegradable light emitters made from organic or hybrid materials to minimize long-term risks. Standardized protocols for cytotoxicity, immunogenicity, and biodistribution should be established to ensure clinical safety in diverse patient populations. Prioritizing alternatives to heavy metal quantum dots containing cadmium or other toxic elements can enhance patient safety and address environmental concerns [99, 102].

- **Enhance Photophysical Properties**

This study focuses on optimizing light emitters for the NIR-II window, addressing photobleaching, and developing smart emission-tuning materials. This emphasizes the importance of high quantum yields and photostability, extending the lifespan of light-emitting materials, and enabling the dynamic adjustment of emission properties in response to environmental or biological stimuli [107].

- **Foster Interdisciplinary Collaboration**

The initiative aims to accelerate the design and integration of multifunctional light emitters by fostering collaboration among various fields; utilizing AI and machine learning to predict optimal material properties; and fostering public–private partnerships between academic institutions, industry, and government agencies to drive innovation and commercialization [78].

- **Innovate Multifunctionality**

Theranostic synergy aims to combine imaging, therapy, and real-time monitoring in a single system. Hybrid technologies merge photonics with magnetic, acoustic, or radiological methods to improve diagnostic and therapeutic outcomes. Multitarget capabilities design systems for detecting and treating multiple biomarkers or disease pathways, addressing multifactorial diseases such as cancer [15, 123].

- **Streamline Scalability and Manufacturing**

Green synthesis methods minimize resource wastage in the large-scale production of light-emitting materials. The modular design standardizes the components of multifunctional light emitters, facilitating their integration into medical devices. Automation and robotics improve reproducibility and efficiency, and ensure consistency across large batches [95].

- **Strengthen Clinical Translation**

This process involves early stage validation, regulatory engagement, and clinical trials to evaluate the safety, efficacy, and scalability of light emitters in biologically relevant models. This involves collaboration with regulatory bodies to establish guidelines for the approval of multifunctional light emitters and designing large-scale trials to validate their performance in diverse patient populations and healthcare settings [72].

- **Expand Accessibility and Affordability**

Invest affordable production by reducing raw material and manufacturing costs, making theranostic technologies accessible in resource-limited settings. Development of portable, user-friendly devices with light emitters for early disease detection and treatment in remote areas. Provide specialized training for healthcare professionals to effectively use theranostic systems in clinical practice [48].

- **Address Environmental and Ethical Concerns**

The use of multifunctional light emitters necessitates sustainable disposal practices, such as the recycling of rare-earth materials and the minimization of electronic waste, to reduce environmental impacts. Ethical frameworks must guide their application, ensure informed consent from patients, and ensure transparency in clinical use. To address global healthcare disparities, collaborative efforts are essential to make these technologies accessible in underserved regions through cost-effective designs and equitable distributions. For example, integrating these emitters into mobile diagnostic units could expand the access to advanced imaging in remote areas. Establishing global ethical guidelines and fostering international cooperation is critical for balancing innovation with social responsibility [17].

- **Encourage Policy and Funding Support**

Government incentives, public awareness campaigns, and venture capital engagement are essential for supporting the research and development of multifunctional light emitters with the potential to revolutionize healthcare. These strategies aim to educate stakeholders and encourage private sector investment in startups and spin-offs [115].

- **Promote Future Innovations**

Advancing future innovations ocuses on the development of self-sustaining emitters, wearable and implantable devices, and disease-specific solutions, with the objective of integrating renewable energy sources, such as solar cells, miniaturizing light emitters for wearable sensors or implantable systems, and customizing them for specific diseases [108, 112].

8 Conclusion

Multifunctional light emitters are a promising solution for theranostics that combines scientific ingenuity and clinical applications. They can intercept diseases at their inception, tailor therapies, and deliver unprecedented outcomes. By addressing the current challenges, these systems could transform theranostics into a cornerstone of modern medicine, promoting a healthier and more equitable world. The promise of these systems is boundless, and with strategic advancements, they will define the future of healthcare.

References

1. Jeong, J., Park, J.H., Jang, C.H., Song, M.H., Woo, H.Y.: Multifunctional charge transporting materials for perovskite light-emitting diodes. Adv. Mater. **32** (2020). https://doi.org/10.1002/adma.202002176
2. Burkett, B.J., Bartlett, D.J., McGarrah, P.W., Lewis, A.R., Johnson, D.R., Berberoğlu, K., et al.: A review of theranostics: perspectives on emerging approaches and clinical advancements. Radiol Imaging Cancer **5** (2023). https://doi.org/10.1148/rycan.220157.
3. Sarbadhikary, P., George, B.P., Abrahamse, H.: Recent advances in photosensitizers as multifunctional theranostic agents for imaging-guided photodynamic therapy of cancer. Theranostics **11**, 9054–88 (2021). https://doi.org/10.7150/thno.62479
4. Chávez-García, D., Guzman, M.: Upconversion luminescent nanoparticles and their biomedical applications in imaging. In: Luminescence–Basic Concepts And Emerging New Applications. IntechOpen (2024). https://doi.org/10.5772/intechopen.1005378
5. Li, J., Li, J., Liu, H., Yi, F.: Phonon-mediated infrared plasmonic metamaterial emitters towards high-capacity multifunctional encoding and display. Opt. Express **32**, 28489 (2024). https://doi.org/10.1364/OE.529006
6. Liu, S., Vaskin, A., Addamane, S., Leung, B., Tsai, M.-C., Yang, Y., et al.: Light-emitting metasurfaces: simultaneous control of spontaneous emission and far-field radiation. Nano Lett. **18**, 6906–14 (2018). https://doi.org/10.1021/acs.nanolett.8b02808
7. Lv, J., Song, S., Li, J., Peng, L., Li, Y., Liu, Y., et al.: High and balanced bipolar-transporting deep-blue HLCT material for efficient monochrome and white OLEDs based on a simple phenanthroimidazole-dibenzothiophene derivative. Adv. Opt. Mater. **12** (2024). https://doi.org/10.1002/adom.202301413

8. Tsamos, D., Krestou, A., Papagiannaki, M., Maropoulos, S.: An overview of the production of magnetic core-shell nanoparticles and their biomedical applications. Metals (Basel) **12**, 605 (2022). https://doi.org/10.3390/met12040605
9. Yang, T., Wang, Y., Liao, L.: Trivalent rare earth ion-doped metal halide perovskite near-infrared semiconductors for high-performance optoelectronic devices. Adv. Funct. Mater. (2024). https://doi.org/10.1002/adfm.202420021
10. Lima, H., Etchebehere, M., Bogoni, M., Torricelli, C., Nogueira-Lima, E., Deflon, V.M., et al.: Theranostics nuclear medicine in prostate cancer. Pharmaceuticals **17**, 1483 (2024). https://doi.org/10.3390/ph17111483
11. Awuah, W.A., Ahluwalia, A., Tan, J.K., Sanker, V., Roy, S., Ben-Jaafar, A., et al.: Theranostics advances in the treatment and diagnosis of neurological and neurosurgical diseases. Arch. Med. Res. **56**, 103085 (2025). https://doi.org/10.1016/j.arcmed.2024.103085
12. Lin, L., Chen, L., Yan, J., Chen, P., Du, J., Zhu, J., et al.: Advances of nanoparticle-mediated diagnostic and theranostic strategies for atherosclerosis. Front. Bioeng. Biotechnol. **11** (2023). https://doi.org/10.3389/fbioe.2023.1268428
13. Hosseini, S.M., Mohammadnejad, J., Salamat, S., Beiram Zadeh, Z., Tanhaei, M., Ramakrishna, S.: Theranostic polymeric nanoparticles as a new approach in cancer therapy and diagnosis: a review. Mater. Today Chem. **29**, 101400 (2023). https://doi.org/10.1016/j.mtchem.2023.101400
14. Kundu, S., Ghosh, M., Sarkar, N.: State of the art and perspectives on the biofunctionalization of fluorescent metal nanoclusters and carbon quantum dots for targeted imaging and drug delivery. Langmuir **37**, 9281–301 (2021). https://doi.org/10.1021/acs.langmuir.1c00732
15. Zorkina, Y., Abramova, O., Ushakova, V., Morozova, A., Zubkov, E., Valikhov, M., et al.: Nano carrier drug delivery systems for the treatment of neuropsychiatric disorders: advantages and limitations. Molecules **25**, 5294 (2020). https://doi.org/10.3390/molecules25225294
16. Agarwal, K., Rai, H., Mondal, S.: Quantum dots: an overview of synthesis, properties, and applications. Mater. Res. Express **10**, 062001 (2023). https://doi.org/10.1088/2053-1591/acda17
17. Nimrawi, S., Gannett, P., Kwon, Y.M.: Inorganic nanoparticles incorporated with transdermal drug delivery systems. Expert Opin. Drug Deliv. **21**, 1349–62 (2024). https://doi.org/10.1080/17425247.2024.2399710
18. Zahed, Z., Hadi, R., Imanzadeh, G., Ahmadian, Z., Shafiei, S., Zadeh, A.Z., et al.: Recent advances in fluorescence nanoparticles "quantum dots" as gene delivery system: a review. Int. J. Biol. Macromol. **254**, 127802 (2024). https://doi.org/10.1016/j.ijbiomac.2023.127802
19. Dheyab, M.A., Aziz, A.A., Khaniabadi, P.M., Jameel, M.S., Oladzadabbasabadi, N., Rahman, A.A., et al.: Gold nanoparticles-based photothermal therapy for breast cancer. Photodiag. Photodyn. Ther. **42**, 103312 (2023). https://doi.org/10.1016/j.pdpdt.2023.103312
20. Paley, M.A., Prescher, J.A.: Bioluminescence: a versatile technique for imaging cellular and molecular features. Medchemcomm **5**, 255–67 (2014). https://doi.org/10.1039/C3MD00288H
21. Kossodo, S.: Bioluminescence imaging: in vivo monitoring of tumor development, disease dissemination and treatment efficacy. Labcorp (2020)
22. Song, W.-J., Zhang, F., Wang, Z.-Y., Wang, Z.-S., Wang, B.-Y., Jia, J.-R.: Colorectal cancer mouse metastasis model combining bioluminescent and micro-computed tomography imaging for monitoring the effects of 5-fluorouracil treatment. Transl. Cancer Res. **12**, 2572–2581 (2023). https://doi.org/10.21037/tcr-23-522
23. Borgarelli, C., Klingl, Y.E., Escamilla-Ayala, A., Munck, S., Van Den Bosch, L., De Borggraeve, W.M., et al.: Lighting up the plasma membrane: development and applications of fluorescent ligands for transmembrane proteins. Chem. Europ. J. **27**, 8605–8641 (2021). https://doi.org/10.1002/chem.202100296
24. Li, J., Li, B., Sun, J., Ma, C., Wan, S., Li, Y., et al.: Engineered near-infrared fluorescent protein assemblies for robust bioimaging and therapeutic applications. Adv. Mater. **32** (2020). https://doi.org/10.1002/adma.202000964

25. Das, S., Dey, M.K., Devireddy, R., Gartia, M.R.: Biomarkers in cancer detection, diagnosis, and prognosis. Sensors **24**, 37 (2023). https://doi.org/10.3390/s24010037
26. Wang, D., Wei, M., Zhao, L., Song, T., Li, Q., Tan, J., et al.: Development of a novel fluorescent protein-based probe for efficient detection of Pb2+ in serum inspired by the metalloregulatory protein PbrR691. Anal. Chim. Acta **1305**, 342580 (2024). https://doi.org/10.1016/j.aca.2024.342580
27. Schupper, A.J., Rao, M., Mohammadi, N., Baron, R., Lee, J.Y.K., Acerbi, F., et al.: Fluorescence-guided surgery: a review on timing and use in brain tumor surgery. Front. Neurol. **12** (2021). https://doi.org/10.3389/fneur.2021.682151
28. Stewart, H.L., Birch, D.J.S.: Fluorescence guided surgery. Methods Appl. Fluoresc. **9**, 042002 (2021). https://doi.org/10.1088/2050-6120/ac1dbb
29. Okay, E., Gonzalez, M.R., Werenski, J.O., Sodhi, A., Ozkan, K., Brookes, M., et al.: What is the diagnostic accuracy of fluorescence-guided surgery for margin assessment in appendicular bone and soft tissue tumors?–a systematic review of clinical studies. Surg. Oncol. **52**, 102030 (2024). https://doi.org/10.1016/j.suronc.2023.102030
30. Fadel, M.G., Zonoobi, E., Rodríguez-Luna, M.R., Mishima, K., Ris, F., Diana, M., et al.: Efficacy and safety of fluorescence-guided surgery compared to conventional surgery in the management of colorectal cancer: a systematic review and meta-analysis. Cancers (Basel) **16**, 3377 (2024). https://doi.org/10.3390/cancers16193377
31. Dai, Z., Wang, Z.: Photoactivatable platinum-based anticancer drugs: mode of photoactivation and mechanism of action. Molecules **25**, 5167 (2020). https://doi.org/10.3390/molecules25215167
32. Kim, H.Y., Baldelli, S., Märtson, A.-G., Stocker, S., Alffenaar, J.-W., Cattaneo, D., et al.: Therapeutic drug monitoring of the echinocandin antifungal agents: is there a role in clinical practice? A position statement of the anti-infective drugs committee of the international association of therapeutic drug monitoring and clinical toxicology. Ther. Drug Monit. **44**, 198–214 (2022). https://doi.org/10.1097/FTD.0000000000000931
33. Lemaitre, F., Budde, K., Van Gelder, T., Bergan, S., Lawson, R., Noceti, O., et al.: Therapeutic drug monitoring and dosage adjustments of immunosuppressive drugs when combined with nirmatrelvir/ritonavir in patients With COVID-19. Ther. Drug Monit. **45**, 191–9 (2023). https://doi.org/10.1097/FTD.0000000000001014
34. Medicinal Chemistry and Synthesis Photopharmacology—photolabile caged compounds. Medicinal Chemistry and Synthesis (2024)
35. Banala, S., Arvin, M.C., Bannon, N.M., Jin, X.-T., Macklin, J.J., Wang, Y., et al.: Photoactivatable drugs for nicotinic optopharmacology. Nat. Methods **15**, 347–50 (2018). https://doi.org/10.1038/nmeth.4637
36. Wang, G., Zhang, M., Lai, W., Gao, Y., Liao, S., Ning, Q., et al.: Tumor microenvironment responsive RNA drug delivery systems: intelligent platforms for sophisticated release. Mol. Pharm. **21**, 4217–37 (2024). https://doi.org/10.1021/acs.molpharmaceut.4c00334
37. Abdelhamid, M.S., Wadan, A.-H.S., Saad, H.A., El-Dakroury, W.A., Hageen, A.W., Mohammed, D.H., et al.: Nanoparticle innovations in targeted cancer therapy: advancements in antibody–drug conjugates. Naunyn Schmiedebergs Arch. Pharmacol. (2025). https://doi.org/10.1007/s00210-024-03764-7
38. Abdurashtov, A.S., Proshin, P.I., Sukhorukov, G.B.: The pursuit of linear dosage in pharmacy: reservoir-based drug delivery systems from macro to micro scale. Expert. Opin. Drug Deliv. 1–20 (2025). https://doi.org/10.1080/17425247.2024.2448026
39. Ighodaro, A., Osarobo, J.A., Onuguh, I.C., Ogbeide, O.K., Ifijen, I.H.: Challenges and future perspectives of biomimetic materials for biomedical applications: bridging the gap between nature and medicine. 877–896 (2024). https://doi.org/10.1007/978-3-031-50349-8_76
40. Gaikwad, S.S., Zanje, A.L., Somwanshi, J.D.: Advancements in transdermal drug delivery: a comprehensive review of physical penetration enhancement techniques. Int. J. Pharm. **652**, 123856 (2024). https://doi.org/10.1016/j.ijpharm.2024.123856
41. Liu, W., Liu, L., Li, H., Xie, Y., Bai, J., Guan, J., et al.: Targeted pathophysiological treatment of ischemic stroke using nanoparticle-based drug delivery system. J. Nanobiotechnol. **22**, 499 (2024). https://doi.org/10.1186/s12951-024-02772-2

42. Li, X., Peng, X., Zoulikha, M., Boafo, G.F., Magar, K.T., Ju, Y., et al.: Multifunctional nanoparticle-mediated combining therapy for human diseases. Signal Transduct. Target. Ther. **9**, 1 (2024). https://doi.org/10.1038/s41392-023-01668-1
43. Deshmukh, R., Sethi, P., Singh, B., Shiekmydeen, J., Salave, S., Patel, R.J., et al.: Recent review on biological barriers and host-material interfaces in precision drug delivery: advancement in biomaterial engineering for better treatment therapies. Pharmaceutics **16**, 1076 (2024). https://doi.org/10.3390/pharmaceutics16081076
44. Pei, J., Yan, Y., Palanisamy, C.P., Jayaraman, S., Natarajan, P.M., Umapathy, V.R., et al.: Materials-based drug delivery approaches: recent advances and future perspectives. Green Proc. Synth. **13** (2024). https://doi.org/10.1515/gps-2023-0094
45. Dachani, S.R., Vashi, A., Mundada, A.B., Mundada, P.A., Rudrangi, S.R.S., Rudrangi, S., et al.: Innovative polymers in pharmaceutical chemistry: revolutionizing drug delivery systems. In: Polymer-Plastics Technology and Materials, pp. 1–23 (2024). https://doi.org/10.1080/25740881.2024.2440531
46. Trucillo, P.: Biomaterials for drug delivery and human applications. Materials **17**, 456 (2024). https://doi.org/10.3390/ma17020456
47. Lobel, B.T., Baiocco, D., Al-Sharabi, M., Routh, A.F., Zhang, Z., Cayre, O.J.: Current challenges in microcapsule designs and microencapsulation processes: a review. ACS Appl. Mater. Interfaces **16**, 40326–55 (2024). https://doi.org/10.1021/acsami.4c02462
48. Sharma, A., Singh, M., Sharma, V., Vashishth, A., Raj, M., Upadhyay, S.K., et al.: Current paradigms in employing self-assembled structures: drug delivery implications with improved therapeutic potential. Colloids Surf. B Biointerfaces **234**, 113745 (2024). https://doi.org/10.1016/j.colsurfb.2024.113745
49. Kallepalli, B., Garg, U., Jain, N., Nagpal, R., Malhotra, S., Tiwari, T., et al.: Intelligent drug delivery: pioneering stimuli-responsive systems to revolutionize disease management- an in-depth exploration. Curr. Drug Deliv. **22**, 195–214 (2025). https://doi.org/10.2174/0115672018278641231221051359
50. Shi, J., Tan, C., Ge, X., Qin, Z., Xiong, H.: Recent advances in stimuli-responsive controlled release systems for neuromodulation. J Mater Chem B **12**, 5769–86 (2024). https://doi.org/10.1039/D4TB00720D
51. Wang, L.L.-W., Gao, Y., Feng, Z., Mooney, D.J., Mitragotri, S.: Designing drug delivery systems for cell therapy. Nat. Rev. Bioeng. **2**, 944–959 (2024). https://doi.org/10.1038/s44222-024-00214-0
52. Pandey, V., Pandey, T.: Mechanistic understanding of pH as a driving force in cancer therapeutics. J. Mater. Chem. B (2025). https://doi.org/10.1039/D4TB02083A
53. Agiba, A.M., Elsayyad, N., ElShagea, H.N., Metwalli, M.A., Mahmoudsalehi, A.O., Beigi-Boroujeni, S., et al.: Advances in light-responsive smart multifunctional nanofibers: implications for targeted drug delivery and cancer therapy. Pharmaceutics **16**, 1017 (2024). https://doi.org/10.3390/pharmaceutics16081017
54. Marques, L., Costa, B., Pereira, M., Silva, A., Santos, J., Saldanha, L., et al.: Advancing precision medicine: a review of innovative in silico approaches for drug development. Clinic. Pharmacol. Pers. Healthcare Pharmaceut. **16**, 332 (2024). https://doi.org/10.3390/pharmaceutics16030332
55. Alavi, S.E., Alharthi, S., Alavi, S.Z., Raza, A., Ebrahimi, S.H.: Bioresponsive drug delivery systems. Drug Discov. Today **29**, 103849 (2024). https://doi.org/10.1016/j.drudis.2023.103849
56. Kashani, G.K., Naghib, S.M., Soleymani, S., Mozafari, M.R.: A review of DNA nanoparticles-encapsulated drug/gene/protein for advanced controlled drug release: current status and future perspective over emerging therapy approaches. Int. J. Biol. Macromol. **268**, 131694 (2024). https://doi.org/10.1016/j.ijbiomac.2024.131694
57. Vasić, K., Knez, Ž, Leitgeb, M.: Multifunctional iron oxide nanoparticles as promising magnetic biomaterials in drug delivery: a review. J Funct. Biomater. **15**, 227 (2024). https://doi.org/10.3390/jfb15080227

58. Shi, Y., Zhang, Y., Zhu, L., Miao, Y., Zhu, Y., Yue, B.: Tailored drug delivery platforms: stimulus-responsive core–shell structured nanocarriers. Adv. Healthcare Mater. **13** (2024). https://doi.org/10.1002/adhm.202301726
59. Dhoundiyal, S., Srivastava, S., Kumar, S., Singh, G., Ashique, S., Pal, R., et al.: Radiopharmaceuticals: navigating the frontier of precision medicine and therapeutic innovation. Eur. J. Med. Res. **29**, 26 (2024). https://doi.org/10.1186/s40001-023-01627-0
60. Elumalai, K., Srinivasan, S., Shanmugam, A.: Review of the efficacy of nanoparticle-based drug delivery systems for cancer treatment. Biomed. Technol. **5**, 109–22 (2024). https://doi.org/10.1016/j.bmt.2023.09.001
61. Zhang, Q., Kuang, G., Wang, L., Fan, L., Zhao, Y.: Tailoring drug delivery systems by microfluidics for tumor therapy. Mater. Today **73**, 151–78 (2024). https://doi.org/10.1016/j.mattod.2024.01.004
62. Prakash, O., Verma, D., Singh, P.C.: Exploring enzyme-immobilized MOFs and their application potential: biosensing, biocatalysis, targeted drug delivery and cancer therapy. J. Mater. Chem. B **12**, 10198–214 (2024). https://doi.org/10.1039/D4TB01556H
63. Desai, N., Sahel, D., Kubal, B., Postwala, H., Shah, Y., Chavda, V.P., et al.: Role of the extracellular matrix in cancer: insights into tumor progression and therapy. Adv. Ther. (Weinh) (2025). https://doi.org/10.1002/adtp.202400370
64. Gamal, O., Agamey, T.A, Mohamed, A.Z, El-Sherbiny, I.M.: Revolutionizing lung cancer treatment with smart pulmonary drug delivery nanosystems. J. Drug Deliv. Sci. Technol. **101**, 106158 (2024). https://doi.org/10.1016/j.jddst.2024.106158
65. Zong, L., Xu, H., Zhang, H., Tu, Z., Zhang, X., Wang, S., et al.: A review of matrix metalloproteinase-2-sensitive nanoparticles as a novel drug delivery for tumor therapy. Int. J. Biol. Macromol. **262**, 130043 (2024). https://doi.org/10.1016/j.ijbiomac.2024.130043
66. Wang, Z., Sun, Y., Shen, Y., Zhou, Z.: Stimuli-responsive nanocarriers for transcytosis-based cancer drug delivery. Adv. Nanobiomed. Res. **4** (2024). https://doi.org/10.1002/anbr.202300125
67. Zhang, H., Song, J., Ward, R., Han, Y., Hunt, A., Shriwas, P., et al.: Diverse temporal and spatial mechanisms work, partially through Stanniocalcin-1, V-ATPase and senescence, to activate the extracellular ATP-mediated drug resistance in human cancer cells. Front. Oncol. **14** (2024). https://doi.org/10.3389/fonc.2024.1276092
68. Meng, X., Shen, Y., Zhao, H., Lu, X., Wang, Z., Zhao, Y.: Redox-manipulating nanocarriers for anticancer drug delivery: a systematic review. J. Nanobiotechnol. **22**, 587 (2024). https://doi.org/10.1186/s12951-024-02859-w
69. Rahimi, M., Gałęziewska, M., Jerczyński, K., Wróbel, S., Pietrasik, J.: Non-linear functional polymers containing selective/cleavable bonds: Synthesis and their biomedical applications. Polym. Adv. Technol. **35** (2024). https://doi.org/10.1002/pat.6387
70. Karthika, V., Sridharan, B., Nam, J.W., Kim, D., Gyun Lim, H.: Neuromodulation by nanozymes and ultrasound during Alzheimer's disease management. J. Nanobiotechnol. **22**, 139 (2024). https://doi.org/10.1186/s12951-024-02406-7
71. Aundhia, C., Parmar, G., Talele, C., kardani, S., Maheshwari, R.: Light-responsive polymers: developments in drug delivery systems. Curr. Org. Chem. **28**, 1179–1189 (2024). https://doi.org/10.2174/0113852728307241240430055059
72. Park, D., Lee, S.J., Park, J.-W.: Aptamer-based smart targeting and spatial trigger-response drug-delivery systems for anticancer therapy. Biomedicines **12**, 187 (2024). https://doi.org/10.3390/biomedicines12010187
73. Fu, Y., Simeth, N.A., Szymanski, W., Feringa, B.L.: Visible and near-infrared light-induced photoclick reactions. Nat. Rev. Chem. **8**, 665–85 (2024). https://doi.org/10.1038/s41570-024-00633-y
74. Rajasekar, M., Kavyashree, V., Sangamithra, E., Baskaran, P., Faustina Maria, M., Mary, J., et al.: Review on biomaterial applications of photoresponsive based chromophore hydrogels: recent developments and future perspectives. Results Chem. **7**, 101462 (2024). https://doi.org/10.1016/j.rechem.2024.101462

75. Feng, Q., Zhou, X., He, C.: <scp>NIR</scp> light-facilitated bone tissue engineering. In: WIREs Nanomedicine and Nanobiotechnology, vol. 16 (2024). https://doi.org/10.1002/wnan.1925
76. Xie, M., Meng, F., Wang, P., Díaz-García, A., Parkhats, M., Santos-Oliveira, R., et al.: Surface engineering of magnetic iron oxide nanoparticles for breast cancer diagnostics and drug delivery. Int. J. Nanomed. **19**, 8437–61 (2024). https://doi.org/10.2147/IJN.S477652
77. Szwed, M., Marczak, A.: Application of nanoparticles for magnetic hyperthermia for cancer treatment—the current state of knowledge. Cancers (Basel) **16**, 1156 (2024). https://doi.org/10.3390/cancers16061156
78. Salmanpour, Z., Abolmaali, S.S., Farahavar, G., Salmanpour, M., Tamaddon, A.M.: Magnetic nanoparticles and their hybrid biomaterials for drug delivery and theranostic applications in cardiovascular diseases. J. Drug Deliv. Sci. Technol. **96**, 105676 (2024). https://doi.org/10.1016/j.jddst.2024.105676
79. Huang, H., Zheng, Y., Chang, M., Song, J., Xia, L., Wu, C., et al.: Ultrasound-based micro-/nanosystems for biomedical applications. Chem. Rev. **124**, 8307–472 (2024). https://doi.org/10.1021/acs.chemrev.4c00009
80. Al Refaai, K.A., AlSawaftah, N.A., Abuwatfa, W., Husseini, G.A.: Drug release via ultrasound-activated nanocarriers for cancer treatment: a review. Pharmaceutics **16**, 1383 (2024). https://doi.org/10.3390/pharmaceutics16111383
81. Hu, H., Busa, P., Zhao, Y., Zhao, C.: Externally triggered drug delivery systems. Smart Mater. Med. **5**, 386–408 (2024). https://doi.org/10.1016/j.smaim.2024.08.004
82. Han, B., Liu, Y., Zhou, Q., Yu, Y., Liu, X., Guo, Y., et al.: The advance of ultrasound-enabled diagnostics and therapeutics. J. Control. Release **375**, 1–19 (2024). https://doi.org/10.1016/j.jconrel.2024.08.039
83. Banerjee, T., Sen, K.: Liposomal encapsulation of different anticancer drugs: an effective drug delivery technique. Bionanoscience **14**, 3476–95 (2024). https://doi.org/10.1007/s12668-024-01580-0
84. Kuperkar, K., Atanase, L., Bahadur, A., Crivei, I., Bahadur, P.: Degradable polymeric bio(nano)materials and their biomedical applications: a comprehensive overview and recent updates. Polymers (Basel) **16**, 206 (2024). https://doi.org/10.3390/polym16020206
85. Samia, S., Sandeep Chary, P., Khan, O., Kumar, M.N.: Recent trends and advances in novel formulations as an armament in Bcl-2/Bax targeted breast cancer. Int. J. Pharm. **653**, 123889 (2024). https://doi.org/10.1016/j.ijpharm.2024.123889
86. Ali, A., Muslim, M., Kamaal, S., Ahmad, M.: Kind and role of linkers for metal–organic frameworks. In: Synthesis of Metal-Organic Frameworks Via Water-based Routes, pp. 35–50. Elsevier (2024). https://doi.org/10.1016/B978-0-323-95939-1.00007-1
87. Vikal, A., Maurya, R., Patel, P., Paliwal, S.R., Narang, R.K., Gupta, G.D., et al.: Exploring metal-organic frameworks (MOFs) in drug delivery: a concise overview of synthesis approaches, versatile applications, and current challenges. Appl. Mater. Today **41**, 102443 (2024). https://doi.org/10.1016/j.apmt.2024.102443
88. Peng, Y., Li, S.J., Yan, J., Tang, Y., Cheng, J.P., Gao, A.J., et al.: Research progress on phytopathogenic fungi and their role as biocontrol agents. Front. Microbiol. **12** (2021). https://doi.org/10.3389/fmicb.2021.670135
89. Pal, P., Sambhakar, S., Paliwal, S.: Revolutionizing ophthalmic care: a review of ocular hydrogels from pathologies to therapeutic applications. Curr. Eye Res. **50**, 1–17 (2025). https://doi.org/10.1080/02713683.2024.2396385
90. Kumar, D., Pandey, S., Shiekmydeen, J., Kumar, M., Chopra, S., Bhatia, A.: Therapeutic potential of microneedle assisted drug delivery for wound healing: current state of the art, challenges, and future perspective. AAPS PharmSciTech **26**, 25 (2025). https://doi.org/10.1208/s12249-024-03017-z
91. Shahi, F., Afshar, H., Dawi, E.A., Khonakdar, H.A.: Smart microneedles in biomedical engineering: harnessing stimuli-responsive polymers for novel applications. Polym. Adv. Technol. **35** (2024). https://doi.org/10.1002/pat.70020

92. Lv, X., Xiang, C., Zheng, Y., Zhou, W.-X., Lv, X.-L.: Recent developments in using microneedle patch technology as a more efficient drug delivery system for treating skin photoaging. Clin. Cosmet. Investig. Dermatol. **17**, 2417–26 (2024). https://doi.org/10.2147/CCID.S492774
93. Oliveira, C., Teixeira, J.A., Oliveira, N., Ferreira, S., Botelho, C.M.: Microneedles' device: design, fabrication, and applications. Macromol **4**, 320–55 (2024). https://doi.org/10.3390/macromol4020019
94. Liu, W., Zhang, B., Liu, T., Jiang, J., Liu, Y.: Artificial intelligence in pancreatic image analysis: a review. Sensors **24**, 4749 (2024). https://doi.org/10.3390/s24144749
95. Umadevi, K., Sundeep, D., Vighnesh, A.R., Misra, A., Krishna, A.G.: Current trends and advances in nanoplatforms-based imaging for cancer diagnosis. Indian J. Microbiol. (2024). https://doi.org/10.1007/s12088-024-01373-9
96. Bischof, J., Fletcher, G., Verkade, P., Kuntner, C., Fernandez-Rodriguez, J., Chaabane, L., et al.: Multimodal bioimaging across disciplines and scales: challenges, opportunities and breaking down barriers. Npj Imaging **2**, 5 (2024). https://doi.org/10.1038/s44303-024-00010-w
97. Khalighi, S., Reddy, K., Midya, A., Pandav, K.B., Madabhushi, A., Abedalthagafi, M.: Artificial intelligence in neuro-oncology: advances and challenges in brain tumor diagnosis, prognosis, and precision treatment. NPJ Precis Oncol. **8**, 80 (2024). https://doi.org/10.1038/s41698-024-00575-0
98. Duan, J., Xiong, J., Li, Y., Ding, W.: Deep learning based multimodal biomedical data fusion: an overview and comparative review. Inform. Fusion **112**, 102536 (2024). https://doi.org/10.1016/j.inffus.2024.102536
99. Alanazi, M.M.F.: Advancements in hybrid imaging techniques: enhancing diagnostic accuracy with PET/MRI and PET/CT. Int. J. Health Sci. (Qassim) **8**, 1800–1811 (2024). https://doi.org/10.53730/ijhs.v8nS1.15396
100. Du, L., Roy, S., Wang, P., Li, Z., Qiu, X., Zhang, Y., et al.: Unveiling the future: advancements in MRI imaging for neurodegenerative disorders. Ageing Res. Rev. **95**, 102230 (2024). https://doi.org/10.1016/j.arr.2024.102230
101. Zuo, C., Ge, J., Wang, J., Watanabe, Y., Tian, M.: Molecular imaging for neurological diseases. In: Transpathology, pp. 247–258. Elsevier (2024). https://doi.org/10.1016/B978-0-323-95223-1.00003-5
102. Akbari, B., Huber, B.R., Sherman, J.H.: Unlocking the hidden depths: multi-modal integration of imaging mass spectrometry-based and molecular imaging techniques. Crit. Rev. Anal. Chem. **55**, 109–38 (2025). https://doi.org/10.1080/10408347.2023.2266838
103. Yu, Y., Feng, T., Qiu, H., Gu, Y., Chen, Q., Zuo, C., et al.: Simultaneous photoacoustic and ultrasound imaging: a review. Ultrasonics **139**, 107277 (2024). https://doi.org/10.1016/j.ultras.2024.107277
104. Kuchimaru, T.: Emerging synthetic bioluminescent reactions for non-invasive imaging of freely moving animals. Int. J. Mol. Sci. **25**, 7338 (2024). https://doi.org/10.3390/ijms25137338
105. Shen, X., Pan, D., Gong, Q., Gu, Z., Luo, K.: Enhancing drug penetration in solid tumors via nanomedicine: evaluation models, strategies and perspectives. Bioact. Mater. **32**, 445–72 (2024). https://doi.org/10.1016/j.bioactmat.2023.10.017
106. Liang, A., Kong, Y., Chen, Z., Qiu, Y., Wu, Y., Zhu, X., et al.: Advancements and applications of single-cell multi-omics techniques in cancer research: unveiling heterogeneity and paving the way for precision therapeutics. Biochem. Biophys. Rep. **37**, 101589 (2024). https://doi.org/10.1016/j.bbrep.2023.101589
107. Liang, Z., Geng, G., Song, Q., Tang, M.: A time-synchronized multimodal monitoring system for general anesthesia. Med. Nov. Technol. Devices **23**, 100324 (2024). https://doi.org/10.1016/j.medntd.2024.100324
108. Kastelik-Hryniewiecka, A., Jewula, P., Bakalorz, K., Kramer-Marek, G., Kuźnik, N.: Targeted PET/MRI imaging super probes: a critical review of opportunities and challenges. Int. J. Nanomed. **16**, 8465–83 (2022). https://doi.org/10.2147/IJN.S336299

109. Boehm, K.M., Khosravi, P., Vanguri, R., Gao, J., Shah, S.P.: Harnessing multimodal data integration to advance precision oncology. Nat. Rev. Cancer **22**, 114–26 (2022). https://doi.org/10.1038/s41568-021-00408-3
110. Hussain, D., Abbas, N., Khan, J.: Recent breakthroughs in PET-CT multimodality imaging: innovations and clinical impact. Bioengineering **11**, 1213 (2024). https://doi.org/10.3390/bioengineering11121213
111. Xue, Q., Yang, Y., Ma, W., Zhang, H., Zhang, D., Lan, X., et al.: Advances in miniaturized computational spectrometers. Adv. Sci. **11** (2024). https://doi.org/10.1002/advs.202404448
112. Calatayud, D.G., Neophytou, S., Nicodemou, E., Giuffrida, S.G., Ge, H., Pascu, S.I.: Nano-theranostics for the sensing, imaging and therapy of prostate cancers. Front. Chem. **10** (2022). https://doi.org/10.3389/fchem.2022.830133
113. Wang, B., Li, Y., Zhou, M., Han, Y., Zhang, M., Gao, Z., et al.: Smartphone-based platforms implementing microfluidic detection with image-based artificial intelligence. Nat. Commun. **14**, 1341 (2023). https://doi.org/10.1038/s41467-023-36017-x
114. Zhang, X., Leng, C., Hong, Y., Pei, Z., Cheng, I., Basu, A.: Multimodal remote sensing image registration methods and advancements: a survey. Remote Sens. (Basel) **13**, 5128 (2021). https://doi.org/10.3390/rs13245128
115. Xu, X., Li, J., Zhu, Z., Zhao, L., Wang, H., Song, C., et al.: A comprehensive review on synergy of multi-modal data and AI technologies in medical diagnosis. Bioengineering **11**, 219 (2024). https://doi.org/10.3390/bioengineering11030219
116. Darzi, F., Bocklitz, T.: A review of medical image registration for different modalities. Bioengineering **11**, 786 (2024). https://doi.org/10.3390/bioengineering11080786
117. Zhang, Z., Du, Y., Shi, X., Wang, K., Qu, Q., Liang, Q., et al.: NIR-II light in clinical oncology: opportunities and challenges. Nat. Rev. Clin. Oncol. **21**, 449–67 (2024). https://doi.org/10.1038/s41571-024-00892-0
118. Tursunalieva, A., Alexander, D.L.J., Dunne, R., Li, J., Riera, L., Zhao, Y.: Making sense of machine learning: a review of interpretation techniques and their applications. Appl. Sci. **14**, 496 (2024). https://doi.org/10.3390/app14020496
119. Altinbasak, I., Alp, Y., Sanyal, R., Sanyal, A.: Theranostic nanogels: multifunctional agents for simultaneous therapeutic delivery and diagnostic imaging. Nanoscale **16**, 14033–56 (2024). https://doi.org/10.1039/D4NR01423E
120. Neilio, J.M., Ginat, D.T.: Emerging head and neck tumor targeting contrast agents for the purpose of CT, MRI, and multimodal diagnostic imaging: a molecular review. Diagnostics **14**, 1666 (2024). https://doi.org/10.3390/diagnostics14151666
121. Mhlanga, N., Mphuthi, N., Van der Walt, H., Nyembe, S., Mokhena, T., Sikhwivhilu, L.: Nanostructures and nanoparticles as medical diagnostic imaging contrast agents: a review. Mater. Today Chem. **40**, 102233 (2024). https://doi.org/10.1016/j.mtchem.2024.102233
122. Al-Thani, A.N., Jan, A.G., Abbas, M., Geetha, M., Sadasivuni, K.K.: Nanoparticles in cancer theragnostic and drug delivery: a comprehensive review. Life Sci. **352**, 122899 (2024). https://doi.org/10.1016/j.lfs.2024.122899
123. Abaei, S., Tarighatnia, A., Mesbahi, A., Aghanejad, A.: Antibody conjugates as CT/MRI Theranostics for diagnosis of cancers: a review of recent trends and advances. Sens. Diagn. **3**, 1428–41 (2024). https://doi.org/10.1039/D4SD00132J
124. Shen, Q., Song, G., Lin, H., Bai, H., Huang, Y., Lv, F., et al.: Sensing, imaging, and therapeutic strategies endowing by conjugate polymers for precision medicine. Adv. Mater. **36** (2024). https://doi.org/10.1002/adma.202310032
125. Wang, J., Jia, R., Wan, W., Han, H., Wang, G., Li, Z., et al.: Drug delivery targeting neuroinflammation to treat brain diseases. Bioconjug. Chem. **35**, 1687–98 (2024). https://doi.org/10.1021/acs.bioconjchem.4c00414
126. Wang, X., Wang, Y.-F., Wang, S.-J.: Value of molecular typing combined with integrated positron emission tomography/magnetic resonance imaging in risk stratification of endometrial cancer. Int. J. Womens Health **16**, 831–42 (2024). https://doi.org/10.2147/IJWH.S444046

Challenges, Future Directions, and Emerging Applications

Regulatory Considerations for Biocompatible Light Emitters

Sumreen Arfan, Rikza Saleem, Laiba Irshad, Muhammad Anas, Waseem Ahmed Khattak, Muhammad Majeed, Jamila Naz, Aftab Umar, Tufail Ahmad, and Muhammad Ramzan

Abstract The creation of innovative biocompatible substances has broadened the range of medical uses, especially in diagnostics, therapeutics, and tissue engineering. Among these, biodegradable polymers show great promise. Regulatory considerations for biocompatible light emitters focus on ensuring the safety and efficacy of these devices in medical applications. This chapter outlines the necessary guidelines and standards that must be adhered to during the development and testing phases, emphasizing the importance of thorough preclinical evaluations and clinical trials. Additionally, it discusses the role of regulatory bodies in overseeing compliance with existing regulations, as well as the need for ongoing monitoring post-approval to address any emerging safety concerns or technological advancements. Effective communication between manufacturers and regulatory agencies is crucial for

S. Arfan · M. Majeed (✉)
Department of Botany, University of Gujrat, Punjab 50700, Pakistan
e-mail: m.majeed@uog.edu.pk; majeedmohal@gmail.com

R. Saleem
Department of Radiology and Imaging Technology, Government College University, Faisalabad, Punjab, Pakistan

L. Irshad
Department of Orthotics and Prosthetics, Government College University, Faisalabad, Punjab, Pakistan

M. Anas · W. Ahmed Khattak
Department of Plant Sciences, Faculty of Biological Sciences, Quaid-I-Azam University, Islamabad, Pakistan

M. Anas
Department of Soil Science and Plant Nutrition, University of Selcuk Campus, Konya, Turkey

J. Naz
Department of Forestry and Range Management, Bahauddin Zakariya University, Multan, Punjab, Pakistan

A. Umar
Department of Botany, University of Agriculture, Faisalabad, Punjab, Pakistan

T. Ahmad · M. Ramzan
Department of Botany, Government Graduate College, Layyah, Punjab, Pakistan

© The Author(s), under exclusive license to Springer Nature Switzerland AG 2025

N. O. Etafo (ed.), *Tailored Light Emitters For Biomedical Applications*, Engineering Materials, https://doi.org/10.1007/978-3-031-88731-4_14

navigating the complex landscape of biocompatible light emitter approval, ensuring that innovations can be safely integrated into clinical practice while maintaining patient safety as a top priority. This collaborative effort will facilitate the establishment of standardized testing protocols and guidelines, ensuring that new innovations meet rigorous safety and performance criteria before reaching the market. Such measures will ultimately lead to greater transparency and accountability in the industry, encouraging further investment and innovation while safeguarding public health.

1 Biocompatibility Testing and Evaluation

The assessment of biocompatibility is crucial in determining the safety and efficacy of materials and devices intended for medical use. This evaluation examines how a medical device or material interacts with the human body to identify potential hazards, including adverse biological responses. A comprehensive evaluation process is essential to ensure these devices comply with necessary safety requirements prior to clinical use [1]. Internationally recognized standards, like ISO 10993, serve as the basis for biocompatibility assessments, offering manufacturers guidance on evaluating biological risks associated with medical devices. ISO 10993 stands as the most widely accepted international standard for biocompatibility testing. It provides a structure for assessing biological risks, focusing on specific evaluations such as cytotoxicity, sensitization, irritation, and systemic toxicity. These assessments aim to verify that a material or device does not cause harmful effects, either locally or systemically, during its intended application [2]. Moreover, these evaluations consider the duration and nature of bodily contact, spanning from brief skin exposure to long-term implantation. The objective is to anticipate and minimize any adverse reactions that could jeopardize patient safety. In the United States, the Food and Drug Administration (FDA) employs ISO 10993 as a fundamental standard but frequently requires additional testing specific to the material, device, and intended use. Likewise, the European Union's Medical Device Regulation (MDR) imposes strict requirements to ensure biocompatibility, making it imperative for manufacturers to adhere to these regulations to obtain market approval. The MDR outlines a risk-based approach that considers the classification of the medical device, demanding comprehensive documentation to demonstrate compliance with safety and performance standards [3].

Throughout the years, biocompatibility evaluation methods have progressed to keep pace with technological advancements and ethical considerations. A significant development in this field is the emphasis on reducing animal testing. Regulatory bodies, such as the FDA and the European Union, urge manufacturers to adopt alternative methods that decrease or eliminate animal studies [4]. In vitro testing, which involves laboratory-based experiments using cells or tissues, has become a preferred alternative. These methods not only align with ethical principles but also provide faster and more cost-effective results compared to traditional animal testing. In vitro techniques include cytotoxicity assays, which measure the toxic effects of materials on cultured cells, and irritation tests, which assess the inflammatory response of cells or tissues to the device. These methods allow researchers to gain valuable insights into the biocompatibility of materials without the ethical concerns associated with animal testing. Furthermore, computational modeling and simulations are increasingly being utilized to predict biological interactions, further diminishing the reliance on in vivo studies [5]. Another notable advancement is the use of existing data to demonstrate equivalence to previously approved devices. This approach involves leveraging historical biocompatibility data for similar materials or devices to establish their safety profile. By demonstrating equivalence, manufacturers can expedite regulatory approval processes while avoiding redundant testing [6]. This strategy is particularly advantageous for iterative improvements of existing devices, as it allows manufacturers to focus on innovation without compromising safety.

The creation of innovative biocompatible substances has broadened the range of medical uses, especially in diagnostics, therapeutics, and tissue engineering. Among these, biodegradable polymers show great promise. These materials safely break down in the body over time, eliminating the necessity for surgical extraction and lowering the risk of long-term issues. Frequently utilized biodegradable polymers include polylactic acid (PLA), polyglycolic acid (PGA), and their copolymers. These substances undergo extensive testing for cytotoxicity, sensitization, and degradation patterns to ensure their safety and effectiveness [7]. Another exciting advancement is biocompatible optical emitters, such as organic light-emitting diodes (OLEDs) and luminescent nanoclusters. These materials are specifically engineered for use in biological settings, where they can function as diagnostic tools or therapeutic devices. For instance, OLEDs can be employed in optogenetics to control neural activity using light, while luminescent nanoclusters can be used for imaging and sensing applications. Assessing the biocompatibility of these materials involves examining their cytotoxicity, optical stability, and interactions with biological tissues. Research has shown that these materials can be engineered to minimize adverse effects, making them suitable for use in sensitive biological environments. The incorporation of biocompatible materials into medical devices has enabled a wide array of applications. Light-emitting devices, like those used in photodynamic therapy (PDT), utilize biocompatible optical materials to provide targeted treatments for conditions such as cancer and bacterial infections [8]. These devices emit specific light wavelengths to activate photosensitive agents, generating reactive oxygen species that destroy diseased cells while preserving healthy tissue. Biocompatibility testing ensures that these devices do not cause unintended harm to surrounding tissues, improving their safety profile. Likewise, biocompatibility testing is crucial for the development of implantable devices, including pacemakers, neural interfaces, and drug delivery systems. These devices often require extended contact with biological tissues, necessitating thorough testing to prevent adverse reactions like inflammation, fibrosis, or device rejection. By adhering to established biocompatibility standards, manufacturers can ensure the reliability and safety of these life-saving devices.

Although significant progress has been made, biocompatibility testing continues to face numerous obstacles. A key challenge is the variation in biological responses stemming from individual genetic differences, immune system function, and underlying health issues. These factors can make it difficult to interpret test results and underscore the necessity for individualized approaches to biocompatibility assessment. Another hurdle is incorporating cutting-edge technologies like nanomaterials and bioelectronics into existing regulatory frameworks. These innovations often involve novel materials and mechanisms of action, necessitating updated guidelines to address their specific risks and benefits. For example, nanomaterials may exhibit distinct biocompatibility profiles due to their high surface area-to-volume ratio and unique interactions with cellular components. Regulatory agencies must adapt to these advancements by developing tailored standards for their evaluation. The future of biocompatibility testing lies in the ongoing development of alternative methods and advanced materials. Innovations in in vitro testing, such as organ-on-chip technologies, offer the potential to replicate complex biological environments and provide more accurate predictions of device performance. Furthermore, integrating artificial intelligence and machine learning into biocompatibility assessment could expedite the analysis of large datasets, enabling quicker and more precise evaluations. Biocompatibility testing is fundamental to medical device development, ensuring that materials and devices are safe and effective for their intended use. By adhering to established standards like ISO 10993 and embracing advancements in testing methods and materials, manufacturers can meet regulatory requirements while minimizing patient risks. The emergence of biocompatible and biodegradable materials, along with innovations in testing methodologies, continues to expand the possibilities for medical applications. As the field evolves, adopting alternative testing methods and developing personalized approaches will be crucial in addressing the challenges of biocompatibility evaluation and advancing the safety and effectiveness of medical devices [9].

2 Regulatory Pathways for Medical Devices

The regulatory pathways for medical devices are intricate and differ significantly across regions, reflecting variations in standards, classifications and approval processes. These pathways aim to ensure that medical devices are safe, effective, and reliable for clinical use, particularly when dealing with technologies such as biocompatible light-emitting devices and other innovative solutions [10]. In the United States, the Food and Drug Administration (FDA) oversees medical devices under the Federal Food, Drug, and Cosmetic Act. The FDA categorizes devices into three classes based on their risk to patients: Class I, Class II, and Class III. Class I devices present the lowest risk and are subject to general controls, such as proper labeling and manufacturing practices. Examples include bandages or tongue depressors. Class II devices carry moderate risks and require additional special controls, such as performance standards and post-market surveillance [11]. Biocompatible light-emitting devices, often used in diagnostic or therapeutic applications, typically fall into Class II and are cleared through the 510(k) premarket notification process. This pathway requires manufacturers to demonstrate that the device is substantially equivalent to a previously approved or legally marketed device (a predicate device). Class III devices, which present the highest risks, such as life-supporting or life-sustaining implants, require premarket approval (PMA). Safety and effectiveness testing along with scientific evaluation regulate the process before approval can be granted. Application for a PMA demands more stringency than 510(k) application through rigorously extensive testing in combination with systematic documentation requirements. To obtain Class III classification for new light-emitting devices and those employing biodegradable polymers or uniquely risky components manufacturers need established predicate devices or must demonstrate device-specific safety advantages. Medical devices receive their biological safety assessment through the globally recognized standard ISO 10993. Through its set of evaluations, the comprehensive framework enables manufacturers to conduct tests for cytotoxicity and sensitization as well as irritation and systemic toxicity assessment [12]. Through standard biocompatibility testing methods established in ISO 10993 manufacturers gain worldwide acceptance along with regulatory compliance for their medical products. Although ISO 10993 establishes the core principles for biological safety assessments it does not eliminate the need for adaptations which particular countries implement to their regulatory systems (Fig. 1).

The Medical Device Regulation (MDR) implemented in 2021 by the European Union (EU) introduces more rigorous regulatory standards compared to the previous Medical Device Directive (MDD). The MDR places greater emphasis on thorough clinical evaluation, post-market monitoring, and transparency throughout a product's lifespan [13]. It also mandates a more comprehensive biocompatibility assessment, particularly for devices intended for long-term use or implantation. For example, light-emitting devices with biocompatible properties marketed in the EU must comply with MDR standards, which require extensive preclinical and clinical data to

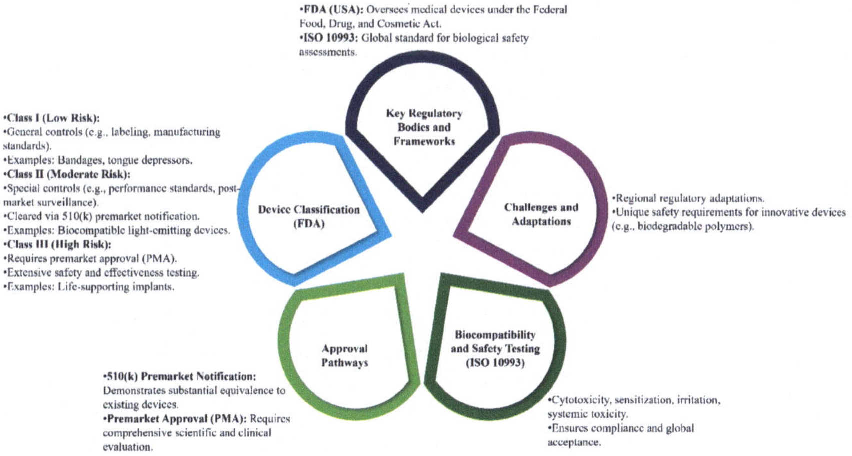

Fig. 1 Regulatory pathways for medical devices

prove safety and efficacy. Other countries, such as Japan and Canada, have their own regulatory bodies and standards, often incorporating ISO guidelines while adding specific requirements. These differences underscore the necessity of understanding regional regulations and adapting development and documentation processes accordingly. Innovative medical products, including 3D-printed and biodegradable devices, present unique regulatory challenges. Unlike conventional manufacturing techniques, 3D printing enables highly customizable and intricate designs. While this technology offers significant benefits, such as patient-specific implants and reduced waste, it also raises concerns about consistency and reproducibility. Regulatory agencies require manufacturers to address these issues through comprehensive design validation and quality control measures. For instance, 3D-printed devices must demonstrate that material properties, layer-by-layer construction, and post-processing techniques meet stringent standards. Biodegradable devices, such as light-emitting materials designed for temporary diagnostic or therapeutic applications, face additional scrutiny due to their interaction with biological systems [14]. These devices must demonstrate biocompatibility not only in their initial state but also as they break down. The evaluation includes testing for cytotoxicity, irritation, and systemic effects of the byproducts released during degradation. Regulatory bodies often require long-term studies to assess these factors and ensure patient safety. Sterilization is another crucial aspect of regulatory compliance for medical devices, especially those intended for implantable or invasive use. Devices must undergo thorough sterilization validation to ensure that manufacturing processes eliminate microbial contaminants without compromising material integrity or functionality [15]. Regulatory authorities require manufacturers to provide detailed documentation of sterilization methods, such as ethylene oxide, gamma radiation, or autoclaving, as well as their impact on device performance. Post-market surveillance is equally important in ensuring ongoing safety and compliance. Manufacturers are obligated to monitor devices after market entry, reporting any adverse events or malfunctions to regulatory authorities. This process helps identify potential issues early and enables corrective actions, such as recalls or design modifications [16].

The global trend of aligning regulatory standards aims to minimize obstacles in worldwide device development and distribution. Organizations like the International Medical Device Regulators Forum (IMDRF) work towards unifying regulatory requirements across different regions, enhancing consistency and efficiency. IMDRF's guidelines on clinical evaluation and risk management, for instance, have contributed to a more streamlined regulatory process for cutting-edge devices. As medical technology advances, regulatory frameworks must evolve to tackle new challenges [17]. Emerging fields such as digital health technologies, artificial intelligence, and nanomaterials will necessitate updated guidelines and evaluation methods [18]. Regulatory bodies are increasingly adopting risk-based approaches, utilizing advanced modeling, simulation, and in vitro testing to decrease dependence on animal studies and expedite device approval. The regulatory pathways for medical devices strive to strike a balance between innovation and safety, ensuring that novel technologies offer concrete benefits without introducing unwarranted risks. While established frameworks like FDA classifications and ISO 10993 provide clear guidance, manufacturers must contend with regional differences and address the unique challenges presented by emerging technologies. For innovative devices, including those that emit light, success hinges on a proactive approach to design validation, biocompatibility evaluation and regulatory compliance [19]. By adhering to stringent standards and embracing harmonization efforts, manufacturers can introduce safe and effective medical devices to the market, ultimately improving healthcare outcomes on a global scale [20].

3 Best Practices for Safety and Compliance

Medical device development needs absolute safety and compliance standards because these devices enter regulated sensitive use environments. The achievement of these intended goals needs holistic best practices combining risk management with adherence to regulatory requirements while conducting standardized testing methods. Followed medical safety guidelines ensure patient protection simultaneously with speedier regulatory review procedures leading to better reliable medical devices. Safety and compliant results depend on an approach based on assessing risk levels. Risk management requires a structured process to discover and assess and solve possible device hazards that persist from product development through all stages of patient use. The ISO 14971 standard provides worldwide guidelines for medical device risk management through evaluation of material risks and process risks and expected use risks. The product-process becomes more manufacturable after manufacturers identify such critical risks as material toxicity and mechanical failure and possible product contamination. Risk assessments start with defining how a device interacts with biological systems [21]. The assessment of light-emitting and biodegradable devices must explore toxicology for cells alongside tissue distress factors and how materials break down with time. Manufacturers use pre-clinical tests to obtain important data about product hazards that they use to rectify design flaws during the early production stages. The selection of safe materials combined with risk reduction methods makes a vital contribution toward reducing complications after device implantation. Medical device compliance together with safety verification requires strict adherence to existing regulatory standards. The ISO 10993 series represent a foundational global standard that checks device compatibility through testing methods designed to assess cytotoxicity sensitization inflammation and DNA damage effects. Manufacturers who implement these guidelines produce devices which fulfill international safety measures and performance standards appropriate for their design purpose. ISO standards stand vital to regulatory approval from the U.S. Food and Drug Administration (FDA) and the European Union's Medical Device Regulation (MDR) because both authorities establish ISO compliance as a mandatory requirement. Both the FDA and MDR regulatory bodies need clinical evaluations to assess device safety through this process. Here the device undergoes testing under

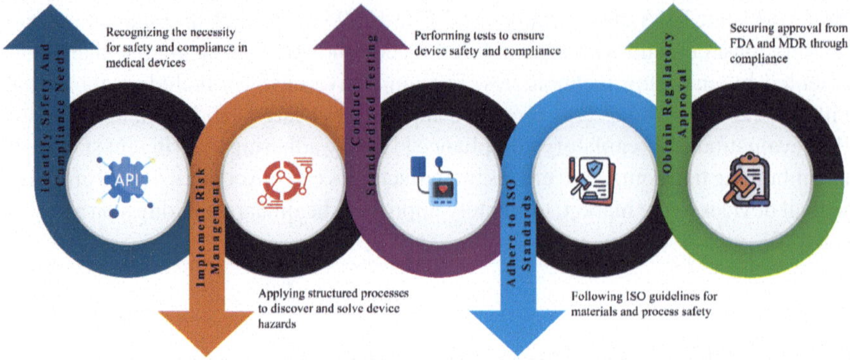

Fig. 2 Medical devices development and compliance process

both simulated and realistic usage environments to verify its secure and productive performance [22]. Clinical trials for light-emitting devices evaluate parameters including heat dissipation together with wavelength safety combined with the assessment of phototoxicity potential. Pre-clinical and clinical evaluations which focus on safety requirements help obtain comprehensive regulatory acceptance through their appropriate execution (Fig. 2).

The implementation of detailed biological evaluation plans based on ISO 10993 standards drastically enhances regulatory ease. Biological evaluation plans consist of three main elements: risk assessment, endpoint identification and proper testing method selection. The assessment of materials with extended tissue or fluid exposure requires performing both long-term toxicity and material degradation studies which are essential components of the evaluation process. Orders that undergo testing require integrated frameworks which manage risks to confirm that testing levels align with actual device risk levels. When manufacturers modify original materials or devices for use they conduct equivalence studies that prove regulatory compliance. Studies which reuse regulatory data demonstrate that new devices act similarly to approved products thus potentially skipping substantial testing requirements. Approval timelines become shorter when manufacturers adopt this method consistent with ISO recommendations to delete repeating information. Device safety depends heavily on sterilization because it applies specifically to devices which must be implanted or used repeatedly [23]. The device becomes suitable for clinical use because proper sterilization protocol enforcement removes dangerous microorganisms. The FDA and ISO establish detailed sterilization validation requirements which specify steam along with ethylene oxide and gamma radiation among possible methods. The method selection must happen after considering device material composition and functional requirements. The evaluation of device physical properties and performance following sterilization takes place through post-sterilization testing protocols [24]. Post-sterilization processes could modify the optical properties as well as mechanical strength of light-emitting devices which would endanger their safety and decrease their performance capabilities. Manufacturers need to create verified sterilization methods that defend both device structural quality and fulfill regulatory safety requirements [25].

The adherence to quality standards including ISO 13485 represents a critical best practice for medical device manufacturing. The standard demands organizations to maintain ongoing documentation linking all processes and maintain consistent control procedures across device production phases. Operating with robust quality management systems enables manufacturers to discover manufacturing problems before production therefore decreasing their chances of producing defective devices. The maintenance of compliance depends heavily on post-market surveillance practices. Regulatory frameworks like MDR require manufacturers to perform ongoing device performance monitoring after release into the market through programs that resolve safety issues which emerge. Healthcare providers together with end-users gather essential feedback which serves to enhance device designs while reducing the potential risks. The implementation of these best practices helps manufacturers overcome substantial regulatory obstacles. The combination of risk assessment methodology and ISO and FDA regulatory standards enables device manufacturers to design safe products which remain compliant [26]. Medical devices achieve enhanced safety through the combination of detailed biological evaluation plans along with validated sterilization procedures and robust post-market surveillance and quality management systems which guarantee long-term reliability.

4 Ethical Considerations for Medical Devices

Ethical priorities guide medical device advancement throughout their development pipeline and subsequent FDA review process leading to final approval while impacting patient treatment and care following deployment. Medical devices spanning basic tools such as syringes to complex biocompatible LEDs and photonic implants directly influence patient medical outcomes and health improvement. Medical devices must meet their regulatory duty along with safety standards that make patients secure while fostering access fairness through societal considerations about technological advancements. Medical device development must follow patient safety as its primary ethical duty [27]. The evaluation process combines pre-clinical assessments with clinical examinations to guarantee device safety when used properly. Increasingly popular biocompatible light-emitting devices require comprehensive evaluations regarding their chemical characteristics alongside potential degradation and tissue engagement effects for use in ontogenetic and therapeutic fields. Failure to recognize and manage product risks leads to patient harm and breaks the "do no harm" medical rule. Strict enforcement of patient safety standards through regulatory frameworks like ISO 10993 and the U.S. FDA's Good Laboratory Practice (GLP) guidance helps safeguard patient health. Manufacturers should advance beyond regulatory compliance by implementing active risk management programs together with real-time performance assessment and solving future safety matters once their devices obtain market authorization [28]. Medical device development requires minimizing risks as an essential ethical principle. Future technological advancements inevitably require products or production methods which are virgin to both regulatory authorities and clinical application frameworks such as biodegradable polymers and advanced photonic systems. New medical device innovations require testing procedures to identify toxicity risks alongside irritations risks and possible long-term systemic consequences. The ethical demand necessitates the reduction of these potential safety threats by using intelligent engineering strategies combined with elaborate testing protocols and regulatory requirements. The medical field works on establishing alternative assessment techniques which help minimize exposure risks to research participants including both human and animal subjects. The development of in vitro testing techniques and computational models now allows scientists to forecast how materials engage with biological processes while performing testing outside of laboratory animals. Scientists can now validate medical device safety by using organ-on-chip technologies alongside 3D cell culture systems that replicate human tissue conditions. The ethical procedure of obtaining informed consent becomes essential when medical devices incorporate new experimental technologies. All medical device users need to grasp all aspects of their potential advantages and disadvantages together with uncertain factors regarding device functionality. Biocompatible LEDs and photonic implants developed for targeted therapies or diagnostics often demonstrate unknown long-term results because of their original design features [29]. Patients must learn about treatment uncertainties according to ethical standards while preserving their right to freely choose medical interventions (Fig. 3).

Transparent communication represents an important requirement across both clinical research and marketing endeavors. Medical device manufacturers and healthcare providers need to deliver precise information about their devices' intended purposes and safety characteristics along with their operational boundaries. Unreliable medical device claims concerning product safety and effectiveness cause damage

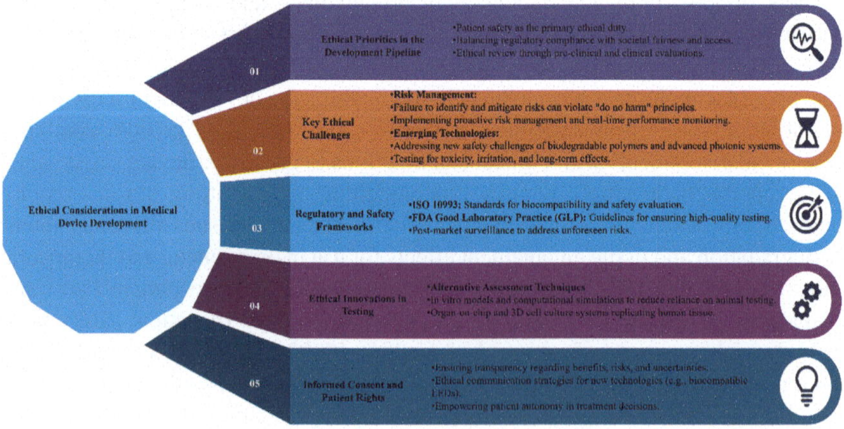

Fig. 3 The figure outlines key ethical priorities in medical device advancement, including

to public trust through ethical misconduct that involved products like metal-on-metal hip replacements. Historically animal testing served as medical device evaluation's foundation but appliance manufacturers and regulators initiate numerous ethical animal welfare approaches to decrease its use [30]. Modern medical device testing must rely on alternative methods according to requirements established by regulatory bodies such as FDA and the European Medicines Agency (EMA). The ISO 10993 guidelines endorse a risk-based strategy which elevates in vitro testing and computational studies above in vivo testing approaches. These alternative testing methods combine ethical compliance with faster and more affordable evaluation processes. When animal testing proves essential for research investigators must establish strict protocols which actively work to reduce both suffering and pain of tested animals [31]. The 3Rs principle functions as a framework for scientists to select non-animal research methods while simultaneously minimizing experimental animal usage through better methods which improve animal wellness. Medical device distribution patterns require equal attention in ethical frameworks of investigation. Average populations within low-income regions lack access to advanced medical technologies because of healthcare inequalities throughout the world. Manufacturers must pursue affordable solution development which maintains safety performance levels while maintaining high efficacy. Unaffordable biocompatible photonic devices may find new market opportunities through their cost-effective versions targeting underserved patient communities [32].

Three strategic initiatives consisting of price tiering, local production alliances and easier medical device designs assist in connecting high-tech innovation with access for underserved countries. Affordable devices reaching low-resource settings receive support from both regulatory entities together with non-governmental organizations through their work in distribution and approval processes. Neomorphic medical device innovations including optogenetics and regenerative medicine along with wearable technologies create distinct ethical dilemmas because of their rapidly evolving nature. Medical device developers need to manage competing demands between achievement of innovation and managing ethical considerations. The implementation of implantable photonic devices in neurological stimulation creates ethical dilemmas which scrutinize patient privacy while questioning both individual autonomy and the risk of device manipulation. Medical device research needs ethical oversight committees to work with multidisciplinary experts who combine scientific expertise with ethical insight and societal concerns [33]. Medical devices provide new ethical dilemmas as we explore their environmental effects during manufacture and use. The medical waste composition is influenced by single-use disposables such as syringes and catheters combined with the energetically demanding processes required to produce medical devices. Manufacturers now focus on developing sustainable materials and production methods which lower their environmental impact as part of their business strategies. Biodegradable materials used for light-emitting devices solve ethical problems by providing both safety for biological systems while concurrently reducing waste production. The development of medical devices gets ethical oversight from two bodies: Institutional Review Boards

(IRBs) and Ethics Committees. The ethical consequences of device trials are evaluated by these bodies who follow Declaration of Helsinki standards for compliance. The Global Harmonization Task Force (GHTF) with other global initiatives work to establish harmonized ethical standards throughout different regions for increasing fairness in device development and approval processes. Every step of medical device development requires ethical considerations that start with design testing and extend through to clinical use and global distribution. Medical advances in healthcare derive from patient-centered safety measures alongside minimized risk assessments and clear processes while eliminating healthcare inequality differences as well as ethical standards systems maintained through regulatory and manufacturing practices [34]. The ongoing development of technology demands persistent ethical observance to maintain innovation versus accountability so healthcare devices serve the needs of every patient without infringing patient rights and health.

5 Future Directions and Challenges

Biocompatible technologies within medical devices face several intriguing challenges along with promising research directions for their future development. The convergence of materials science technology, engineering capabilities and regulatory policies leads to future medical devices that will enhance clinical results through advanced safety and regulatory compliance systems. The speedy progression of innovation exceeds regulatory systems' capacity to transform thus creating challenges which need precise navigation. The development of biocompatible emerging materials including biodegradable polymers and hybrid composites explores new possibilities for medical device construction. Biocompatible materials combine effortlessly with biological structures to advance devices which improve therapeutic delivery of drugs as well as regenerate tissues and conduct photonic treatments [35]. The evaluation of long-term safety along with effectiveness of these materials remains difficult to conduct. The existing healthcare regulations including ISO 10993 and FDA guidelines prioritize preclinical testing alongside clinical examinations while failing to capture the complete complexity aspect of new materials. The full understanding of biodegradable device degradation products represents a critical requirement to prevent unexpected toxic effects which demands better evaluation approaches. Regulatory pathways become more complex because of modern manufacturing approaches including 3D bio-printing [36]. These technologies allow customized medical devices with anatomically matched characteristics but introduce operational variability that becomes difficult to control for quality assurance. The regulatory mechanisms established for standardized mass-produced products fail to adapt properly to managing the personalized nature of products developed through 3D printing. The exploration of adaptive regulatory frameworks by authorities faces an ongoing struggle to establish proper balance between system flexibility and maintaining rigorous standards.

The medical field experiences fundamental transformation through artificial intelligence (AI) and machine learning (ML) that leads to better predictive analysis and tailored remedies and diagnostic advancements. Companies which integrate AI/ML technology face new regulatory hurdles for data privacy standards as well as demands for algorithm transparency and cybersecurity risks. The reliable functioning of AI-enabled medical devices across different populations depends on accessible big datasets that represent various populations [37]. Many cases exist where representative datasets remain inaccessible to such devices. The adoption of new regulations starts to tackle safety challenges of AI/ML technology but worldwide standardization remains essential for borderless deployment of these systems. Medical device accessibility gaps between different global regions pose major challenges from both ethical and practical visibility requirements. Medical devices that show advances remain restricted to high-income nations but resource-deprived settings entirely miss out on accessing even standard healthcare equipment. To fill this gap, we need creative solutions starting with multilevel pricing models alongside production facilities based locally together with building technology-specific medical devices that perform reliably under harsh situations [38]. To provide worldwide patients with reliable medical treatment we must align our medical innovation with restrictive safety protocols and quality guidelines (Fig. 4).

The force with which regulatory frameworks adapt to technological developments remains a fundamental necessity. The EU Medical Device Regulation (MDR) pioneered new requirements to secure patient safety by enhancing clinical evidence standards together with post-market surveillance requirements [39]. New regulatory requirements have imposed elevated costs and procedural complexities on compliance processes especially for small and medium-sized enterprises (SMEs) who generate crucial innovative advancements. The challenge lies in achieving cohesive measures between disciplined supervisory requirements and innovation drive through strong cooperation among regulators manufacturers and other key players. Future medical device progress will greatly depend on innovations that combine better biocompatibility with sustainability standards and advances in regulatory science [40]. The growth of environmental concerns will require sustainable design to focus on biodegradable devices alongside energy-efficient manufacturing methods. Moreover, the integration of biocompatible materials with wireless technologies and energy-harvesting systems holds the potential to create fully autonomous devices that minimize invasiveness while maximizing functionality [41].

6 Conclusion

Regulatory considerations for biocompatible light emitters are crucial in ensuring their safety and efficacy, ultimately paving the way for innovative applications in medical technology and beyond. As the field continues to evolve, it is essential for regulatory frameworks to adapt accordingly, fostering collaboration between researchers, manufacturers, and regulatory bodies to address emerging challenges

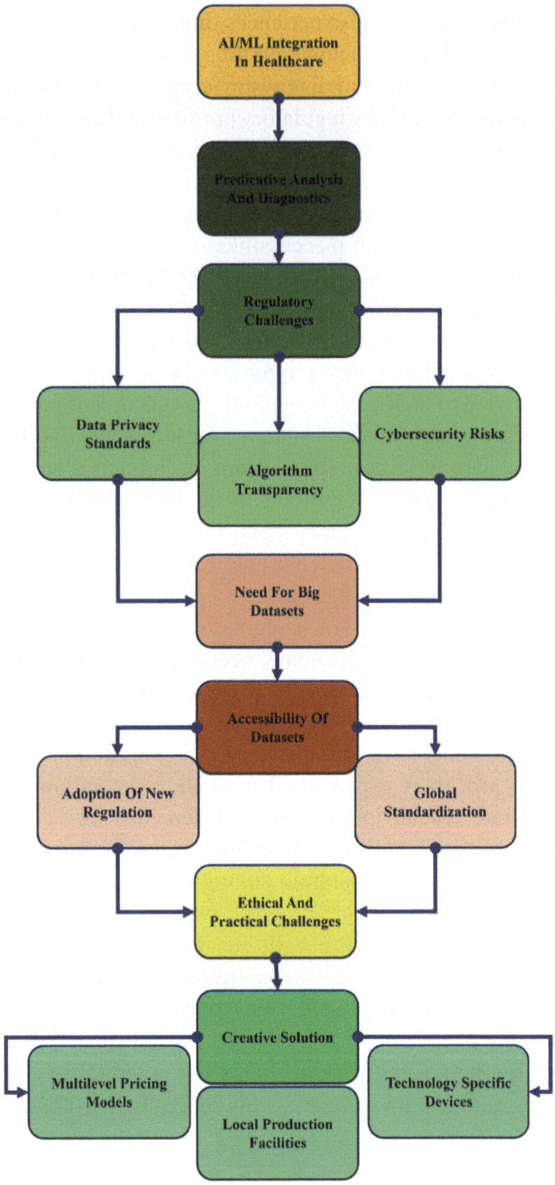

Fig. 4 Integration of AI/ML in healthcare

and promote public trust in these advanced technologies. In summary, a proactive approach to regulation will not only enhance the development of biocompatible light emitters but also ensure that their integration into clinical practice is both safe and beneficial for patients, thereby driving forward the future of medical advancements. This collaborative effort will facilitate the establishment of standardized testing protocols and guidelines, ensuring that new innovations meet rigorous safety and performance criteria before reaching the market. Such measures will ultimately lead to greater transparency and accountability in the industry, encouraging further investment and innovation while safeguarding public health. This commitment to regulatory excellence will also foster a culture of continuous improvement, where stakeholders can adapt swiftly to new findings and evolving technologies in the field. Such a proactive approach not only enhances patient outcomes but also instills confidence among healthcare providers and patients alike, paving the way for broader acceptance of advanced medical technologies. By prioritizing collaboration between regulatory bodies, industry leaders, and healthcare professionals, the path towards a more efficient and effective healthcare system can be achieved, ultimately benefiting society as a whole. This holistic strategy will ensure that the healthcare ecosystem remains responsive to emerging challenges, driving advancements that align with both ethical standards and patient needs. Emphasizing education and training for all participants in the healthcare system will further empower them to embrace innovation, leading to a more knowledgeable workforce capable of navigating the complexities of modern medical practices. Investing in continuous professional development and fostering a culture of lifelong learning will not only enhance the skills of healthcare providers but also improve patient outcomes by ensuring that the latest evidence-based practices are implemented effectively.

References

1. Cai, Y., Lv, Z., Chen, X., Jin, K., Mou, X.: Recent advances in biomaterials based near-infrared mild photothermal therapy for biomedical application: a review. Int. J. Biol. Macromol. 134746 (2024)
2. Cha, G.D., Kim, D.-H., Kim, D.C.: Wearable and implantable light-emitting diodes and their biomedical applications. Korean J. Chem. Eng. **41**, 1–24 (2024)
3. Cho, Y., Park, S., Lee, J., Yu, K.J.: Emerging materials and technologies with applications in flexible neural implants: a comprehensive review of current issues with neural devices. Adv. Mater. **33**, 2005786 (2021)
4. El Guerraf, A., Ziani, I., Ben Jadi, S., El Bachiri, A., Bazzaoui, M., Bazzaoui, E.A., et al.: Smart conducting polymer innovations for sustainable and safe food packaging technologies. Compr. Rev. Food Sci. Food Saf. **23**, e70045 (2024)
5. Meskher, H., Sharifianjazi, F., Tavamaishvili, K., Irandoost, M., Nejadkoorki, D., Makvandi, P.: Limitations, challenges and prospective solutions for bioactive glasses-based nanocomposites for dental applications: a critical review. J. Dent. 105331 (2024)
6. Emiliani, V., Entcheva, E., Hedrich, R., Hegemann, P., Konrad, K.R., Lüscher, C., et al.: Optogenetics for light control of biological systems. Nat. Rev. Methods Prim. **2**, 55 (2022)
7. Alexandre-Franco, M.F., Kouider, R., Kassir Al-Karany, R., Cuerda-Correa, E.M., Al-Kassir, A.: Recent advances in polymer science and fabrication processes for enhanced microfluidic applications: an overview. Micromachines **15**, 1137 (2024)
8. Fidan, I., Huseynov, O., Ali, M.A., Alkunte, S., Rajeshirke, M., Gupta, A., et al.: Recent inventions in additive manufacturing: holistic review. Inventions **8**, 103 (2023)
9. Islam, A., Shah, S.H.U., Haider, Z., Imran, M., Amin, A., Haider, S.K., et al.: Biological interfacial materials for organic light-emitting diodes. Micromachines (Basel) **14**, 1171 (2023)
10. Jayan, K.D., Babu, K.: Luminescent perovskite quantum dots: progress in fabrication, modelling and machine learning approaches for advanced photonic and quantum computing applications. J. Lumin. 120906 (2024)

11. Khonina, S.N., Kazanskiy, N.L., Skidanov, R.V., Butt, M.A.: Advancements and applications of diffractive optical elements in contemporary optics: a comprehensive overview. Adv. Mater. Technol. 2401028 (2024)
12. Kong, D., Zhang, K., Tian, J., Yin, L., Sheng, X.: Biocompatible and biodegradable light-emitting materials and devices. Adv. Mater. Technol. **7**, 2100006 (2022)
13. Liu, K., Yao, Y., Xue, S., Zhang, M., Li, D., Xu, T., et al.: Recent advances of tumor microenvironment-responsive nanomedicines-energized combined phototherapy of cancers. Pharmaceutics **15**, 2480 (2023)
14. Liu, Z.: Visualized medicine: emerging techniques and developing. Frontiers (2023)
15. Liu, G., Lv, Z., Batool, S., Li, M., Zhao, P., Guo, L., et al.: Biocompatible material-based flexible biosensors: from materials design to wearable/implantable devices and integrated sensing systems. Small **19**, 2207879 (2023)
16. Tropp, J., Rivnay, J.: Design of biodegradable and biocompatible conjugated polymers for bioelectronics. J. Mater. Chem. C **9**, 13543–56 (2021)
17. Abernethy, A., Adams, L., Barrett, M., Bechtel, C., Brennan, P., Butte, A., et al.: The promise of digital health: then, now, and the future. NAM Perspectives (2022)
18. Molani, A., Pennati, F., Ravazzani, S., Scarpellini, A., Storti, F.M., Vegetali, G., et al.: Advances in portable optical microscopy using cloud technologies and artificial intelligence for medical applications. Sensors **24**, 6682 (2024)
19. Murawski, C., Gather, M.C.: Emerging biomedical applications of organic light-emitting diodes. Adv. Opt. Mater. **9**, 2100269 (2021)
20. Patel, V., Chaurasia, V., Siddiqui, E.A., Patole, S.P., Mahadeva, R.: Machine learning solutions in smart healthcare: features, applications, and challenges. Open AI Comput. Intell. Soc. **50**, 291–314 (2025)
21. Pelucchi, E., Fagas, G., Aharonovich, I., Englund, D., Figueroa, E., Gong, Q., et al.: The potential and global outlook of integrated photonics for quantum technologies. Nat. Rev. Phys. **4**, 194–208 (2022)
22. Ran, C., Pu, K.: Molecularly generated light and its biomedical applications. Angew. Chem. Int. Ed. **63**, e202314468 (2024)
23. Righini, G.C., Krzak, J., Lukowiak, A., Macrelli, G., Varas, S., Ferrari, M.: From flexible electronics to flexible photonics: a brief overview. Opt. Mater. (Amst) **115**, 111011 (2021)
24. Shi, S., Chen, J., Wang, X., Xiao, M., Chandrasekaran, A.R., Li, L., et al.: Biointerface engineering with nucleic acid materials for biosensing applications. Adv. Funct. Mater. **32**, 2201069 (2022)
25. Kutner, N., Kunduru, K.R., Rizik, L., Farah, S.: Recent advances for improving functionality, biocompatibility, and longevity of implantable medical devices and deliverable drug delivery systems. Adv. Func. Mater. **31**, 2010929 (2021)
26. Wang, Y., Wen, Y., Zhuang, X., Liu, S., Zhang, L., Xie, W.: Flexible organic optoelectronic devices: design, fabrication, and applications. APL Photonics 9 (2024)
27. Williamson, S.M., Prybutok, V.: Balancing privacy and progress: a review of privacy challenges, systemic oversight, and patient perceptions in AI-driven healthcare. Appl. Sci. **14**, 675 (2024)
28. Yadav, S., Mittal, P., Negi, S.: Recent advancements over a decade for organic light-emitting diodes: from structural diversity, role of layers, colour emission, material classification, performance improvement, fabrication to applications. Bull. Mater. Sci. **45**, 109 (2022)
29. Han, Y., Ceross, A., Bergmann, J.: Regulatory frameworks for AI-enabled medical device software in China: comparative analysis and review of implications for global manufacturer. JMIR AI **3**, e46871 (2024)
30. Yang, D., Lee, Y., Kang, H., Vu, Q.H., Kang, G., Lee, S.E., et al.: Green manufacturing of electrically-tunable smart light-weight planar optics: a review. Int. J. Prec. Eng. Manuf. Green Technol. 1–23 (2024)
31. Haleem, A., Javaid, M., Singh, R.P., Suman, R.: Medical 4.0 technologies for healthcare: features, capabilities, and applications. Internet Things Cyber-Phys. Syst. **2**, 12–30 (2022)
32. Matin, A., Islam, M.R., Wang, X., Huo, H., Xu, G.: AIoT for sustainable manufacturing: overview, challenges, and opportunities. Internet of Things 100901 (2023)

33. Yang, Y., Jiang, Q., Zhang, F.: Nanocrystals for deep-tissue in vivo luminescence imaging in the near-infrared region. Chem. Rev. **124**, 554–628 (2023)
34. Zheludev, N.I., Yuan, G.: Optical superoscillation technologies beyond the diffraction limit. Nat. Rev. Phys. **4**, 16–32 (2022)
35. Han, W.B., Yang, S.M., Rajaram, K., Hwang, S.: Materials and fabrication strategies for biocompatible and biodegradable conductive polymer composites toward bio-integrated electronic systems. Adv. Sustain. Syst. **6**, 2100075 (2022)
36. Thakur, M., Modi, V.K.: Biocolorants in food: sources, extraction, applications and future prospects. Crit. Rev. Food Sci. Nutr. **64**, 4674–713 (2024)
37. Arif, Z.U., Khalid, M.Y., Sheikh, M.F., Zolfagharian, A., Bodaghi, M.: Biopolymeric sustainable materials and their emerging applications. J. Environ. Chem. Eng. **10**, 108159 (2022)
38. Afolabi, O.A., Ndou, N.: Synergy of hybrid fillers for emerging composite and nanocomposite materials—a review. Polymers **16**, 1907 (2024)
39. Reis, O., Eneh, N.E., Ehimuan, B., Anyanwu, A., Olorunsogo, T., Abrahams, T.O.: Privacy law challenges in the digital age: a global review of legislation and enforcement. Int. J. Appl. Res. Soc. Sci. **6**, 73–88 (2024)
40. Singh, A.V., Chandrasekar, V., Prabhu, V.M., Bhadra, J., Laux, P., Bhardwaj, P., et al.: Sustainable bioinspired materials for regenerative medicine: balancing toxicology, environmental impact, and ethical considerations. Biomed. Mater. **19**, 060501 (2024)
41. Rasool, A., Sri, S., Zulfajri, M., Krismastuti, F.S.H.: Nature inspired nanomaterials, advancements in green synthesis for biological sustainability. Inorgan. Chem. Commun. 112954 (2024)

Challenges, Future Perspectives and Emerging Applications

Daniel Gbenga Adekanmi, Samuel Ebenezer Kayode, Olaolu Samuel Awobifa, Femi Tope Adefemisoye, Ayodunmomi Esther Adekanmi, Ayobamiji Emmanuel Olowofoyeku, and Oluwakemi Susan Nelson-Etafo

Abstract The design of light emitters for biomedical applications necessitates a careful balance of technical performance, biological safety, and environmental sustainability. These devices must deliver precise functionality while minimizing toxicity, particularly from heavy metals, and ensuring biocompatibility to prevent adverse immune responses. Optimizing wavelengths in the red and near-infrared spectrum for effective bioimaging and biosensing is crucial for enhanced tissue penetration and therapeutic efficacy. Additionally, controlling light intensity is essential to protect healthy tissues. The push for personalized medicine drives the miniaturization of these devices, complicating innovations in nanoscale materials and flexible substrates while maintaining efficiency and managing heat in compact designs. Future advancements in biodegradability, using eco-friendly materials like chitosan or silk fibroin, offer promising solutions for temporary electronics and medical implants, addressing electronic waste concerns. Moreover, integrating bioenergy harvesting with microfluidic systems will lead to energy-efficient, minimally invasive solutions. Wearable technologies and implantable emitters designed for personalized

D. G. Adekanmi (✉) · S. E. Kayode · O. S. Awobifa
Facultad de Ciencias Químicas, Universidad Autónoma de Coahuila, 25280 Saltillo, Coahuila, Mexico
e-mail: danieladekanmi@uadec.edu.mx

F. T. Adefemisoye
Facultad de Producción Agropecuaria, Universidad Autónoma Agraria Antonio Narro, Torreon, Coahuila, Mexico

A. E. Adekanmi
Department of Environmental Sciences, Pan African University of Life and Health Sciences, University of Ibadan, Ibadan, Nigeria

A. E. Olowofoyeku
Faculty of Chemical Science, Olusegun Agagu University of Science and Technology, Ondo, Nigeria

O. S. Nelson-Etafo
College of Plant Science and Crop Production, Federal University of Agriculture Abeokuta, Abeokuta, Nigeria

© The Author(s), under exclusive license to Springer Nature Switzerland AG 2025

N. O. Etafo (ed.), *Tailored Light Emitters For Biomedical Applications*, Engineering Materials, https://doi.org/10.1007/978-3-031-88731-4_15

medicine aim to provide precise biosensing and targeted therapies. Beyond healthcare, applications such as artificial photosynthesis utilize advanced light emitters to improve sunlight absorption and energy conversion, contributing to sustainable energy solutions. Thus, light emitters are poised to revolutionize both biomedical and technological fields.

Keywords Light emitters · Biomedical applications · Microfluidic devices · Artificial photosynthesis · Biodegradable light emitters

1 Challenges of the Light Emitter Designs

Biomedical applications present unique challenges for light emitters, encompassing technical and biological aspects. These challenges demand precision and safety in light emitters used in biomedical devices, whether for internal or external applications, while ensuring energy efficiency and environmental sustainability. A detailed exploration of these challenges follows below [1, 2].

1.1 Biocompatibility and Safety

Materials used in contact with living systems must prioritize biocompatibility. Light emitters designed for use in or on the body must avoid triggering immune responses or releasing harmful substances. Those containing heavy metals can pose significant toxicity risks. Achieving biocompatibility often involves identifying biocompatible alternatives or employing encapsulation techniques to ensure safety. However, these alternatives or protective layers mustn't compromise the light emitter's effectiveness in its intended application. Striking the right balance between safety and functionality is essential [3, 4].

1.2 Wavelength Optimization and Tissue Penetration

Different wavelengths have varying levels of tissue penetration, with red and near-infrared (NIR) light being the most effective. These wavelengths penetrate deeper into tissues, are safe, and are rapidly absorbed by melanin and blood. Consequently, light emitters used in such applications must optimally produce light within this usable spectrum. In phototherapies, precision and tunability in wavelength are crucial, as the light must align with the absorption peak of the drugs or agents involved to maximize effectiveness [5, 6].

1.3 Control of Light Intensity and Dosage

Achieving precise dosage is critical, as light intensity directly affects treatment outcomes. Insufficient intensity may fail to activate the treatment, while excessive intensity can damage healthy tissues. This presents challenges in avoiding hotspots and preventing device overheating. To maintain this delicate balance, light emitters must deliver consistent and adjustable intensity levels. Additionally, managing heat generation is essential, particularly for implantable devices, to ensure comfort and safety.

1.4 Miniaturization Without Sacrificing Performance

Miniaturizing devices to create compact and flexible implantable or wearable medical solutions introduce challenges such as reduced performance and overheating, often requiring trade-offs between efficiency and size. To overcome these limitations, advancements in light emitter designs are essential to achieve optimal performance and compactness. Solutions include the use of nanoscale materials, flexible substrates, and advanced photonic materials, though these innovations add complexity to the design process [7] and the design of devices [8].

1.5 Energy Efficiency and Power Management

Effective power management is critical for the longevity and performance of implantable and wearable devices, which rely on small batteries. Achieving energy efficiency ensures longer battery life and sustained functionality. This requires the integration of highly efficient photoluminescent materials that consume minimal power, as well as the exploration of innovative power replenishment methods, such as wireless charging or energy harvesting.

1.6 Heat Management in Compact Designs

Light emission inherently generates heat, making thermal management crucial for light-emitting devices, particularly in biomedical applications. Excess heat can damage surrounding tissues and shorten device lifespan, challenges that are exacerbated in miniaturized and implantable systems. Current research focuses on advanced solutions, including thermally conductive substrates, microfluidic cooling channels, and phase-change materials, to address these issues effectively [9].

1.7 Ensuring Longevity and Durability

Biomedical applications demand devices that maintain longevity and consistent performance despite exposure to body fluids and complex physiological environments. Sustained reliability over extended use is critical. However, photomaterials can degrade over time due to contact with fluids, posing a significant challenge. To mitigate this, encapsulation techniques are employed to protect the materials. These encapsulation methods must be both transparent and highly effective to preserve the device's functionality without altering its output [9].

1.8 Precision and Targeted Light Emission

Precision is crucial in applications like targeted tumor ablation or localized therapies. Advanced technologies, such as photonic crystals or waveguides, enhance specificity but introduce challenges, including greater design complexity and the potential for bulkier, less flexible devices.

1.9 Integration with Medical Systems and Cost Considerations

Light emitters in biomedical applications often operate in conjunction with other systems, such as sensors, drugs, or devices, as part of a comprehensive diagnostic, therapeutic, or monitoring process. Ensuring seamless integration without interference among components is essential but poses challenges related to hybridization and compatibility. These demands can lead to increased device size and higher manufacturing costs, further complicating their design and production [2, 10].

Designing light emitters for biomedical applications requires balancing biocompatibility, compactness, energy efficiency, and precise control over light properties, all while minimizing trade-offs. Despite these challenges, the ongoing pursuit of improved health outcomes and patient care continues to drive innovation and solutions in this field [11].

2 Future Perspective

Transitioning from the challenges posed by traditional light emitters in biomedical applications necessitates the development of biocompatible materials that are biodegradable and free from heavy metals. Such photopolymers would not only minimize toxicity but also provide sufficient photoluminescence tailored to specific applications. Smart coatings offer dual advantages: enhanced safety to prevent adverse immune responses and the ability to dynamically adapt emitters to physiological conditions, broadening the scope of safe applications.

The discovery of more tunable materials will enable greater precision in the emission properties of photonic materials, including improved wavelength control and intensity adjustments for specific therapeutic needs. This adaptability is especially beneficial for treatments like photodynamic therapy, which rely on targeted and responsive emissions. Additionally, advancements in miniaturization driven by nanoscale engineering and flexible electronics will lead to the development of more compact, high-performing wearable and implantable devices.

The potential for bioenergy harvesting promises greater energy efficiency by utilizing piezoelectric or thermoelectric materials, thus reducing reliance on batteries. These devices would harness energy from body movements and heat, providing a sustainable, maintenance-free power source. Additionally, advancements in heat management solutions, such as innovative cooling channels, will enable more compact designs, making implantable emitters more viable for sensitive applications.

Self-healing materials and encapsulation will improve device durability by promoting recovery and preventing damage from bodily fluids. New approaches to integrating emitters into complex biomedical systems will lead to better outcomes, minimizing interference with other treatments. With AI-driven innovations on the horizon, personalized light-based therapies are set to be optimized, with real-time adjustments based on continuous patient data.

These developments suggest a future where affordable, standardized, AI-powered biomedical light emitters lead to safer, more adaptable, and precise diagnostics and therapies, transforming healthcare delivery.

3 Emerging Applications of the Light Emitter Designs

Over the past five decades, biomedical applications have progressed rapidly, with advancements in light emitters bringing substantial advantages to diagnostics (Fig. 1), therapeutic interventions, and patient monitoring [12]. Innovations in biophotonics, like in many other fields, reflect technological progress and a shift toward more efficient, effective, and safer options as presented in Table 1 [13–15]. The introduction of the biocompatible advanced light emitter has substituted many ineffective methods such as using organic dyes which are limited because of photobleaching

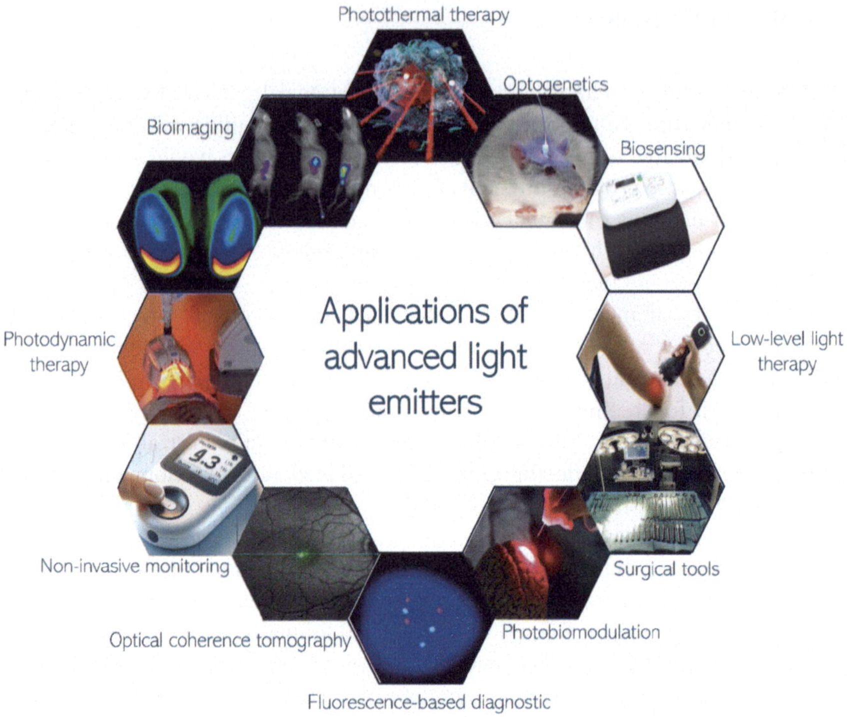

Fig. 1 Applications of advanced light emitters in biomedicine

and low sensitivity [16, 17]. Light emitters have various functions in biomedicine as summarized in the table below.

Innovations in light emitters for biomedical applications result from many factors. One of these is the need for less invasive medical procedures [13, 18]. Another is the drive for miniaturized devices for compactness and adaptability [19]. The flexibility of technologies like OLEDs and LEDs allow them to fit seamlessly into wearable devices for continuous health monitoring [20, 21]. Additionally, the fine tunability of these light sources enables precise diagnostics and targeted therapies, resulting in better treatment outcomes [22]. These innovations improve patient comfort and encourage them to adhere to treatment plans.

There are various perspectives on the evolution of light emitters in biomedical applications, but we can frame the discussion around three main areas: technological innovations in light emission, advancements in material properties and functional efficiency, and innovative designs for safety and monitoring. While these areas are interrelated, they highlight the unique contributions of different types of emitters and the interconnected roles of technology, material science, and design in improving healthcare outcomes.

Technological innovations in light emission focus on developing new methods and technologies for light generation, enabling more refined and innovative applications.

Table 1 Advanced light emitters and their functions in biomedicine

Biomedical application	Light emitters	References
Bioimaging	- Upconversion nanoparticles (UCNPs) - Plasmonic nanoparticles - Phosphorescent probes and nanophosphors - Carbon dots - X-ray scintillators - Laser diodes - Superluminescent diodes (SLDs)	[23, 23–29]
Photodynamic therapy (PDT)	- Organic Light-Emitting Diodes (OLEDs) - Light-Emitting Diodes (LEDs) - Upconversion nanoparticles (UCNPs) - Laser diodes - Plasmonic nanoparticles	[5, 27, 28, 20, 30–33]
Photothermal therapy	- Plasmonic nanoparticles	[1–3]
Optogenetics	- Organic Light-Emitting Diodes (OLEDs) Light -Emitting Diodes (LEDs)	[4, 5]
Biosensing	- Plasmonic nanoparticles	[6, 7]
Low-level light therapy (LLLT)	- Organic Light-Emitting Diodes (OLEDs)	[8, 9]
Surgical tools	- Laser diodes	[10, 11]
Photobiomodulation (PBM)	- Organic Light-Emitting Diodes (OLEDs) Light-Emitting Diodes (LEDs)	[12, 13]
Fluorescence-based diagnostics	- Organic Light-Emitting Diodes (OLEDs) - Light-Emitting Diodes (LEDs) - Plasmonic nanoparticles - Carbon dots - Phosphorescent probes and nanophosphors	[5, 14]
Optical coherence tomography (OCT)	- Superluminescent diodes (SLDs)	[15, 16]
Non-invasive monitoring	- Organic Light-Emitting Diodes (OLEDs) - Light-Emitting Diodes (LEDs)	[13, 17]

This progression leverages the potential of advanced light-emitting systems to be integrated into medical practices, offering higher success rates through continuous health monitoring. Organic Light-Emitting Diodes (OLEDs) and Light-Emitting Diodes (LEDs) are prime examples in this category. These technologies enable portable, energy-efficient devices that provide flexible lighting solutions for wearable health devices and biosensing applications [4, 9, 34, 35].

Material enrichment and functional efficiency involve the use of advanced materials that improve imaging clarity and enable more precise surgical procedures. These enhancements directly affect clinical efficacy by boosting the performance of light emitters. Laser diodes and Superluminescent Diodes (SLDs) are important examples since they are made from materials that improve coherence and brightness. These innovations are integral to imaging techniques like confocal microscopy, where high resolution is essential for detailed cellular analysis [12, 27].

Finally, innovative designs for safety and monitoring cover light emitters that are compatible with living systems. The focus is low toxicity and lasting emissions for safer in vivo applications. They are more effective for monitoring therapeutic responses without compromising patient health. Phosphorescent probes and carbon dots are typical examples. They are designed for the safety of use and offer non-toxic alternatives in suitable situations [36, 37].

3.1 Light-Delivering and Light-Responsive Materials

Light-emitting materials play a crucial role in the development of light-based healthcare devices that function deep within biological tissues. These light sources work alongside optical waveguides, which channel and transmit light with minimal loss. Optical waveguides are typically made from materials with a high refractive index and are coated with lower refractive index materials to efficiently confine and guide the light. While silica fibers are commonly used in traditional applications, there is growing interest in creating flexible, biocompatible, and biodegradable waveguides designed for implantable healthcare devices. The core of these waveguides typically has a refractive index greater than 1.47, which is the refractive index of biological tissues [38–40].

Light-responsive materials sometimes play complementary roles to light emitters but have significant roles due to their ability to absorb light and exhibit various optical responses, including fluorescence, phosphorescence, and photothermal effects. The advancements in the understanding, design, and production of these materials have made them raw materials in the design of innovative implantable and wearable diagnostic and therapeutic systems. Examples of such materials include quantum dots (QDs), transition-metal dichalcogenides, plasmonic gold nanostructures, upconversion nanoparticles, and organic and integrated semiconductors [40–44].

3.2 *Advanced Light Emitters*

Advanced light emitters (Fig. 2) represent a class of technological materials that are becoming relevant in many advanced biomedical and diagnostic applications. These emitters range from organic light-emitting diodes (OLEDs) and light-emitting diodes (LEDs) to advanced nanoscale solutions like upconversion nanoparticles (UCNPs) and plasmonic materials. They are tailor-made for precision and adaptable use. Their unique optical properties enable diverse functionalities, from non-invasive imaging and targeted therapies to real-time biosensing and disease monitoring. This section delves into the mechanisms, material compositions, and cutting-edge biomedical applications of these emitters, emphasizing their potential to revolutionize healthcare and diagnostics.

3.2.1 Organic Light-Emitting Diodes (OLEDs) and Light-Emitting Diodes (LEDs)

These have distinct yet similar features in terms of flexibility (Fig. 2), energy efficiency, and precise light emission. Both OLEDs and LEDs produce light when electrical current passes through specific materials, however the materials and mechanisms involved differentiate their applications and synthesis [4].

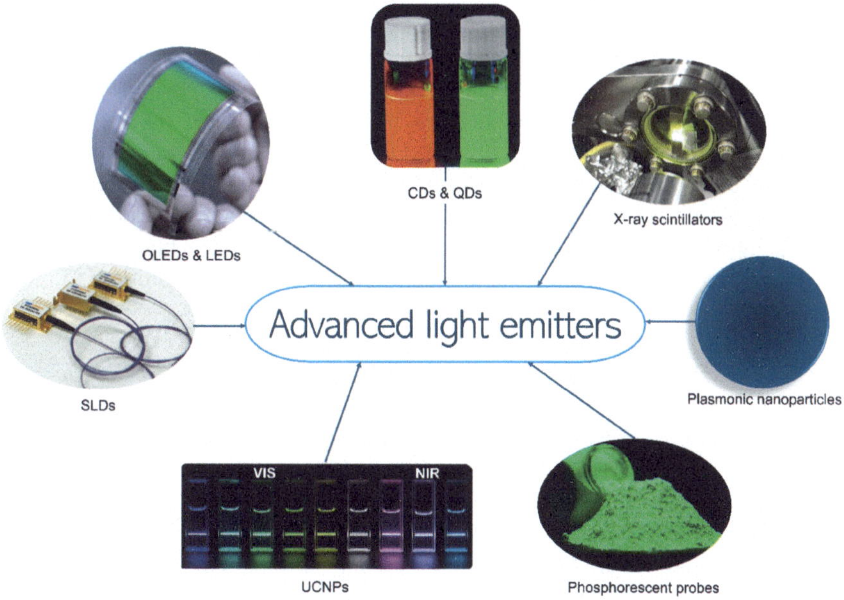

Fig. 2 Advanced light emitters

OLEDs utilize biocompatible organic compounds that emit light when an electric current flows through them. The organic materials are placed between electrodes, which initiate the recombination of electrons and holes and in the process, light is released. OLED materials include Alq3 (tris(8-hydroxyquinolinato)aluminum), polyfluorene, poly(phenylene vinylene), fluorescent dyes and polymer [45–47]. Specifically, OLEDs are flexible and emit light across a wide spectrum and are made through scalable and cost-effective solution-based techniques. In biomedical applications, OLEDs are essential in the production of wearable health monitoring systems, such as flexible patches for tracking heart rate and oxygen levels. They are also used in optogenetics, photodynamic therapy (PDT), and photobiomodulation (PBM) procedures. Attili et al. have reported that using OLEDs for PDT improves comfort during treatment and is effective in antimicrobial PDT against *Staphylococcus aureus* with minimal power consumption. Morton et al. also studied the use of OLEDs in neuronal activation. However, OLEDs are susceptible to moisture, which degrades their performance. Various forms of encapsulation techniques are being explored to counter this limitation [4, 48, 49].

LEDs, on the other hand, are made from inorganic semiconductor materials. Materials like Gallium Nitride (for blue and UV LEDs), Aluminum Gallium Arsenide (AlGaAs) (for red LEDs), Gallium Arsenide (GaAs) (for infrared LEDs), and Indium Gallium Nitride (InGaN) (for green and blue light) emit light when electrons pass through their p–n junction. LEDs are durable and energy efficient. They emit light ranging from ultraviolet (UV) to infrared (IR) [33, 50]. Their precise control over light limits the potential for phototoxicity thereby encouraging their use in biomedical diagnostics and therapeutics. For instance, LEDs are used in fluorescence microscopy for detailed cellular imaging and for detecting pathogenic organisms and molecules in diagnostic tests [51]. Therapeutically, LEDs are effective in phototherapy treatments of conditions like neonatal jaundice in infants. Also, red and near-infrared (NIR) producing LEDs are used in low-level light therapy (LLLT) to reduce inflammation and accelerate tissue healing [52, 53]. In optogenetics, LEDs provide precise light pulses used to control neuron activity in genetically modified organisms [54]. Micro-LED offer more flexibility and can be chip-based, or thin film-based. They have potential for use in biomedical implants because of their capabilities [55, 56].

3.2.2 Laser Diodes and Superluminescent Diodes (SLDs)

Laser diodes produce consistent light with precision and intensity. They are effective in procedures requiring focused and directed light. Laser diodes operate by stimulated emission. This occurs through the excitation of electrons in semiconductor materials which then release photons in a synchronized phase [57–59]. The resulting beam is highly focused and intense. Semiconductors used include gallium arsenide or indium gallium nitride [60, 61]. This precision of laser diodes is beneficial in imaging techniques like confocal and two-photon microscopy since the beams provide deep penetration and enhanced cellular visualization [62, 63]. They are also used for making incisions, cauterizing vessels, and treating skin conditions in minimally invasive procedures. Lasers are used in photodynamic therapy for cancer treatments [64–66].

Superluminescent diodes (SLDs) are hybrids of LEDs and lasers. They combine high brightness with versatility because they can reduce feedback. They are advanced imaging tools used for optical coherence tomography (OCT) to provide non-invasive, well-resolved images of tissues like the retina or vascular structures. Their broad spectral output produces images with depth and better resolution [30, 61, 67].

3.2.3 Upconversion Nanoparticles (UCNPs)

Emerging nanoscale emitters like upconversion nanoparticles (UCNPs) convert low-energy near-infrared (NIR) light into higher-energy visible or ultraviolet (UV) light. NIR light penetrates tissues more effectively than visible or UV light while causing minimal damage. In simple terms, UCNPs can absorb and convert low-energy photons to higher-energy photons. Most UCNPs have rare-earth ions in their matrix [68, 69]. The choice of the host materials and dopants affects the efficiency of the upconversion process and the attributes of the emitted light. Rare earth elements considered for up-conversion doping must produce lasting and highly stable sharp narrow emissions in lower wavelength regions when they absorb NIR. Although UCNPs are hydrophobic they are coated with hydrophilic polymers, fibers, or silica to increase biocompatibility [70]. Synthesis methods include co-precipitation, sol–gel processes, or hydrothermal synthesis [35, 68]. In their study, Gupta et al. observed that Er^{3+}/Yb^{3+} codoped $LaZr_2O_7$ produced emission at 1540 nm when excited at 980 nm [71]. Similarly, Zhang et al. observed up-conversion in Yb^{3+}-Er^{3+}/Ho^{3+}co-doped $Ca_2Gd_8(SiO_4)_6O_2$ phosphor [72]. They are fast becoming non-invasive imaging materials to monitor biological processes and diseases as well as in photodynamic therapy (PDT) [5, 23, 24, 73–75].

3.2.4 Plasmonic Nanoparticles

Plasmon is a phenomenon observed in noble metals like silver and gold and some materials like graphene, molybdenum oxide, tungsten oxide, copper, aluminum, and transparent conducting oxides. They have been studied for possible biomedical plasmonic applications [25, 76–78]. Plasmonic nanoparticles absorb and scatter light when the incident radiation interacts with the electrons on their surfaces. This produces enhanced electromagnetic fields around the particles. Apart from light, other triggers like heat, pH changes, and enzymes have also been used to activate plasmonic particles [79, 80]. Plasmonic nanomaterials are effective for detecting small quantities of molecular analytes in real-time [31, 81, 82]. Typically, plasmonic nanoparticles are produced through chemical reduction methods. Biosynthesis and extract-mediated synthesis are becoming popular alternative routes. Gold nanoparticles for example can be synthesized from gold chloride through reduction with stabilizing agents. Plasmonic properties are highly dependent on the dimensions and morphology of the particles [83–86]. Biomedical applications include cancer treatment in photothermal therapy of cancer where they convert NIR light to heat that selectively destroys cancer cells. The light scattering ability of plasmonic nanoparticles is beneficial in biosensing as enhanced light scatters for the detection of very low concentrations of disease markers or pathogens [79]. Kim et al. showed that mesenchymal stem cells could enhance PTT by assembling pH-responsive AuNPs for better tumor targeting [87].

3.2.5 Phosphorescent Probes and Nanophosphors

Phosphorescent probes and nanophosphors are useful in biosensing and multiplexed bioimaging. Phosphorescent probes are used for measuring oxygen levels in biological systems by providing long-lived light emission. These probes in their excited state emit light for extended periods which in the presence of oxygen quenchers diminish in intensity. This relationship is used to establish oxygen concentrations in tissues or cellular environments [88–92]. Phosphorescent probes often contain transition metal complexes in polymer or silica matrices. They are also referred to as persistent luminescent materials [93]. They are effective in the study of metabolic states, hypoxic conditions, and cancer studies [94, 95]. Maldiney et al., reported the drug delivery and photodetection properties of chromium-doped zinc gallate core that was coated with mesoporous silica [96]. The synthesis of phosphorescent material is carried out through many routes, including sol–gel, co-precipitation, solid-state synthesis, and combustion synthesis. Advanced methods like layer-by-layer assembly are used to achieve precise control over the thickness and composition of the probes for better stability and performance in biological environments [97, 98].

Nanophosphors, on the other hand, are suited for high-contrast labeling in bioimaging, biosensing, and theranostics [28]. Materials used as nanophosphors have a stable, intense, lasting, and renewable afterglow. This glow is a result of intersystem crossing. Rare-earth-doped oxides and transition metal-doped garnets offer improved efficiency and tunability. Nanophosphors can emit distinct wavelengths which can be used to differentiate various markers within a single sample for better diagnostics. Their synthesis route is like phosphorescent probes [99–102].

3.2.6 X-ray Scintillators

X-ray scintillators are designed to convert high-energy X-rays into visible light for biomedical imaging [103]. Since traditional photosensitizers do not fully utilize the X-rays, transducers, also called scintillators, are used to maximize the high energy provided. Scintillation is the process in which visible light is emitted from scintillators when they are exposed to high-energy X-ray photons. This conversion process converts X-ray radiation into light that can be easily analyzed and visualized in diagnostic imaging. Materials used as scintillators must have high light yield, high x-ray absorption properties, and adequate size [14, 104].

X-ray scintillators contain elements with high atomic numbers, such as cesium iodide (CsI), sodium iodide (NaI), and bismuth germanate ($Bi_4Ge_3O_{12}$). Their high density and atomic composition make it possible to efficiently absorb X-ray photons. Common synthesis routes include the melt-growth method and hydrothermal synthesis. Doping scintillator materials with activator ions, such as thallium (Tl^+) or europium (Eu^{2+}) improves light output and increases the scintillation response speed in real-time imaging applications [105–107]. In computed tomography, the light produced by scintillators provides images of human internal structures and organs for the detection of abnormalities [6, 108, 109].

3.2.7 Carbon Dots and Quantum Dots

The optical properties of carbon dots stem from their nanoscale size and quantum confinement effects, which enhance their fluorescence. This feature is particularly beneficial for real-time imaging of biological processes at the cellular level. Carbon dots can fluoresce when exposed to specific excitation wavelengths. Additionally, they are biocompatible and non-toxic, making them a superior alternative to conventional semiconductor quantum dots [110–113]. Carbon dots are synthesized using both top-down and bottom-up approaches. Top-down methods involve breaking down larger carbon materials into nanoscale particles through techniques such as laser ablation, chemical oxidation, electrochemical exfoliation, ultrasonication, and hydrothermal treatment. In contrast, bottom-up methods produce carbon dots from smaller precursors like organic molecules or biomass. These precursors are subjected to high-temperature and pressure conditions, such as hydrothermal synthesis and pyrolysis, to form carbon nanoparticles. The bottom-up approach plays a key role in determining the size, surface properties, and fluorescent characteristics of the resulting carbon dots [114–116]. Their biocompatibility and solubility are enhanced through surface functionalization. Biomedical applications include tracking biological processes with high spatial and temporal resolution [117–119]. Quantum dots are like carbon dots but differ in that they consist of light-emitting semiconductor nanoparticles whose light emission is influenced by their size and chemical composition. They typically exhibit narrower emission spectra than carbon dots and are often coated with shells to enhance their stability. These dots are synthesized using high-temperature methods that accelerate the dissolution of precursors, promoting the nucleation and growth of nanocrystals. Their optical properties arise from quantum confinement, making them ideal for applications in light-based diagnostic and therapeutic technologies [120–123].

3.3 Integration with Microfluidic Devices

Microfluidic devices (Fig. 3) are microscale systems designed to work with liquids at the microliter or nanoliter level. The liquids travel through channels that are just

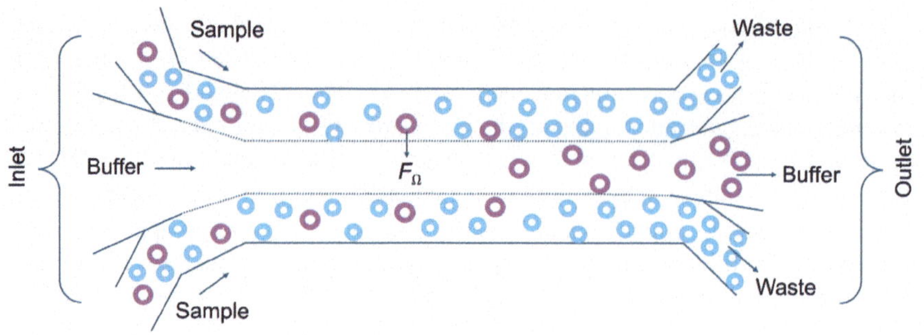

Fig. 3 A simple schematic representation of microfluidic device

a few micrometers wide. For perspective, the channels are only a fraction of the width of a human hair [124, 125]. These devices precisely control fluid dynamics, enabling efficient mixing, separation, or detection of substances within liquids. Key benefits include the use of smaller liquid volumes and high sensitivity. They are lightweight and require minimal power to operate. The miniaturization of traditional biochemical laboratory processes through microchannel networks in microfluidics offers an efficient and cost-effective solution in the biomedical field. Microfluidic devices encompass micro- and nano-sized integrated systems and platforms for particle manipulation and sensing. Additionally, they are used to produce micro- and nanomaterials for biomedical applications [126–131]. Broadly, microfluidics can be classified into passive and active devices based on their ability to operate with or without external influence [132]. Table 2 presents more information about the types, fabrication methods, and biomedical applications of microfluidic devices.

Passive devices depend on internal forces, diffusion, and geometrical design to combine and manipulate materials. The mechanism in passive devices is relevant in organ-on-a-chip technology. Inertial micromixers are also examples of passive microfluidics that utilize channel design to improve mixing efficiency through secondary flows in curved microchannels [132–134]. Common techniques used in passive microfluidics include sorting and separating specific cell types from complex samples using methods like microfiltration and deterministic lateral displacement (DLD). DLD devices separate particles based on size by guiding them through specially designed micro-post arrays. Other methods, such as pinched flow fractionation, use sheath flows to direct particles based on their size in laminar flow conditions [135–137]. Droplet microfluidics involves precisely creating and manipulating small volumes of immiscible liquids for high-efficiency applications in fields such as microbiology and drug delivery. This technology is used to produce uniform droplets through careful channel design. Different configurations, including crossflow, co-flow, and flow-focusing geometries, affect the characteristics and efficiency of droplet production. In crossflow setups, two immiscible liquids are introduced through junctions, while flow-focusing designs generate smaller droplets with minimal wall contact [138–141].

Table 2 Overview of microfluidic device types, fabrication methods, and biomedical applications

Category	Subcategory/ technique	Principles	Key advantages	Limitations	Biomedical applications	References
Microfluidic devices	Passive	Relies on internal forces and geometry	Low-cost, minimal input	Limited particle control	Organs-on-a-chip, droplet microfluidics	[132, 136, 139]
	Active	Uses external fields (acoustic, magnetic, thermal)	Precise control over particles	High power needs, design complexity	Particle sorting, drug delivery	[132, 134, 136]
Fabrication methods	Soft lithography	PDMS casting from a master mold	High fidelity, low cost	Swelling in solvents	Cell culturing, tissue engineering	[144]
	3D printing	Layer-by-layer additive manufacturing	Rapid prototyping, complex designs	Limited resolution, post-processing needed	Custom microfluidic devices, lab-on-chip	[124, 144, 145]
	Hot embossing	Imprints mold shapes on thermoplastics	High detail, moderate production	Cycle delays, limited to thermoplastics	Diagnostic microchannels, drug delivery	[124, 146]
	Injection molding	Injects melted polymer into molds	Cost-effective for high volumes	Material restrictions, mold costs	Diagnostic kits, microfluidic platforms	[3, 146, 147]
Biomedical applications	Drug delivery	Encapsulated carriers for targeted release	Precise, reduced side effects	Complex production	Tumor-targeted chemotherapy, liposome formulations	[148, 149]
	Diagnostic devices	Biomarker detection with minimal sample volume	Portable, fast	Risk of contamination in small channels	COVID-19 POC tests, cardiovascular diagnostics	[40, 136]

(continued)

Table 2 (continued)

Category	Subcategory/ technique	Principles	Key advantages	Limitations	Biomedical applications	References
	Tissue engineering	Mimics physiological environments for cell cultures	Simulates real conditions, higher accuracy	Scalability issues for larger tissues	Gut, liver, and brain-on-a-chip models	[148, 150]
	Biosensors	Rapid biological molecule detection	High sensitivity, low reagent use	Sensor limitations	Glucose monitors, SARS-CoV-2 antibody tests	[8, 136, 151]
	Cryopreservation	Controls freeze–thaw cycles to reduce damage	Minimizes osmotic stress, preserves cells	Needs high precision in fluid control	Bioengineered cell cryopreservation	[152, 153]

Active microfluidic devices depend on external forces like electric, acoustic, magnetic, optical fields, and thermal gradients for operation so they are categorized based on the external energy used [132, 137]. The sample materials' properties are crucial to these devices' effectiveness. Typically, acoustic transducers can influence the movement of diverse particles, while electric and magnetic fields are more suited for submicron particles. Acoustic field-driven micromixers use acoustic streaming to achieve high mixing efficiency and at optimal conditions can attain 100% efficiency. Electric field-driven mixers leverage techniques like electrophoresis and dielectrophoresis to mix materials based on particle properties. Magnetic field-driven mixers can rapidly and efficiently mix fluids by applying magnetic forces to nanoparticles. Thermal field micromixers use temperature gradients to control fluid dynamics effectively, unlike pressure field mixers, which use pulsatile flow for enhanced mixing [127, 132, 134, 136, 142, 143].

3.3.1 Production of Microfluidics

As with any fabrication process, the selection of the appropriate method depends on factors such as material properties, application needs, production scale, precision, resolution, and cost. Early microfluidic devices were constructed using materials like glass, silicon, and quartz, with design processes involving photolithography and etching. For instance, wet etching of silicon and quartz is typically performed with potassium hydroxide and hydrofluoric acid, respectively, or reactive ion etching for dry etching of silicon. However, traditional materials and techniques have limitations, including high substrate costs, lengthy fabrication times, restricted design options with shallow channels, and a tendency for substrates to attract contaminants [124, 154–156]. More recent microfluidic devices have embraced the use of polymer substrates due to affordability and variety of options. Polymers can also be tailored for optimal performance in terms of optical, porosity, and insulation characteristics while offering relative ease of mass production. With the use of polymer materials, there are many ways of fabricating microfluidic devices [3, 146, 157].

Molding is a highly suited process for the rapid production of articles. In the context of microfluidics, replica molding is common [3, 136]. This method uses soft lithography to fabricate biomedical devices. The advantage of this approach for creating microstructures is its cost-effectiveness and time efficiency, as it eliminates the need to individually fabricate each structure. Once the template is designed as a mold or master, multiple duplicates can be produced. Great care is taken in crafting the master, which holds the negative of the desired pattern, ensuring it can be easily detached from the replicas without distortion. This requires minimizing friction and other factors that could cause deformation during production. The master consists of two components: structural support and the interchangeable mold inserts that imprint the desired features. The use of interchangeable mold inserts further reduces production costs. These inserts are etched and lithographed with the negative pattern of the design and are typically made from traditional materials like metal, glass, silicon, or polymers, chosen for their ability to detach easily [3, 136, 146, 158]. Injection molding is a method that allows high-volume fabrication with a good degree of accuracy, though limited by material restrictions and mold fabrication costs. It involves injecting the hot melted polymer at high pressure into a mold, cooling it, and then removing the finished product. Its advantages are cost-effectiveness for disposable medical products and full automation that reduces cycle times. It can be categorized into three types: micro-injection molding for small features, reaction injection molding that combines two polymer components, and injection compression molding that merges the benefits of both techniques [3, 144, 146].

Casting is applicable when working with silicone-based elastomers through soft lithography to produce features smaller than 100 nm. Soft lithography is ideal for small-scale prototyping due to its cost-effectiveness, ease, and high fidelity. Polydimethylsiloxane (PDMS) is a widely used material because of its flexibility, optical transparency, and gas permeability. It is ideal for applications like cell culturing although limited by its swelling in some organic solvents [124, 146, 148].

Microfluidic devices designed by laminate manufacturing are created by stacking layers of structures together. This method takes advantage of various techniques and materials with each bringing their specific benefits. It works with polymers like polycarbonate and polymethyl methacrylate [124, 154, 158, 159].

Laser engraving techniques are preferred for patterning polyimide for flexible sensor applications. UV and femtosecond lasers offer high precision and resolutions, though they are expensive to acquire and maintain. In contrast, CO_2 lasers provide lower resolution due to higher heat concentration, which can limit their applications [124, 146, 154, 160].

Three-dimensional printing is a reasonably new technique that builds microfluidic devices layer by layer. 3D printing in microfluidic design produces three-dimensional objects through an additive layer-on-layer process. It makes rapid prototyping easy, especially when the structures are complex. 3D printing technologies such as fused deposition modeling (FDM) and selective laser sintering (SLS) can be used to fabricate microfluidic devices with intricate features where soft lithography may be inapplicable [124, 157, 158, 161–163].

Hot embossing imprints mold shapes on thermoplastics at high temperature and pressure. It introduces a degree of flexibility in the geometric designs of the system although it is limited by the attribute of substrate material. Hot embossing is better achieved in a vacuum and requires optimum pressure for the features to be properly set on a substrate. First, the polymer is placed between the heated molds in a vacuum, then the mold is pressed on the softened polymer and then product is allowed to cool. Though there is a time lag between each cycle, this is compensated for by the high-volume capacity of the process and the capacity to produce parts with higher aspect ratios and finer features [124, 146, 164].

Thin foil methods which use thin substrates are also becoming popular. The thin foils protect sensitive contents and allow easy puncturing for reagent transfer. They require quick heat transfer and lower stiffness due to their reduced mass. In terms of cost, using thin films minimizes material usage, making production more economical, especially in large volumes. Foil materials can be either metals, paper, or polymers [124, 154].

3.3.2 Biomedical Applications

Microfluidics plays a vital role in diagnosis for better treatment outcomes which in a way increases the precision of medical diagnosis and treatments. They are used for studying drug resistance, and complex disease mechanisms and for evaluating therapeutic responses. They are also used to control theranostic nanoparticles in both treatment and diagnosis of cancer which increases efficacy while minimizing systemic toxicity. In cardiovascular disease detection, microfluidic platforms are often used as quick and compact diagnostic kits for biomarkers associated with heart conditions. During the COVID-19 pandemic, many point-of-care testing kits were products of microfluidic platforms which saved lives with easy scalability [136, 139, 165–168].

Traditional drug administration methods often require high doses to increase bioavailability which results in many side effects. Microfluidics enhances drug bioavailability, specificity, and precise control over drug delivery. They offer the advantage of targeted and controlled drug release, utilizing nanotechnology to encapsulate drugs within carriers like liposomes, dendrimers, and polymers. Using microfluidic fabrication techniques tailor-made nanoparticles with desired properties can be synthesized which enhances their effectiveness in drug delivery. For example, Doxil, a PEGylated liposomal carrier, has been successful in reducing side effects while delivering chemotherapy directly to tumor cells. Microfluidics also offer the potential for successful personalized medicine based on individual patient profiles and to better [149, 169–172].

Microfluidics have advanced tissue engineering and disease modeling by providing realistic biological environments for better therapeutic performance and effective predictive models. The use of microfluidics in tissue repair creates dynamic environments that better simulate natural physiological conditions by enhancing normal cell behavior and biochemical signaling. Microfluidics designs and principles have helped in fabricating better-performing extracellular matrixes. For instance, microfluidic platforms have been used to create magnetic chitosan microspheres for wound healing. Similarly, organ-on-a-chip (OoC) systems are built using microfluidic technology and they mimic the specific functions of human organs. They are used to studying complex bodily processes and provide a more accurate alternative to traditional animal testing in a controlled miniaturized environment. Typical examples are gut-on-a-chip platforms that simulate gut dynamics and microbial interactions, while bone-on-a-chip systems are used to study the relationship between breast cancer cells and bone cells. Liver-on-a-chip models can provide more information on pathological conditions like non-alcoholic fatty liver disease, while brain disorders like epilepsy are studied using brain-on-a-chip platforms [127, 136, 138, 171].

Microfluidics-based biosensors are clean, easy-to-deploy alternatives, being capable of rapidly analyzing biological molecules using minimal reagents thereby reduces byproducts and costs. These biosensors are categorized based on the type of bioelements used: nanozyme-based, enzyme-based, nucleic acid-based, and antibody- and sensors. Nanozyme-based biosensors are based on synthetic enzymes-imitating nanomaterials and are more stable and resistant to harsh conditions but limited in specificity. Enzyme-based microfluidic biosensors utilize enzymes to catalyze reactions and are capable of continuous monitoring activity with high selectivity and detection although limited by harsh conditions and loss of stability over time. The use of non-invasive flexible microfluidic system capable of measuring glucose levels from body fluids has expanded their potential. Nucleic acid-based biosensors work by identifying specific nucleic acid sequences which make them highly specific with the ability to regenerate layers of identification. Antibody-based microfluidic biosensors consist of immobilized antibodies for rapid detection and were effective during the COVID-19 pandemic for detecting SARS-CoV-2 antibodies using pharyngeal swabs. They tend to give false positives and may have stability issues [130, 136, 173–177].

Effective cryopreservation prevents cell damage due to osmotic shock and ice crystal formation. Microfluidics offers significant advantages in this regard, especially for preserving bioengineered materials. Microfluidic devices have enabled automated freeze–thaw cycle control and precise control over cryoprotective agent loading which minimizes osmotic stress on cells. Additionally, microfluidics is integral in the development of artificial cells and optimizing cryopreservation techniques. For instance, microfluidic platforms have been designed to preserve adherent cells on sensor surfaces which facilitate "ready-to-use" applications in various fields [152, 153, 178].

3.4 Personalized Medicine with Tailored Light Emitters

Personalized health care using light-based systems has transformed healthcare through minimal invasiveness and better performance of light emitters. In personalized medicine, the use of light emitters can be in the form of technological gadgets that interact with biological tissues for various medical purposes. These technological gadgets could be implanted or wearable medical devices and are now popular as a noninvasive means to track health metrics for daily living and in hospitals or for other self-administered procedures. Common metrics like heart rate and peripheral oxygen saturation are now at the fingertips of patients being made available using these devices [40, 43, 138, 179].

3.4.1 Personalized Devices in Biosensing and Imaging

Biosensing and molecular imaging use radiation emitted and reflected from biological tissues to obtain biometric information such as molecular content and microstructure. For example, wearable functional near-infrared (NIR) spectroscopy provides noninvasive neuroimaging for tracking brain activity. Similarly, wearable pulse oximeters measure blood oxygen levels based on the oxygenation and deoxygenation of hemoglobin. There are also photonic materials triggered biologically that are used in bioimaging [40, 177, 180]. An example is luciferin, which is a light-emitting compound that becomes oxidized and produces light in the presence of luciferase enzymes. This reaction requires oxygen and is found in various organisms such as fireflies and certain bacteria. The development of d-luciferin variants that emit different colors has enhanced bioimaging capabilities. Luciferins and mutant luciferases are being customized to improve stability and bioavailability for practical applications [40, 181]. Bioluminescent materials rely on bioluminescence resonance energy transfer (BRET) which is a phenomenon that occurs in biologically triggered materials when energy is transferred from a bioluminescent donor substance to an acceptor molecule without radioactive emissions [2, 40, 151, 179–183] (Table 3).

3.4.2 Personalized Devices in Phototherapy

In simple terms, phototherapy is based on delivering precise wavelengths for therapeutic effects using light emitters. There are different light-based therapies, each having its unique approach and purpose. Photothermal therapy (PTT) is a thermal therapy that uses light to generate heat in targeted tissues most time to kill cancer cells. The agents used for this procedure absorb near-infrared light and convert it into heat through non-radiative transitions. Similarly, photodynamic therapy (PDT) operates by using light-activated photosensitizers to produce reactive oxygen species (ROS) that can kill cancer cells [74, 184, 185]. These two therapies are often used together for better outcomes. Photobiomodulation (PBM) uses red or NIR light to stimulate physiological processes such as wound healing and tissue regeneration. PBM primarily involves cytochrome c oxidase which is a mitochondrial chromophore that enhances mitochondrial metabolism upon absorption of light. This process leads to increased production of adenosine triphosphate (ATP) which promotes cellular repair and regeneration[40, 43, 186–188]. Optogenetics involves optical control of cellular functions and is applicable in neurology and immunology. Implantable optogenetic devices have μLEDs embedded in hydrogel waveguides to stimulate specific cells or monitor biological responses in real time. Fluorescence is emitted in response to harmful substances and this phenomenon is used as in situ toxicity detection in living systems. The capabilities of optogenetic devices have been included to include stimulation, sensing, and wireless control[23, 42, 48, 54].

3.4.3 Implanted and Wearable Devices

The materials used and structural design of personalized medical devices are critical to their functionality [2, 40, 189]. Personalized medical devices are created using stretchable electronic materials that enable repeated use. These materials are essential in the design of implantable and wearable photonic healthcare devices due to their conformability, durability, and reliable performance. Their stretchability allows them to deform while adapting to biological systems, maintaining functionality and integrity. This feature also enables them to accommodate the elasticity of surrounding organs and tissues. Biocompatible elastomers, often used as substrates and insulating layers, are a key component of these materials. Common elastomers include

Table 3 Applications of light emitters in personalized medicine

Application area	Functionality	Device examples	Mechanism	Outcome	Benefits	Limitations	References
Biosensing and imaging	Data collection	NIR spectrometers	Tissue interaction for molecule detection	Brain, oxygen tracking	Non-invasive, real-time	Depth limit, movement sensitivity	[23, 24]
Bioimaging	Diagnostics	Bioluminescent probes	Light from luciferin-luciferase reaction	High-res imaging	High specificity	Limited to certain organisms	[25, 18, 26]
Photothermal therapy (PTT)	Cancer cell destruction	NIR-emitting devices	NIR light absorption heats and kills cells	Tumor targeting	Precise, minimally invasive	Risk to nearby tissues	[27, 28]
Photodynamic therapy (PDT)	Cancer treatment	Photosensitizers	Light-activated ROS kills cells	Tumor targeting	Targeted, low side effects	Limited penetration, ROS-dependent	[28, 29]
Photobiomodulation (PBM)	Tissue repair	LEDs	Red/NIR light boosts ATP for healing	Pain relief, regeneration	Noninvasive, natural healing	Limited depth, wavelength sensitivity	[20, 30]
Optogenetics	Cell control in brain research	μLED implants	Light activates modified neurons	Real-time brain studies	High control, specificity	Genetic modification required	[4, 31]
Wearables	Health monitoring	Smart lenses, glucose monitors	Sensors track markers like glucose	Continuous health tracking	Noninvasive, long-term wear	Battery life, irritation risk	[32, 33]
Implantables	Long-term monitoring	Cochlear implants, pacemakers	Wireless energy enables minimal invasiveness	Ongoing therapy or monitoring	No removal needed, wireless	Condition-specific, complex tech	[19, 21]

Ecoflex, poly(dimethylsiloxane), and polyurethane [189–192]. Stretchable conductors can withstand substantial strain without compromising their electrical performance. They are created using conductive materials or inks embedded within flexible substrates. Stretchable interconnections are typically formed from serpentine metal electrodes. The structural design of these materials is crucial to their adaptability and functionality. Effective structural configurations, such as island-interconnect designs, wavy patterns, and kirigami structures, help reduce stiffness and enhance mechanical performance. The concept of self-healing devices is based on their inherent ability to restore functionality independently after damage. This self-repair capability arises from dynamic molecular interactions, including metal–ligand coordination, π–π interactions, hydrogen bonding, and electrostatic interactions [191–195].

New generations of implanted devices are often designed with comfort, biocompatibility, and biodegradability in mind. They are made from materials that can degrade within the body which eliminates the need for removal of devices after they have performed their intended function in the body. Biodegradable materials are in essence bioabsorbable or excretable without leaving toxic remnants in the body. Biopolymers such as silk, gelatin, and cellulose, and synthetic polymers like poly(lactic-co-glycolic acid) (PLGA) and poly(1,8-octanediol-co-citrate), have been used in this wise [8, 196–199]. Organic materials derived from imine compounds and Iron and magnesium-based inorganic materials are also popular [8]. Implantable devices are now miniaturized, and their fabrication often means designing micro emitters and photodetectors. Implantable devices can be powered by electrochemical systems or wireless energy transfer systems. Electrochemical systems such as batteries are not as favored because of their space requirement and toxicity. Wireless power transfer methods such as near-field resonant inductive coupling, ultrasonic transcutaneous energy transfer, and far-field electromagnetic coupling are preferred. Such systems have been successfully implemented in commercially available devices like cochlear implants [8, 200, 201].

Wearable biomedical devices are popular for health monitoring and intervention including skin rejuvenation, wound care, mental health support, and therapies for brain diseases. There are myriads of products such as wristbands, patches, smart glasses, and contact lenses, all aimed at achieving seamless integration with the human body. Recent smart contact lenses, for example, offer continuous monitoring capabilities for glucose levels in tears. By integrating glucose sensors that utilize glucose oxidase, they can measure glucose concentrations in tears, which correlate closely with blood glucose levels. The μLEDs embedded within these lenses also serve as visual indicators that are activated when glucose levels drop below a specified threshold [202–204].

3.5 Artificial Photosynthesis

Artificial photosynthesis seeks to reproduce natural photosynthesis by converting sunlight into chemical energy as a means towards sustainable energy production. This process takes place in photochemical cells which are composed of photosensitizers, catalysts, and redox mediators that facilitate the necessary chemical reactions [205, 206]. An ecological benefit of the process is the mitigation of climate challenges by offsetting CO_2 emissions. The light emitters used determine the efficiency of these systems for maximizing sunlight capture and enhancing the efficiency of associated reactions. Advanced materials such as plasmonic nanoparticles and organic light emitters improve light absorption and charge separation efficiency. Multi-junction light-emitting systems can capture a broader spectrum of sunlight which closely resembles the layered absorption found in plants [207–211].

Advancements in photocatalysts and emitters have improved the prospect of hydrogen production and CO_2 reduction by using lower energy thresholds. Integrating light-emitting devices with two-dimensional materials like graphene or transition metal dichalcogenides improves efficiency by improving charge carrier mobility. Stability under prolonged light exposure is important and is important for ensuring that artificial photosynthesis can serve as a reliable alternative to traditional fuels. Photochemical cell performance can be improved by broadening absorption spectra, enhancing light absorption, and optimization of charge transport. The charge separation process in photochemical cells is a crucial step for converting light energy into chemical energy and preventing energy loss by recombination. The separate charges are responsible for the water oxidation which produces oxygen gas and protons. Separate charges also drive carbon dioxide reduction leading to the production of carbon monoxide and methanol. The role of redox mediators is to minimize energy loss during the electron transfer process and influence carbon dioxide reduction selectivity. The final products of artificial photosynthesis include hydrogen gas and various fuels [212–215].

3.6 Biodegradable Light Emitters

The growing concern about environmental footprints drives the push for biodegradability in technological inventions while maintaining performance excellence. The fabrication of biodegradable light emitters increases the possibility of sustainability. Recent advancements in material science have enabled the creation of biodegradable materials that exhibit excellent light-emitting properties, and they are equally as effective as conventional ones. In the biomedical implant space, this will eliminate the electronic waste generated by conventional light emitters [8, 36, 196].

Since biodegradable or bio-based materials can decompose, they present opportunities for applications in temporary electronics, eco-friendly sensors, and disposable diagnostic tools. For example, plant or protein-based organic light-emitting diodes (OLEDs) provide tunable emission properties and ensure environmental safety after use through natural decomposition. When used as biomedical implants, they can degrade after their functional life removing the need for surgery. By taking advantage of eco-friendly substrates like cellulose, silk fibroin, and chitosan, light emitters with excellent optical properties and stability have been developed. Biodegradable electronic devices can be protected from harsh conditions by encapsulations with biopolymers like carbohydrate-based sugars and starch. These biopolymers are also used as insulation materials between device components [8, 197].

3.6.1 Inorganic, Synthetic Polymers and Naturally Derived Semiconductors

Biodegradable electronics are often made of inorganic materials like silicon (Si) and metal oxides. Silicon is a core element in the semiconductor industry. Since nanosized silicon can undergo total hydrolysis its use in biodegradable materials has become popular. For instance, the use of nanosized silicon in biodegradable elastomer substrates to develop stretchable electrophysiology sensors that dissolve uniformly within hours has been carried out [147, 196, 216, 217].

Semiconducting polymers, such as polythiophenes and donor–acceptor copolymers, provide mechanical flexibility than inorganic options at a cheaper cost. Semiconducting polymers can be processed for custom-made applications and their conductivity is a function of the degree of π-conjugation because a higher level of conjugation improves charge transport. Partial degradability in these synthetic polymers is often accomplished by blending them with biodegradable insulating materials and natural fibers while completely degradable polymers are made by incorporating hydrolyzable linkages into the polymer backbone [196, 218–220].

Naturally occurring conjugated molecules and dyes, such as indigo have semiconductor properties and stable exciton transfer because of their strong intermolecular hydrogen bonding. Other naturally inspired synthetic dyes also show promise for biocompatible and biodegradable applications [196, 221–223].

3.6.2 Electrode Materials

Electrodes used in biodegradable light emitters can be noble metals, polymers, or carbon-based. Noble metals like gold and silver are used as electrode materials because of their conductivity and corrosion resistance. They are limited by their scarcity and the danger of bioaccumulation from long-term use. The potential of biodegradable metals such as magnesium and zinc is being explored because of their ease of processing and biocompatibility. Organic polymer and their doped derivatives being flexible are used especially in monitoring devices and stretchable electronics. Graphite and carbon nanotubes are carbon-based materials with good charge transfer attributes and flexibility and are choice materials for various sensor applications [1, 216, 224, 225].

Physical Sensors and chemical sensors in biodegradable devices play crucial roles in monitoring devices. Physical sensors are used to monitor changes in physical parameters such as pressure and temperature and so on while chemical sensors monitor changes in chemical properties, such as pH or concentration of compounds. Some physical sensors are used in capacitive structures filled with biodegradable materials that respond to pressure changes. For example, a wireless capacitive pressure sensor made of Zn/Fe bilayers exhibited sensitivity in the 0–20 kPa range and degraded over time in saline solutions. Temperature sensors made of piezoresistive materials such as functionalized silkworm fibers and carbon nanotubes with enhanced sensitivity have been developed. Chemical sensing materials can be made of polymers such as mesoporous chitosan which was developed for dopamine detection. They also provide non-invasive monitoring for biomarkers in biomedical devices [1, 196, 198, 226–230].

Soon, the integration of biodegradable light emitters with flexible electronics and energy-harvesting systems is expected to accelerate the adoption of sustainable, temporary electronic devices. These innovations could support the principles of a circular economy, ensuring that the entire life cycle of electronic products, from creation to disposal, remains fully sustainable. By focusing on both functionality and environmental impact, biodegradable light emitters represent a significant advancement in developing greener technologies for a wide range of applications.

4 Conclusion

Advanced light emitters are transformative elements shaping the future of medicine, sustainability, and technology. Their precise light delivery and exceptional control over parameters make them indispensable in diagnostics, personalized therapies, and emerging biodegradable applications that prioritize both functionality and environmental responsibility. In medicine, emitters like LEDs, OLEDs, and upconversion nanoparticles provide effective means for treating hard-to-reach areas with minimal invasiveness. The development of biodegradable light emitters further extends their impact, offering sustainable solutions for temporary implants and disposable medical devices that align innovation with environmental accountability goals. Beyond healthcare, light emitters are crucial parts of artificial photosynthesis systems and are enabling efficient sunlight-to-fuel conversion as solutions to global energy challenges. By mimicking natural processes and integrating with advanced catalysts, these systems hold the potential to capture carbon and produce renewable fuels. Innovation and research are further extending the precision, adaptability, and sustainability of light emitters for solving urgent and relevant global issues.

References

1. Zhang, P., Zhu, B., Du, P., Travas-Sejdic, J.: Electrochemical and electrical biosensors for wearable and implantable electronics based on conducting polymers and carbon-based materials. Chem. Rev. (2023). https://doi.org/10.1021/acs.chemrev.3c00392
2. Cha, G.D., Kim, D.-H., Kim, D.C.: Wearable and implantable light-emitting diodes and their biomedical applications. Korean J. Chem. Eng. **41**, 1–24 (2024). https://doi.org/10.1007/s11814-023-00006-z

3. Alexandre-Franco, M.F., Kouider, R., Kassir Al-Karany, R., Cuerda-Correa, E.M., Al-Kassir, A.: Recent advances in polymer science and fabrication processes for enhanced microfluidic applications: an overview. Micromachines **15**, 1137 (2024). https://doi.org/10.3390/mi15091137
4. Murawski, C., Gather, M.C.: Emerging biomedical applications of organic light-emitting diodes. Adv. Opt. Mater. **9** (2021). https://doi.org/10.1002/adom.202100269.
5. Rezende, T.K.L., Barbosa, H.P., dos Santos, L.F., de Lima, O.K., Alves de Matos, P., Tsubone, T.M., et al.: Upconversion rare earths nanomaterials applied to photodynamic therapy and bioimaging. Front. Chem. **10** (2022). https://doi.org/10.3389/fchem.2022.1035449.
6. Sun, W., Zhou, Z., Pratx, G., Chen, X., Chen, H.: Nanoscintillator-mediated X-ray induced photodynamic therapy for deep-seated tumors: from concept to biomedical applications. Theranostics **10**, 1296–318 (2020). https://doi.org/10.7150/thno.41578
7. Chelushkin, P.S., Shakirova, J.R., Kritchenkov, I.S., Baigildin, V.A., Tunik, S.P.: Phosphorescent NIR emitters for biomedicine: applications, advances and challenges. Dalton Trans. **51**, 1257–80 (2022). https://doi.org/10.1039/D1DT03077A
8. Alam, F., Ashfaq Ahmed, M., Jalal, A., Siddiquee, I., Adury, R., Hossain, G., et al.: Recent progress and challenges of implantable biodegradable biosensors. Micromachines **15**, 475 (2024). https://doi.org/10.3390/mi15040475
9. Sudheendran Swayamprabha, S., Dubey, D.K., Shahnawaz, Yadav, R.A.K., Nagar, M.R., Sharma, A., et al.: Approaches for long lifetime organic light emitting diodes. Adv. Sci. **8**, 1–29 (2021). https://doi.org/10.1002/advs.202002254
10. Kim, J.A., Wales, D.J., Yang, G.-Z.: Optical spectroscopy for in vivo medical diagnosis—a review of the state of the art and future perspectives. Prog. Biomed. Eng. **2**, 042001 (2020). https://doi.org/10.1088/2516-1091/abaaa3
11. Gomez Palacios, L.R., Bracamonte, A.G.: Development of nano- and microdevices for the next generation of biotechnology, wearables and miniaturized instrumentation. RSC Adv. **12**, 12806–22 (2022). https://doi.org/10.1039/D2RA02008D
12. Yun, S.H., Kwok, S.J.J.: Light in diagnosis, therapy and surgery. Nat. Biomed. Eng. **1**, 0008 (2017). https://doi.org/10.1038/s41551-016-0008
13. Chehelgerdi, M., Chehelgerdi, M., Allela, O.Q.B., Pecho, R.D.C., Jayasankar, N., Rao, D.P., et al.: Progressing nanotechnology to improve targeted cancer treatment: overcoming hurdles in its clinical implementation. Mol. Cancer **22** (2023). https://doi.org/10.1186/s12943-023-01865-0
14. Zhao, W., Huang, X., Hu, S., Yang, F., Zhong, J.: Rare-earth nanocrystalline scintillators for biomedical application: a review. Ceram. Int. (2024). https://doi.org/10.1016/j.ceramint.2024.08.149
15. Hong, Z., Chen, Z., Chen, Q., Yang, H.: Advancing X-ray luminescence for imaging, biosensing, and theragnostics. Acc. Chem. Res. **56**, 37–51 (2023). https://doi.org/10.1021/acs.accounts.2c00517
16. Wagner, A.M., Knipe, J.M., Orive, G., Peppas, N.A.: Quantum dots in biomedical applications. Acta Biomater. **94**, 44–63 (2019). https://doi.org/10.1016/j.actbio.2019.05.022
17. Vasilopoulou, M., Fakharuddin, A., García de Arquer, F.P., Georgiadou, D.G., Kim, H., Mohd Yusoff, A.R.B., et al.: Advances in solution-processed near-infrared light-emitting diodes. Nat. Photonics **15**, 656–669 (2021). https://doi.org/10.1038/s41566-021-00855-2
18. Jin, H., Jiang, X., Sun, Z., Gui, R.: Phosphorescence-based ratiometric probes: design, preparation and applications in sensing, imaging and biomedicine therapy. Coord. Chem. Rev. **431**, 213694 (2021). https://doi.org/10.1016/j.ccr.2020.213694
19. Mehta, P.P.: Miniaturized devices: a silk route for innovative commercial prospects. Lab-on-a-chip devices for advanced biomedicines. R. Soc. Chem. 615–648 (2024). https://doi.org/10.1039/9781837673476-00615
20. Pode, R.: Organic light emitting diode devices: an energy efficient solid state lighting for applications. Renew. Sustain. Energy Rev. **133**, 110043 (2020). https://doi.org/10.1016/j.rser.2020.110043

21. Zhang, J., Han, M., Xu, M., Zhang, L., Liu, S., Xie, W.: Color-tunable organic light-emitting devices and their applications. Cell Rep. Phys. Sci. **5**, 101764 (2024). https://doi.org/10.1016/j.xcrp.2023.101764
22. Chen, F.: Emerging organic and organic/inorganic hybrid photovoltaic devices for specialty applications: low-level-lighting energy conversion and biomedical treatment. Adv. Optic. Mater. **7** (2019). https://doi.org/10.1002/adom.201800662
23. Mahata, M.K., De, R., Lee, K.T.: Near-infrared-triggered upconverting nanoparticles for biomedicine applications. Biomedicines **9**, 1–26 (2021). https://doi.org/10.3390/biomedicines9070756
24. Osuchowski, M., Osuchowski, F., Latos, W., Kawczyk-Krupka, A.: The use of upconversion nanoparticles in prostate cancer photodynamic therapy. Life **11**, 360 (2021). https://doi.org/10.3390/life11040360
25. Divya, J., Selvendran, S., Raja, A.S., Sivasubramanian, A.: Surface plasmon based plasmonic sensors: a review on their past, present and future. Biosens. Bioelectron. X **11**, 100175 (2022). https://doi.org/10.1016/j.biosx.2022.100175
26. Jiang, M., Deng, Z., Zeng, S., Hao, J.: Recent progress on lanthanide scintillators for soft X-ray-triggered bioimaging and deep-tissue theranostics. View **2**, 1–9 (2021). https://doi.org/10.1002/VIW.20200122
27. Michalik, M., Szymańczyk, J., Stajnke, M., Ochrymiuk, T., Cenian, A.: Medical applications of diode lasers: pulsed versus continuous wave (cw) regime. Micromachines **12** (2021). https://doi.org/10.3390/mi12060710
28. Mushtaq, U., Ayoub, I., Kumar, V., Sharma, V., Swart, H.C., Chamanehpour, E., et al.: Persistent luminescent nanophosphors for applications in cancer theranostics, biomedical, imaging and security. Mater. Today Bio **23**, 100860 (2023). https://doi.org/10.1016/j.mtbio.2023.100860
29. Xiao, D., Qi, H., Teng, Y., Pierre, D., Kutoka, P.T., Liu, D.: Advances and challenges of fluorescent nanomaterials for synthesis and biomedical applications. Nanoscale Res. Lett. **16** (2021). https://doi.org/10.1186/s11671-021-03613-z.
30. Lu, H., Alkhazragi, O., Wang, Y., Almaymoni, N., Yan, W., Gunawan, W.H., et al.: Low-coherence semiconductor light sources: devices and applications. Npj Nanophotonics **1**, 9 (2024). https://doi.org/10.1038/s44310-024-00005-w
31. Armstrong, R.E., Horáček, M., Zijlstra, P.: Plasmonic assemblies for real-time single-molecule biosensing. Small **16** (2020). https://doi.org/10.1002/smll.202003934
32. Barbora, A., Bohar, O., Sivan, A.A., Magory, E., Nause, A., Minnes, R.: Higher pulse frequency of near-infrared laser irradiation increases penetration depth for novel biomedical applications. PLoS ONE **16**, 1–11 (2021). https://doi.org/10.1371/journal.pone.0245350
33. Hidayat, W., Usman, M.: Applications of molecular beam epitaxy in optoelectronic devices: an overview. Phys. Scr. **99**, 112002 (2024). https://doi.org/10.1088/1402-4896/ad8318
34. Anand, V., Mishra, R., Barot, Y.: Recent advances in the development of pure organic white light emitters. Dyes Pigm. **191**, 109390 (2021). https://doi.org/10.1016/j.dyepig.2021.109390
35. Kaur, S., Kaur, H., Rao, A.S., Prakash, G.V.: A review on photoluminescence phosphors for biomedical, temperature sensing, photovoltaic cell, anti-counterfeiting and white LED applications. Physica B **690**, 416224 (2024). https://doi.org/10.1016/j.physb.2024.416224
36. Kong, D., Zhang, K., Tian, J., Yin, L., Sheng, X.: Biocompatible and biodegradable light-emitting materials and devices. Adv. Mater. Technol. **7**, 1–17 (2022). https://doi.org/10.1002/admt.202100006
37. Guo, K., Righetto, M., Minotto, A., Zampetti, A., Cacialli, F.: Non-toxic near-infrared light-emitting diodes. IScience **24**, 102545 (2021). https://doi.org/10.1016/j.isci.2021.102545
38. Yew, P.Y.M., Chee, P.L., Lin, Q., Owh, C., Li, J., Dou, Q.Q., et al.: Hydrogel for light delivery in biomedical applications. Bioactive Mater. **37**, 407–23 (2024). https://doi.org/10.1016/j.bioactmat.2024.03.031
39. Sahoo, P.R.: Light responsive materials: properties, design, and applications. 101–27 (2023). https://doi.org/10.1021/bk-2023-1436.ch005

40. Lee, G.H., Moon, H., Kim, H., Lee, G.H., Kwon, W., Yoo, S., et al.: Multifunctional materials for implantable and wearable photonic healthcare devices. Nat. Rev. Mater. **5**, 149–65 (2020). https://doi.org/10.1038/s41578-019-0167-3
41. Lee, H.P., Gaharwar, A.K.: Light-responsive inorganic biomaterials for biomedical applications. Adv. Sci. **7** (2020). https://doi.org/10.1002/advs.202000863
42. Chen, L., Liu, Y., Guo, W., Liu, Z.: Light responsive nucleic acid for biomedical application. Exploration **2** (2022). https://doi.org/10.1002/EXP.20210099
43. Sia, C.S., Tey, B.T., Low, L.E.: Light-responsive nanoassemblies: advancing biomedical innovation. Adv. Funct. Mater. **34** (2024). https://doi.org/10.1002/adfm.202314278
44. Koryakina, I., Kuznetsova, D.S., Zuev, D.A., Milichko, V.A., Timin, A.S., Zyuzin, M.V.: Optically responsive delivery platforms: from the design considerations to biomedical applications. Nanophotonics **9**, 39–74 (2020). https://doi.org/10.1515/nanoph-2019-0423
45. Haque, S., Sher Shah, M.S.A., Rahman, M., Mohiuddin, M.: Biopolymer composites in light emitting diodes. In: Biopolymer Composites in Electronics, pp. 277–310. Elsevier (2017). https://doi.org/10.1016/B978-0-12-809261-3.00010-3
46. Zampetti, A., Minotto, A., Cacialli, F.: Near-Infrared (NIR) Organic light-emitting diodes (OLEDs): challenges and opportunities. Adv. Funct. Mater. **29** (2019). https://doi.org/10.1002/adfm.201807623
47. Chen, Z., Obaid, S.N., Lu, L.: Recent advances in organic optoelectronic devices for biomedical applications. Optic. Mater. Express **9**, 3843 (2019). https://doi.org/10.1364/OME.9.003843
48. Morton, A., Murawski, C., Pulver, S.R., Gather, M.C.: High-brightness organic light-emitting diodes for optogenetic control of Drosophila locomotor behaviour. Sci. Rep. **6**, 31117 (2016). https://doi.org/10.1038/srep31117
49. Attili, S.K., Lesar, A., McNeill, A., Camacho-Lopez, M., Moseley, H., Ibbotson, S., et al.: An open pilot study of ambulatory photodynamic therapy using a wearable low-irradiance organic light-emitting diode light source in the treatment of nonmelanoma skin cancer. Br. J. Dermatol. **161**, 170–3 (2009). https://doi.org/10.1111/j.1365-2133.2009.09096.x
50. Rahman, T., Raza, S., Saeed, M., Jameel, S.: An emerging white LED technology and associated thermal issues—a review. J. Appl. Emerg. Sci. 106–120 (2019). https://doi.org/10.36785/BUITEMS.JAES.301
51. Mukunda, D.C., Rodrigues, J., Joshi, V.K., Raghushaker, C.R., Mahato, K.K.: A comprehensive review on LED-induced fluorescence in diagnostic pathology. Biosens. Bioelectron. **209**, 114230 (2022). https://doi.org/10.1016/j.bios.2022.114230
52. Glass, G.E.: Photobiomodulation: the clinical applications of low-level light therapy. Aesthetic Surg. J. **41**, 723–38 (2021). https://doi.org/10.1093/asj/sjab025
53. Oyama, J., Fernandes Herculano Ramos-Milaré, Á.C., Lopes Lera-Nonose, D.S.S., Nesi-Reis, V., Galhardo Demarchi, I., Alessi Aristides, S.M., et al.: Photodynamic therapy in wound healing in vivo: a systematic review. Photodiagn. Photodyn. Therapy **30**, 101682 (2020). https://doi.org/10.1016/j.pdpdt.2020.101682
54. Hee Lee, J., Lee, S., Kim, D., Jae, L.K.: Implantable micro-light-emitting diode (μLED)-based optogenetic interfaces toward human applications. Adv. Drug Deliv. Rev. **187**, 114399 (2022). https://doi.org/10.1016/j.addr.2022.114399
55. Zhang, H., Peng, Y., Zhang, N., Yang, J., Wang, Y., Ding, H.: Emerging optoelectronic devices based on microscale LEDs and their use as implantable biomedical applications. Micromachines **13**, 1069 (2022). https://doi.org/10.3390/mi13071069
56. Lee, H.E., Shin, J.H., Park, J.H., Hong, S.K., Park, S.H., Lee, S.H., et al.: Micro light-emitting diodes for display and flexible biomedical applications. Adv. Funct. Mater. **29** (2019). https://doi.org/10.1002/adfm.201808075
57. Gunnarsson, W.B., Roh, K., Zhao, L., Murphy, J.P., Grede, A.J., Giebink, N.C., et al.: Toward nonepitaxial laser diodes. Chem. Rev. **123**, 7548–84 (2023). https://doi.org/10.1021/acs.chemrev.2c00721
58. Insero, G., Fusi, F., Romano, G.: The safe use of lasers in biomedicine: principles of laser-matter interaction. J. Publ. Health Res. **12** (2023). https://doi.org/10.1177/22799036231187077

59. Chamkouri, H., Si, J., Chen, P., Niu, C., Chen, L.: Biomedical optics and photonics for advanced clinical technologies. Opt. Laser Technol. **179**, 111265 (2024). https://doi.org/10.1016/j.optlastec.2024.111265
60. Baten, M.Z., Alam, S., Sikder, B., Aziz, A.: III-nitride light-emitting devices. Photonics **8**, 430 (2021). https://doi.org/10.3390/photonics8100430
61. Ng, T.K., Holguin-Lerma, J.A., Kang, C.H., Ashry, I., Zhang, H., Bucci, G., et al.: Group-III-nitride and halide-perovskite semiconductor gain media for amplified spontaneous emission and lasing applications. J. Phys. D Appl. Phys. **54**, 143001 (2021). https://doi.org/10.1088/1361-6463/abd65a
62. Ishii, H., Takahashi, T., Yamaguchi, K., Nemoto, T.: Advanced observation of brain and nerve cells using two-photon microscopy with novel techniques. Microscopy **72**, 144–50 (2023). https://doi.org/10.1093/jmicro/dfac047
63. Sanderson, J.: Multi-photon microscopy. Curr. Protoc. **3** (2023). https://doi.org/10.1002/cpz1.634
64. Nazar, J., Nibin, T.N.: LASER in oral and maxillofacial surgery- review of literature. Int. J. Sci. Res. Sci. Technol. 87–112 (2023). https://doi.org/10.32628/IJSRST52310612
65. Huang, A., Nguyen, J.K., Jagdeo, J.: Light-emitting diode-based photodynamic therapy for photoaging, scars, and dyspigmentation: a systematic review. Dermatol. Surg. **46**, 1388–94 (2020). https://doi.org/10.1097/DSS.0000000000002351
66. Mosaddad, S.A., Namanloo, R.A., Aghili, S.S., Maskani, P., Alam, M., Abbasi, K., et al.: Photodynamic therapy in oral cancer: a review of clinical studies. Med. Oncol. **40**, 91 (2023). https://doi.org/10.1007/s12032-023-01949-3
67. Cattini, S., Rovati, L.: A review on guided optical feedback in super-luminescence diodes for metrological purposes. J. Lightwave Technol. **39**, 3771–80 (2021). https://doi.org/10.1109/JLT.2020.3035565
68. Ansari, A.A., Sillanpää, M.: Advancement in upconversion nanoparticles based NIR-driven photocatalysts. Renew. Sustain. Energy Rev. **151**, 111631 (2021). https://doi.org/10.1016/j.rser.2021.111631
69. Francés-Soriano, L., Ferrera-González, J., González-Béjar, M., Pérez-Prieto, J.: Near-infrared excitation/emission microscopy with lanthanide-based nanoparticles. Anal. Bioanal. Chem. **414**, 4291–310 (2022). https://doi.org/10.1007/s00216-022-03999-4
70. Zhang, Z., Chen, Y., Zhang, Y.: Self-assembly of upconversion nanoparticles based materials and their emerging applications. Small **18** (2022). https://doi.org/10.1002/smll.202103241.
71. Gupta, S.K., Penilla Garcia, M.A., Zuniga, J.P., Abdou, M., Mao, Y.: Visible and ultraviolet upconversion and near infrared downconversion luminescence from lanthanide doped La2Zr2O7 nanoparticles. J. Lumin. **214**, 116591 (2019). https://doi.org/10.1016/j.jlumin.2019.116591
72. Zhang, J., Jin, C.: Electronic structure, upconversion luminescence and optical temperature sensing behavior of Yb3+-Er3+/Ho3+ doped NaLaMgWO6. J. Alloy. Compd. **783**, 84–94 (2019). https://doi.org/10.1016/j.jallcom.2018.12.281
73. Wang, C., Cheng, L., Liu, Z.: Upconversion nanoparticles for photodynamic therapy and other cancer therapeutics. Theranostics **3**, 317–30 (2013). https://doi.org/10.7150/thno.5284
74. Lee, S.Y., Lee, R., Kim, E., Lee, S., Park II, Y.: Near-infrared light-triggered photodynamic therapy and apoptosis using upconversion nanoparticles with dual photosensitizers. Front. Bioeng. Biotechnol. **8** (2020). https://doi.org/10.3389/fbioe.2020.00275
75. Naher, H.S., Al-Turaihi, B.A.H., Mohammed, S.H., Naser, S.M., Albark, M.A., Madlool, H.A., et al.: Upconversion nanoparticles (UCNPs): synthesis methods, imaging and cancer therapy. J. Drug Deliv. Sci. Technol. **80**, 104175 (2023). https://doi.org/10.1016/j.jddst.2023.104175
76. Hang, Y., Wang, A., Wu, N.: Plasmonic silver and gold nanoparticles: shape- and structure-modulated plasmonic functionality for point-of-caring sensing, bio-imaging and medical therapy. Chem. Soc. Rev. **53**, 2932–71 (2024). https://doi.org/10.1039/D3CS00793F
77. Yuan, Y., Peng, X., Weng, X., He, J., Liao, C., Wang, Y., et al.: Two-dimensional nanomaterials as enhanced surface plasmon resonance sensing platforms: design perspectives and illustrative

applications. Biosens. Bioelectron. **241**, 115672 (2023). https://doi.org/10.1016/j.bios.2023.115672
78. Ta, N., Huang, J.-Y., He, S., Hanggai, W., Chao, L.-M.: Applications of optical control materials based on localized surface plasmon resonance effect in smart windows. Tungsten **6**, 711–31 (2024). https://doi.org/10.1007/s42864-024-00273-1
79. Fu, Q., Li, Z., Fu, F., Chen, X., Song, J., Yang, H.: Stimuli-responsive plasmonic assemblies and their biomedical applications. Nano Today **36**, 101014 (2021). https://doi.org/10.1016/j.nantod.2020.101014
80. Philip, A., Kumar, A.R.: The performance enhancement of surface plasmon resonance optical sensors using nanomaterials: a review. Coord. Chem. Rev. **458**, 214424 (2022). https://doi.org/10.1016/j.ccr.2022.214424
81. Jin, C., Wu, Z., Molinski, J.H., Zhou, J., Ren, Y., Zhang, J.X.J.: Plasmonic nanosensors for point-of-care biomarker detection. Mater. Today Bio **14**, 100263 (2022). https://doi.org/10.1016/j.mtbio.2022.100263
82. Sharma, S., Swami, S., Sharma, N., Saini, A.: Recent trends in plasmonic silver nano-sensors development for copper metal ion sensing in aqueous medium: a comprehensive review. Plasmonics (2024). https://doi.org/10.1007/s11468-024-02409-y
83. Yu, X., Wang, Z., Cui, H., Wu, X., Chai, W., Wei, J., et al.: A review on gold nanotriangles: synthesis, self-assembly and their applications. Molecules **27**, 8766 (2022). https://doi.org/10.3390/molecules27248766
84. Coviello, V., Forrer, D., Amendola, V.: Recent developments in plasmonic alloy nanoparticles: synthesis, modelling, properties and applications. ChemPhysChem **23** (2022). https://doi.org/10.1002/cphc.202200136
85. Wei, Z., Janczarek, M., Wang, K., Zheng, S., Kowalska, E.: Morphology-governed performance of plasmonic photocatalysts. Catalysts **10**, 1070 (2020). https://doi.org/10.3390/catal10091070
86. Chupradit, S., Kavitha, M., Suksatan, W., Ansari, M.J., Al Mashhadani, Z.I., Kadhim, M.M., et al.: Morphological control: properties and applications of metal nanostructures. Adv. Mater. Sci. Eng. **2022**, 1–15 (2022). https://doi.org/10.1155/2022/1971891
87. Kim, J., Piao, Y., Hyeon, T.: Multifunctional nanostructured materials for multimodal imaging, and simultaneous imaging and therapy. Chem. Soc. Rev. **38**, 372–90 (2009). https://doi.org/10.1039/B709883A
88. Wang, Y., Pan, M., Yu, X., Xu, L.: The recent advances of fluorescent sensors based on molecularly imprinted fluorescent nanoparticles for pharmaceutical analysis. Curr. Med. Sci. **40**, 407–21 (2020). https://doi.org/10.1007/s11596-020-2195-z
89. Zhen, X., Qu, R., Chen, W., Wu, W., Jiang, X.: The development of phosphorescent probes for in vitro and in vivo bioimaging. Biomater. Sci. **9**, 285–300 (2021). https://doi.org/10.1039/D0BM00819B
90. Ding, C., Ren, T.: Near infrared fluorescent probes for detecting and imaging active small molecules. Coord. Chem. Rev. **482**, 215080 (2023). https://doi.org/10.1016/j.ccr.2023.215080
91. Zhao, S., Chen, L., Yang, Y., Liu, X.: Research progress of phosphorescent probe for biological imaging. J. Mol. Struct. **1269**, 133855 (2022). https://doi.org/10.1016/j.molstruc.2022.133855
92. Kwon, N., Kim, D., Swamy, K.M.K., Yoon, J.: Metal-coordinated fluorescent and luminescent probes for reactive oxygen species (ROS) and reactive nitrogen species (RNS). Coord. Chem. Rev. **427**, 213581 (2021). https://doi.org/10.1016/j.ccr.2020.213581
93. Lécuyer, T., Bia, N., Burckel, P., Loubat, C., Graillot, A., Seguin, J., et al.: Persistent luminescence nanoparticles functionalized by polymers bearing phosphonic acid anchors: synthesis, characterization, and in vivo behaviour. Nanoscale **14**, 1386–94 (2022). https://doi.org/10.1039/D1NR07114A
94. Borghei, Y.S., Hosseinkhani, S., Ganjali, M.R.: "Plasmonic Nanomaterials": an emerging avenue in biomedical and biomedical engineering opportunities. J. Adv. Res. **39**, 61–71 (2022). https://doi.org/10.1016/j.jare.2021.11.006
95. Akgönüllü, S., Denizli, A.: Plasmonic nanosensors for pharmaceutical and biomedical analysis. J. Pharmaceut. Biomed. Anal. **236** (2023). https://doi.org/10.1016/j.jpba.2023.115671

96. Maldiney, T., Bessière, A., Seguin, J., Teston, E., Sharma, S.K., Viana, B., et al.: The in vivo activation of persistent nanophosphors for optical imaging of vascularization, tumours and grafted cells. Nat. Mater. **13**, 418–26 (2014). https://doi.org/10.1038/nmat3908
97. Jin, M., Shi, P., Sun, Z., Zhao, N., Shi, M., Wu, M., et al.: Advancements in polymer-assisted layer-by-layer fabrication of wearable sensors for health monitoring. Sensors **24**, 2903 (2024). https://doi.org/10.3390/s24092903
98. Zhu, H., Ding, X., Wang, C., Cao, M., Yu, B., Cong, H., et al.: Preparation of rare earth-doped nano-fluorescent materials in the second near-infrared region and their application in biological imaging. J. Mater. Chem. B **12**, 1947–72 (2024). https://doi.org/10.1039/D3TB01987J
99. Parauha, Y.R., Sahu, V., Dhoble, S.J.: Prospective of combustion method for preparation of nanomaterials: a challenge. Mater. Sci. Eng., B **267**, 115054 (2021). https://doi.org/10.1016/j.mseb.2021.115054
100. Rahman, J.U., Khan, S., Jain, V., Rajiv, A., Dasi, S., Fawy, K.F., et al.: Exploring inorganic phosphors: basics, types, fabrications and their luminescence properties for LED/WLED/displays. Rev. Inorg. Chem. (2024). https://doi.org/10.1515/revic-2024-0044
101. Gupta, S.K., Sudarshan, K., Kadam, R.M.: Optical nanomaterials with focus on rare earth doped oxide: a review. Mater. Today Commun. **27**, 102277 (2021). https://doi.org/10.1016/j.mtcomm.2021.102277
102. Li, H., Wang, Y., Liao, L.: Near-infrared luminescent materials incorporating rare earth/transition metal ions: from materials to applications. Adv. Mater. **36** (2024). https://doi.org/10.1002/adma.202403076
103. Chen, M.-H., Jenh, Y.-J., Wu, S.-K., Chen, Y.-S., Hanagata, N., Lin, F.-H.: Non-invasive photodynamic therapy in brain cancer by use of Tb3+-doped LaF3 nanoparticles in combination with photosensitizer through X-ray irradiation: a proof-of-concept study. Nanoscale Res. Lett. **12**, 62 (2017). https://doi.org/10.1186/s11671-017-1840-3
104. Michail, C., Liaparinos, P., Kalyvas, N., Kandarakis, I., Fountos, G., Valais, I.: Phosphors and scintillators in biomedical imaging. Crystals **14** (2024). https://doi.org/10.3390/cryst14020169
105. Kumar, V., Luo, Z.: A review on X-ray excited emission decay dynamics in inorganic scintillator materials. Photonics **8**, 71 (2021). https://doi.org/10.3390/photonics8030071
106. Jayaprakash Saiji, S., Tang, Y., Wu, S.-T., Stand, L., Tratsiak, Y., Dong, Y.: Metal halide perovskite polymer composites for indirect X-ray detection. Nanoscale **16**, 17654–82 (2024). https://doi.org/10.1039/D4NR02716G
107. Mukhopadhyay, S., Maurer, R.J., Guss, P.P.: Modern trends in gamma detection systems for emergency response. In: Fiederle, M., Burger, A., Payne, S.A. (eds.) Hard X-Ray, Gamma-Ray, and Neutron Detector Physics XXII, SPIE, p. 10. (2020). https://doi.org/10.1117/12.2560115
108. Wehrse, E., Klein, L., Rotkopf, L.T., Wagner, W.L., Uhrig, M., Heußel, C.P., et al.: Photon-counting detectors in computed tomography: from quantum physics to clinical practice. Radiologe **61**, 1–10 (2021). https://doi.org/10.1007/s00117-021-00812-8
109. Lu, L., Sun, M., Lu, Q., Wu, T., Huang, B.: High energy X-ray radiation sensitive scintillating materials for medical imaging, cancer diagnosis and therapy. Nano Energy **79** (2021). https://doi.org/10.1016/j.nanoen.2020.105437
110. Baig, N., Kammakakam, I., Falath, W., Kammakakam, I.: Nanomaterials: a review of synthesis methods, properties, recent progress, and challenges. Mater. Adv. **2**, 1821–71 (2021). https://doi.org/10.1039/d0ma00807a
111. Liu, M.: Optical properties of carbon dots: a review. Nanoarchitectonics **1**, 1–12 (2020). https://doi.org/10.37256/nat.112020124.1-12
112. Zhao, Q., Song, W., Zhao, B., Yang, B.: Spectroscopic studies of the optical properties of carbon dots: recent advances and future prospects. Mater. Chem. Front. **4**, 472–88 (2020). https://doi.org/10.1039/C9QM00592G
113. Bhattacharya, T., Preetam, S., Mukherjee, S., Kar, S., Roy, D.S., Singh, H., et al.: Anticancer activity of quantum size carbon dots: opportunities and challenges. Discover Nano **19**, 122 (2024). https://doi.org/10.1186/s11671-024-04069-7

114. Alafeef, M., Srivastava, I., Aditya, T., Pan, D.: Carbon dots: from synthesis to unraveling the fluorescence mechanism. Small **20** (2024). https://doi.org/10.1002/smll.202303937
115. Döring, A., Ushakova, E., Rogach, A.L.: Chiral carbon dots: synthesis, optical properties, and emerging applications. Light Sci. Appl. **11**, 75 (2022). https://doi.org/10.1038/s41377-022-00764-1
116. Kuang, T., Jin, M., Lu, X., Liu, T., Vahabi, H., Gu, Z., et al.: Functional carbon dots derived from biomass and plastic wastes. Green Chem. **25**, 6581–602 (2023). https://doi.org/10.1039/D3GC01763J
117. Cohen, E.N., Kondiah, P.P.D., Choonara, Y.E., du Toit, L.C., Pillay, V.: Carbon dots as nanotherapeutics for biomedical application. Curr. Pharm. Des. **26**, 2207–21 (2020). https://doi.org/10.2174/1381612826666200402102308
118. Wang, B., Cai, H., Waterhouse, G.I.N., Qu, X., Yang, B., Lu, S.: Carbon dots in bioimaging, biosensing and therapeutics: a comprehensive review. Small Sci. **2** (2022). https://doi.org/10.1002/smsc.202200012
119. Ge, G., Li, L., Wang, D., Chen, M., Zeng, Z., Xiong, W., et al.: Carbon dots: synthesis, properties and biomedical applications. J. Mater. Chem. B **9**, 6553–75 (2021). https://doi.org/10.1039/D1TB01077H
120. Alaghmandfard, A., Sedighi, O., Tabatabaei Rezaei, N., Abedini, A.A., Malek Khachatourian, A., Toprak, M.S., et al.: Recent advances in the modification of carbon-based quantum dots for biomedical applications. Mater. Sci. Eng. C **120**, 111756 (2021). https://doi.org/10.1016/j.msec.2020.111756
121. Vibhute, A., Patil, T., Gambhir, R., Tiwari, A.P.: Fluorescent carbon quantum dots: synthesis methods, functionalization and biomedical applications. Appl. Surf. Sci. Adv. **11**, 100311 (2022). https://doi.org/10.1016/j.apsadv.2022.100311
122. Iravani, S., Varma, R.S.: Green synthesis, biomedical and biotechnological applications of carbon and graphene quantum dots. A review. Environ. Chem. Lett. **18**, 703–27 (2020). https://doi.org/10.1007/s10311-020-00984-0
123. Abdellatif, A.A., Younis, M.A., Alsharidah, M., Al Rugaie, O., Tawfeek, H.M.: Biomedical applications of quantum dots: overview, challenges, and clinical potential. Int. J. Nanomed. **17**, 1951–70 (2022). https://doi.org/10.2147/IJN.S357980
124. Scott, S.M., Ali, Z.: Fabrication methods for microfluidic devices: an overview. Micromachines **12** (2021). https://doi.org/10.3390/mi12030319
125. Whitesides, G.M.: The origins and the future of microfluidics. Nature **442**, 368–73 (2006). https://doi.org/10.1038/nature05058
126. Zhang, X., Xu, X., Wang, J., Wang, C., Yan, Y., Wu, A., et al.: Public-health-driven microfluidic technologies: from separation to detection. Micromachines **12**, 391 (2021). https://doi.org/10.3390/mi12040391
127. Nasiri, R., Shamloo, A., Ahadian, S., Amirifar, L., Akbari, J., Goudie, M.J., et al.: Microfluidic-based approaches in targeted cell/particle separation based on physical properties: fundamentals and applications. Small **16** (2020). https://doi.org/10.1002/smll.202000171
128. Hettiarachchi, S., Cha, H., Ouyang, L., Mudugamuwa, A., An, H., Kijanka, G., et al.: Recent microfluidic advances in submicron to nanoparticle manipulation and separation. Lab Chip **23**, 982–1010 (2023). https://doi.org/10.1039/D2LC00793B
129. Măriuţa, D., Colin, S., Barrot-Lattes, C., Le Calvé, S., Korvink, J.G., Baldas, L., et al.: Miniaturization of fluorescence sensing in optofluidic devices. Microfluid. Nanofluid. **24**, 65 (2020). https://doi.org/10.1007/s10404-020-02371-1
130. Wang, L., Zhu, W., Zhang, J., Zhu, J.-J.: Miniaturized microfluidic electrochemical biosensors powered by enzymatic biofuel cell. Biosensors **13**, 175 (2023). https://doi.org/10.3390/bios13020175
131. Fu, X., Sun, J., Liang, R., Guo, H., Wang, L., Sun, X.: Application progress of microfluidics-integrated biosensing platforms in the detection of foodborne pathogens. Trends Food Sci. Technol. **116**, 115–29 (2021). https://doi.org/10.1016/j.tifs.2021.07.006

132. Zhang, Y., Zheng, T., Wang, L., Feng, L., Wang, M., Zhang, Z., et al.: From passive to active sorting in microfluidics: a review. Rev. Adv. Mater. Sci. **60**, 313–24 (2021). https://doi.org/10.1515/rams-2020-0044
133. Bayareh, M.: An updated review on particle separation in passive microfluidic devices. Chem. Eng. Proc. Process Intensificat. **153**, 107984 (2020). https://doi.org/10.1016/j.cep.2020.107984
134. Ju, T.: Working principle and applications of active and passive microfluidic valves. J. Phys: Conf. Ser. **2230**, 012013 (2022). https://doi.org/10.1088/1742-6596/2230/1/012013
135. Zhang, T., Di Carlo, D., Lim, C.T., Zhou, T., Tian, G., Tang, T., et al.: Passive microfluidic devices for cell separation. Biotechnol. Adv. **71**, 108317 (2024). https://doi.org/10.1016/j.biotechadv.2024.108317
136. Gharib, G., Bütün, İ., Muganlı, Z., Kozalak, G., Namlı, İ., Sarraf, S.S., et al. Biomedical applications of microfluidic devices: a review. Biosensors **12** (2022). https://doi.org/10.3390/bios12111023
137. Shiri, F., Feng, H., Gale, B.K.: Passive and active microfluidic separation methods. In: Particle Separation Techniques, pp. 449–484. Elsevier (2022). https://doi.org/10.1016/B978-0-323-85486-3.00013-5
138. Mudugamuwa, A., Roshan, U., Hettiarachchi, S., Cha, H., Musharaf, H., Kang, X., et al.: Periodic flows in microfluidics. Small (2024). https://doi.org/10.1002/smll.202404685
139. Tang, H., Niu, J., Jin, H., Lin, S., Cui, D.: Geometric structure design of passive label-free microfluidic systems for biological micro-object separation. Microsyst. Nanoeng. **8**, 62 (2022). https://doi.org/10.1038/s41378-022-00386-y
140. Azimi-Boulali, J., Madadelahi, M., Madou, M.J., Martinez-Chapa, S.O.: Droplet and particle generation on centrifugal microfluidic platforms: a review. Micromachines **11**, 603 (2020). https://doi.org/10.3390/mi11060603
141. Moragues, T., Arguijo, D., Beneyton, T., Modavi, C., Simutis, K., Abate, A.R., et al.: Droplet-based microfluidics. Nat. Rev. Methods Prim. **3**, 32 (2023). https://doi.org/10.1038/s43586-023-00212-3
142. Yang, M., Gao, Y., Liu, Y., Yang, G., Zhao, C.-X., Wu, K.-J.: Integration of microfluidic systems with external fields for multiphase process intensification. Chem. Eng. Sci. **234**, 116450 (2021). https://doi.org/10.1016/j.ces.2021.116450
143. Afsaneh, H., Mohammadi, R.: Microfluidic platforms for the manipulation of cells and particles. Talanta Open **5**, 100092 (2022). https://doi.org/10.1016/j.talo.2022.100092
144. Pelin, G., Sonmez, M., Pelin, C.-E.: The use of additive manufacturing techniques in the development of polymeric molds: a review. Polymers **16**, 1055 (2024). https://doi.org/10.3390/polym16081055
145. Mohd, N., Razali, M., Ghazali, M.J., Kasim, N.H.A.: 3D-printed hydroxyapatite and tricalcium phosphates-based scaffolds for alveolar bone regeneration in animal models: a scoping review. Materials **15** (2022). https://doi.org/10.3390/ma15072621
146. Juang, Y.-J., Chiu, Y.-J.: Fabrication of polymer microfluidics: an overview. Polymers **14**, 2028 (2022). https://doi.org/10.3390/polym14102028
147. Vinet, L., Zhedanov, A.: A "missing" family of classical orthogonal polynomials. J. Phys. A Math. Theor. **44**, 149–200 (2011). https://doi.org/10.1088/1751-8113/44/8/085201
148. Damiati, L.A., El-Yaagoubi, M., Damiati, S.A., Kodzius, R., Sefat, F., Damiati, S.: Role of polymers in microfluidic devices. Polymers **14**, 5132 (2022). https://doi.org/10.3390/polym14235132
149. Rawas-Qalaji, M., Cagliani, R., Al-hashimi, N., Al-Dabbagh, R., Al-Dabbagh, A., Hussain, Z.: Microfluidics in drug delivery: review of methods and applications. Pharm. Dev. Technol. **28**, 61–77 (2023). https://doi.org/10.1080/10837450.2022.2162543
150. Hiromoto, S., Itoh, S., Noda, N., Yamazaki, T., Katayama, H., Akashi, T.: Osteoclast and osteoblast responsive carbonate apatite coatings for biodegradable magnesium alloys. Sci. Technol. Adv. Mater. **21**, 346–58 (2020). https://doi.org/10.1080/14686996.2020.1761237
151. Garzón, V., Bustos, R.-H., Pinacho, G.D.: Personalized medicine for antibiotics: the role of nanobiosensors in therapeutic drug monitoring. J. Personal. Med. **10**, 147 (2020). https://doi.org/10.3390/jpm10040147

152. Casciani, V., Galliano, D., Franasiak, J.M., Mariani, G., Meseguer, M.: Are we approaching automated assisted reproductive technology? Embryo culture, metabolomics, and cryopreservation. F&S Rev. **2**, 251–64 (2021). https://doi.org/10.1016/j.xfnr.2021.08.001
153. Fang, Y., Wu, R., Lee, J.M., Chan, L.H.M., Chan, K.Y.J.: Microfluidic in-vitro fertilization technologies: transforming the future of human reproduction. TrAC, Trends Anal. Chem. **160**, 116959 (2023). https://doi.org/10.1016/j.trac.2023.116959
154. Niculescu, A.-G., Chircov, C., Bîrcă, A.C., Grumezescu, A.M.: Fabrication and applications of microfluidic devices: a review. Int. J. Mol. Sci. **22**, 2011 (2021). https://doi.org/10.3390/ijms22042011
155. Aralekallu, S., Boddula, R., Singh, V.: Development of glass-based microfluidic devices: a review on its fabrication and biologic applications. Mater. Des. **225**, 111517 (2023). https://doi.org/10.1016/j.matdes.2022.111517
156. Shubhava, Jayarama, A., Kannarpady, G.K., Kale, S., Prabhu, S., Pinto, R.: Chemical etching of glasses in hydrofluoric acid: a brief review. Mater. Today Proc. **55**, 46–51 (2022). https://doi.org/10.1016/j.matpr.2021.12.110
157. Mehta, V., Rath, S.N.: 3D printed microfluidic devices: a review focused on four fundamental manufacturing approaches and implications on the field of healthcare. Bio-Design Manuf. **4**, 311–43 (2021). https://doi.org/10.1007/s42242-020-00112-5
158. Gale, B.K., Jafek, A.R., Lambert, C.J., Goenner, B.L., Moghimifam, H., Nze, U.C., et al.: A review of current methods in microfluidic device fabrication and future commercialization prospects. Inventions **3** (2018). https://doi.org/10.3390/inventions3030060
159. Ali@Hasim, N.R., Ahaitouf, A., Abdullah, M.Z.: Irreversible bonding techniques for the fabrication of a leakage-free printed circuit board-based lab-on-chip in microfluidic platforms—a review. Meas. Sci. Technol. **32**, 052001 (2021). https://doi.org/10.1088/1361-6501/abeb92
160. Bogdanowicz, R., Jönsson-Niedziółka, M., Vereshchagina, E., Dettlaff, A., Boonkaew, S., Pierpaoli, M., et al.: Microfluidic devices for photo-and spectroelectrochemical applications. Curr. Opin. Electrochem. **36**, 101138 (2022). https://doi.org/10.1016/j.coelec.2022.101138
161. Guo, Z., Zhao, Y., Jin, Z., Chang, Y., Wang, X., Guo, G., et al.: Monolithic 3D nanoelectrospray emitters based on a continuous fluid-assisted etching strategy for glass droplet microfluidic chip-mass spectrometry. Chem. Sci. **15**, 7781–8 (2024). https://doi.org/10.1039/d4sc01700e
162. Gonzalez, G., Roppolo, I., Pirri, C.F., Chiappone, A.: Current and emerging trends in polymeric 3D printed microfluidic devices. Addit. Manuf. **55**, 102867 (2022). https://doi.org/10.1016/j.addma.2022.102867
163. Milton, L.A., Viglione, M.S., Ong, L.J.Y., Nordin, G.P., Toh, Y.-C.: Vat photopolymerization 3D printed microfluidic devices for organ-on-a-chip applications. Lab Chip **23**, 3537–60 (2023). https://doi.org/10.1039/D3LC00094J
164. Shakeri, A., Khan, S., Jarad, N.A., Didar, T.F.: The fabrication and bonding of thermoplastic microfluidics: a review. Materials **15**, 6478 (2022). https://doi.org/10.3390/ma15186478
165. Bakhshi, A., Pandey, A., Kharaba, Z., Razlansari, M., Sargazi, S., Behzadmehr, R., et al.: Microfluidic-based nanoplatforms for cancer theranostic applications: a mini-review on recent advancements. OpenNano **15**, 100197 (2024). https://doi.org/10.1016/j.onano.2023.100197
166. Venkatesalu, S., Dilliyappan, S., Satish Kumar, A., Palaniyandi, T., Baskar, G., Ravi, M., et al.: Prospectives and retrospectives of microfluidics devices and lab-on-A-chip emphasis on cancer. Clin. Chim. Acta **552**, 117646 (2024). https://doi.org/10.1016/j.cca.2023.117646
167. Ayuso, J.M., Virumbrales-Muñoz, M., Lang, J.M., Beebe, D.J.: A role for microfluidic systems in precision medicine. Nat. Commun. **13**, 3086 (2022). https://doi.org/10.1038/s41467-022-30384-7
168. Mahhengam, N., fahem ghetran Khazaali, A., Aravindhan, S., Olegovna Zekiy, A., Melnikova, L., Siahmansouri, H.: Applications of microfluidic devices in the diagnosis and treatment of cancer: a review study. Critic. Rev. Anal. Chem. **52**, 1863–1877 (2022). https://doi.org/10.1080/10408347.2021.1922870
169. Shepherd, S.J., Issadore, D., Mitchell, M.J.: Microfluidic formulation of nanoparticles for biomedical applications. Biomaterials **274**, 120826 (2021). https://doi.org/10.1016/j.biomaterials.2021.120826

170. Arduino, I., Liu, Z., Rahikkala, A., Figueiredo, P., Correia, A., Cutrignelli, A., et al.: Preparation of cetyl palmitate-based PEGylated solid lipid nanoparticles by microfluidic technique. Acta Biomater. **121**, 566–78 (2021). https://doi.org/10.1016/j.actbio.2020.12.024
171. Lacombe, J., Soldevila, M., Zenhausern, F.: From organ-on-chip to body-on-chip: the next generation of microfluidics platforms for in vitro drug efficacy and toxicity testing. Prog. Mol. Biol. Transl. Sci. **187**, 41–91 (2022). https://doi.org/10.1016/bs.pmbts.2021.07.019
172. Maurya, R., Gohil, N., Bhattacharjee, G., Khambhati, K., Alzahrani, K.J., Ramakrishna, S., et al.: Advances in microfluidics devices and its applications in personalized medicines. Prog. Mol. Biol. Transl. Sci. **186**, 191–201 (2022). https://doi.org/10.1016/bs.pmbts.2021.07.012
173. Zhang, X., Zhu, D., Yang, X., Man, C., Jiang, Y., Zhao, Q., et al.: Nanozyme-enabled microfluidic biosensors: a promising tool for on-site food safety analysis. Trends Food Sci. Technol. **148**, 104486 (2024). https://doi.org/10.1016/j.tifs.2024.104486
174. Yamaguchi, H., Miyazaki, M.: Enzyme-immobilized microfluidic devices for biomolecule detection. TrAC, Trends Anal. Chem. **159**, 116908 (2023). https://doi.org/10.1016/j.trac.2022.116908
175. Hamed, R.E.: Emerging trends in computational biosensors: challenges and future directions. J. Surv. Fish. Sci. (2023). https://doi.org/10.53555/sfs.v10i1.1280
176. Amreen, K., Guha, K., Goel, S.: An Overview of Integrated Miniaturized/Microfluidic Electrochemical Biosensor Platforms for Health Care Applications, pp. 81–101. (2023). https://doi.org/10.1007/978-981-19-7107-5_5
177. Kulkarni, M.B., Ayachit, N.H., Aminabhavi, T.M.: A short review on miniaturized biosensors for the detection of nucleic acid biomarkers. Biosensors **13**, 412 (2023). https://doi.org/10.3390/bios13030412
178. Jiang, B., Huang, B., Cai, G., Chen, Y., Wu, T.: Facile and highly efficient loading and freezing of cryoprotectants for oocyte vitrification based on planar microfluidics. Microfluid. Nanofluid. **25**, 63 (2021). https://doi.org/10.1007/s10404-021-02462-7
179. Wang, J., Dong, J.: Optical waveguides and integrated optical devices for medical diagnosis, health monitoring and light therapies. Sensors (Switzerland) **20**, 1–33 (2020). https://doi.org/10.3390/s20143981
180. Liu, Y., Li, J., Xiao, S., Liu, Y., Bai, M., Gong, L., et al.: Revolutionizing precision medicine: exploring wearable sensors for therapeutic drug monitoring and personalized therapy. Biosensors **13**, 726 (2023). https://doi.org/10.3390/bios13070726
181. Pirovano, G., Roberts, S., Kossatz, S., Reiner, T.: Optical imaging modalities: principles and applications in preclinical research and clinical settings. J. Nucl. Med. **61**, 1419–27 (2020). https://doi.org/10.2967/jnumed.119.238279
182. Radhakrishnan, A., Kuppusamy, G., Ponnusankar, S., Mutalik, S.: Towards next-generation personalization of tacrolimus treatment: a review on advanced diagnostic and therapeutic approaches. Pharmacogenomics **22**, 1151–75 (2021). https://doi.org/10.2217/pgs-2021-0008
183. Huang, Y., Qiu, F., Chen, R., Yan, D., Zhu, X.: Fluorescence resonance energy transfer-based drug delivery systems for enhanced photodynamic therapy. J. Mater. Chem. B **8**, 3772–88 (2020). https://doi.org/10.1039/D0TB00262C
184. Wang, Y., Staudinger, J.N., Mindt, T.L., Gasser, G.: Theranostics with photodynamic therapy for personalized medicine: to see and to treat. Theranostics **13**, 5501–44 (2023). https://doi.org/10.7150/thno.87363
185. Yang, J., Fu, Q., Jiang, H., Li, Y., Liu, M.: Progress of phototherapy for osteosarcoma and application prospect of blue light photobiomodulation therapy. Front. Oncol. **12** (2022). https://doi.org/10.3389/fonc.2022.1022973
186. Yi, J., Liu, L., Gao, W., Zeng, J., Chen, Y., Pang, E., et al.: Advances and perspectives in phototherapy-based combination therapy for cancer treatment. J. Mater. Chem. B **12**, 6285–304 (2024). https://doi.org/10.1039/D4TB00483C
187. Overchuk, M., Weersink, R.A., Wilson, B.C., Zheng, G.: Photodynamic and photothermal therapies: synergy opportunities for nanomedicine. ACS Nano **17**, 7979–8003 (2023). https://doi.org/10.1021/acsnano.3c00891

188. Agwa, M.M., Elmotasem, H., Moustafa, R.I., Abdelsattar, A.S., Mohy-Eldin, M.S., Fouda, M.M.G.: Advent in proteins, nucleic acids, and biological cell membranes functionalized nanocarriers to accomplish active or homologous tumor targeting for smart amalgamated chemotherapy/photo-therapy: a review. Int. J. Biol. Macromol. **253**, 127460 (2023). https://doi.org/10.1016/j.ijbiomac.2023.127460
189. Wang, L., Jiang, K., Shen, G.: Wearable, implantable, and interventional medical devices based on smart electronic skins. Adv. Mater. Technol. **6** (2021). https://doi.org/10.1002/admt.202100107
190. Qi, D., Zhang, K., Tian, G., Jiang, B., Huang, Y.: Stretchable electronics based on PDMS substrates. Adv. Mater. **33** (2021). https://doi.org/10.1002/adma.202003155
191. Bubniene, U.S., Ratautaite, V., Ramanavicius, A., Bucinskas, V.: Conducting polymers for the design of tactile sensors. Polymers **14**, 2984 (2022). https://doi.org/10.3390/polym14152984
192. Turner, B., Ramesh, S., Menegatti, S., Daniele, M.: Resorbable elastomers for implantable medical devices: highlights and applications. Polym. Int. **71**, 552–61 (2022). https://doi.org/10.1002/pi.6349
193. Jin, L., Yang, S.: Engineering Kirigami frameworks toward real-world applications. Adv. Mater. **36** (2024). https://doi.org/10.1002/adma.202308560
194. Kothawade, S., Shende, P.: Coordination bonded stimuli-responsive drug delivery system of chemical actives with metal in pharmaceutical applications. Coord. Chem. Rev. **510**, 215851 (2024). https://doi.org/10.1016/j.ccr.2024.215851
195. Wan, Y., Li, X., Yuan, H., Liu, D., Lai, W.: Self-healing elastic electronics: materials design, mechanisms, and applications. Adv. Funct. Mater. **34** (2024). https://doi.org/10.1002/adfm.202316550
196. Hosseini, E.S., Dervin, S., Ganguly, P., Dahiya, R.: Biodegradable materials for sustainable health monitoring devices. ACS Appl. Bio Mater. **4**, 163–94 (2021). https://doi.org/10.1021/acsabm.0c01139
197. Baburaj, A., Banerjee, S., Aliyana, A.K., Shee, C., Banakar, M., Bairagi, S., et al.: Biodegradable based TENGs for self-sustaining implantable medical devices. Nano Energy **127**, 109785 (2024). https://doi.org/10.1016/j.nanoen.2024.109785
198. Morsada, Z., Hossain, M.M., Islam, M.T., Mobin, M.D.A., Saha, S.: Recent progress in biodegradable and bioresorbable materials: From passive implants to active electronics. Appl. Mater. Today **25**, 101257 (2021). https://doi.org/10.1016/j.apmt.2021.101257
199. Ershad-Langroudi, A., Babazadeh, N., Alizadegan, F., Mehdi Mousaei, S., Moradi, G.: Polymers for implantable devices. J. Ind. Eng. Chem. **137**, 61–86 (2024). https://doi.org/10.1016/j.jiec.2024.03.030
200. Zhou, J., Zhou, S., Fan, P., Li, X., Ying, Y., Ping, J., et al.: Implantable electrochemical microsensors for in vivo monitoring of animal physiological information. Nano-Micro Lett. **16**, 49 (2024). https://doi.org/10.1007/s40820-023-01274-4
201. Dei, M., Muñoz, X.: Electrochemical miniaturized devices. In: Micro- and Nanotechnology Enabled Applications for Portable Miniaturized Analytical Systems, pp. 109–140. Elsevier (2022). https://doi.org/10.1016/B978-0-12-823727-4.00014-6
202. Kazanskiy, N.L., Khonina, S.N., Butt, M.A.: Smart contact lenses—a step towards non-invasive continuous eye health monitoring. Biosensors **13**, 933 (2023). https://doi.org/10.3390/bios13100933
203. Ma, X., Ahadian, S., Liu, S., Zhang, J., Liu, S., Cao, T., et al.: Smart contact lenses for biosensing applications. Adv. Intell. Syst. **3** (2021). https://doi.org/10.1002/aisy.202000263
204. Seçkin, M., Seçkin, A.Ç., Gençer, Ç.: Biomedical sensors and applications of wearable technologies on arm and hand. Biomed. Mater. & Dev. **1**, 443–55 (2023). https://doi.org/10.1007/s44174-022-00002-7
205. Zhang, D., Tung, C., Wu, L.: Artificial photosynthesis. Prog. Chem. **34**, 1590–9 (2022). https://doi.org/10.7536/PC220323
206. Machín, A., Cotto, M., Ducongé, J., Márquez, F.: Artificial photosynthesis: current advancements and future prospects. Biomimetics **8** (2023). https://doi.org/10.3390/biomimetics8030298

207. Ruffini, A., Sandri, M., Dapporto, M., Campodoni, E., Tampieri, A., Sprio, S.: Nature-inspired unconventional approaches to develop 3d bioceramic scaffolds with enhanced regenerative ability. Biomedicines **9** (2021). https://doi.org/10.3390/biomedicines9080916
208. Lim, J.W.: Polymer materials for optoelectronics and energy applications. Materials **17**, 3698 (2024). https://doi.org/10.3390/ma17153698
209. Hannappel, T., Shekarabi, S., Jaegermann, W., Runge, E., Hofmann, J.P., van de Krol, R., et al.: Integration of multijunction absorbers and catalysts for efficient solar-driven artificial leaf structures: a physical and materials science perspective. Solar RRL **8** (2024). https://doi.org/10.1002/solr.202301047
210. Chandran, B., Oh, J.-K., Lee, S.-W., Um, D.-Y., Kim, S.-U., Veeramuthu, V., et al.: Solar-driven sustainability: III–V semiconductor for green energy production technologies. Nano-Micro Lett. **16**, 244 (2024). https://doi.org/10.1007/s40820-024-01412-6
211. Wei, S., Xia, X., Bi, S., Hu, S., Wu, X., Hsu, H.-Y., et al.: Metal–insulator–semiconductor photoelectrodes for enhanced photoelectrochemical water splitting. Chem. Soc. Rev. **53**, 6860–916 (2024). https://doi.org/10.1039/D3CS00820G
212. Zhou, X., Zeng, Y., Lv, F., Bai, H., Wang, S.: Organic semiconductor-organism interfaces for augmenting natural and artificial photosynthesis. Acc. Chem. Res. **55**, 156–70 (2022). https://doi.org/10.1021/acs.accounts.1c00580
213. Wang, Z., Hu, Y., Zhang, S., Sun, Y.: Artificial photosynthesis systems for solar energy conversion and storage: platforms and their realities. Chem. Soc. Rev. **51**, 6704–37 (2022). https://doi.org/10.1039/D1CS01008E
214. Nguyen, V.-H., Nguyen, B.-S., Jin, Z., Shokouhimehr, M., Jang, H.W., Hu, C., et al.: Towards artificial photosynthesis: sustainable hydrogen utilization for photocatalytic reduction of CO_2 to high-value renewable fuels. Chem. Eng. J. **402**, 126184 (2020). https://doi.org/10.1016/j.cej.2020.126184
215. Yoshino, S., Takayama, T., Yamaguchi, Y., Iwase, A., Kudo, A.: CO_2 reduction using water as an electron donor over heterogeneous photocatalysts aiming at artificial photosynthesis. Acc. Chem. Res. **55**, 966–77 (2022). https://doi.org/10.1021/acs.accounts.1c00676
216. Li, W., Liu, Q., Zhang, Y., Li, C., He, Z., Choy, W.C.H., et al.: Biodegradable materials and green processing for green electronics. Adv. Mater. **32** (2020). https://doi.org/10.1002/adma.202001591
217. Ko, G., Naganaboina, V.R., Goda, E.S., Dutta, A., Cheng, H., Hwang, S.: Towards polymer composite-based transient electronic systems. Adv. NanoBiomed Res. (2024). https://doi.org/10.1002/anbr.202400126
218. Samir, A., Ashour, F.H., Hakim, A.A.A., Bassyouni, M.: Recent advances in biodegradable polymers for sustainable applications. Npj Mater. Degrad. **6**, 68 (2022). https://doi.org/10.1038/s41529-022-00277-7
219. Nandi, A.K.: A review on self-assembly driven optoelectronic properties of polythiophene-peptide and polythiophene-polymer conjugates. Langmuir **40**, 9385–405 (2024). https://doi.org/10.1021/acs.langmuir.4c00713
220. Liu, C., Shao, L., Chen, S., Hu, Z., Cai, H., Huang, F.: Recent progress in π-conjugated polymers for organic photovoltaics: solar cells and photodetectors. Prog. Polym. Sci. **143**, 101711 (2023). https://doi.org/10.1016/j.progpolymsci.2023.101711
221. Fallon, K.J., Bronstein, H.: Indolonaphthyridine: a versatile chromophore for organic electronics inspired by natural indigo dye. Acc. Chem. Res. **54**, 182–93 (2021). https://doi.org/10.1021/acs.accounts.0c00601
222. Trinh, C.K., Abdo, N.I.: A Mini-Review: Intermolecular interactions of small molecules containing amide groups-based organic semiconductors and their applications†. J. Mol. Struct. **1269**, 133764 (2022). https://doi.org/10.1016/j.molstruc.2022.133764
223. Xing, L., Luscombe, C.K.: Advances in applying C-H functionalization and naturally sourced building blocks in organic semiconductor synthesis. J. Mater. Chem. C **9**, 16391–409 (2021). https://doi.org/10.1039/D1TC04128B
224. Min J, Jung Y, Ahn J, Lee JG, Lee J, Ko SH (2023) Recent advances in biodegradable green electronic materials and sensor applications. Adv Mater **35** (2023). https://doi.org/10.1002/adma.202211273

225. Fritea, L., Banica, F., Costea, T., Moldovan, L., Dobjanschi, L., Muresan, M., et al.: Metal nanoparticles and carbon-based nanomaterials for improved performances of electrochemical (Bio)Sensors with biomedical applications. Materials **14**, 6319 (2021). https://doi.org/10.3390/ma14216319
226. Yang, X.-C., Wang, X.-X., Wang, C.-Y., Zheng, H.-L., Yin, M., Chen, K.-Z., et al.: Silk-based intelligent fibers and textiles: structures, properties, and applications. Chem. Commun. **60**, 7801–23 (2024). https://doi.org/10.1039/D4CC02276A
227. Lakard, S., Pavel, I.-A., Lakard, B.: Electrochemical biosensing of dopamine neurotransmitter: a review. Biosensors **11**, 179 (2021). https://doi.org/10.3390/bios11060179
228. Zhang, Y., Lee, G., Li, S., Hu, Z., Zhao, K., Rogers, J.A.: Advances in bioresorbable materials and electronics. Chem. Rev. **123**, 11722–73 (2023). https://doi.org/10.1021/acs.chemrev.3c00408
229. De Santis, M., Cacciotti, I.: Wireless implantable and biodegradable sensors for postsurgery monitoring: current status and future perspectives. Nanotechnology **31**, 252001 (2020). https://doi.org/10.1088/1361-6528/ab7a2d
230. Li, Y., Chen, W., Lu, L.: Wearable and biodegradable sensors for human health monitoring. ACS Appl. Bio Mater. **4**, 122–39 (2021). https://doi.org/10.1021/acsabm.0c00859

The manufacturer's authorised representative in the EU is Springer Nature Customer Service Centre GmbH, Europaplatz 3, 69115 Heidelberg, Germany. If you have any concerns regarding our products, please contact ProductSafety@springernature.com

Printed and bound by CPI Group (UK) Ltd, Croydon, CR0 4YY
01/10/2026
02225949-0015